# allergic
# skin
# disease

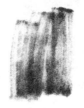

# allergic
# skin
# disease

## A MULTIDISCIPLINARY APPROACH

**EDITED BY**

DONALD Y. M. LEUNG

*National Jewish Center for Immunology
and Respiratory Medicine
Denver, Colorado*

MALCOLM W. GREAVES

*United Medical and Dental School of
Guy's and St. Thomas's Hospitals
King's College
London, England*

MARCEL DEKKER, INC.          NEW YORK · BASEL

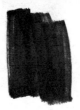

ISBN: 0-8247-0287-5

This book is printed on acid-free paper.

**Headquarters**
Marcel Dekker, Inc.
270 Madison Avenue, New York, NY 10016
tel: 212-696-9000; fax: 212-685-4540

**Eastern Hemisphere Distribution**
Marcel Dekker AG
Hutgasse 4, Postfach 812, CH-4001 Basel, Switzerland
tel: 41-61-261-8482; fax: 41-61-261-8896

**World Wide Web**
http://www.dekker.com

The publisher offers discounts on this book when ordered in bulk quantities. For more information, write to Special Sales/Professional Marketing at the headquarters address above.

Current printing (last digit):
10 9 8 7 6 5 4 3 2 1

**PRINTED IN THE UNITED STATES OF AMERICA**

# Preface

Allergic skin diseases—particularly atopic dermatitis, urticaria, and contact dermatitis—are extremely common, affecting over 20% of the general population at some point during their lifetime. Population studies since World War II have documented a continuous rise in the prevalence of allergic skin diseases. In those patients afflicted with these skin disorders, involvement can be lifelong, causing significant interference with education, occupations, and overall quality of life. The economic impact of allergic skin diseases is also enormous, with atopic hand dermatitis representing a major cause of occupation-related disability.

In recent years, there has been an explosion of knowledge concerning immune responses in the skin and their role in the pathogenesis of allergic skin diseases. Key cell types, effector molecules, cytokines, mediators, chemokines, cell adhesion molecules, and immunogenetic mechanisms that determine the final clinical phenotype of various allergic skin disorders are rapidly being delineated. These advances have led to new paradigms for the mechanisms of these skin disorders and the development of new approaches to their management.

*Allergic Skin Diseases* is aimed at updating the reader on the pathophysiology of allergic skin responses, the mechanisms underlying specific allergic skin diseases, their socioeconomic impact, and new treatment approaches that take advantage of emerging concepts of the pathobiology of these diseases. An outstanding group of allergists, immunologists, and dermatologists, who are acknowledged leaders in their fields, has been assembled in this book to discuss this important and rapidly changing area of medicine. Every effort has been made to achieve prompt publication of this book, thus ensuring that the content of each chapter is ''state of the art.'' Part One presents general principles critical to an understanding of the impact and causes of allergic skin diseases. These include a discussion of epidemiology and socioeconomic impact, quality-of-life issues, molecular and cellular mechanisms of skin responses, the role of adhesion molecules, and the pathophysiology of pruritus. Part Two examines the clinical features and pathophysiology of specific allergic skin diseases, emphasizing the role of immune mechanisms in accounting for the clinical course of each illness. Part Three underpins the clinical relevance of understanding mechanisms of allergic skin diseases in the context of their differential diagnoses, evaluations, environmental triggers, and concepts of emerging and established treatments.

We would like to thank each of the contributors for their time and invaluable expertise, which were vital to the success of this book. We hope that this new text will provide a valuable resource for dermatologists, allergists, internists, pediatricians, basic and clinical immunologists; and graduate students interested in the immunological basis and treatment of allergic skin diseases.

*Donald Y. M. Leung*
*Malcolm W. Greaves*

# Contents

**PART THREE: MANAGEMENT OF ALLERGIC SKIN DISEASE**

# Contributors

**Werner Aberer, M.D.**   Department of Dermatology, University of Graz Medical School, Graz, Austria

**John L. Aeling, M.D.**   Department of Dermatology, University of Colorado Health Sciences Center, Denver, Colorado

**Cem Akin, M.D., Ph.D.**   National Institute of Allergy and Infectious Diseases, National Institutes of Health, Bethesda, Maryland

**Roger T. Anderson, Ph.D.**   Department of Public Health Services, Wake Forest University School of Medicine, Winston-Salem, North Carolina

**Ole Baadsgaard, M.D.**   Department of Dermatology, Gentofte Hospital, University of Copenhagen, Hellerup, Denmark

**Lisa A. Beck, M.D.**   The Johns Hopkins University School of Medicine, Baltimore, Maryland

**Vincent S. Beltrani, M.D.**   Department of Dermatology, College of Physicians and Surgeons, Columbia University, New York, New York; and Division of Allergy, Immunology, and Rheumatology, Department of Medicine, University of Medicine and Dentistry of New Jersey, Newark, New Jersey

**David Bickers, M.D.**   Department of Dermatology, Columbia-Presbyterian Medical Center, New York, New York

**Bruce S. Bochner, M.D.**   Clinical Immunology Unit, The Johns Hopkins University School of Medicine, Baltimore, Maryland

**Mark Boguniewicz, M.D.**   National Jewish Medical and Research Center, Denver, Colorado

**B. Lauren Charous**   Milwaukee Medical Clinic, Milwaukee, Wisconsin

**Kevin D. Cooper, M.D.**   Department of Dermatology, University Hospitals of Cleveland and Case Western Reserve University, Cleveland, Ohio

**Ulf Darsow, M.D.**   Department of Dermatology and Allergy Biederstein, Technical University Munich, Munich, Germany

**Vincent DeLeo, M.D.**   Department of Dermatology, Roosevelt Hospital, New York, New York

**Pamela W. Ewan**   Molecular Immunopathology Unit, MRC Centre & Addenbrooke's Hospital, University of Cambridge Clinical School, Cambridge, United Kingdom

**Robert C. Fuhlbrigge, M.D., Ph.D.**   Department of Medicine, Harvard Institutes of Medicine, Boston, Massachusetts

**Malcolm W. Greaves, M.D., Ph.D.**   United Medical and Dental School of Guy's and St. Thomas' Hospitals, King's College, London, England

**Rebecca S. Gruchalla, M.D., Ph.D.**   Department of Internal Medicine, University of Texas Southwestern Medical Center, Dallas, Texas

**John L. M. Hawk**   St. Thomas' Hospital, London, England

**Kefai Kang, M.D.**   University Hospitals of Clevaland and Case Western Reserve University, Cleveland, Ohio

**Thomas S. Kupper, M.D.**   Dermatology Services, Brigham and Women's Hospital, Boston, Massachusetts

**Finn Schultz Larsen, M.D., Ph.D.**   Dermatology Clinic, Fredericia, Denmark

**E. Frances Lawlor, M.D.**   St. John's Institute of Dermatology, St. Thomas' Hospital, and Newham Healthcare, St. Andrews Hospital, London, England

**Yung-Hian Leow, M.D.**   National Skin Centre, Singapore, Singapore

**Donald Y. M. Leung, M.D., Ph.D.**   Department of Pediatrics, National Jewish Center for Immunology and Respiratory Medicine, Denver, Colorado

**Daniel H. Maes**   The Estee Lauder Companies, New York, New York

**Howard I. Maibach, M.D.**   University of California School of Medicine, San Francisco, California

**Kenneth D. Marenus**   The Estee Lauder Companies, New York, New York

**Mary Steidl Matsui**   Biological Research Division, The Estee Lauder Companies, and Columbia University, New York, New York

**Jeffery S. McBride**   Wake Forest University School of Medicine, Winston-Salem, North Carolina

**John McFadden**   St. John's Institute of Dermatology, St. Thomas' Hospital, London, England

**Hélène du Peloux Menagé, M.D.**   Lewisham University Hospital and St. John's Institute of Dermatology, St. Thomas' Hospital, London, England

**Dean D. Metcalfe, M.D.**   Laboratory of Allergic Diseases, National Institute of Allergy and Infectious Diseases, National Institutes of Health, Bethesda, Maryland

**Dennis Ownby, M.D.**   Department of Pediatrics, Medical College of Georgia, Augusta, Georgia

**Thomas A. E. Platts-Mills, M.D., Ph.D.**   Department of Internal Medicine, University of Virginia Health Sciences Center, Charlottesville, Virginia

**Rukmini Rajagopalan, Ph.D.**   Dermatology Clinical Research, Glaxo Wellcome, Inc., Research Triangle Park, North Carolina

**Johannes Ring**   Department of Dermatology and Allergy Biederstein, Technical University Munich, Munich, Germany

**Hugh A. Sampson, M.D.**   Mount Sinai School of Medicine, New York, New York

**Scott H. Sicherer, M.D.**   Division of Pediatric Allergy and Immunology, Mount Sinai School of Medicine, New York, New York

**F. Estelle R. Simons, M.D.**   Section of Allergy and Clinical Immunology, Department of Pediatrics and Child Health, University of Manitoba, Winnipeg, Manitoba, Canada

**Lone Skov, M.D., Ph.D.**   Gentofte Hospital, University of Copenhagen, Hellerup, Denmark

**Nicholas A. Soter, M.D.**   Department of Dermatology, New York University School of Medicine, Charles C. Harris Skin and Cancer Pavilion, and Tisch Hospital—The University Hospital of New York University, New York, New York

**Seth R. Stevens**   University Hospitals of Cleveland and Case Western Reserve University, Cleveland, Ohio

**Matthew Stiller, M.D.**   Department of Dermatology, Columbia-Presbyterian Medical Center, New York, New York

**James S. Taylor, M.D.**   Department of Dermatology, Cleveland Clinic, Cleveland, Ohio

**Penpun Wattanakrai**   Cleveland Clinic, Cleveland, Ohio

**Richard W. Weber, M.D.**   National Jewish Medical and Research Center and University of Colorado Health Sciences Center, Denver, Colorado

**Lisa M. Wheatley, M.D.**   Department of Internal Medicine and The Asthma and Allergic Diseases Center, University of Virginia Health Sciences Center, Charlottesville, Virginia

**Klaus Wolff, M.D.**   Department of Dermatology, University of Vienna, Vienna, Austria

# 1

## Epidemiology and Socioeconomic Impact of Allergic Skin Diseases

**Finn Schultz Larsen**
*Dermatology Clinic, Fredericia, Denmark*

In recent years allergic skin diseases have attracted an increasing amount of public attention. The reason for this is obvious. They have become more and more common and are an economic threat to the health system. Every year alarming news about the occurrence of allergic disorders is broadcast. This chapter is intended to outline and interpret the relevant and available recent sources on the extent and burden of allergic skin diseases, in particular, atopic dermatitis.

## I. ATOPIC DERMATITIS

Atopic dermatitis is one of the most frequently diagnosed dermatoses in many parts of the western World, and in retrospect we are able to comprehend that the rising occurrence of both atopic dermatitis and respiratory atopy took place starting in the beginning of the 1960s [1,2]. Bearing in mind the shortcomings in measuring and comparing disease frequencies from different studies, this chapter will mainly concentrate on the outcome of recently published population-based surveys. For those born before 1960 the lifetime prevalence in well-conducted and even clinical studies has been estimated to be approximately 3% in England and Scandinavia [1], which is in sharp contrast to the recent reported frequencies in children born after 1980 (Table 1). Furthermore, several studies using identical or almost identical procedures and assessments indicate a definite time trend in the occurrence of atopic dermatitis during recent decades (Table 2).

Newer epidemiological investigations of atopic dermatitis from western countries show that:

1. The frequency has increased since 1960.
2. There are geographical variations in occurrence.
3. This skin disease is still uncommon in certain Mediterranean countries.
4. The increased frequency is even more marked at higher latitudes of the Northern hemisphere [3,25,27]. In fact, in 7- to 12-year-old schoolchildren in a rural community in northern Norway, 33% of the boys and 41% of the girls clinically

**Table 1**  Recent Prevalence Surveys on Atopic Dermatitis in Western Countries

| Country/ County/Town | Year of birth | Year of age | Instrument | Lifetime prevalence (%) | Ref. |
|---|---|---|---|---|---|
| Australia and New Zealand | | | | | |
| Wagga Wagga | 1982–84 | 8–10 | E | 31.9 | 3 |
| Belmont | 1982–84 | 8–10 | E | 24.4 | 3 |
| Hastings | ~1980 | 12 | Q | 15.9 | 4 |
| Europe | | | | | |
| Spain | 1974–88 | 4–17 | Q | 1.3 | 5 |
| Sardinia | 1979–80 | 6–7 | Q | 2.4 | 6 |
| France | 1970–80 | 4–14 | Q | 10.3 | 7 |
| Italy | 1988–89 | 6–7 | Q | 13.2 | 8 |
| England | | | | | |
| Birmingham | 1979–86 | 3–11 | Q | 20.2 | 9 |
| Wales | ~1980 | 12 | Q | 15.9 | 4 |
| Leicester | ~1989–92 | 1–4 | E | 14.0* | 10 |
| London | 1982–90 | 3–11 | E | 11.7* | 11 |
| Nottingham | ~1991–95 | 1–5 | E | 16.5** | 12 |
| Germany | | | | | |
| Freiburg | ~1982–84 | 6–8 | Q | 17.3 | 13 |
| Munich | 1979–80 | 9–11 | Q | 13.9 | 14 |
| Hanover | 1983–84 | 6–7 | Q | 11.8 | 15 |
| Erlangen | 1985 | 7 | Q | 13.1 | 16 |
| Bavaria | 1978–80 | 9–11 | Q | 17.9 | 17 |
| Bavaria | 1983–85 | 5–6 | Q | 7.9–15.5 | 18 |
| Scandinavia | | | | | |
| Denmark | 1983–85 | 5–7 | Q | 9.8** | 19 |
| Denmark | 1985 | 7 | Q | 22.9 | 16 |
| Denmark | 1984–86 | 7 | Q | 18.7 | 20 |
| Finland | 1973–75 | 15–16 | E | 17.8 | 21 |
| Finland | 1980–82 | 13–14 | Q | 17.0** | 22 |
| Sweden | 1968–72 | 10–14 | E | 18.6 | 23 |
| Sweden | 1974–75 | 11 | Q | 21.2 | 24 |
| Sweden | ~1980 | 12 | Q | 22.0 | 4 |
| Sweden | 1985 | 7 | Q | 15.5 | 16 |
| Sweden | 1982–84 | 7 | E | 30.9** | 25 |
| Norway | 1978–84 | 7–13 | Q | 13.2 | 26 |
| Norway | 1980–86 | 7–12 | E | 36.8 | 27 |

E = examination; Q = questionnaire; * = point prevalence; ** = 1-year prevalence; ~ = approximately.

examined presented with past or present atopic dermatitis [27], and at the same time and almost the same northern latitude in Kiruna, Sweden, an interview study resulted in a 1-year prevalence of 31% in 7-year-olds (Table 3).

5. There is quite good agreement between the questionnaire studies and the surveys with subsequent clinical examination, some of which result in even higher figures in the clinical setting [11,16,25].

**Table 2** Trends in the Frequency of Atopic Dermatitis

| Country/Town | Year of birth | Year of age | Instrument | Lifetime prevalence (%) | Ref. |
|---|---|---|---|---|---|
| England | -1976 | All | E | 9.3 | 28 |
| | -1979 | ages | E | 11.9 | |
| England | 1946 | 5–7 | Q | 5.1 | 29 |
| | 1970 | 5–7 | Q | 12.2 | |
| Switzerland | 1962–64 | 4–6 | E | 2.2 | 30 |
| | 1975–77 | 4–6 | E | 2.8 | |
| Denmark | 1960–64 | 7 | E | 3.2 | 31 |
| | 1970–74 | 7 | E | 10.2 | |
| England | 1961 | 12 | Q | 4.8 | 32 |
| | 1976 | 12 | Q | 15.9 | |
| Scotland (Aberdeen) | 1951–56 | 8–13 | Q | 5.3 | 33 |
| | 1976–81 | 8–13 | Q | 12.0 | |
| Denmark | 1965–69 | 7 | Q | 5.9 | 34 |
| | 1975–79 | 7 | Q | 11.5 | |
| Sweden (Göteborg) | 1972 | 7 | Q | 6.8 | 25 |
| | 1984 | 7 | Q | 16.3 | |
| Norway (Oslo) | 1969–74 | 7–12 | Q | 8.6 | 35 |
| | 1981–86 | 7–12 | Q | 9.6 | |
| Scotland (Aberdeen) | 1976–81 | 8–13 | Q | 12.0 | 36 |
| | 1981–86 | 8–13 | Q | 17.7 | |
| Scotland (Highland) | 1979–80 | 12 | Q | 14.1 | 37 |
| | 1981–82 | 12 | Q | 17.7 | |
| Norway (Oslo) | 1964–74 | 6–16 | Q | 9.7 | 38 |
| | 1978–88 | 6–16 | Q | 17.1 | |
| Germany (Leipzig) | 1981–82 | 9–11 | Q | 12.1 | 39 |
| | 1985–86 | 9–11 | Q | 14.2 | |

E = examination; Q = questionnaire.

**Table 3** Epidemiology of Atopic Dermatitis[a]

| | Göteborg | Kiruna |
|---|---|---|
| 1979—Questionnaire Lifetime prevalence | 6.8% | 10.1% |
| 1991—Questionnaire Lifetime prevalence | 16.3% | 22.1% |
| 1991—Examination 1-year prevalence | 27.3% | 30.9% |

[a] Questionnaire study in 7-year-old schoolchildren in Göteborg and Kiruna in 1979 (N = 4682) and in 1991 (N = 2481), and a subsequent interview on a subsample in 1991 (N = 409).
*Source*: Ref. 25.

**Table 4** Recent Prevalence Surveys on Atopic Dermatitis in Non-Western Countries

| Region | Country/county/town | Year of birth | Year of age | Instrument | Lifetime prevalence (%) | Ref. |
|---|---|---|---|---|---|---|
| Africa | | | | | | |
| | Cape Town | ~1980 | 12 | Q | 11.1 | 4 |
| | Tanzania | ~1975–86 | 7–18 | E | 0.7 | 41 |
| Turkey | | | | | | |
| | Ankara | 1980–86 | 6–12 | Q | 6.1 | 42 |
| | Ankara | 1978–86 | 6–13 | Q | 2.6 | 43 |
| | Edirne | 1982–87 | 7–12 | Q | 2.2 | 44 |
| | Izmir | 1979–87 | 6–13 | Q | 13.6 | 45 |
| East Europe | | | | | | |
| | Czech Rep. | ~1989–91 | 3–5 | Q | ~5.1** | 46 |
| | Romania | 1983–89 | 6–12 | E | 2.4* | 47 |
| Asia | | | | | | |
| | China | 1972–81 | 11–20 | Q | 10.4 | 48 |
| | Malasia | 1972–81 | 11–20 | Q | 7.6 | 49 |
| | Hong Kong | 1972–81 | 11–20 | Q | 20.1 | 49 |
| | Hong Kong | 1979–86 | 3–10 | Q | 6.8 | 50 |
| | Singapore | 1979–88 | 6–15 | Q | 6.9 | 51 |
| | Japan | ~1980–86 | 6–12 | Q | 9.5* | 52 |
| | Japan | 1988–89 | 5–6 | E | 24.0 | 53 |

E = examination; Q = questionnaire; * = point prevalence; ** = 1-year prevalence; ~ = approximately.

Surveys from nonwestern countries indicate that the occurrence of atopic dermatitis is almost nonexistent in Central Africa, rare or modest in eastern Europe, and similar to that of north European estimates in urban areas of Asia such as Hong Kong and Japan (Table 4).

The political reunification of Germany in 1990 provided an opportunity to explore the impact of eastern and western European lifestyles and living conditions on the prevalence of respiratory and allergic disorders in two ethnically similar populations. The studies can be summarized as follows: Bronchitis and chronic cough were more prevalent in children in the former East Germany, while asthma, hay fever, positive skin prick tests, and increased specific IgE to standard allergens were more frequent in West Germany [2]. The interpretation of studies on atopic dermatitis is not as clear-cut (Table 5). Although

**Table 5** Comparative Prevalence Surveys on Atopic Dermatitis in East and West Germany

| Author [Ref.] | East/West Germany | Lifetime prevalence Eastern (%) | Western (%) |
|---|---|---|---|
| Mutius [14] | Leipzig/Munich (urban areas) | 13.0 | 13.9 |
| Krämer [54] | Saxony/North Rhine-Westphalia (urban areas) | ~15 | ~8 |
| Englert [55] | Berlin/Berlin (urban areas) | 12.9 | 11.2 |
| Schäfer [56] | Halle/North Rhine-Westphalia | 17.5 | 5.7–15.3 |
| Krämer [57] | Saxony/North Rhine-Westphalia (urban areas) | 14.6 | 10.3 |

there seemed to be an excess of atopic dermatitis in East Germany, the studies do not support the idea that $SO_2$ and airborne particles in the highly polluted areas of East Germany were a major cause of atopic sensitization or influenced the occurrence of atopic dermatitis to any great extent; they suggest that different causative agents or mechanisms are operating in respiratory atopy and atopic dermatitis.

So far, relatively few established risk factors for the development of atopic dermatitis have been identified: genetics, female sex, maternal atopy, maternal smoking, urbanization, high social class, decreasing family size, and decreased microbial stimulation. It seems logical to hypothesize that environmental factors operating in utero and in early life work side by side with a still noncharacterized genetic make-up that favors disease expression [58]. However, the recognized risk factors do not explain the change in the prevalence [2], and it is reasonable to speculate that still unheeded elements of the western lifestyle must have affected the occurrence of atopic dermatitis [59]. Some newly proposed explanations include house dust mite allergens [60,61], increasing maternal age [62], increased intake of polyunsaturated fats (margarine, vegetables oil, linoleic acid) [39,63], chemical damage to the epidermal and mucosal barriers [64], and hard water [65].

There is a surprising paucity of epidemiological studies on atopic dermatitis from North America. From vital and health statistics it can be extracted that about 2% of children in the United States suffered from atopic dermatitis in 1977 [66,67]. In European countries, validated strategies of data collection have been successfully applied to clinically examined schoolchildren [11] or, more simply and cost-effectively, with a purely questionnaire instrument [16]. It is of course much more informative to compare the outcome of the same survey technique applied in different areas, at different times, or at different levels of exposure.

These ideas have been followed in a recent paper from the International Study of Asthma and Allergies in Childhood (ISAAC) [68]. Almost a half million 13- to 14-year-olds (born 1980–1982) in 56 countries worldwide participated in the study, with a response rate of more than 80% in 96% of the centers. The survey concentrated on respiratory atopy and the questions on atopic dermatitis were based on the U.K. Refinement of the Hanifin and Rajka Diagnostic Criteria [40]. These criteria have been validated in a questionnaire version (i.e., without visible flexural dermatitis), which resulted in lower specificity (93%) and an unsatisfactory positive predictive value of 47% [11]. In addition, the questions are different from the U.K. Criteria both in wording and content (widened definition of history of flexural rash, lack of questions on dry skin, and new questions on sleep disturbances and clearance rate), and no other validation procedure seems to have been done before this important study [69]. Thus, although valid criticism can be directed at this part of the ISAAC study, this international, systematic, and standardized comparison sheds some new light on our knowledge of the occurrence of atopic dermatitis. One of the most important and not quite unexpected findings was that the lowest prevalence of flexural eczema was reported from former socialist countries with a lifestyle most different from that of western countries, i.e., Albania, Georgia, Russia, and Uzbekistan. It is also interesting to note that the study confirms the high 1-year prevalence of atopic eczema symptoms in Scandinavia and England, and that a U.S. frequency of about 10% was calculated in Seattle (in, however, fewer than 10 schools). The questions seem to work fairly well in English-speaking countries, but there are quite surprising estimates from some countries. In Nigeria the 1-year prevalence is supposedly about 18%. This is striking in light of a previous communication from the Lagos University Teaching Hospital showing that atopic dermatitis was rare in the clinical setting and that a significant proportion of the patients with atopic dermatitis were born in England while their parents were study-ing there and their eczema had been diagnosed and treated there *before* they moved to Nigeria [70]. Thus, more detailed information is indispensable to test the validity of several of the assessments of this large-scaled study. The investigators have chosen to publish the 1-year prevalence as the measure of disease frequency. This appears to be a suitable unit of measurement for the actual societal impact of this fluctuating disease. In some new studies in schoolchildren the point prevalence is about half the lifetime prevalence, and it has to be anticipated that the 1-year prevalence is somewhere in between, depending on the age at examination [9,13,21].

This brings us to another area of concern. Has the natural history of atopic dermatitis changed in recent decades? Is it mostly milder cases that are responsible for the increasing prevalence, or has the chronicity changed [53,71]? For the time being we have no definitive answer even though the prognosis seems to be slightly more unfavorable than hitherto believed based on record information from a British 1958 birth cohort study. That study reported clearance rates of 65–74% for 16-year-olds, but those children were born before the rising occurrence of atopic dermatitis in the 1960s [71,72].

While the prevalence of atopic dermatitis will soon have been mapped worldwide, there has as yet been only sparse research into the economic burden of this common disease. The high prevalence in most of the developed countries implies that health-care resources and expenditure are considerable. Based on the 1990–1991 billing record from the Children's Hospital in Philadelphia, the U.S. cost of atopic dermatitis in those 16 years and under has been estimated to be $364 million annually, one third of which was spent on pharmaceutical remedies [73]. Although it is difficult to compare these results with those from European countries because of the differences in health-care systems, the out-come of a more recent study from Scotland indicates that the financial burden of atopic dermatitis is higher than in the United States. In a semi-rural general practice of about 10,000 patients, Herd and coworkers [74] identified and examined all possible cases and contacted every family with a patient less than 2 years of age. The overall 1-year preva-lence, age standardized to the Scottish population, was calculated to 2.3%—highest under the age of 2 (9.8%) and lowest over the age of 40 (0.2%). It is worthy of note that persons over the age of 16 years made up 38% of the patients with atopic dermatitis. The annual costs to patients and health services in the practice were £50,000, making the total national expenditure (including lost working days) £465 million, or a per capita cost of £7.38 per annum in 1992 in the United Kingdom. Although any projection is subject to error, this corresponds to a total annual spending of $3.9 billion in United States. It should be remem-bered that the study from Philadelphia only dealt with children, that the treatment in the community was not included, and that the cost to the patients (other than medication) were omitted [73]. A recently published abstract of a study of 1760 preschool children from four urban and semi-rural general practices in Nottingham recorded a mean treatment cost for each child with atopic dermatits of £37.70 annually [74]. As the 1-year prevalence was 16.5%, confirmed by a dermatologist at a clinical examination, it means a per capita cost of £6.22, which is not grossly different from the findings in Scotland [75]. Both British studies indicate that the U.S. estimate may be an underestimate, even if the prevalence of atopic dermatitis is markedly lower in the United States than in the United Kingdom.

Not only do more and more children suffer from atopic dermatitis, it also has a profound impact on the child's quality of life. The introduction of disability measures such as the Children's Dermatology Life Quality Index (CDLQI) has been a major step forward [76]. The questionnaire consists of 10 questions (maximum score 30) about how much the skin disease has influenced the patient's daily life during the previous week. The questions concern itchiness, embarrassment, friendships, clothes, hobbies, sports, schoolwork, teasing, sleep, and treatment. Based on 233 dermatology pediatric outpatients, the mean CDLQI score for atopic dermatitis was 7.7 and was significantly higher than for acne (5.7) and psoriasis (5.4). Preschool children with severe atopic dermatitis (defined as eczema over at least 10% of the skin surface area) exhibit an excess of dependency/clinginess and fearfulness in comparison with a control group [77]. The psychological effect of scratching, sleep loss, and visible skin disease may also stress the families in parenting and social functioning; moderate and severe atopic dermatitis have a significantly higher impact on family life than does insulin-dependent diabetes [78,79]. When the skin problem persists in adulthood, U.K. patients with severe atopic dermatitis believe that having diabetes or hypertension would be far better than having eczema, and 49% of them would be prepared to pay £10,000 or more for a cure for atopic dermatitis [80]. Perhaps more important, this disease in advanced cases may affect children at a critical stage in their emotional and social development with unknown and unexplored psychosocial implications for their future lives [81].

## II. URTICARIA

Although urticaria, or nettle rash, is rarely a serious illness, it is a common complaint; it is difficult, however, to obtain precise figures on its occurrence. Many cases are probably not seen by doctors and the majority are treated in primary care. Therefore, hospital-based information is misleading; in several series papular urticaria caused by insect bite is included. Furthermore, the number of newer unselected studies are limited (Table 6), and for the time being it seems that about 5–10% of the population will have an episode of urticaria during their lifetime. There is no comparative data that allow evaluation of a trend over time regarding a general increase or decrease in the prevalence of urticaria.

**Table 6** Prevalence Surveys on Urticaria in the General Population

| Author [Ref.] | Country | Year of age | Instrument | Lifetime prevalence (%) |
|---|---|---|---|---|
| Service [82] | US (Colorado) | 0–60 | Q | 3.2 |
| Eriksson-Lihr [83] | Finland | 8–13 | Q | 2.2 |
| Lomholt [84] | Faeröer Islands | All ages | E | 0.1 |
| Freeman [85] | US (Colorado) | 14–18 | Q | 2.1 |
| Hellgren [86] | Sweden | All ages | E | 0.1* |
| Kjellman [87] | Sweden | 7 | Q | 2.0 |
| Weeke [88] | Denmark | 16–60+ | Q | 11.1 |
| Varonier [30] | Switzerland | 4–6 | E | 0.4–0.9 |
| Storm [89] | Denmark | 7 | E | 2.0 |
| Agnoni [6] | Sardinia | 6–7 | Q | 1.9 |
| Åberg [90] | Sweden | 7–14 | Q | 8.3 |
| Bakke [91] | Norway | 15–70 | Q | 9.0 |
| Keiding [92] | Denmark | 16–65+ | Q | 4.2 |

E = examination; Q = questionnaire; * = point prevalence.

**Table 7**  Prevalence Surveys of Special Forms of Urticaria

| Author [Ref.] | Form | Year of age | Instrument | Lifetime prevalence (%) | Comments |
|---|---|---|---|---|---|
| Ebken [93] | Dermographism | ? | E | 1.5 | 200 controls in good health |
| Kirby [94] | Dermographism | All ages | E | 4.2 | General practice, routinely examined patients |
| Zuberbier [95] | Cholinerg | 15–35 | Q | 11.2 | High school and university students, 22% previously seen by doctors |
| Möller [96] | Cold | All ages | E | 0.1 | Dermatology clinic, 23% suffered from other types of urticaria |

Q = questionnaire; E = examination.

The newest and most thoroughly conducted studies point to a female: male ratio of about 1.5:1.0 (just as in atopic dermatitis) and positive and negative predictive values of answers about urticaria defined as a periodic, localized puritic edema of the skin of 95% and 86%, respectively [88,91]. A representative sample of the adult Danish population revealed that the incidence of nettle rash (defined as a rather sudden flushing, itching, and edema of the skin at the same time) was highest in the 16- to 29-year age group, and that the 1-year prevalence was almost the same in the different adult age groups (5.2%). The age of onset with the highest frequency was 10–19 years (32.4%), and 78.0% had an onset of urticaria before 30 years of age [88]. A more recent similar investigation from 1994 reported a lifetime prevalence of 4.2% [92]. A few investigations give some idea of the occurrence of special forms of urticaria (Table 7).

## III.  ALLERGIC CONTACT DERMATITIS

Information on the prevalence of allergic contact dermatitis in the population is scarce. A few major studies on hand eczema in adulthood have been performed in northern Europe (Table 8) indicating that the point prevalence of allergic hand eczema is about 1%, whereas figures regarding other skin sites are lacking. Although the partial correlation between positive patch test and clinical allergic contact dermatitis is well known, it is surprising that 10–15% of healthy individuals have one or more positive patch tests [100–102]. In addition, a population-based study showed that 45% of nickel-sensitive individuals reported past or present relevant eczema, indicating a higher incidence of allergic contact dermatitis in the general population [103].

Two recently conducted surveys on asthma, allergy, and other types of hypersensitivity from the Danish Institute for Clinical Epidemiology (DICE) of a representative sample of the adult Danish population reveal some new and suggestive data [92]. DICE's nationwide surveys in 1987 and 1994 were based on a random sample of about 6000 Danes (≥16 years of age) identified by the Danish personal numbering system. The data collection was carried out by trained interviewers, and the participation rates were 80%

**Table 8** Prevalence Surveys of Allergic Hand Dermatitis

| Country | Point prevalence (%) | Comments | Ref. |
|---|---|---|---|
| Sweden | 0.4 | Questionnaire + patch testing of patients | 97 |
| Netherlands | 1.0** | Clinical exam. + patch testing of patients | 98 |
| Sweden | ~2.0* | Questionnaire + patch testing of patients | 99 |

* = 1-year prevalence; ** = 3-year prevalence.

and 78%, respectively. Subjects were asked about "allergic eczema on the skin," and in the accompanying instruction to the interviewer, the condition was described as follows: "in this context allergic eczema on the skin does not include atopic eczema, but for example eczema caused by contact with cosmetic, nickel, plaster, etc. Not UV-induced eczema." An explanation was given to participants who were in doubt about the meaning of "allergic eczema on the skin." The 1994 investigation showed that allergic eczema occurred for the first time within the previous year (the incidence) in 1.6% persons and in up to 3.0% of 16- to 24-year-old women, whereas the total 1-year prevalence was calculated to be 7.8% and the lifetime prevalence 12.9%. About 20% of those reporting allergic eczema experienced onset within the previous year (1.6:7.8). It is even more interesting that, with the same survey procedure and the same working definition, the 1-year prevalence increased from 6.1% in 1987 to 7.8% in 1994. However, the above-mentioned figures are most likely overestimated, as it might be difficult or even impossible for participants and interviewers to differentiate between endogenous hand eczema, atopic hand eczema, irritant skin reaction, and allergic contact dermatitis, but even then this well-conducted and representative study of the adult Danish population clearly indicates an increasing trend over time and that a point prevalence of 1% and a 1-year prevalence of 2% is an underestimation of the occurrence of allergic contact dermatitis, at least in Denmark. The higher prevalence of allergic contact dermatitis in relation to sex, age, and in some professional groups is discussed in more detail in Chapter 10.

The socioeconomic costs of allergic contact dermatitis include hospital and medical billings, treatment remedies, sickness benefits, rehabilitation, and in some cases compensation for loss of earning capacity and/or permanent injury. In Denmark, with about 5 million inhabitants and a working force of 2.6 million people, insurance companies paid compensation rates of $3 million a year from 1991 through 1995. Comparable spending in the United States would cost, conservatively, $160 million [104,105]. These amounts represent the tip of the iceberg of health-care costs related to allergic contact dermatitis.

## IV.  PHOTODERMATITIS/PHOTOALLERGY

Abnormal response to ultraviolet radiation includes polymorphous light eruption in which sunlight is thought to induce a neoantigen and a subsequent delayed hypersensitivity reaction by continuous light exposure (see Chap. 11). The few population-based studies indicate that 10–21% of fair-skinned adults have a history suggestive of polymorphous light eruption [106,107]. However, in light of the difficulty in distinguishing between sunburn and polymorphous light eruption in questionnaire investigations, it seems reasonable to assume that the incidences are overestimated. Other photodermatoses, such as hydroa vacciniforme, are very rare disorders.

Although the list of photoallergenic reactions as a result of systemically administrated drugs increases every year, such reactions affect less than 1% of the population [108], and the photodermatoses that result from topical photo-allergens are likely to be included in surveys on contact dermatitis.

## V. LATEX ALLERGY

Since the first report in 1979 of a glove-related case of contact urticaria due to natural rubber, latex allergy has reached almost epidemic proportions in the medical professions [109]. Investigations during the 1990s reveal that about 10–15% of tested regular users of latex gloves on hospital staffs show evidence of sensitivity (Table 9). About one third of skin prick–positive subjects, however, do not at the time of testing have symptoms of latex allergy [124], and, importantly, people without symptoms are less likely to answer questionnaires and undergo testing. Several of the studies cited in Table 9 had a low response rate, and the figures certainly represent an overestimation of the actual occurrence of latex sensitivity among health-care workers. It has been estimated that 250,000–500,000 U.S. health-care workers have latex allergy [125]. Allergic reactions may also be induced by latex products such as balloons, condoms, catheters, etc., and in addition to health professionals, workers in the rubber industry and patients exposed to multiple mucosal and/or surgical procedures have been found to be at special risk for latex allergy. Other

**Table 9** Prevalence of Latex Sensitivity in Health-Care Workers in the 1990s

| Author [Ref.] | Positive skin prick test (%) | Comments |
|---|---|---|
| Arellano [110] | 10 | Anesthesiologists, Toronto |
| Lagier [111] | 11 | Operating room nurses, France |
| Yassin [112] | 17 | Hospital employees, Ohio |
| Turjanmaa [113] | 8 | Nurses, New Orleans, Louisiana |
| Vandenplas [114] | 5 | Nurses, Belgium |
| Kaczmarek [115] | 6 | Hospital employees, 9 hospitals in US |
| Grzybowsky [116] | 9 | Nurses, Michigan |
| Leung [117] | 7 | Hospital employees, Hong Kong |
| Sussman [118] | 12 | Hospital employees, Pennsylvania |
| Harfi [119] | 19 | Hospital employees, Saudi Arabia |
| Tarlo [120] | 10 | Dental students, Toronto |
| Douglas [121] | 22 | Nurses, Australia |
| deGroot [122] | 8 | Laboratory workers, Netherlands |
| Handfield-Jones [123] | 14 | Hospital employees, England |

recognized risk factors include atopic predisposition, previous hand eczema, and use of powdered gloves. Of 6720 patients referred to a contact dermatitis clinic in England, 2.3% were thought to have an allergic contact dermatitis to an allergen (mostly rubber chemicals) present in rubber gloves, and in the subsequent 6-month period the overall prevalence of latex allergy by prick and patch testing was 1.9% in 822 patients [126]. Although some studies from blood donors (often hospital staff) indicate a higher rate of sensitivity, the prevalence of clinical allergy to latex in the general population is most likely far less than 1% [127].

## VI. REACTION TO STINGING AND BITING INSECTS

Allergic reactions to insects are predominantly caused by members of the Hymenoptera family—bees, wasps, and ants. These insects are well known for their painful stings, which may in rare cases be associated with anaphylactic reactions. The mortality from insect stings in the United States and Europe since 1960 is at most 1 death per year per 4 million inhabitants [128,129]. The prevalence of Hymenoptera sting allergy may be estimated from the history of allergic sting reaction and from determination of specific IgE in serum or skin prick tests (Tables 10, 11). Allergic reaction to Hymenoptera stings has been reported in 4–22%, while positive venom-specific IgE serum antibodies were observed in 12–18% of unselected samples of the general population. However, it should be noted that in surveys with diagnostic tests, the history of sting allergy is always less than the percentage of positive specific IgE, probably because an allergic sting reaction has not been clinically evident because many people lose their sensitivity before they are restung [133]. And of course, it has to be expected that the prevalence varies geographically corresponding to amount of stinging Hymenoptera in the region, outdoor wook activities, and degree of exposure. In fact, about 20% of beekeepers have a history of systemic allergic reaction after bee sting, indicating that the risk of developing an allergic reaction increases with the number of stings received [133]. This figure should be related to the 1–3% systemic allergic reaction reported in the general population (Table 10), and it appears to be a plausible assumption that, at most, 5–10% of the population in the temperate zone will have an allergic and mostly local reaction to Hymenoptera during their lifetime.

**Table 10**  Prevalence of Hymenoptera Sting Allergy

| Author [Ref.] | Year of age | Instrument | Lifetime prevalence (%) | Comments |
|---|---|---|---|---|
| Stuckey [130] | adults | Q | 7 | Western Australia |
| Herbert [131] | male adults | Q | 4* | Canada |
| Wüthrich [132] | 10–74 | Q | 5 | Switzerland |
| Golden [133] | adults | Q | 22** | Industrial workers, US |
| Charpin [134] | adults | Q | 11* | South France |

\* = 1% systemic allergic reaction; \*\* = 3% systemic allergic reaction.

**Table 11**  Prevalence of Hymenoptera Sting Allergy and Venom-Specific Serum Antibodies

| Author [Ref.] | Age | Lifetime prevalence (%) | Positive RAST (%) | Comments |
|---|---|---|---|---|
| Stuckey [130] | Adults | 7 | 16 | Western Australia |
| Herbert [131] | Male adults | 4 | 12 | Canada |
| Golden [133] | Adults | 22 | 17* | Industrial workers, US |
| Müller [134] | Adults | 12 | 18 | Blood donors, Switzerland |

* = 23% positive venom skin prick test.

## VII.  DRUG REACTIONS

Although adverse drug reaction is a daily problem in medical practice, it is difficult to get a clear picture from the available literature. Investigations of intensively treated inpatients may indicate a relatively high incidence, while more or less voluntarily reporting systems underestimate the occurrence of drug reactions. In fact, a database on adverse cutaneous reactions established in the United Kingdom in 1988 was closed in 1990 due to an unacceptably small number of reports received; the offer of a small fee has been shown to increase the rate of reporting almost 50-fold [136,137]. About 10–20% of patients develop an adverse drug reaction during hospital stay, whereas about 5% of hospital admissions are a direct consequence of drug reactions. In multicenter general practice study from the United Kingdom, the percentage of consultations involving drug reactions increased from 0.6% for patients ≤20 years of age to 2.7% for patients >50 years of age [138]. At present, hardly any systematic studies describe the incidence and prevalence of allergic adverse drug reactions in the general population. A recent reported computerized comprehensive hospital drug-monitoring program in Switzerland during a 20-year period (1974–1993) showed that 1,317 of 48,005 drug-receiving patients had definite or probable drug-induced skin reactions during hospitalization, corresponding to an overall frequency of 2.7% in divisions of internal medicine in cooperation with consultant dermatologists [139]. The above-mentioned Danish survey on allergy included the following question: "Are you allergic or hypersensitive to any drug or medical product?" [92]. A total of 5.1% of respondents answered positively (women 6.8%; men 3.3%), and when adjusted to those who at the same time reported that they had suffered from an allergic disease, the figures reveal an increasing prevalence from 1.7% in 1987 to 2.9% in 1994 [92]. Thus, the lifetime prevalence of allergic drug reactions seems to be in the region of 3–5% in the adult population and increasing slightly. The differential risks in relation to sex, age, particular drugs, and diseases are dealt with in Chapter 15.

## VIII.  CONCLUSIONS

The available data confirm that allergic skin disease is a growing socioeconomic problem that has a major impact on occupational performance and the quality of life of millions of people. A rather conservative estimate of 25–40% of humans will suffer from one or more allergic skin diseases during their lifetime. Moreover, data confirm that the incidence of allergic skin disorders rose during recent decades and that the total U.S. costs reached $5 billion annually. If the rising frequency of allergic skin diseases continues, it seems that in the future every human being will suffer from a more or less distressing allergic skin problem during his or her lifetime. As we march into the twenty-first century, it must be hoped that a combination of public awareness, responsible decision makers, and medical expertise may slow down or even reverse the epidemic of allergy and especially allergic skin disorders that has affected the western world and prevent or at least postpone a similar scenario in the developing countries.

## REFERENCES

1. Schultz Larsen F. The epidemiology of atopic dermatitis. In: Burr ML, ed. Epidemiology of Clinical Allergy. Monogr Allergy 31. Basel: Karger, 1993:9–28.
2. Wichmann HE. Environment, life-style and allergy: the German answer. Allergy J 1995; 4: 315–316.
3. Peat JK, Berg RH van den, Green WF, Mellis CM, Leeder SR, Woolcock AJ. Changing prevalence of asthma in Australian children. BMJ 1994; 308:1591–1596.
4. Burr ML, Limb ES, Andrae S, Barry DM, Nagel F. Childhood asthma in four countries: a comparative survey. Int J Epidemiol 1994; 23:341–347.
5. Lopez FM, Alcolea MR. Epidemiological study of allergic pathology in the general childhood population in Spain. Socioeconomic impact. Rev Esp Alergol Immunol Clin 1994; 9:23–35.
6. Angioni AM, Fanciulli G, Corchia C. Frequency of and risk factors for allergy in primary school children: results of a population survey. Pediatr Perinatal Epidemiol 1989; 3:248–255.
7. Moneret-Vautrin DA, Schiele F, Locuty J, Mikstacki T, Galteau MM, Grilliat JP. Etude épidémiologique du terrain atopigue en Lorraine. Allerg Immunol 1986; 18:4–12.
8. Peroni DG, Piacentini GL, Zizzo MG, Boner AL. Prevalence of wheezing, rhinitis and eczema in 6-7 years old children resident in northeastern Italy. Eur Respir J 1996; 9(suppl 23): 233.
9. Kay J, Gawkrodger DJ, Mortimer MJ, Jaron AG. The prevalence of childhood atopic eczema in a general population. J Am Acad Dermatol 1994; 30:35–39.
10. Neame RL, Berth-Jones J, Kurinczuk JJ, Graham-Brown RAC. Prevalence of atopic dermatitis in Leicester: a study of methodology and examination of possible ethnic variation. Br J Dermatol 1995; 132:772–777.
11. Williams HC, Burney PGJ, Pembroke AC, Hay RJ. Validation of the U.K. diagnostic criteria for atopic dermatitis in a population setting. Br J Dermatol 1996; 135:12–17.
12. Emerson RM, Williams HC, Allen BR. Severity distribution of atopic dermatitis in the community and its relationship to secondary referral. Br J Dermatol 1998; 139:73–76.
13. Kuehr J, Frischer T, Karmaus W, Meinert R, Barth R, Urbanek R. Clinical atopy and associated factors in primary-school pupils. Allergy 1992; 47:650–655.
14. von Mutius E, Fritzsch C, Weiland SK, Röll G, Magnussen H. Prevalence of asthma and allergic disorders among children in united Germany: a descriptive comparison. Br Med J 1992; 305:1395–1399.
15. Buser K, Bohlen F von, Werner P, Gernhuber E, Robra B-P. Neurodermitis—Prävalenz bei Schulkindern im Landkreis Hannover. Dtsch Med Wschr 1993; 118:1141–1145.
16. Schultz Larsen F, Diepgen T, Svensson Å. The occurrence of atopic dermatitis in North Europe: an international questionnaire study. J Am Acad Dermatol 1996; 34:760–764.

17. von Mutius E, Illi S, Nicolai T, Martinez FD. Relation of indoor heating with asthma, allergic sensitisation and bronchial responsiveness: survey of children in south Bavaria. Br Med J 1996; 312:1448–1450.

18. Schäfer T, Dirschedl P, Kunz B, Ring J, Überla K. Maternal smoking during pregnancy and lactation increases the risk for atopic eczema in the offspring. J Am Acad Dermatol 1997; 36:550–556.

19. Saval P, Fuglsang G, Madsen C, Østerballe O. Prevalence of atopic disease among Danish school children. Pediatr Allergy Immunol 1993; 4:117–122.

20. Olesen AB, Ellingsen AR, Olesen H, Juul S, Thestrup-Pedersen K. Atopic dermatitis and birth factors: historical follow up by record linkage. Br Med J 1997; 314:1003–1008.

21. Varjonen E, Kalimo K, Lammintausta K, Terho P. Prevalence of atopic disorders among adolescent in Turku, Finland. Allergy 1992;47:243–248.

22. Remes ST, Korppi M, Kajosaari M, Koivikko A, Soininen L, Pekkanen J. Prevalence of allergic rhinitis and atopic dermatitis among children in four regions of Finland. Allergy 1998; 53:682–689.

23. Hattevig G, Kjellman B, Björkstén B, Johansson SGO. The prevalence of allergy and IgE antibodies to inhalant allergens in Swedish school children. Acta Pediatr Scand 1987; 76: 349–355.

24. Croner S, Kjellman N-IM. Development of atopic disease in relation to family history and cord blood IgE levels. Pediatr Allergy Immunol 1990; 1:14–20.

25. Åberg N, Hesselmar B, Åberg B, Eriksson B. Increase of asthma, allergic rhinitis and eczema in Swedish school children between 1979 and 1991. Clin Exp Allergy 1995; 25:815–819.

26. Steen-Johnsen J, Bolle R, Holt J, Benan K, Magnus P. Impact of pollution and place of residence on atopic diseases among school children in Telemark County, Norway. Pediatr Allergy Immunol 1995; 6:192–199.

27. Dotterud LK, Kvammen B, Lund E, Falk E. Prevalence and some clinical aspects at atopic dermatitis in the community of Sørvaranger. Acta Derm Venereol (Stockh) 1995; 75:50–53.

28. Eaton KK. The incidence of allergy—Has it changed? Clin Allergy 1982; 12:107–110.

29. Taylor B, Wadworth J, Wadworth M, Peckham C. Changes in the reported prevalence of childhood eczema since the 1939–45 war. Lancet 1984; ii:1255–1257.

30. Varonier HS, Haller J de, Schopfer C. Prévalence de l'allergie chez les enfants et les adolescents. Helv Paediatr Acta 1984; 39:129–136.

31. Schultz Larsen F, Holm NV, Henningsen K. Atopic dermatitis. A genetic-epidemiologic study in a population-based twin sample. J Am Acad Dermatol 1986; 15:487–494.

32. Burr ML, Butland BK, King S, Vaughan-Williams E. Changes in asthma prevalence: two surveys 15 years apart. Arch Dis Child 1989; 64:1452–1456.

33. Ninan TK, Russell G. Respiratory symptoms and atopy in Aberdeen school children: Evidence from two surveys 25 years apart. Br Med J 1992; 304:873–875.

34. Schultz Larsen F. Atopic dermatitis: a genetic-epidemiological study in a population-based twin sample. J Am Acad Dermatol 1993; 28:719–723.

35. Skjønsberg OH, Clench-Aas J, Leegaard J, Skarpaas IJK, Giæver P, Bartonova A, Moseng J. Prevalence of bronchial asthma in Oslo, Norway. Comparison of data obtained in 1993 and 1981. Allergy 1995; 50:806–810.

36. Omran M, Russell G. Continuing increase in respiratory symptoms and atopy in Aberdeen school children Br Med J 1996; 312:34.

37. Austin JB, Russell G. Wheeze, cough, atopy and indoor environment in the Scottish Highlands. Arch Dis Child 1997; 76:22–26.

38. Nystad W, Magnus P, Gulsvik A, Skarpas IJK, Carlsen K-H. Changing prevalence of asthma in school children: evidence for diagnostic changes in asthma in two surveys 13 yrs apart. Eur Respir J 1997; 10:1046–1051.

39. von Mutius E, Weiland SK, Fritzsch C, Duhme H, Keil U. Increasing prevalence of hay fever and atopy among children in Leipzig, East Germany. Lancet 1998; 351:862–866.
40. Williams HC, Burney PGJ, Pembroke AC, Hay RJ. The U.K. working part's diagnostic criteria for atopic dermatitis. III. Independent hospital validation. Br J Dermatol 1994; 131: 406–416.
41. Henderson CA. The prevalence of atopic eczema in two different villages in rural Tanzania. Br J Dermatol 1995; 133(suppl 45):50.
42. Kalyoncu AF, Selsuk ZT, Karakoca Y, Emri AS, Cöplü L, Sahin AA, Baris YI. Prevalence of childhood asthma and allergic diseases in Ankara, Turkey. Allergy 1994; 49:485–488.
43. Saraclar Y, Yigit S, Adalioglu G, Tuncer A, Tuncbilek E. Prevalence of allergic diseases and influencing factors in primary school children in Ankara Region of Turkey. J Asthma 1997; 34:23–30.
44. Selcuk ZT, Caglar T, Enûnlü T, Topal T. The prevalence of allergic diseases in primary school children in Edirne, Turkey. Clin Exp Allergy 1997; 27:262–269.
45. Karaman Ö, Türkmen M, Uzuner N. Allergic disease prevalence in Izmir. Allergy 1997; 52: 689–690.
46. Bobák M, Koupilová I, Williams HC, Leon DA, Dánová J, Kriz B. Prevalence of asthma, atopic eczema and hay fever in five Czech towns with different levels of air pollution. Epidemiology 1995; 6(suppl 35):s35.
47. Popescu CM, Popescu R, Williams HC, Forsea D. Community validation of the United Kingdom diagnostic criteria for atopic dermatitis in Romanian school children. Br J Dermatol 1998; 138:436–442.
48. Leung R, Jenkins M. Asthma, allergy and atopy in southern Chinese school students. Clin Exp Allergy 1994; 24:353–358.
49. Leung R, Ho P. Asthma, allergy and atopy in three southeast Asian populations. Thorax 1994; 49:1205–1210.
50. Lau YL, Karlberg J, Yeung CY. Prevalence of and factors associated with childhood asthma in Hong Kong. Acta Pædiatr 1995; 84:820–822.
51. Goh DYT, Chew FT, Quek SC, Lee BW. Prevalence and severity of asthma, rhinitis and eczema in Singapore school children. Arch Dis Child 1996; 74:131–135.
52. Okuma M. Prevalence rate of allergic diseases among school children in Okinawa. Jpn J Allergol (Arerugi) 1994; 43:492–500.
53. Sugiura H, Umemoto N, Deguchi H, Tanaka K, Sawai T, Omoto M, Uchiyama M, Kiriyama T, Uehara M. Prevalence of childhood and adolescent atopic dermatitis in a Japanese population. Comparison with the disease frequency examined 20 years ago. Acta Derm Venereol (Stockh) 1998; 78:293–294.
54. Krämer U, Altus C, Behrendt H, Dolgner R, Gutsmuths FJ, Hille J, Hinrichs J, Mangold M, Paetz B, Ranft U, Röpke H, Teichmann S, Willer H-J, Schlipköter H-W. Epidemiologische Untersuchungen zur Auswirkung der Luftverschmutzung auf die Gesundheit von Schulanfängern. Forum Städte-Hygiene 1992; 43:82–87.
55. Englert N, Babisch W. Lungenfunktionsuntersuchungen bei Schulkindern in Berlin während der Wintermonate 1992/93. Institut für Wasser-, Boden- und Lufthygiene des Umweltbundesamtes Berlin, WaBoLu Heft 1/95, 1995.
56. Schäfer T, Vieluf D, Behrendt H, Krämer U, Ring J. Atopic eczema and other manifestation of atopy: results of a study in East and West Germany. Allergy 1996; 51:532–539.
57. Krämer U, Behrendt H, Ring J. Air pollution as a risk factor for allergy: the East-West German experience. In: Ring J, Behrendt H, Vieluf D, eds. New Trends in Allergy IV. Berlin: Springer, 1997:25–35.
58. Schultz Larsen F. Genetic epidemiology of atopic dermatitis. In: Williams HC, ed. Epidemiology of Atopic Eczema. Cambridge: Cambridge University Press. In press.
59. Schultz Larsen F. Atopic Dermatitis. Etiological Studies Based on a Twin Population. Copenhagen: Lægeforeningens Forlag, 1985.

60. Platts-Mills TAE, Mitchell EB, Rowntree S, Chapman MD, Wilkins SR. The role of dust mite allergens in atopic dermatitis. Clin Exp Dermatol 1983; 8:233–247.

61. Tan BB, Weald D, Strickland I, Friedman PS. Double-blind controlled trial of effect of housedust-mite allergen avoidance on atopic dermatitis. Lancet 1996; 347:15–18.

62. Olesen AB, Ellingsen AR, Olesen H, Juul S, Thestrup-Pedersen K. Atopic dermatitis and birth factors: Historical follow up by record linkage. Br Med J 1997; 314:1003–1008.

63. Black PN, Sharpe S. Dietary fat and asthma: Is there a connection? Eur Respir J 1997; 10: 6–12.

64. Traupe H, Menge G, Kandt I, Karmaus W. Higher frequency of atopic dermatitis and decrease in viral warts among children exposed to chemicals liberated in a chemical accident in Frankfurt, Germany. Dermatology 1997; 95:112–118.

65. McNally NJ, Williams HC, Philips DR, Smallman-Raynor M, Lewis S, Venn A, Britton J. Atopic eczema and domestic water hardness. Lancet 1998; 352:527–531.

66. Johnson M-LT. Prevalence of dermatological disease among persons 1–74 years of age: United States. Advance data from vital and health statistics of the National Center for Health Statistics, Rockville, Maryland, 1977, pp. 1–7.

67. Massicot JG, Cohen SG. Epidemiologic and socioeconomic aspects of allergic diseases. J Allergy Clin Immunol 1986; 78:954–958.

68. Beasley R, Keil U, von Mutius E, Pearce N, ISAAC Steering Committee. Worldwide variation in prevalence of symptoms of asthma, allergic rhinoconjunctivitis and atopic eczema: ISAAC. Lancet 1998; 351:1225–1232.

69. Asher MI, Keil U, Anderson HR, Beasley R, Crane J, Martinez F, Mitchell EA, Pearce N, Sibbald B, Stewart AW, Strachan D, Weiland SK, Williams HC. International study of asthma and allergies in childhood (ISAAC): rationale and methods. Eur Respir J 1995; 8: 483–491.

70. Olumide YM. The incidence of atopic dermatitis in Nigeria. Int J Dermatol 1986; 25:367–368.

71. Vickers CFH. The natural history of atopic eczema. Acta Derm Venereol (Stockh) 1980; suppl 92:113–115.

72. Williams HC, Strachan DP. The natural history of childhood eczema: observations from the British 1958 birth cohort study. Br J Dermatol 1998; 139:834–839.

73. Lapidus CS, Schwartz DF, Honig PJ. Atopic dermatitis in children: Who cares? Who pays? J Am Acad Dermatol 1993; 28:699–703.

74. Herd RM, Tidman MJ, Prescott RJ, Hunter JAA. The cost of atopic eczema. Br J Dermatol 1996; 135:20–23.

75. Emerson RM, Williams HC, Allen BR. What are the prescribing costs for atopic dermatitis in young children? Br J Dermatol 1998; 139(suppl 51):21–22.

76. Lewis-Jones MS, Finley AY. The children's dermatology life quality index (CDLQI): initial validation and practical use. Br J Dermatol 1995; 132:942–949.

77. Daud LR, Garralda ME, David TJ. Psychosocial adjustment in preschool children with atopic eczema. Arch Dis Child 1993; 69:670–676.

78. Lawson V, Lewis-Jones MS, Finley AY, Reid P, Owens RG. The family impact of childhood atopic dermatitis: the dermatitis family impact questionnaire. Br J Dermatol 1998; 138:107–113.

79. Su JC, Kemp AS, Varigos GA, Nolan TM. Atopic eczema: its impact on the family and financial cost. Arch Dis Child 1997; 76:159–162.

80. Finley AY. Measures of the effect of adult severe atopic eczema on quality of life. J Eur Acad Dermatol Venereol 1996; 7:149–154.

81. Absolon CM, Cottrell D, Eldridge SM, Glover MT. Psychological disturbance in atopic eczema: the extent of the problem in school-aged children. Br J Dermatol 1997; 137:241–245.

82. Service WC. The incidence of major allergic diseases in Colorado Springs. JAMA 1939; 112:2034–2037.

83. Eriksson-Lihr Z. Incidence of allergic diseases in childhood. Acta Allergol 1955; 8:289–313.

84. Lomholt G. Psoriasis: Prevalence, Spontaneus Course and Genetics. A Census Study on the Prevalence of Skin Disease on the Faröer Islands. Copenhagen: Gads Forlag, 1963.

85. Freeman GL, Johnson S. Allergic diseases in adolescents. Am J Dis Child 164; 107:549–559.

86. Hellgren L, Hersle K. Acute and chronic urticaria. Acta Allergol 1964; 9:406–420.

87. Kjellman N-IM. Atopic disease in seven-year-old children. Acta Pædiatr Scand 1977; 66: 465–471.

88. Weeke ER, Kamper-Jørgensen F, Pedersen PA. Incidences of nettle-rash and hypersensitivity in the adult Danish population. Ugeskr Læg 1980; 142:3340–3343.

89. Storm K, Haahr J, Kjellman N-IM, Østerballe O. The occurrence of asthma and allergic rhinitis, atopic dermatitis and urticaria in Danish children born in one year. Ugeskr Læg 1986; 148:3295–3299.

90. Åberg N, Engström I, Lindberg U. Allergic diseases in Swedish school children. Acta Pædiatr Scand 1989; 78:246–252.

91. Bakke P, Gulsvik A, Eide GE. Hay fever, eczema and urticaria in southwest Norway. Allergy 1990; 45:515–522.

92. Keiding L. Asthma, Allergy and Other Types of Hypersensitivity in Denmark—and the Development 1987–1994. Copenhagen: Danish Institute for Clinical Epidemiology (DICE), 1997.

93. Ebken RK, Bauschard FA, Levine MI. Dermographism: its definition, demonstration and prevalence. J Allergy 1968; 41:338–343.

94. Kirby JD, Matthews CNA, James J, Duncan EHL, Warin RP. The incidence and other aspects of factitious wealing (dermographism). Br J Dermatol 1971; 85:331–335.

95. Zuberbier T, Althaus C, Chantraine-Hess S, Czarnetzki BM. Prevalence of cholinergic urticaria in young adults. J Am Acad Dermatol 1994; 31:978–981.

96. Möller A, Henning M, Zuberbier T, Czarnetzki-Henz BM. Epidemiologie und Klinik der Kälteurtikaria. Hautarzt 1996; 47:510–514.

97. Agrup G. Hand eczema and other dermatoses in south Sweden. Acta Derm Venereol (Stockh) 1969; 49(suppl 61):1–91.

98. Lantinga H, Nater JP, Coenraads PJ. Prevalence, incidence and course of eczema on the hands and forearms in a sample of the general population. Contact Dermatitis 1984; 10:135–139.

99. Meding B. Epidemiology of hand eczema in an industrial city. Acta Derm Venereol (Stockh) 1990; 70(suppl 153):1–43.

100. Magnusson B, Möller H. Contact allergy without skin disease. Acta Derm Venereol (Stockh) 1979; 59(suppl 85):113–115.

101. Seidenari S, Manzini BM, Danese P, Motolese A. Patch and prick test study of 593 healthy subjects. Contact Dermatitis 1990; 23:162–167.

102. Nielsen NH, Menné T. Allergic contact sensitization in an unselected Danish population. Acta Derm Venereol (Stockh) 1992; 72:456–460.

103. Peltonen L. Nickel sensivity in the general population. Contact Dermatitis 1979; 5:27–32.

104. Mathias CGT. The cost of occupational skin disease. Arch Dermatol 1985; 121:332–334.

105. Halkier-Sørensen L. Occupational skin diseases: reliability and utility of the data in the various registers; the course from notification to compensation and the costs. Contact Dermatitis 1998; 39:71–78.

106. Morison WL, Stern RS. Polymorphous light eruption: a common reaction uncommonly recognized. Acta Derm Venereol (Stockh) 1982; 62:237–240.

107. Ros A-M, Wennersten G. Current aspects of polymorphous light eruption in Sweden. Photodermatology 1986; 3:298–302.

108. Selvaag E. Clinical drug photosensitivity. A retrospective analysis of reports to the Norwe-

gian Adverse Drug Reactions Committee from years 1970–1994. Photodermatol Photoimmunol Photomed 1997; 13:21–23.

109. Nutter AF. Contact urticaria to rubber. Br J Dermatol 1979; 101:597–598.

110. Arellano R, Bradley J, Sussman G. Prevalence of latex sensitization among hospital physicians occupationally exposed to latex gloves. Anesthesiology 1992; 77:905–908.

111. Lagier F, Vervloet D, Lhemet I, Poyen D, Charpin D. Prevalence of latex allergy in operating room nurses. J Allergy Clin Immunol 1992; 90:319–322.

112. Yassin MS, Lierl MB, Fischer TJ, O'Brian K, Cross J, Steinmetz C. Latex allergy in hospital employees. Ann Allergy 1994; 72:245–249.

113. Turjanmaa K, Cacioli P, Thompson RL, Simlote P, Lopez M. Frequency of natural rubber latex allergy among US operating room nurses using skin prick testing. J Allergy Clin Immunol 1995; 95:214.

114. Vandenplas O, Delwiche J-P, Evrard G, Aimont P, Brempt X van der, Jamart J, Delaunois L. Prevalence of occupational asthma due to latex among hospital personnel. Am J Respir Crit Care Med 1995; 151:54–60.

115. Kaczmarek RG, Silverman BG, Gross TP, Hamilton RG, Kessler E, Arrowsmith-Lowe JT, Moore RM. Prevalence of latex-specific IgE antibodies in hospital personnel. Ann Allergy Asthma Immunol 1996; 76:51–56.

116. Grzybowski M, Ownby DR, Peyser PA, Johnson CC, Schork MA. The prevalence of anti-latex IgE among registered nurses. J Allergy Clin Immunol 1996; 98:535–544.

117. Leung R, Ho A, Chan J, Choy D, Lai CKW. Prevalence of latex allergy in hospital staff in Hong Kong. Clin Exp Allergy 1997; 27:167–174.

118. Sussman GL, Liss GM. Latex allergy: epidemiologic study of 1351 hospital workers. J Allergy Clin Immunol 1997; 99:344.

119. Harfi H, Tirpirneni P, Mohammed GH, Lonnevig VG. Latex hypersensitivity: prevalence among health care personnel, as measured by skin prick test (SPT), CAP and challenge. J Allergy Clin Immunol 1997; 99:160.

120. Tarlo SM, Sussmman GL, Holness DL. Latex sensitivity in dental students and staff: a cross-sectional study. J Allergy Clin Immunol 1997; 99:396–401.

121. Douglas R, Czarny D, Morton J, O'Hehir RE. Prevalence of IgE-mediated allergy to latex in hospital nursing staff. Aust NZ J Med 1997; 27:165–169.

122. Groot H de, Jong NW de, Duijster E, Wijk RG van, Vermeulen A, Toorenenbergen AW van, Geursen L, Joost T van. Prevalence of natural rubber latex allergy (Type I and Type IV) in laboratory workers in the Netherlands. Contact Dermatitis 1998; 38:159–163.

123. Handfield-Jones SE. Latex allergy in health-care workers in an English district general hospital. Br J Dermatol 1998; 138:273–276.

124. Sussman GL, Beezhold DH. Allergy to latex rubber. Ann Intern Med 1995; 122:43–46.

125. Frankland AW. Latex allergy. Clin Exp Allergy 1995; 25:199–201.

126. Wilkinson SM, Beck MH. Allergic contact dermatitis from latex rubber. Br J Dermatol 1996; 134:910–914.

127. Turjanmaa K. Allergy to natural rubber latex: a growing problem. Ann Med 1994; 26:297–300.

128. Nall TM. Analysis of 667 death certificates and 168 autopsies of stinging insect deaths. J Allergy Clin Immunol 1985; 75:207.

129. Mosbech H. Death resulting from bee and wasp stings in Denmark 1960–1980. Ugeskr Læger 1983; 145:1757–1760.

130. Stuckey M, Cobain T, Sears M, Cheney J, Dawkins RL. Bee venom hypersensitivity in Busselton. Lancet 1982; ii:41.

131. Herbert FA, Salkie ML. Sensitivity to Hymenoptera in adult males. Ann Allergy 1982; 48:12–13.

132. Wüthrich B, Schnyder U, Henauer S, Heller A. Häufigkeit der Pollinosis in der Schweiz. Schweiz Med Wochenschr 1986; 116:909–917.

133. Golden DBK, Marsh DG, Kagey-Sobotka A, Freidhoff L, Szklo M, Valentine MD, Lichtenstein LM. Epidemiology of insect venom sensitivity. JAMA 1989; 262:240–244.

134. Charpin D, Vervloet D, Haddi E, Segalen C, Tafforeau M, Birnbaum J, Lanteaume A, Charpin J. Prevalence of allergy to Hymenoptera stings. Allergy Proc 1990; 11:29–32.

135. Müller UR. Insect Sting Allergy: Clinical Picture, Diagnosis and Treatment. Stuttgart: Fischer, 1990.

136. Black AK, Greaves MW. Cutaneous reactions database closure. Br J Dermatol 1990; 123: 277.

137. Feely J, Moriarty S, O'Connor P. Stimulating reporting of adverse drug reactions by using a fee. Br Med J 1990; 300:22–23.

138. Lumley CE, Walker SR, Hall GC, Staunton N, Grob PR. The under-reporting of adverse drug reactions seen in general practice. Pharmaceut Med 1986; 1:205–212.

139. Hunziker T, Künzi U-P, Braunschweig S, Zehnder D, Hoigné R. Comprehensive hospital drug monitoring (CHDM): adverse skin reactions, a 20-year survey. Allergy 1997; 52:388–393.

# 2
## Economic Evaluations in Allergic Skin Diseases

**Rukmini Rajagopalan**
*Glaxo Wellcome, Inc., Research Triangle Park, North Carolina*

## I. OVERVIEW

Allergy has been identified as the underlying etiological factor in skin disorders such as atopic dermatitis (AD) and allergic contact dermatitis (ACD). Even though AD can be associated with immunological deficiencies related back to genetic origin, exposure to certain trigger factors such as air pollutants, food items, and clothing items (e.g., wool) can cause exacerbation and give rise to an acute episode. In this age of industrial explosion, a large proportion of subjects afflicted with allergic contact dermatitis are exposed to a variety of allergenic material in their occupational settings. When disease invades innocent individuals in their workplace, the burden of disease for those individuals and their families will be enormous. For these subjects, going to work is like buying trouble through their labor; they not only become diseased but also are financially penalized by the direct and indirect costs of the disease and its treatment, not to mention the impact on the quality of life for themselves and their family.

In spite of the double jeopardy that befalls the subjects with allergic skin diseases, there have not been many studies demonstrating the extent and value of economic impact these diseases have on their victims. In the last two decades, dermatologists and immunologists have, through their intense efforts in research, been able to quantify to a certain extent the tremendous repercussions of allergic skin diseases. Arikian et al. [1] provided a detailed plan for a prospective program of economic evaluation for the treatment of atopic dermatitis and analysis methods using decision analysis modeling. In this chapter, a review of the studies that have attempted to gauge the burden of disease in subjects with AD and in those with ACD will be presented. Table 1 summarizes the plan.

## II. ATOPIC DERMATITIS

Management of AD for the most part consists of understanding the individual patient's disease pattern followed by identifying and reducing exacerbating factors as much as possible. In fact, the first-line therapy recently suggested [2] gives utmost importance to

**Table 1**  Studies and Audiences

| | | Audiences | |
|---|---|---|---|
| Stage | Study type | Internal | External[a] |
| Preclinical | Cost of illness | Strategic R&D Planning | Government |
| Phase I | Preliminary model | Strategic R&D Planning | Scientists, clinicians |
| Phase II | Detailed model for validation | R&D Marketing | Clinicians Health-care managers |
| Phase III | Piggyback study Validated model Management trial | Marketing R&D | Clinicians Health-care managers |
| Phase IV | Comparative management trials Comparative models | Marketing | Clinicians Health-care managers Formulary managers |

[a] Audiences external to the organization involved with the evaluation.

avoiding irritants and allergens, eliminating stress factors, and educating patients (Table 2).

The factors to consider in assessing the cost of AD management include drug costs, physician costs, procedures, laboratory tests, and hospitalization. Health economic evaluations are designed to examine resource consumption and consequences of alternative therapies. The design of a particular study may be determined by the perspective chosen, as these studies may be conducted from various perspectives such as payers/providers, administrators, government/society, or patients. Whatever the perspective, the overall aim of the study is to quantify the costs associated with care (tangible and intangible) and to establish objective criteria for the valuation of this investment.

Health economic research can help decision makers address such questions as:

What is the impact of the disease and treatment on the patient's economic (not to mention social and emotional) status?
What is the best drug for treating a particular disease?
What are the clinical outcomes associated with various therapies?

**Table 2**  First-Line Therapy for Atopic Dermatitis

Avoidance of irritants
Elimination of proven food and inhalant allergens
Stress reduction
Patient and family education
Hydration
Occlusives and moisturizers
Topical corticosteroids
Antimicrobials
Antihistamines

*Source*: Ref. 2.

What is the cost per quality-adjusted life-year extended by a particular therapy? How do two clinical pharmacy services compare?

In 1984 it was estimated that more than $300 million is spent annually in managing dermatitis in the US [3]. In 1995, the National Center for Health Statistics (NCHS) survey recorded that 7.6 million office visits were due to ACD, AD, and other eczema [4]. A recent estimation of occurrence rate shows an increase of up to 20% for atopic eczema, which was previously thought to be 10–15% [5]. In the past 2–3 years, the disease burden due to AD has been studied in depth in the United States [6], United Kingdom [7], and Australia [8]. Dermatologists in all three countries expressed similar concerns regarding the inadequate processes followed to diagnose and treat AD patients and children, suboptimal therapies available to treat them, and incomplete records available on the occurrence and prevalence of AD. The details of these three studies are discussed here.

## A. United States

Lapidus et al. [6] have expressed great concern about the fact that, despite the escalating prevalence and associated morbidity of AD, there is no systematic approach documented to deliver care and manage AD, particularly in urban children.

In the United States, 60% of AD cases occur in the first year of life and 90% in the first 5 years of life [9]. The prevalence of AD over the past three decades has more than tripled from 3 to 10% and seems to be even higher in some heavily populated urban areas [10,11]. In the absence of documentation for care delivery, local institution-specific data provided information on service use and expense of care for children with atopic dermatitis and national data sets were used to estimate the direct cost for care of children with AD in the United States.

The hospital data revealed that 63% of the outpatient visits occurred in the emergency department setting and 37% in other practice setting throughout the hospital. Further, it was interesting to note that 60% of emergency department visits for AD occurred during regular clinic hours. In just one urban children's hospital, approximately $410,000 was incurred in annual medical reimbursement cost for AD.

The total estimated cost for treatment of AD is $364 million annually in the United States. This includes inpatient and outpatient care (office visits and emergency department visits). AD definitely carries a high cost for the nation. As its prevalence continues to increase and funding for research and health care continues to decrease, the cycle of unending issues can be broken only by organizing the management of diagnosis and care in innovative and efficient ways, such as directing these children to dermatology clinics and family guidance, including home care. A recent study [12] showed that use of an emollient as an adjunctive therapy—reduced by half the amount of steroid used daily in a once-daily rather than twice-daily regimen—not only offers a steroid-sparing alternative for the treatment of mild to moderate AD, but may provide the added benefit of potentially reducing the cost of treatment.

## B. United Kingdom

According to Herd et al. [7], atopic eczema (AE) affects 2–3% of the UK population. The objective of the Lothian Atopic Dermatitis study was to estimate the costs associated with treatment of AE patients of all ages in the United Kingdom. They studied a sample of 155 patients randomly selected from the computerized records of eight general practitioners in Livingston, West Lothian. Diagnostic coding for various forms of eczema was used for easy identification. Patients were selected in stages:

1. All subjects satisfied the diagnostic criteria.
2. All families in the practice who were known to have children under the age of 2 years were questioned and examined.
3. A random sample of families were chosen and were contacted on the phone, and each adult in the family was interviewed to obtain information on any child in the family known to have a complaint or history of itchy skin.
4. All members in a family of six that denied the presence of an itchy member at stage 3 were individually examined to avoid oversight of an AE-afflicted subject.

To calculate the cost of disease and treatment prospectively, clear instructions were given to the patients to provide data on direct costs such as purchase of drugs and medical costs, office visits and procedures, costs of nonmedical purchases due to the disease, indirect costs such as loss of salary, absence from school or work, and any other expenses directly or indirectly resulting from the skin condition. The costs were monitored for a 2-month period.

Personal costs were as follows:

1. The mean personal expenditure by patients over the 2-month period was £25.90 and the maximum spent was £546, 81% of which was due to salary loss.
2. Forty-five percent of patients under the age of 16 and 26% over the age of 16 had no expenditure because they were in remission.
3. Patients aged 2–15 years incurred significantly less expenses than those over the age of 16,* and those under the age of 2 years had significantly less expenses than the former group.

Health service costs were as follows:

1. The mean health service cost was £16.20 and the maximum attributable to one patient was £177.07. The median cost for the group 2–15 years of age was significantly higher than that for the group over 16 years of age. The group under the age of 2 had significantly higher expenses than the former group.
2. The majority of health service costs were on treatments: 38% on emollients or bath additives, 32% on topical steroids, 10% on bandages, and the remaining 20% on antihistamines, shampoos, antibiotics, and evening primrose oil.

Hospital costs included the 2-month cost of the more severely affected cohort of patients attending hospital to the health service, which was up to £1500 per patient (mean £415), 63% of which was incurred by the hospital and 34% by the GPs. The maximum personal cost was £1225 (mean £325) over 2 months, 75% of which was due to loss of salary.

Extrapolation from the above data collection and analysis projected a total annual expenditure in the United Kingdom of £297 million by patients, an estimated annual cost to the health service of £125 million, and the cost to the society in lost working days of

---

* Patients below the age of 16 do not pay for prescriptions.

£43 million for a grand total of £465 million. The authors have cautioned the readers regarding some limitations of the data. The final estimate of the cost is likely to be an underestimate for the following reasons:

1. The prevalence of AE in Scotland is less than in the rest of the United Kingdom.
2. The GPs in the study practice are low prescribers.
3. None of the patients in the study population required hospital treatment during the study.
4. Patients lived within walking distance of the health center, which reduced travel costs.
5. The cost of the time of caretakers of dependents is not included in the calculation.

The data do give an indication of the magnitude of the problem in the United Kingdom. Patients' readiness to spend large sums of money for relief from their skin disease is demonstrated by 10 patients in the sample paying more than £100 in 2 months. To compare the burden of this disease on society with a few other diseases, annual per capita cost of treating AE (£7.38) was examined, as was treating venous ulcers (£6.73), stroke in Scotland (£18.78), and benign prostatic hypertrophy (£1.04–1.53).

The financial cost of severe AE undoubtedly has considerable impact on the sufferers. The burden is heavy and the ceiling of expenditure high. In an effort to measure the effect of adult severe atopic eczema on quality of life, Finaly [13] found out that 32% of patients had lost a median income of £5,000 over a 1-year period because of their eczema, and those patients who were working had lost a median of 5 days from work over a year period. Fifty percent of patients would be prepared to give up 2 hours or more a day in order to have normal skin, and 74%/49% of patients would be prepared to pay £1000/£10,000 or more for a cure.

## C. Australia

Su et al. [8] have found that some 25–50% of children suffering from AD develop asthma and 30% develop allergic rhinitis. AD is the single most common skin condition in children less than 11 years of age, and it is also an important cause of morbidity in adults. [14]. They decided to evaluate the impact of childhood AD of varying severity on families and assess the personal financial cost of its management by cross-sectional survey.

Infants and children presenting with AD to the dermatology clinic at the Royal Children's Hospital between March and August, 1995, and their families were studied. Forty-eight children were selected sequentially, and their eczema was categorized as mild, moderate, or severe by assessing the percent body surface area involved, the course of the illness, and intensity of itching.

The impact-on-family questionnaire of Stein and Riessman [15] was administered by a single researcher. This questionnaire, which has been used to assess the impact of several other chronic conditions, has four subscales assessing (1) financial burden, (2) familial/social impact, (3) personal strain, and (4) mastery, as perceived by the parent.

A control population of 46 children with insulin-dependent diabetes also enrolled sequentially from the diabetes clinic at the same hospital was also studied using the same questionnaire. This group was compared with an eczema group by a two-sample *t*-test. Analysis of covariance was performed to adjust for age as a covariate.

Impact-on-family scores were compared between the diabetes group and the eczema group (mild, moderate, and severe eczema children separately):

1. Impact-on-family scores: Children with moderate or severe eczema had higher scores than those with diabetes after adjusting for age differences, meaning that eczema had higher impact.
2. Community costs: The annual cost to the community of medical consultations for each child in the mild, moderate, and severe groups (calculated from the medical benefits schedule book) was Aus$209, 389, and 642, respectively. The annual cost to the community of hospitalization for each child in these three groups was Aus$453, 1,523, and 2,912, respectively.
3. Direct financial costs: The mean annual cost of eczema was related to the severity of eczema. The total mean costs of medication, dressings, diet, other eczema-management strategies, and medical consultations for the mild, moderate, and severe groups were Aus$330, 818, and 1,255, respectively. The major costs were for medication and dressings. Other expenses included change of carpets, purchase of dust mite–free covers, and purchase of extra nonirritant clothing. Comparable costs for 22 diabetic children averaged Aus$444.
4. Indirect costs: Only time off from work to care for the sick child was included. The potential income loss due to employment reduced, ceased, or not started for parents was not estimated. The cost and time to travel to and from the provider's office or clinic were not determined. Therefore the indirect costs were considerably underestimated.

The social, family, and emotional effects and personal financial costs of eczema have never been quantified. The impact on family scores was higher in the moderate and severe eczema groups compared with scores for the type I diabetes group. It is very clear that this common disorder has a profound impact on families, a fact that is underappreciated in view of the lack of support for families of children with eczema compared with that for families of children with diabetes or asthma. Even in the mild eczema group, the family score was equivalent to that for children with insulin-dependent diabetes.

Management of AD in children is complex and costly, often requiring a well-planned multifaceted approach for optimal care. There is a great impact on the quality of life in children and families. There is a real need for doctors and health-care managers to recognize that eczema is not merely a minor skin disorder, but a major handicap with a major personal, social, and financial burden on the family.

## III. ALLERGIC CONTACT DERMATITIS

ACD is caused by either irritants or allergens. ACD is a common allergic condition affecting the skin. It presents as an acute or subacute eruption characterized by erythema, vesicles, and scaling after exposure to the contact allergen. The first-line therapy suggested for AD (Table 1) is appropriate for ACD also. However, history of the disease is important to obtain and confirm the diagnosis. In 1989, Rietschel [16] demonstrated that patch testing is a valuable tool in providing an accurate, relatively simple means of diagnosis that allows the physician to initiate appropriate management to alleviate patients' suffering without losing precious time.

In a prospective study to evaluate the benefits of patch testing in suspected ACD subjects [17], it was found that patch testing is considered worthwhile by patients in spite of the discomfort caused and the additional cost involved. Patch testing also helps to confirm diagnosis at a higher rate and at an earlier time point than no-patch testing. In general, patients who were patch tested in the first week had greater quality-of-life benefits than those who were patch tested at later times, although cost-effectiveness ratios were less favorable with early patch testing in mild ACD subjects. The study also predicted a savings of about $700 million in the national expenditure using patch testing and confirming early diagnosis, assuming that a million subjects in the United States suffer from moderate to severe ACD—extrapolated from the NCHS data [3] on annual physician visits for AD, eczema, and ACD. (This did not take into account the cost of actual patch-test packages, which could range from $90 to $520 per patient.)

The study also demonstrated that the improvement in quality of life was greater in patients who had their diagnosis confirmed earlier with patch testing than in those who were not patch tested or who were patch tested later. In terms of dermatology-specific quality of life (DSQL) [18], patients who were patch tested in the first week had the greatest quality-of-life benefits and, in general, had greater economic benefits than those who were patch tested at later times.

## IV.  CONCLUSION

From the literature reviewed here, it is strikingly evident that a number of activities—such as avoidance of irritants, elimination of proven food and inhalant allergies, stress reduction, patient and family education, and hydration—to reduce the rigors of the diseases caused or triggered by allergy can be accomplished with no or minimum financial involvement. Patients and family should be educated to include these activities in their regular routine with strict adherence. Such a discipline can, for most patients, reduce the severity of the disease to a manageable level and contain the costs of pharmaceuticals and hospital services within reasonable limits.

## REFERENCES

1.  Arikian S, Einarson TR, Doyle JJ. Atopic Dermatitis: Economic evaluation of treatments for eczema and atopic dermatitis. In Rajagopalan R, Sherertz EF, Anderson RT, eds. Care and Management of Skin Diseases—Life Quality and Economic Impact. New York: Marcel Dekker, 1998:317–340.
2.  Boguniewicz M, Leung DYM. New concepts in atopic dermatitis. Compr Ther 1996; 22(3): 144–151.
3.  Johnson ML, Johnson KG, Engel A. Prevalence, morbidity and cost of dermatologic disease. J Am Acad Dermatol 1984; 11:930–936.
4.  Office visits to dermatologists: National Ambulatory Medical Care Survey, United States, 1991–92. In: Advanced Data, 1996. Division of Health Care Statistics. National Center for Health Statistics. Hyattsville, MD.
5.  Kay J, Gawkrodger DJ, Martimer MJ, Jaron AG. The prevalence of childhood atopic eczema in a general population. J Am Acad Dermatol 1994; 30:35–39.
6.  Lapidus CS, Schwartz FD, Honig PJ. Atopic dermatitis in children: Who cares? Who pays? J Am Acad Dermatol 1993; 28(5):699–703.

7.  Herd RM, Tidman MJ, Prescott RJ, Hunter JAA. The cost of atopic eczema. Br J Dermatol 1996; 135:20–23.
8.  Su JC, Kemp AS, Varigos GA, Terence MN. Atopic eczema: its impact on the family and financial cost. Arch Dis Childhood 1997; 76:159–162.
9.  Rajka G. Atopic dermatitis. In: Rook A, ed. Major Problems in Dermatology. London: W.B. Saunders, 1975:3.
10. Larsen FS, Holm NV, Henningsen K. Atopic dermatitis. J Am Acad Dermatol 1986; 15:487–494.
11. Hannifin JM. Epidemiology of atopic dermatitis. Monogr Allergy 1987; 21:116–131.
12. Lucky WL, Leach AD, Laskarzewski P, Wenck H. Use of an emollient as a steroid-sparing agent in the treatment of mild to moderate atopic dermatitis in children. Pediatr Dermatol 1997; 14(4):321–324.
13. Finlay AY. Measures of the effect of adult severe atopic eczema on quality of life. Eur Acad Dermatol Venereol 1996; 7:149–154.
14. Hanifin JM, Rajka G. Diagnostic features of atopic dermatitis. Acta Derm Venereol (Stockholm) 1980; 92(Suppl):44.
15. Stein REK, Riessman CK. The development of an impact-on-family scale: preliminary findings. Med Care 1980; 28:462–472.
16. Rietschel RL. Human and economic impact of allergic contact dermatitis and the role of patch testing. J Am Acad Dermatol 1995; 21:812–815.
17. Rajagopalan R, Anderson RT, Sarma S, Retchin C, Jones J. The use of decision-analytical modeling in economic evaluation of patch testing in allergic contact dermatitis. Pharmacoeconomics 1998; 14(1):79–95.
18. Anderson RT, Rajagopalan R. Development and validation of a quality of life instrument for cutaneous diseases. J Am Acad Dermatol 1997; 37:41–50.

# 3

## Molecular Mechanisms of Allergic Skin Responses

**Robert C. Fuhlbrigge**
*Harvard Institutes of Medicine, Boston, Massachusetts*

**Thomas S. Kupper**
*Brigham and Women's Hospital, Boston, Massachusetts*

## I. INTRODUCTION

The skin, as the body's principal interface with the environment, plays a crucial role in protecting us from a variety of potential pathogens. The skin is often viewed as simply a passive barrier, limiting invasion by interposing a layer of dead keratinocytes (stratum corneum) between the fragile live tissues and the hostile environment. The speed at which infection develops when this barrier is disrupted, as in a burn victim, emphasizes this role and confirms its effectiveness. It is increasingly apparent, however, that these mechanical aspects of epidermal defense are backed up by an immunosurveillance and rapid response mechanism that is crucial in maintaining homeostasis [1]. The influence of this more subtle function of skin is made evident by the dramatic increase in the frequency and severity of cutaneous tumors and infections observed when immune function is limited, as among patients with genetic and acquired immunodeficiency disorders and those receiving immunosuppressive medications following organ transplantation [2,3]. Excessive immune function is also detrimental and drives the pathogenesis of a remarkable variety of acquired inflammatory skin disorders including psoriasis, atopic and allergic contact dermatitis, lichen planus, alopecia areata, and vesiculo-bullous disorders [4–10]. The role of immune dysfunction in these conditions is reflected in their response to immunosuppressive therapeutic interventions, with the most effective therapies either directly or indirectly targeting T-cell function [11–15]. While the lesions of a particular condition may differ between individuals with respect to gross phenotype and physical location, immunohistology often reveals characteristic structural changes and cellular infiltrates that are constant between individuals with the same disorder and can serve to confirm or disprove the diagnosis [16]. For example, although a minor population in peripheral blood, eosinophils are often prominent in chronic allergic inflammatory reactions (e.g., reactive airways, allergic rhinitis) [17,18]. These common features reflect common mechanisms of immune activation leading to the attraction and accumulation of unique and characteristic subsets of inflammatory cells according to the mode of stimulation. In this review we describe the components of the cutaneous immune system and discuss the elements regulating its function, with particular regard to the development of allergic skin inflammation.

## II. IMMUNE EFFECTOR CELLS OF THE SKIN

Many of the cellular elements of skin have been shown to mediate immune functions directly or to produce proinflammatory cytokines and chemical mediators in response to stimulation that can act to modify the immune functions of other cells. It is evident from the breadth of recent reports that a complex interplay of stimulatory and control signals exists between the various cellular elements of skin and regulates the patterns of cellular infiltration and growth observed in particular disorders. Both passive (e.g., release of pre-formed mediators in response to injury) and active (e.g., recruitment of restricted circulating leukocyte subpopulations) mechanisms for the induction and maintenance of immune responses exist and contribute to the development and maintenance of cutaneous immune responses. We will highlight some of the most prominent aspects of this process below.

The cellular components of skin can be divided primarily into structural elements, or semi-permanent residents of the skin, versus cells that are actively recruited from the blood in response to inflammatory stimuli (Table 1). Immunohistology of inflammatory

**Table 1** Immune Functions of Skin Elements

| Cell type | Immune functions |
|---|---|
| Tissue resident cells | |
| Keratinocyte | Production/Release of IL-1 in response to injury |
| | Cytokine production in situ |
| Intraepidermal lymphocytes | Cytokine production |
| | Cell-mediated cytotoxic effects |
| Dendritic cells (Langerhans) | Antigen processing and presentation |
| | Cytokine production |
| | Antigen transport to lymph nodes |
| Dermal macrophage | Phagocytosis |
| | Antigen processing and presentation |
| | Cytokine production |
| Fibroblasts | Cytokine production |
| | Production of keratinocyte growth factor |
| Mast cells | Production/Release of anaphylactic mediators |
| | Production of chemokines |
| Endothelial cells | Regulation of leukocyte trafficking |
| | Production/Presentation of selectins, chemo-kines, integrin receptors, etc. |
| Cells trafficking through skin | |
| Granulocytes | Phagocytosis/Pathogen degradation |
| Neutrophils | Production/Release of inflammatory mediators |
| Eosinophils | Production/Release of cytokines |
| Lymphocytes | Cytokine production |
| | Cell-mediated cytotoxic effects |
| | Immunoregulatory/Suppressor effects |
| Monocytes | Antigen processing and presentation |
| | Cytokine production |
| Blood dendritic cells | Antigen processing and presentation |
| | Cytokine production |
| | Antigen transport to lymph nodes |

skin lesions reveals patterns of involvement of these elements that are quite variable between disorders but are often characteristic for specific disorders [16,19].

## A. Keratinocytes

Keratinocytes (KC) are an important and often underappreciated participant in cutaneous immune responses. KC produce and store large quantities of interleukin (IL)-1$\alpha$, which is released in response to a variety of stimuli, including kinetic and thermal trauma, ultraviolet (UV) irradiation, IL-1$\beta$, interferon gamma (IFN-$\gamma$), IL-17, substance P, and alpha melanocyte-stimulating hormone ($\alpha$MSH) [20–24]. IL-1$\alpha$, in turn, acts as a potent and immediate nonspecific initiator and facilitator of local immune function [25]. KC also produce a large number of chemokines and other immunoregulatory cytokines in response to stimulation (Table 2) [26–29]. These products attract various subpopulations of circulating leukocytes to the site and promote the immune function of these leukocytes and the other skin elements. The conspicuous lack of IFN-$\gamma$ and IL-12 production by KC biases many cutaneous inflammatory responses toward T helper type 2 (Th2) responses (discussed in further detail below). In addition to the production of soluble immune mediators, dysregulation of KC proliferation and differentiation is also often characteristic for particular cutaneous inflammatory lesions and can be used as an independent diagnostic feature.

## B. Fibroblasts

Fibroblasts (Fb) also play an important role in cutaneous immune responses via their production of growth factors and a range of cytokines and chemokines [30]. Fibroblasts

**Table 2** Immunoregulatory Mediators Produced by Keratinocytes

Cytokines
    IL-1$\alpha$ (preformed and released in response to
      injury)
    IL-1$\beta$, IL-1ra
    IL-3, 6, 7, 10, 12, 15, 18
    TGF-$\alpha$, TGF-$\beta$
    TNF-$\alpha$
Chemokines
    RANTES
    IL-8
    IP-10
Growth factors
    GM-CSF
    G-CSF
    M-CSF
    KGF
    PDGF
    VEGF
Others
    Acetylcholine
    ICAM-1 and other adhesion molecules
    Superoxide
    $\alpha$MSH

produce a variety of chemokines, including monocyte chemotactic protein-1 (MCP-1), RANTES, eotaxin, IL-8, and fractalkine, in response to IL-1 and other pro-inflammatory cytokines. The products of Th2 infiltrates (e.g., IL-4) are thought to be especially important in the recruitment of eosinophils to atopic skin [31]. Fibroblasts also produce an assortment of growth factors, including keratinocyte growth factor (KGF), platelet-derived growth factor (PDGF), tumor growth factor β (TGF-β) and granulocyte-monocyte colony-stimulating factor (GM-CSF), that have autocrine effects and may also support the local proliferation and differentiation of other cellular elements [32–36].

## C. Dendritic Cells and Macrophages

Dendritic cells (DC) and macrophages are potent bone marrow–derived antigen-processing cells that can be found in most tissues, where they perform diverse functions involved in antigen processing and presentation and immune regulation [37]. Langerhans cells are a specialized population of dendritic cells found only in skin that possesses unique intracellular inclusions, called Birbeck granules, and a distinct pattern of differentiation markers [38,39]. Dermal DC cells are similar in appearance but lack the characteristic granules of Langerhans cells. DC form a crucial link between the innate and acquired aspects of immune function [40–43]. DC exposed to antigen in skin migrate to the local lymphatics and carry antigen fragments from the local site of inflammation to the draining lymph nodes [44]. Here they are able to present antigen to naïve T cells and promote the development of memory T-cell responses. Dermal DC and macrophages can also process and present antigen and remain in the skin to promote the development of local immune responses [45]. Dendritic cells and macrophages produce multiple inflammatory cytokines and co-stimulatory molecules important in promoting T-cell proliferation, maturation, and function [46,47]. Depending on the context of stimulation, Langerhans cells are capable of expressing co-stimulatory molecules and cytokines that can support differentiation of T cells into either Th1 (e.g., via expression of IL-12) or Th2 (e.g., via expression of IL-1) phenotype [48,49]. The high frequency of skin infections in patients lacking the ability to phagocytose pathogens or to produce a respiratory burst highlights the importance of these cells in cutaneous surveillance for invading organisms [50]. Circulating populations of monocytes and CD34+ DC precursors can also be actively recruited from the blood to inflammatory sites to provide additional immunoregulatory support [43]. At each stage of differentiation, from bloodborne precursor to tissue DC to lymph node antigen-presenting cell (APC), DC express different chemokine receptors and respond to distinct subsets of chemoattractants. This allows precise control over the migration of DC and their participation in various aspects of the immune response.

## D. Lymphocytes

T cells also exist in stable resident populations and as recirculating elements of the cutaneous immune system [51]. Intraepidermal T cells reside in the basal epidermis and are thought to provide primarily an immunoregulatory or suppressive influence [31,42,52–54]. Both αβ and γδ T-cell receptor (TCR)–bearing populations are found in the skin, where their relative role in innate immune responses is the subject of intense investigation [55]. Circulating αβ memory T cells form the primary antigen-specific defense element of skin, migrating into tissues under the direction of adhesion molecules and chemokines expressed on the local endothelial surfaces (discussed in greater detail below). T cells trafficking through a tissue that encounter their cognate antigen can proliferate and participate in the local inflammatory response, while those that do not encounter their antigen will move on into the lymphatics and return to the circulation.

## E. Mast Cells

Mast cells reside primarily in the superficial dermis and closely opposed to blood vessels and nerves. They possess high-affinity surface receptors for IgE and play an important role in the development of allergic disease. Mast cells release a number of preformed immune modulators and produce additional products in response to stimulation. In addition to antigen/IgE, skin mast cells respond to a large number of nonimmunological products including poly-L-lysine, morphine, substance P, vasoactive intestinal peptide, and somatostatin. Preformed proinflammatory and vasoactive products available for rapid release include histamine, tryptase, chymase, heparins, chondroitin sulfate, and tumor necrosis factor $\alpha$ (TNF-$\alpha$). Cytokines produced by mast cells in response to stimulation include TNF-$\alpha$, IL-4, IL-5, IL-6, and prostaglandin $D_2$. These, in turn, can stimulate the expression of endothelial adhesion molecules and activate other immune effector cells attracted to the site.

## F. Granulocytes

Neutrophils are acute inflammatory response elements, providing nonspecific control of pathogens by phagocytosis and release of oxygen radicals and other cytotoxic products [56,57]. Neutrophils are not found in the resident population of uninflamed skin, but emigrate rapidly from blood in response to acute inflammatory mediators. Neutrophils are unique in their expression of the CXCR1 and CXCR2 chemokine receptors and, therefore, in their ability to migrate in response to the family of chemokines that bind to these receptors (e.g., IL-8, Gro-$\alpha$, LIX, etc.)(see below). While neutrophils are often an element of early cutaneous inflammatory lesions, chronic allergic skin conditions are typically characterized by lymphocytic and/or eosinophilic infiltration. Eosinophils are attracted and promoted by cytokines and chemokines (e.g., IL-5 and eotaxin) produced by mast cells and Th2 type memory T cells in response to inflammation. Eosinophil products implicated in the maintenance of chronic allergic dermatitis include major basic protein, eosinophil cationic protein, IL-3, IL-5, GM-CSF, leukotriene C4, and TGF.

## G. Endothelial Cells

The role of endothelium in the recruitment of leukocytes to inflammatory lesions has been recognized for over 100 years [58]. Adhesion molecules and chemokines presented on the endothelial surfaces direct the recruitment of specific leukocyte subpopulations through a well-described sequence of interactions with counterreceptors presented on the circulating leukocytes [59,60]. This multistep model of leukocyte-endothelial interactions has been well supported in cutaneous inflammatory responses, with a number of molecules specifically involved in cutaneous responses identified. This interface between the circulating immune elements and the local tissue sites serves several functions critical to the development and regulation of cutaneous immune responses and will be discussed in greater detail.

## III.  REGULATION OF LEUKOCYTE TRAFFICKING TO SKIN

The regulation of leukocyte accumulation in tissues is fundamental to both the initiation of appropriate immune responses and the suppression of inappropriate immune responses. As the largest environmental interface, the skin is subject to many insults and susceptible to many disorders. It is clearly desirable to be able to direct a relevant subset of memory T cells to skin whenever this environmental interface is breached. Indeed, the importance of normal T-cell function at the skin environmental interface has been highlighted in tragic fashion by the HIV pandemic. As CD4 counts fall in such patients, novel presentations of infectious skin diseases, as well as exaggerated iterations of known skin diseases, emerged with high frequency [2]. These events suggest that the CD4 lymphopenia induced by AIDS reveals in a more obvious fashion what is normally an ongoing but invisible subclinical battle between host and pathogen in skin. Increasing evidence suggests that cell surface adhesion molecules expressed on subclasses of memory T cells mediate their accumulation in inflamed skin [60,61]. The mechanisms by which neutrophils, monocytes, and individual memory T cells, including the effector cells of antigen-specific cutaneous allergic responses, target to skin has been the subject of numerous investigations and a source of extensive speculation.

### A.  Multistep Model of Leukocyte-Endothelial Interaction

Substantial data support a multistep model of leukocyte trafficking from blood to tissue involving, sequentially, reversible selectin-mediated attachment, chemokine-stimulated activation, and integrin-dependent firm-adhesion followed by transmigration across vessel walls (Fig. 1). This model predicts that each vascular site will display a unique "address code" formed by the combinatorial expression of the leukocyte adhesion molecule receptors, chemoattractants, and regulatory cytokines produced in response to a given inflammatory stimulus. The particular effector molecules present direct the local margination and transmigration of the subset of circulating leukocytes with the best "fit," as determined by their complement of surface adhesion molecules and chemoattractant counterreceptors. While each leukocyte has its best vascular "address," substantial overlap allows recruitment of more or less broad cell populations in response to individual and varying degrees of stimuli.

Clearly, identification of the specific "homing" mechanism regulating inflammation in any particular tissue bed will have important implications for the study of disease pathophysiology and the development of therapeutic strategies for disorders affecting that tissue. While considerable effort has been directed toward identifying various components of this pathway, no one set of ligands and receptors has been identified that definitively directs the accumulation of a unique subset of leukocytes in a particular tissue bed. However, the identification of a putative T-cell skin-homing receptor, called the cutaneous lymphocyte-associated antigen (CLA), has spurred recent advances in our understanding of these processes in skin.

### B.  Cutaneous Lymphocyte-Associated Antigen

Cutaneous lymphocyte-associated antigen (CLA) is a surface carbohydrate epitope, identified by reactivity with a unique monoclonal antibody called HECA-452, that is found on

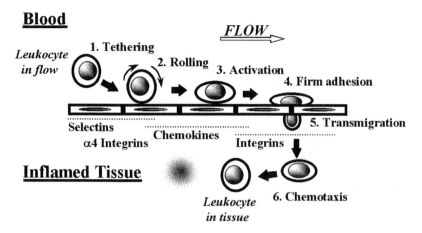

**Figure 1** Multistep model of leukocyte endothelial interaction. In order to enter an inflammatory site, leukocytes moving in the blood flow must successfully negotiate a sequential series of intermediate steps. Cells in flow first tether to the vessel wall and roll across the venular endothelium via the interaction of endothelial selectins with leukocyte selectin ligands (e.g., CLA/PSGL-1) and/or endothelial VCAM-1 with leukocyte $\alpha4$ integrins (e.g., VLA-4). Rolling cells that express counterreceptors for the chemokines and activating cytokines presented at the site of inflammation become activated and form firm adhesions via the binding of leukocyte integrins (e.g., LFA-1, Mac-1) to vascular Ig superfamily ligands (e.g., ICAM-1, ICAM-2). Firmly bound cells can then transmigrate into the underlying tissue and participate in local immune responses. Each step is required for successful leukocyte entry into a given tissue. Cells lacking appropriate receptors for the particular adhesion molecules and chemokines expressed in response to a stimulus will pass through the vessel and remain in the general circulation.

approximately 15% of circulating memory T cells and is virtually absent on naïve T cells [62]. Nearly all T cells found in inflammatory skin lesions are CD45RO+, and the majority of these are CLA+. In contrast, very few T cells accumulating in noncutaneous inflammatory sites express CLA [62,63]. There is additional evidence that T cells specific for skin disease–related antigens in patients with inflammatory skin disorders bear CLA when circulating in peripheral blood [61,64–67]. In cutaneous T-cell lymphoma (CTCL) biopsies, both the malignant and reactive T cells in the skin lesion are CLA+. CLA appears to be a good marker of CTCL cells in peripheral blood, and the CLA+ fraction contains the malignant clone [68].

## C. Structure, Function, and Regulation of CLA

The CLA epitope recognized by mAb HECA-452 has recently been identified as an inducible carbohydrate modification of a known adhesion molecule, the P-selectin glycoprotein ligand-1 (PSGL-1) [69]. PSGL-1 is constitutively expressed on all T cells and myeloid lineage cells as a disulfide-linked homodimer that is extensively decorated with O-linked polysaccharides (Fig. 2). Electron microscopy studies indicate that PSGL-1 is found exclusively at the tips of microvilli, where it is in prime position to interact with blood vessel walls [70]. Published reports from several laboratories have led to the hypothesis that PSGL-1 is synthesized as a non–selectin-binding precursor, which can be modified to bind P-selectin and/or E-selectin via separate, posttranslational pathways [69,71–75].

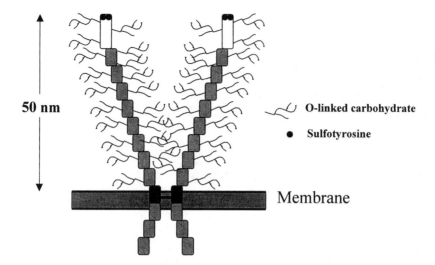

50 nm

O-linked carbohydrate

Sulfotyrosine

Membrane

**Figure 2** Structure of CLA/PSGL-1: PSGL-1 is a disulfide-linked homodimeric glycoprotein with an extensively O-glycosylated mucin-like extracellular domain. The P-selectin binding site is contained in the most N-terminal nine amino acids and is dependent on three sulfated tyrosine residues and an adjacent O-linked carbohydrate chain. The E-selectin–binding elements and HECA-452 Ab-binding epitopes that define the CLA are not dependent on the protein backbone and likely include several, if not all, of the available O-linked carbohydrate residues.

P-selectin and E-selectin binding function has also been reported to be differentially expressed on T cells of Th1 versus Th2 phenotype, although the actual ligands involved remain incompletely defined [76–78].

Recent studies have provided some insight into potential mechanisms for the production of independent selectin-binding sites on this single glycoprotein. P-selectin binding has been convincingly demonstrated to arise from a combinatorial domain near the amino terminus of PSGL-1 that is composed of a trio of sulfated tyrosine residues and an adjacent O-linked carbohydrate [74,79–81]. PSGL-1 is the only glycoprotein currently recognized as able to support high-affinity P-selectin binding. E-selectin binding is less well defined, in that multiple glycoproteins have been identified with E-selectin ligand activity without a clear indication as to which is/are physiologically relevant. At one extreme, E-selectin can be demonstrated to be able to bind sLex and related carbohydrates on a number of surface glycoproteins and probably on glycolipids as well. PSGL-1 itself contains a large number of O-linked carbohydrate chains, any one, or even all, of which could be decorated with sLex and potentially serve as an effective E-selectin binding site.

Investigation of the carbohydrate elements of E- and P-selectin ligands has identified the function of $\alpha(1,3)$-fucosyltransferase VII (FucTVII) and core 2 $N$-acetylglucosamine transferase (C2 GlcNAc T) as essential steps in the biosynthesis of the carbohydrate elements involved in selectin binding [74,82]. Although multiple fucosyltransferases have been described, FucTVII is the only candidate known to be expressed in leukocytes that is capable of producing the relevant structures. Most informative has been the production of a mouse strain with homozygous deletion of the FucTVII gene, which results in a near complete lack of demonstrable selectin ligands and a profound defect in leukocyte localization in tissues [83]. The recent demonstration of a mouse deficient in core 2 activity has also clarified the role of this modifying enzyme in the formation of selectin ligands [84]. Loss of core 2 oligosaccharides reduced neutrophil binding to E- and P-selectins in vitro and neutrophil recruitment to sites of inflammation but did not affect L-selectin–mediated homing to lymph nodes.

These studies highlight an intriguing hypothesis—that the regulation of leukocyte homing behavior, may be mediated in part by posttranslational modification of the carbohydrates expressed on surface glycoproteins.

## D. Chemokines

As outlined above, leukocyte extravasation from blood into tissues is a multistep process involving sequential coordinated interactions between leukocytes and endothelial cells. As the ligands for the endothelial selectins (e.g., PSGL-1 and CLA) and the various leukocyte integrins (e.g., LFA-1, VLA-4) are expressed on relatively large, overlapping fractions of circulating leukocytes, these alone would not be able to direct the highly specific cellular accumulations seen in many inflammatory disease responses. This specificity is increasingly recognized to depend on the local production of chemotactic cytokines, termed chemokines [85,86]. Chemokines are small 8–10 kDa proteins produced by virtually every cell population present in skin, including keratinocytes, fibroblasts, dermal macrophages, and Langerhans cells, and endothelial cells in response to inflammatory stimuli. More than 40 chemokines have been identified, representing at least four families of molecules related by structure and function (Table 3). The α-chemokines (or CXC chemokines) are comprised of two main subgroups. Those that contain the sequence glutamic acid–leucine–arginine near the N-terminus (e.g., IL-8) are chemotactic for neutrophils, while those lacking this sequence (e.g., IP-10, SDF-1) act on lymphocytes. The β-chemokines (or CC chemokines), in general, do not act on neutrophils, but attract other leukocytes with variable efficacy. They can also be divided into two subgroups based on sequence homology: one consisting of the five monocyte chemotactic proteins and eotaxin and the other containing all of the other CC chemokines. Lymphotactin (C chemokine) and fractalkine (CXXXC chemokine) are structurally dissimilar from the α and β chemokines and may represent their own families. Another way to divide chemokines is between (1) those that are constitutively expressed (e.g., TARC, ELC, SLC, SDF-1, and BCA-1) and appear to be involved in baseline trafficking and (2) those that are inducible and appear to direct accumulation of specific cell subsets in response to inflammation. The main stimuli for chemokine production are the primary pro-inflammatory cytokines (e.g., IL-1 and TNF-α), lipopolysaccharide from bacterial degradation, and viral infection of somatic cells. Chemokines produced in inflamed skin are transported across the endothelial surface and presented to rolling leukocytes. On cells bearing the appropriate counterreceptors, chemokines act to upregulate integrin adhesive functions leading to firm adhesion and directional migration of leukocytes across endothelium and into the underlying tissue [59]. The type of inflammatory infiltrate that characterizes a specific disease is, thus, directly related to the subgroup of cytokines and chemokines expressed in the diseased tissue. The population of cells that respond to an initial stimulus can also modify the pattern of cytokines produced (e.g., production of IL-5 by infiltrating T cells of the Th2 phenotype will favor the subsequent accumulation of eosinophils). The capacity of small numbers of activated T cells to recruit large inflammatory infiltrates of specific cellular composition is a fundamental feature of the cutaneous immune response.

**Table 3** Chemokines Implicated in Leukocyte Migration to Skin

| Cell type operant chemokines | Receptor |
|---|---|
| Neutrophil | |
|    IL-8; GCP-2 | CXCR1 |
|    IL-8; GCP-2; GRO-α, -β, -γ; ENA-78; NAP-2; LIX | CXCR2 |
| Eosinophil | |
|    MCP-3, -4; MIP-1α; RANTES | CCR1 |
|    MCP-3, -4; Eotaxin-1, -2; RANTES | CCR3 |
| T cell | |
|   Activated | |
|     MCP-3, -4; MIP-1α; RANTES | CCR1 |
|     MCP-1, -2, -3, -4, -5 | CCR2 |
|     TARC | CCR4 |
|     MIP-1α; MIP-1β; RANTES | CCR5 |
|     MIP-3β (ELC) | CCR7 |
|     PARC, SLC, 6Ckine (Exodus-2) | ? |
|     Fractalkine | CX$_3$CR1 |
|     IP-10; MIG; I-TAC | CXCR3 |
|   Resting | |
|     PARC; DC-CK1 | ? |
|     Lymphotactin | ? |
|     SDF-1 | CXCR4 |
| Dendritic cells | |
|    MCP-3, -4; MIP-1α; RANTES | CCR1 |
|    MCP-1, -2, -3, -4, -5 | CCR2 |
|    MCP-3, -4; Eotaxin-1, -2; RANTES | CCR3 |
|    TARC | CCR4 |
|    MIP-1α; MIP-1β; RANTES | CCR5 |
|    MIP-3α (LARC, Exodus-1) | CCR6 |
|    MDC; TECK | ? |
|    SDF-1 | CXCR4 |

*Source*: Adapted from Ref. 86.

## E.  Chemokine Receptors

The chemokines bind to specific G-protein coupled cell surface receptors leading to a cascade of cellular activation including inositol-triphosphate generation, release of intracellular calcium, and activation of protein kinase C [86,87]. These mediators, in turn, regulate the intracellular machinery involved in directed cell migration [60]. Four different CXC chemokine receptors (CXCR1-4), eight different CC chemokine receptors (CC1-8), and a single CXXXC chemokine receptor have been identified to date (see Table 3). While most chemokine receptors are known to bind more than one chemokine, CC chemokine receptors will bind only CC chemokines and CXC receptors will bind only CXC chemokines. Expression of individual receptors is determined by a variety of factors. While some are expressed only by specific cell types (e.g., CXCR1 is expressed exclusively on neutrophils), others are broadly expressed on multiple lineages (e.g., CCR2 is expressed on T cells, natural killer cells, monocytes, dendritic cells, and basophils). Chemokine receptors can also be constitutively expressed on one cell population but inducible on others (e.g., CCR1 is constitutively expressed on monocytes and induced on lymphocytes by IL-2) or restricted to particular states of activation or differentiation (e.g., CXCR3 is expressed by activated T cells of the Th1 phenotype, while CCR3 is expressed by cells of the Th2 phenotype) [88]. Naïve T cells, in general, express receptors for constitutively expressed chemokines [e.g., CCR7 (receptor for SLC) and CXCR4 (receptor for SDF-1)], while activation and polarization of T cells into Th1 and Th2 phenotype results in expression of chemokine receptors for inducible chemokines [89] (Th1 and Th2 T cell polarization will be discussed in greater detail below). CXCR3 (receptor for IP-10, Mig, and I-TAC), is expressed on all memory T cells, but at much higher levels on Th1 than on Th2 cells, and leads to Th1 cell activation at much lower concentrations of chemokine. This variety of receptors, ligand specificities, and adaptable expression patterns provides a mechanism by which selective subpopulations of cells are enabled to accumulate in response to specific patterns of chemokines expressed in diseased tissues.

## F. Integrins

Firm adhesion is mediated by integrins activated by the action of chemokines and inflammatory cytokines. Neutrophils, eosinophils, and lymphocytes all express LFA-1 ($\alpha_L\beta_2$), which mediates binding to vascular endothelia via ICAM-1. Eosinophils and lymphocytes also express VLA-4 ($\alpha_4\beta_7$), which mediates adhesion to endothelial VCAM-1 [90]. The $\alpha_4$ integrins also contribute to tethering and rolling interactions of eosinophils in vivo [91,92]. These data suggest that local endothelial expression of VCAM-1 may be an important factor in the selective recruitment of eosinophils to allergic inflammatory sites.

Natural and experimental deletions of the individual components of the leukocyte adhesion cascade highlight the importance of each step and confirm their interdependence. Two children have been identified that lack the ability to incorporate fucose into carbohydrate structures [93–95]. This defect, termed LAD II, results in the complete absence of leukocyte ligands for endothelial selectins and HEV ligands for L-selectin. These children also have markedly elevated peripheral blood counts and fail to recruit significant numbers of leukocytes to sites of inflammation. Targeted disruption of the FucTVII gene in mice results in a similar phenotype [83]. Deletion of either the E-selectin or P-selectin gene results in a delay in recruitment, but some level of overlap in function is evident [96]. Numerous chemokine receptor knockout strains have been produced in mice, with variable, but generally only partial, specific loss of function in tissue specific homing [97,98]. Leukocyte adhesion deficiency (LAD I) results from the lack of expression of functional $\beta_2$-integrin chain, resulting in the simultaneous loss of LFA-1, Mac-1, and P150, 95 [99,100]. These patients also have markedly elevated peripheral blood leukocyte counts, experience frequent infections, and have severe dental caries. Mice engineered to lack relevant integrin or Ig superfamily receptors (e.g., ICAM-1) are quite similar [101].

## G. Th1 Versus Th2 Lymphocyte-Driven Responses

When naïve T cells are activated by antigen presented by DC and differentiate into memory cells, the pattern of co-stimulatory molecules and cytokines they are exposed to causes polarization into one of two phenotypes, termed type 1 and type 2, defined by the pattern

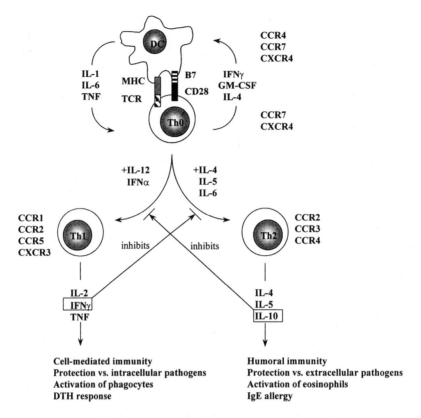

**Figure 3**  Th1 versus Th2 memory T-cell differentiation. Naïve (Th0) cells bind antigen in the context of MHC on DC in association with surface co-stimulatory molecules (e.g., B7) and regulatory cytokines. T cells stimulated in the presence of IL-12, and the absence of IL-4, differentiate to produce IL-2 and IFNγ (Th1 phenotype) and express chemokine receptors CCR1, CCR2, CCR5, and CXCR3. These cells primarily support cell-mediated immune responses (cytotoxic T-cell activity), and defense against intracellular pathogens. In contrast, T cells stimulated in the presence of IL-4, and the absence of IL-12, differentiate to produce IL-4, IL-5, and IL-10 (Th2 phenotype). These cells primarily support humoral immune responses (B-cell responses) and defense against extracellular pathogens.

of cytokines and cytokine receptors that the T cells express (Fig. 3) [88,102,103]. This polarization, in turn, influences all subsequent functions of the T cells involved and, thus, represents a crucial feature of virtually all immune responses. Type 1 and type 2 T-cell polarization is seen with both MHC class II–restricted helper T-cell functions and MHC class I–restricted CD8+ cytotoxic T-cell responses. Influential cytokines are produced by the APC, the responding T cells themselves, and any of a number of potential bystander cell populations. Stimulation of CD4+ T cells in the presence of IL-12 and the absence of IL-4 results in Th1 phenotype cells that produce IFN-γ in addition to various other cytokines (see Fig. 3). These secondary cytokines can activate local mononuclear phagocytes to enhance antimicrobial immune activity and stimulate increased expression of adhesion molecules on adjacent endothelia. Similarly, stimulation in the presence of IL-4 and the absence of IL-12 leads to the development of Th2 phenotype cells that produce

IL-4 and IL-5. These cytokines regulate the development of immune reactions involving eosinophils, basophils, and IgE [102,104,105]. Cells of each Th phenotype also produce one or more products that inhibit the development of the alternate phenotype, thus perpetuating the polarization of a cellular infiltrate once a pattern is established. While IL-12 and IL-4 are important mediators in determining Th phenotype, the presence of IFN-α and TGF-β can significantly modulate the end result. IFN-α drives T cells toward a Th1 phenotype even in the absence of IL-12 or in the presence of IL-4. TGF-β, in contrast, maintains T cells in an undifferentiated state [106]. These cells can be subsequently polarized toward either phenotype by appropriate stimulation.

## IV.  MOLECULAR MECHANISMS OF ALLERGIC
## SKIN RESPONSES

Given these experimental observations, a paradigm emerges defining the regulation of cutaneous immune responses (see Fig. 4). These responses are naturally divided into primary, or antigen-independent, responses, encompassing the innate immune mechanisms employed in the organism's first encounter with an antigen, and secondary responses, in which antigen-specific memory immune mechanisms dominate [107].

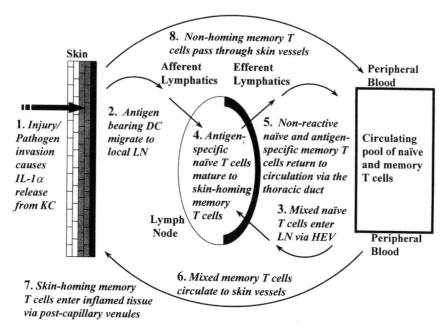

**Figure 4**  Leukocyte recirculation in primary and secondary immune responses. Skin injury (1) leads to release of pro-inflammatory cytokines that activate skin DC to process antigen and migrate local draining LN (2). Naïve T cells enter the LN via HEV (3) and encounter antigen-bearing DC. Ag-reactive T cells proliferate and mature into tissue-specific memory T cells (4), which then reenter the peripheral blood pool (5) and circulate to sites of cutaneous inflammation (6). Skin-specific T cells of mixed antigen-specificity enter sites of skin inflammation via interaction with specific adhesion molecules and chemokines expressed by the postcapillary venules (7), while non–skin-homing cells pass through and recirculate to other tissue sites (8).

The primary cutaneous immune response to a specific antigen is initiated upon introduction of antigen into the skin. Antigenic material is taken up nonspecifically by resident Langerhans cells and dermal DC and processed for presentation to T cells. The initial immune response is greatly enhanced by proinflammatory cytokines released as a result of keratinocyte injury or inclusion of a nonspecific inflammatory activator (i.e., adjuvant) such as LPS with the antigen. Keratinocyte injury results in the release of performed proinflammatory cytokines (e.g., IL-1$\alpha$, TNF-$\alpha$) and neutrophil chemoattractants (e.g., IL-8, LIX). IL-1 and TNF-$\alpha$ activate Langerhans cells and dermal DC, enhancing their phagocytic, antigen processing, and presenting capacity, and stimulate these and other skin resident cells to produce secondary cytokines (e.g., IL-1$\beta$, IL-6, IL-12) and various chemokines. Proinflammatory cytokines (especially IL-1 and TNF-$\alpha$) also upregulate the expression of E-selectin, P-selectin, and the integrin ligands ICAM-1 and VCAM-1 on the adjacent postcapillary venules. Circulating cells bearing functional E- or P-selectin ligands (e.g., CLA/PSGL-1) will tether and roll on the venular endothelium. Chemokines produced in the inflamed tissue are presented to the rolling leukocytes by the venular endothelia. Leukocytes with appropriate corresponding chemokine receptors are induced to form firm attachments and transmigrate into the dermis. In the initial stages, this infiltrate will be dominated by cells responding to IL-8 (CXCR1 and CXCR2: neutrophils) and to RANTES/MCP-1 (CCR1 and CCR2: monocytes, blood dendritic cells, and previously activated T cells). The populations of leukocytes infiltrating the site change with time, as the resident and infiltrating cells produce additional secondary cytokines and chemokines [e.g., eotaxin (ligand for CCR3), attracts Th2 memory cells, eosinophils, and basophils].

Langerhans cells and dermal DC, in response to antigen and cytokine stimulation, downregulate certain surface receptors (e.g., CCR1 and CCR2) and upregulate others (e.g., CCR7; receptor for SLC) and migrate into the afferent lymphatics and to the paracortical areas of local draining lymph nodes [108]. The chemokines SLC and SDF-1, which bind to CCR7 and CXCR4, respectively, are expressed constitutively in secondary lymphoid structures and appear important in directing the transmigration of DC and naïve T cells into lymph nodes. Naïve T cells (CD45RA+, CD62L+, CCR7+, CXCR4+) enter the lymph node via specialized high-endothelial venules (HEV). In lymph nodes, the Langerhans cells and other DC produce ELC and DC-CK 1, chemokines that attract naïve T cells to the DC, where they can interact with antigen presented on MHC class I and class II surface molecules. T cells that recognize their cognate antigen via their TCR can be induced to proliferate and differentiate. The expression of co-stimulator molecules (e.g., B7, CD40) and modulatory cytokines (e.g., IL-6, IL-12) by the APC influences the subsequent development of the T cells toward different helper and effector phenotypes, as discussed above. Antigen-stimulated T cells downregulate expression of CD45RA, CD62L, and CCR7 and upregulate expression of the "memory T cell" marker CD45RO [109]. In skin-draining nodes, memory T cells are also stimulated to express the "skin-homing receptor" CLA and specific chemokine receptors that will allow them to preferentially home to vessels in cutaneous inflammatory sites (e.g., CCR4 receptor for TARC and CXCR3 receptor for IP-10, I-TAC) [110,111]. In the secondary lymphoid structures of other organs, other homing receptors and patterns of cytokine receptors may be induced [112,113]. Thus, there is immunological memory not only for the antigen, but also for the anatomic context in which it was first encountered.

The newly differentiated memory T cells, along with naïve T cells that did not recognize antigen, move through the node into the efferent lymphatics and back into the peripheral circulation via the thoracic duct. Memory T cells are, thus, available to participate in secondary immune responses anywhere in the body. Naïve cells, in contrast, continuously traffic through secondary lymphoid organs, providing access to the pool of available TCR to APC from all tissues.

Subsequent exposure to the same antigen results in the development of secondary, antigen-specific, immune responses. The release of proinflammatory cytokines from the epidermis in response to injury or inflammation activates resident APC, as in the primary response, upregulates the expression of adhesion molecules on the venular endothelium, and induces secondary cytokine and chemokine production by cells resident in both the dermis and the epidermis [21,114]. T cells trafficking to the inflammatory site must bear the appropriate counterreceptors for the particular molecules produced in the affected tissue. Cells bearing functional PSGL-1 or CLA can bind to endothelial P-selectin or E-selectin, respectively. Alternatively, eosinophils and T cells expressing VLA-4 may also be able to tether and roll via VCAM-1 on the venular endothelium. The production of chemokines by skin involved in inflammatory responses (e.g., MIP-1α, MCP-1, IP-10, TARC) directs the accumulation of leukocyte subpopulations (including CLA+ memory T cells) that express the appropriate chemokine receptors and integrins for transmigration into the inflammatory site. Skin inflammation will lead to a polyclonal influx of CLA-positive memory T cells bearing a variety of distinct antigen-specific TCR. The circulating pool of CLA+ T cells represents a mixture of all those clones of memory T cells previously stimulated in skin-draining peripheral lymph nodes. Thus, the cells recruited to a cutaneous inflammatory sites comprise, in effect, a representative sample from a library of T cells specific for all antigens previously encountered at the skin-environmental interface. Those memory T cells that reencounter their cognate antigen presented by local APC are stimulated to proliferate and will influence the subsequent development of the lesion by production of their own cytokine and chemokine profiles. Those that do not encounter their specific antigen will eventually exit the skin passively via afferent lymphatics and traffic proximally through lymph nodes to the thoracic duct and ultimately back to the circulating peripheral blood pool.

## V. MODEL MECHANISMS OF CUTANEOUS INFLAMMATION

While the highly adaptive process outlined above is designed to protect the host from pathogenic infection at the earliest stages, subversion of the process may cause chronic and debilitating skin disease. Repeated exposure to antigen, or cross-reactivity of exogenous stimuli with autologous tissue components, may result in chronic inflammation. In a similar fashion, inherited or acquired loss of control elements may also lead to unrestricted stimulation. As outlined above, the histological phenotype of chronic allergic or inflammatory skin disorders generally reflects the dominant pattern of cytokines and growth factors produced by the secondary (memory) immune response pathways, which is modified in turn by the host genetic background and antigen exposure history. While the specific pathogenesis of a particular inflammatory disorder may be difficult to ascertain, some common themes can be identified that may be amenable to therapeutic intervention.

As discussed above, the primary immune response to epicutaneous allergens represents the connections of the innate, or antigen-independent, immune response to the development of acquired, or antigen-specific, immune responses [107]. Trauma or nonspecific inflammation causes increased expression of adhesion molecules on local endothelial surfaces and production of chemokines, increased leukocyte adhesion and transmigration into the inflammatory site, and ultimately an antigen-specific response. The combinatorial interaction of leukocyte and endothelial adhesion molecules and the subgroup of chemokines expressed determine the composition of the inflammatory infiltrate that characterizes a specific disease. The selective accumulation and activation of eosinophils is a hallmark of many allergic disorders, including allergic contact dermatitis. Recent studies have revealed that many CC chemokines, including RANTES, MCP-3, MCP-4, and eotaxin, are potent and selective chemoattractants for eosinophils [86].

Eotaxin also binds with high fidelity to CCR3, which is selectively expressed on Th2 cells versus Th1 cells. Th2 cells, in turn, produce eosinophil growth factors (e.g., Il-5) supporting a positive feedback loop. The MCPs and eotaxin are also potent histamine-releasing factors and, thus, are strong candidates for a central role in the pthogenesis of disorders involving mast cell degranulation.

## A. Contact Hypersensitivity

Contact hypersensitivity (CHS) is an exceedingly common skin disorder, affecting a sizeable fraction of the population on an intermittent basis. While rarely life threatening, allergic contact dermatitis and irritant contact dermatitis cause significant morbidity and cost society millions of dollars per year in treatment costs and lost revenue [115]. Immunologically, CHS is a prototypic delayed-type hypersensitivity (DTH) reaction to an epicutaneously encountered hapten antigen with a classically defined primary immune response (sensitization) phase and a secondary immune response (elicitation or effector) phase. The hapten antigen or its vehicle typically causes, or is encountered in the context of, some local epidermal injury resulting in the release and production of primary proinflammatory cytokines. In the sensitization phase, antigen-independent inflammation, or direct hapten binding itself, causes upregulation of antigen processing and presentation by resident APC and their migration to local draining nodes. In the secondary phases, local inflammation also causes induction of endothelial selectins, chemokines, and CAMs and, thus, the nonspecific accumulation of CLA+ memory T cells [116–118]. The activation of antigen-specific T cells will lead to secondary cytokine production and the accumulation of additional leukocyte subpopulations. Contact hypersensitivity lesions often contain mixed elements of Th1 and Th2 memory T cells and are dominated by CD8+, MHC class I–restricted, hapten-specific T-cell infiltrates. Classic DTH lesions are almost exclusively CD4+ MHC class II–restricted T-cell infiltrates with a strong predominance of Th1 type cytokines [107].

## B. Atopy

Atopic patients express a spectrum of disease encompassing varying degrees of atopic dermatitis (AD), asthma, and allergic rhinitis. AD is exceedingly common and may result in significant morbidity [119,120]. Elevated serum IgE levels and a high incidence of immediate skin test reactivity to allergens support an allergic basis for the initiation and/ or exacerbation of AD and other manifestations of atopic disease [121]. Although histologically similar to DTH reactions, the T cells from acute AD lesions do not produce IFN-γ and, accordingly, there is minimal upregulation of class II MHC in acute AD lesions compared with allergic contact dermatitis [122]. T cells isolated from acute inflammatory sites in atopic patients are predominantly Th2 phenotype, expressing high levels of IL-4 and IL-5. These cytokines, in turn, are instrumental in directing the accumulation and activation, respectively, of eosinophils. CC chemokines that bind CCR3 (e.g., RANTES, MCP-3, MCP-4, and eotaxin) are also strong eosinophil chemoattractants and are abundantly expressed in atopic skin lesions, suggesting that they play a role linking antigen-specific immune activation and the migration of eosinophils into skin [17,86]. While intact eosinophils are infrequent in stable AD lesions, eosinophil major basic protein is found throughout the dermis, indicating that eosinophils have transmigrated into the tissue and degranulated [123,124].

## C. Psoriasis

Psoriatic lesions are characterized by the activation and exuberant proliferation of keratinocyte, as well as the accumulation of neutrophils and activated T cells [16]. The progression of psoriatic plaques is thought to result from a positive feedback loop between infiltrating T cells and KC. According to this model, keratinocyte activation results in the expression and release of pro-inflammatory cytokines (e.g., IFN-$\alpha$, IL-6, and TGF-$\alpha$), as well as T-cell (e.g., MCP-1 and IP-10) and neutrophil (e.g., IL-8 and GRO-$\alpha$) chemoattractants. The infiltrating T cells of a psoriatic plaque are predominantly Th1 phenotype, as in a delayed-type hypersensitivity (DTH) reaction, which produce large quantities of IFN-$\gamma$. This, in turn, stimulates the local production of keratinocyte growth factors resulting in keratinocyte overgrowth and increased production of proinflammatory cytokines. IL-12 is also produced at high levels by mononuclear cells in psoriatic plaques, supporting the T-cell bias toward a Th1 phenotype. In psoriatic patients, this cycle appears to persist in an unregulated fashion, leading to overgrowth of keratinocytes and development of the characteristic plaques. Many of the therapeutic modalities employed in treatment of psoriasis appear to act via depletion of one or more of the cell populations implicated in this positive feedback loop (e.g., UV exposure and PUVA deplete Langerhans cells, cyclosporin limits T-cell proliferation, etc.) and, thus, break the cycle of self-activation. Successful treatment of psoriasis has also been associated with a decrease in IP-10 and an increase in IL-10 measured in diseased skin [125,126].

## VI. CONCLUSION

Substantial progress has been made in recent years in regard to elucidation of the mechanisms regulating the development of allergic skin responses. Both positive and negative regulation occurs at all stages of development, from the stimulation of initial antigen-nonspecific innate inflammatory responses to the development and accumulation of antigen-specific T cells. The multistep nature of leukocyte-endothelial interactions provides both a mechanism for generating highly specific inflammatory infiltrates and a framework for the investigation and development of targeted therapeutic strategies.

## REFERENCES

1. Bos JD. The skin as an organ of immunity. Clin Exp Immunol 1997; 107(suppl 1):3–5.
2. Uthayakumar S, Nandwani R, Drinkwater T, Nayagam AT, Darley CR. The prevalence of

skin disease in HIV infection and its relationship to the degree of immunosuppression. Br J Dermatol 1997; 137:595–598.

3. Lugo-Janer G, Sánchez, JL, Santiago-Delpin E. Prevalence and clinical spectrum of skin diseases in kidney transplant recipients. J Am Acad Dermatol 1991; 24:410–414.

4. Kadunce DP, Krueger GG. Pathogenesis of psoriasis. Dermatol Clin 1995; 13:723–737.

5. Bos JD, Wierenga EA, Sillevis Smitt JH, van der Heijden FL, Kapsenberg ML. Immune dysregulation in atopic eczema. Arch Dermatol 1992; 128:1509–1512.

6. Leung DY. The immunologic basis of atopic dermatitis. Clin Rev Allergy 1993; 11:447–469.

7. González FJ, et al. Participation of T lymphocytes in cutaneous allergic reactions to drugs. Clin Exp Allergy 1998; 28(suppl 4):3–6.

8. Porter SR, Kirby A, Olsen I, Barrett W. Immunologic aspects of dermal and oral lichen planus: a review. Oral Surg Oral Med Oral Pathol Oral Radiol Endod 1997; 83:358–366.

9. McDonagh AJ, Messenger AG. The pathogenesis of alopecia areata. Dermatol Clin 1996; 14:661–670.

10. Boh EE, Millikan LE. Vesiculobullous diseases with prominent immunologic features. JAMA 1992; 268:2893–2898.

11. Cooper KD, et al. Effects of cyclosporine on immunologic mechanisms in psoriasis. J Am Acad Dermatol 1990; 231:1318–1326.

12. Wong RL, Winslow CM, Cooper KD. The mechanisms of action of cyclosporin A in the treatment of psoriasis. Immunol Today 1993; 14:69–74.

13. Krueger JG, Wolfe JT, Nabeya RT. Successful ultraviolet B treatment of psoriasis is accompanied by a reversal of keratinocyte pathology and by selective depletion of intraepidermal T cells. J Exp Med 1995; 182:2057–2068.

14. Gottlieb SL, Gilleaudeau P, Johnson R. Response of psoriasis to be lymphocyte-selective toxin (DAB389IL-2) suggests a primary immune, but not keratinocyte, pathogenic basis. Nature Med 1995; 1:442–447.

15. Lim KK, et al. Cyclosporine in the treatment of dermatologic disease: an update. Mayo Clin Proc 1996; 71:1182–1191.

16. Lever WF, Schaumberg-Lever G, eds. Histopathology of the Skin. Philadelphia: JB Lippincott, 1990.

17. Garcia-Zepeda EA, et al. Human eotaxin is a specific chemoattractant for eosinophil cells and provides a new mechanism to explain tissue eosinophilia. Nature Med 1996; 2:449–456.

18. Martin LB, Kita H, Leiferman KM, Gleich GJ. Eosinophils in allergy: role in disease, degranulation, and cytokines. Int Arch Allergy Immunol 1996; 109:207–215.

19. Christophers E. The immunopathology of psoriasis. Int Arch Allergy Immunol 1996; 110:199–206.

20. Didierjean L, Saurat J-H, Ucia C, Mach B, Dayer J-M. Expression of interleukin-1 mRNA is regulated by UVB in normal human skin. J Invest Dermatol 1987; 89(3):322.

21. Kupper TS, Groves RW. The Interleukin-1 axis and cutaneous inflammation. J Invest Dermatol 1995; 105:62S–66S.

22. Wood LC, Elias PM, Calhoun C. Barrier disruption stimulates interleukin-1α expression and release from a pre-formed pool in murine epidermis. J Invest Dermatol 1996; 106:397–403.

23. Lee R, et al. IL-1 alpha, a cytokine which lacks a secretory leader sequence, is released from cytoplasmic stores by mechanical deformation. J Immunol 1997; 159:5084–5088.

24. Luger TA, Scholzen T, Grabbe S. The role of alpha-melanocyte-stimulating hormone in cutaneous biology. J Invest Dermatol Symp Proc 1997; 2:87–93.

25. Dinarello CA. Biologic basis for interleukin-1 in disease. Blood 1996; 87:2095–2147.

26. Takashima A, Bergstresser PR. Cytokine-mediated communication by keratinocytes and Langerhans cells with dendritic epidermal T cells. Semin Immunol 1996; 8:333–339.

27. Pastore S, Cavani A, Girolomoni G. Epidermal cytokine and neuronal peptide modulation of contact hypersensitivity reactions. Immunopharmacology 1996; 31:117–130.
28. Dahl M. Clinical Immunodermatology. St. Louis: Mosby, 1996.
29. Stoll S, et al. Production of IL-18 (IFN-gamma-inducing factor) messenger RNA and functional protein by murine keratinocytes. J Immunol 1997; 159:298–302.
30. Smith RS, Smith TJ, Blieden TM, Phipps RP. Fibroblasts as sentinel cells. Synthesis of chemokines and regulation of inflammation. Am J Pathol 1997; 151:317–322.
31. Mochizuki M, Bartels J, Mallet AI, Christophers E, Schröder JM. IL-4 induces eotaxin: a possible mechanism of selective eosinophil recruitment in helminth infection and atopy. J Immunol 1998; 160:60–68.
32. Werner S, et al. Large induction of kerantinocyte growth factor expression in the dermis during wound healing. Proc Natl Acad Sci USA 1992; 89:6896–6900.
33. Le Panse R, Bouchard B, Lebreton C, Coulomb B. Modulation of keratinocyte growth factor (KGF) mRNA expression in human dermal fibroblasts grown in monolayer or within a collagen matrix. Exp Dermatol 1996; 5:108–114.
34. de Boer WI, Schuller AG, Vermey M, van der Kwast TH. Expression of growth factors and receptors during specific phases in regenerating urothelium after acute injury in vivo. Am J Pathol 1994; 145:1199–1207.
35. Antoniades HN, Galanopoulos T, Neville-Golden J, Kiritsy CP, Lynch SE. Expression of growth factor and receptor mRNAs in skin epithelial cells following acute cutaneous injury. Am J Pathol 1993; 142:1099–1110.
36. Maas-Szabowski N, Fusenig NE. Interleukin-1-induced growth factor expression in postmitotic and resting fibroblasts. J Invest Dermatol 1996; 107:849–855.
37. Banchereau J, Steinman RM. Dendritic cells and the control of immunity. Nature 1998; 392: 245–252.
38. Strobl H, Riedl E, Bello-Fernandez C, Knapp W. Epidermal Langerhans cell development and differentiation. Immunobiology 1998; 198:588–605.
39. Ebner S, et al. Expression of maturation-/migration-related molecules on human dendritic cells from blood and skin. Immunobiology 1998; 198:568–587.
40. Belsito DV. The rise and fall of allergic contact dermatitis. Am J Contact Dermatitis 8:193–201.
41. Kimber I, Dearman RJ, Cumberbatch M, Huby RJ. Langerhans cells and chemical allergy. Curr Opin Immunol 1998; 10:614–619.
42. Takashima A, Kitajima T. T cell-mediated terminal maturation of dendritic cells, a critical transition into fully potent antigen presenting cells. Pathol Biol (Paris) 1998; 46:53–60.
43. Robert C, et al. Interaction of dendritic cells with skin endothelium: a new perspective on immunosurveillance. J Exp Med 1999; 189:627–636.
44. Steinman R, Hoffman L, Pope M. Maturation and migration of cutaneous dendritic cells. J Invest Dermatol 1995; 105:2S–7S.
45. Nestle FO, Filgueira L, Nickoloff BJ, Burg G. Human dermal dendritic cells process and present soluble protein antigens. J Invest Dermatol 1998; 110:762–766.
46. Morhenn VB. Langerhans cells may trigger the psoriatic disease process via production of nitric oxide. Immunol Today 1997; 18:433–436.
47. Kawamura T, Furue M. Comparative analysis of B7-1 and B7-2 expression in Langerhans cells: differential regulation by T helper type 1 and T helper type 2 cytokines. Eur J Immunol 1995; 25:1913–1917.
48. Chang CH, Furue M, Tamaki K. B7-1 expression of Langerhans cells is up-regulated by proinflammatory cytokines, and is down-regulated by interferon-gamma or by interleukin-10. Eur J Immunol 1995; 25:394–398.
49. Kang K, et al. IL-12 synthesis by human Langerhans cells. J Immunol 1996; 156:1402–1407.

50. Dohil M, Prendiville JS, Crawford RI, Speert DP. Cutaneous manifestations of chronic granu-
    lomatous disease. A report of four cases and review of the literature. J Am Acad Dermatol
    1997; 36:899–907.

51. Spetz AL, Strominger J, Groh-Spies V. T cell subsets in normal human epidermis. Am J
    Pathol 1996; 149:665–674.

52. Bata-Csorgo Z, Hammerberg C, Voorhees JJ, Cooper KD. Intralesional T-lymphocyte activa-
    tion as a mediator of psoriatic epidermal hyperplasia. J Invest Dermatol 1995; 105:89S–94S.

53. Boismenu R, Hobbs MV, Boullier S, Havran WL. Molecular and cellular biology of dendritic
    epidermal T cells. Semin Immunol 1996; 8:323–331.

54. Kitajima T, Ariizumi K, Bergstresser PR, Takashima A. A novel mechanism of glucocorti-
    coid-induced immune suppression: the inhibition of T cell-mediated terminal maturation of
    a murine dendritic cell line. J Clin Invest 1996; 98:142–147.

55. Boismenu R, Feng L, Xia YY, Chang JC, Havran WL. Chemokine expression by intraepithe-
    lial gamma delta T cells. Implications for the recruitment of inflammatory cells to damaged
    epithelia. J Immunol 1996; 157:985–992.

56. Dallegri F, Ottonello L. Tissue injury in neutrophilic inflammation. Inflamm Res 1997; 46:
    382–391.

57. Brown E. Neutrophil adhesion and the therapy of inflammation. Semin Hematol 1997; 34:
    319–326.

58. Cohnheim J. Lectures on General Pathology: A Handbook for Practitioners and Students.
    London: The New Sydenham Society, 1889.

59. Springer TA. Traffic signals on endothelium for lymphocyte recirculation and leukocyte emi-
    gration. Ann Rev Physiol 1995; 57:827–872.

60. Butcher E, Picker L. Lymphocyte homing and homeostasis. Science 1996; 272:60–66.

61. Picker L, et al. Differential expression of lymphocyte homing receptors by human memory/
    effector T cells in pulmonary versus cutaneous immune effector sites. Eur J Immunol 1994;
    24:1269–1277.

62. Picker LJ, Michie SA, Rott LS, Butcher EC. A unique phenotype of skin-associated lympho-
    cytes in human. Preferential expression of the HECA-452 epitope by benign and malignant
    T cells at cutaneous sites. Am J Pathol 1990; 136:1053–1068.

63. Pitzalis C, et al. Cutaneous lymphocyte antigen-positive T lymphocytes preferentially migrate
    to the skin but not to the joint in psoriatic arthritis. Arthritis Rheum 1996; 39:137–145.

64. Abernathy-Carver K, Sampson H, Picker L, Leung D. Milk-induced eczema is associated
    with the expansion of T cells expressing cutaneous lymphocyte antigen. J Clin Invest 1995;
    95:913–918.

65. Leung DY, et al. Bacterial superantigens induce T cell expression of the skin-selective hom-
    ing receptor, the cutaneous lymphocyte-associated antigen, via stimulation of interleukin 12
    production. J Exp Med 1995; 181:747–753.

66. Rossiter H, et al. Skin disease-related T cells bind to endothelial selectins: expression of
    cutaneous lymphocyte antigen (CLA) predicts E-selectin but not P-selectin binding. Eur J
    Immunol 1994; 24:205–210.

67. Santamaria Babi L, et al. Circulating allergen-reactive T cells from patients with atopic der-
    matitis and allergic contact dermatitis express the skin-selective homing receptor, the cutane-
    ous lymphocyte-associated antigen. J Exp Med 1995; 181:1935–1940.

68. Rook AH, Heald P. The immunopathogenesis of cutaneous T-cell lymphoma. Hematol Oncol
    Clin North Am 1995; 9:997–1010.

69. Fuhlbrigge RC, Kieffer JD, Armerding D, Kupper TS. Cutaneous lymphocyte antigen is a
    specialized form of PSGL-1 expressed on skin-homing T cells. Nature 1997; 389:978–981.

70. Bruehl R, et al. Leukocyte activation induces surface redistribution of P-selectin glycoprotein
    ligand-1. J Leukoc Biol 1997; 61:489–499.

71. Asa D, et al. The P-selectin glycoprotein ligand functions as a common human leukocyte
    ligand for P- and E-selectins. J Biol Chem 1995; 270:11662–11670.

72. Diacovo T, et al. Interactions of human alpha/beta and gamma/delta T lymphocyte subsets in shear flow with E- and P-selectin. J Exp Med 1996; 183:1193–1203.
73. Fujimoto T, et al. Expression and functional characterization of the P-selectin glycoprotein ligand-1 in various cells. Int J Hematol 1996; 64:231–239.
74. Li F, et al. Post-translational modifications of recombinant P-selectin glycoprotein ligand-1 required for binding to P- and E-selectin. J Biol Chem 1996; 271:3255–3264.
75. Borges E, et al. The binding of T cell-expressed P-selectin glycoprotein ligand-1 to E- and P-selectin is differentially regulated. J Biol Chem 1997; 272:28786–28792.
76. Austrup F, et al. P- and E-selectin mediate recruitment of T-helper-1 but not T-helper-2 cells into inflamed tissues. Nature 1997; 385:81–83.
77. van Wely C, Blanchard A, Britten C. Differential expression of alpha3 fucosyltransferases in Th1 and Th2 cells correlates with their ability to bind P-selectin. Biochem Biophys Res Commun 1998; 247:307–311.
78. Austrup F, et al. P- and E-selectin mediate recruitment of T-helper-1 but not T-helper-2 cells into inflammed tissues. Nature 1997; 385:81–83.
79. Pouyani T, Seed B. PSGL-1 recognition of P-selectin is controlled by a tyrosine sulfation consensus at the PSGL-1 amino terminus. Cell 1995; 83:333–343.
80. Sako D, et al. A sulfated peptide segment at the amino terminus of PSGL-1 is critical for P-selectin binding. Cell 1995; 83:323–331.
81. Liu W, et al. Identification of N-terminal residues on P-selectin glycoprotein ligand-1 required for binding to P-selectin. J Biol Chem 1998; 273:7078–7087.
82. Lowe JB. In: Fukuda M, ed. Frontiers in Molecular Biology. Oxford: Oxford University Press, 1994:163–205.
83. Maly P, et al. The alpha(1,3)fucosyltransferase Fuc-TVII controls leukocyte trafficking through an essential role in L-, E-, and P-selectin ligand biosynthesis. Cell 1996; 86:643–653.
84. Ellies L, et al. Core 2 oligosaccharide biosynthesis distinguishes between selectin ligands essential for leukocyte homing and inflammation. Immunity 1998; 9:881–890.
85. Baggiolini M, Dewald B, Moser B. Human chemokines: an update. Ann Rev Immunol 1997; 15:675–705.
86. Luster AD. Chemokines: chemotactic cytokines that mediate inflammation. N Engl J Med 1998; 338:436–445.
87. Moser B, Loetscher M, Piali L, Loetscher P. Lymphocyte responses to chemokines. Int Revi Immunol 1998; 16:323–344.
88. Sallusto F, Lanzavecchia A, Mackay CR. Chemokines and chemokine receptors in T-cell priming and Th1/Th2-mediated responses. Immunol Today 1998; 19:568–574.
89. Sallusto F, Lenig D, Mackay CR, Lanzavecchia A. Flexible programs of chemokine receptor expression on human polarized T helper 1 and 2 lymphocytes. J Exp Med 1998; 187:875–883.
90. Bochner BS, et al. Adhesion of human basophils, eosinophils, and neutrophils to interleukin 1-activated human vascular endothelial cells: Contributions of endothelial cell adhesion molecules. J Exp Med 1991; 173:1553–1556.
91. Sriramarao P, von Andrian UH, Butcher EC, Bourdon MA, Broide DH. L-selectin and VLA-4 integrin mediate early events of eosinophil adhesion at physiologic shear rates in vivo. J Immunol 1994; 153:4238–4246.
92. Kitayama J, Fuhlbrigge RC, Puri KD, Springer TA. P-selectin, L-selectin, and alpha 4 integrin have distinct roles in eosinophil tethering and arrest on vascular endothelial cells under physiological flow conditions. J Immunol 1997; 159:3929–3939.
93. Etzioni A, et al. Leukocyte adhesion deficiency (LAD) II: a new adhesion defect due to absence of sialyl Lewis X, the ligand for selectins. Immunodeficiency 1993; 4:307–308.
94. Kuijpers T, Etzioni A, Pollack S, Pals S. Antigen-specific immune responsiveness and lymphocyte recruitment in leukocyte adhesion deficiency type II. Int Immunol 1997; 9:607–613.

95. von Andrian UH, et al. In vivo behavior of neutrophils from two patients with distinct inherited leukocyte adhesion deficiency syndromes. J Clin Invest 1993; 91:2893–2897.

96. Frenette PS, Wagner DD. Insights into selectin function from knockout mice. Thromb Haemostasis 1997; 78:60–64.

97. Bacon KB, Oppenheim JJ. Chemokines in disease models and pathogenesis. Cytokine Growth Factor Rev 1998; 9:167–173.

98. Ward SG, Westwick J. Chemokines: understanding their role in T-lymphocyte biology. Biochem J 1998; 333 (Pt 3):457–470.

99. Boxer LA, Blackwood RA. Leukocyte disorders: quantitative and qualitative disorders of the neutrophil, part 2. Pediatr Rev 1996; 17:47–50.

100. Malech HL, Nauseef WM. Primary inherited defects in neutrophil function: etiology and treatment. Semin Hematol 1997; 34:279–290.

101. Hynes RO, Wagner DD. Genetic manipulation of vascular adhesion molecules in mice. J Clin Invest 1997; 100:S11–13.

102. Romagnani S. Biology of human TH1 and TH2 cells. J Clin Immunol 1995; 15:121–129.

103. Mosmann TR, et al. Differentiation and functions of T cell subsets. Ciba Foundation Symposium 204, 1997, discussion 154-8.

104. Kay AB, et al. Messenger RNA expression of the cytokine gene cluster, interleukin 3 (IL-3), IL-4, IL-5, and granulocyte/macrophage colony-stimulating factor, in allergen-induced late-phase cutaneous reactions in atopic subjects. J Exp Med 1991; 173:775–778.

105. Ohmen JD, et al. Overexpression of IL-10 in atopic dermatitis. Contrasting cytokine patterns with delayed-type hypersensitivity reactions. J Immunol 1995; 154:1956–1963.

106. Sad S, Mosmann TR. Single IL-2-secreting precursor CD4 T cell can develop into either Th1 or Th2 cytokine secretion phenotype. J Immunol 1994; 153:3514–3522.

107. Grabbe S, Schwarz T. Immunoregulatory mechanisms involved in elicitation of allergic contact hypersensitivity. Immunol Today 1998; 19:37–44.

108. Saeki H, Moore AM, Brown MJ, Hwang ST. Cutting edge: secondary lymphoid-tissue chemokine (SLC) and CC chemokine receptor 7 (CCR7) participate in the emigration pathway of mature dendritic cells from the skin to regional lymph nodes. J Immunol 1999; 162:2472–2475.

109. Mackay C, Marston W, Dudler L. Naive and memory T cells show distinct pathways of lymphocyte recirculation. J Exp Med 1990; 171(3):801–817.

110. Imai T, et al. The T cell-directed CC chemokine TARC is a highly specific biological ligand for CC chemokine receptor 4. J Biol Chem 1997; 272:15036–15042.

111. Tensen CP, et al. Epidermal interferon-gamma inducible protein-10 (IP-10) and monokine induced by gamma-interferon (Mig) but not IL-8 mRNA expression is associated with epidermotropism in cutaneous T cell lymphomas. J Invest Dermatol 1998; 111:222–226.

112. Mackay CR. Migration pathways and immunologic memory among T lymphocytes. Semin Immunol 1992; 4(1):51–58.

113. Abitorabi MA, et al. Differential expression of homing molecules on recirculating lymphocytes from sheep gut, peripheral, and lung lymph. J Immunol 1996; 156:3111–3117.

114. Williams IR, Kupper TS. Immunity at the surface: homeostatic mechanisms of the skin immune system. Life Sci 1996; 58:1485–1507.

115. Rietschel RL. Human and economic impact of allergic contact dermatitis and the role of patch testing. J Am Acad Dermatol 1995; 33:812–815.

116. Kupper TS. Immune and inflammatory processes in cutaneous tissues: mechanisms and speculations. J Clin Invest 1990; 86:1783–1789.

117. Kalish RS. Recent developments in the pathogenesis of allergic contact dermatitis. Arch Dermatol 1991; 127:1558–1563.

118. Katz SI, Aiba S, Cavani A, Enk AH. Early events in contact sensitivity. Adv Exp Med Biol 1995; 378:497–500.

119. Keil JE, Shmunes E. The epidemiology of work-related skin disease in South Carolina. Arch Dermatol 1983; 119:650–654.

120. Shmunes E, Keil JE. Occupational dermatoses in South Carolina: a descriptive analysis of cost variables. J Am Acad Dermatol 1983; 9:861–866.
121. Boguniewicz M, Nicol NH, Leung DYM. In: Charlesworth EN, ed. Cutaneous Allergy. Cambridge: Blackwell Science, 1996:209–231.
122. Barker JN, Ophir J, MacDonald DM. Products of class II major histocompatibility complex gene subregions are differentially expressed on keratinocytes in cutaneous disease. J Am Acad Dermatol 1988; 19:667–672.
123. Leiferman KM. Eosinophils in atopic dermatitis. J Allergy Clin Immunol 1994; 94:1310–1317.
124. Cheng JF, et al. Dermal eosinophils in atopic dermatitis undergo cytolytic degeneration. J Allergy Clin Immunol 1997; 99:683–692.
125. Gottlieb AB, et al. Studies of the effect of cyclosporine in psoriasis in vivo: combined effects on activated T lymphocytes and epidermal regenerative maturation. J Invest Dermatol 1992; 98:302–309.
126. Ockenfels HM, Schultewolter T, Ockenfels G, Funk R, Goos M. The antipsoriatic agent dimethylfumarate immunomodulates T-cell cytokine secretion and inhibits cytokines of the psoriatic cytokine network. Br J Dermatol 1988; 139:390–395.

# 4

# Cellular Mechanisms of Allergic Skin Responses

**Kefei Kang, Seth R. Stevens, and Kevin D. Cooper**
*University Hospitals of Cleveland and Case Western Reserve University, Cleveland, Ohio*

Tremendous progress in immunology and related basic sciences has been made in recent decades. The development of technical tools such as monoclonal antibodies used for immunostaining and flow cytometry has been essential to the understanding of immune cells. Such innovation has allowed for the identification of cell surface antigens, such as accessory molecules, and characterization of their function, which in turn provides better insight into the cell-mediated mechanisms of allergic responses. Due to the complexity of the interrelationship and interaction among immunocompetent cells, in this chapter we will first delineate the specific cells that mediate these responses, followed by an introduction of the major pathomechanisms of allergic conditions. Finally we will illustrate possible sites for therapeutic intervention.

## I. CELLS INVOLVED IN ALLERGIC SKIN RESPONSES

### A. Antigen-Presenting Cells

The skin is a rich source of antigen-presenting cells (APC), which are bone marrow–derived MHC class II molecule-bearing accessory cells such as dendritic cells, monocytes/macrophages, and B cells, that have the capacity to present antigen to antigen-specific T cells. Although not professional APC, keratinocytes can function in immune responses and immunomodulation, both mainly through their production of cytokines and chemokines after activation by such stimuli as superantigens and by providing co-stimulatory signals. Thus, under certain circumstances, keratinocytes, a major component of epidermis, can function as accessory cells for T-cell proliferation [1].

Langerhans cells (LC) are the predominant dendritic APCs residing in the epidermis. Dendritic cells are in general characterized by (1) their dendritic morphology, (2) the expression of CD1a, (3) high levels of MHC class II antigens (HLA-DR), FcγRII(CD32) and accessory molecules, such as CD40, CD54(ICAM-1), CD58(LFA-3), CD80(B7-1), and CD86(B7-2), (4) the presence of Birbeck granules, which are formed in the course of receptor-mediated endocytosis [2] and specifically in epidermal LC, (5) low adherent and phagocytic activity, and (6) induction of the proliferation of allogeneic resting naïve

T cells. By contrast, another specialized dendritic APC exists in the B-cell areas of lymph nodes, called follicular dendritic cells, which present native antigen to B cells and are likely to be involved in the affinity maturation of antibodies and maintenance of humoral immune response [3]. For nominal antigens, dendritic cells are the most potent APC (10- to 50-more potent than monocytes or B cells) in inducing T-cell responses to microbial superantigens [4].

Two distinct forms of LC exist based on their phenotypic, developmental, and functional characteristics [5–7]. Freshly isolated, immature resident LC as a rule are excellent in antigen processing but poor in stimulating resting T cells because, despite high expression of CD1a and FcγRII(CD32), they exhibit low expression of accessory molecules. By contrast, after encountering and processing antigens, resident LC are activated and migrate to draining lymph nodes as lymphoid dendritic cells. This latter process is modeled in vitro by culturing ex vivo, upon which LC markedly reduce their expression of CD1a and FcγRII(CD32) and increase their expression of HLA-DR and accessory/co-sitmulatory molecules along with their functional changes. In the process, mature LC become excellent in stimulating resting T cells but poor in antigen processing [8]. In addition, in dermis, a distinct group of LC-like interstitial dendritic APC, which are distinct from dermal macrophages, has been found that exhibit potent antigen processing and presenting activity [9–11].

In addition to FcγR expression on LC, an important finding is that the high-affinity IgE receptor, FcεRI, is expressed on LC [12,13] in addition to its usual expression on basophils and mast cells. Differences from the latter are its lack of the classical β chain and highly variable expression dictated by the microenvironment of the cells [4]. The consequences of LC having FcεRI may be envisaged in two ways. LC that express only low amounts of FcεRI can capture allergens via specific IgE, leading to secondary and possibly primary immune responses, but without alteration of their cytokine-secretion program; LC expressing high amounts of FcεRI not only efficiently capture and internalize allergens, but are also activated upon receptor ligation, with subsequent modification of their cytokine secretion, resulting in skewing of T-cell function. However, neither normal epidermal LC nor dermal DR$^{high}$ CD1a$^+$ dendritic cells change their intracellular calcium level after FcεRI cross-linking [15]. Furthermore, LC bearing FcεRI as triggers for IgE-mediated delayed-type hypersensitivity have also been postulated. It has been suggested that LC bearing FcεRI is a prerequisite to provoking eczematous skin lesions after application of aeroallergens to clinically uninvolved skin of atopic patients [14]. The low-affinity IgE receptor (FcεRIIa/FcεRIIb, CD23), which is not evidently expressed on normal epidermal LC, can be induced by stimulation with IL-4 and/or IFN-γ and further released by them as a soluble CD23(IgE-binding protein) [16]. Thus, LC IgE receptors can function to focus allergens for processing and presentation but also may facilitate clearing allergens as well.

Other recent findings shed light on the nature of LC localization and travel through the epidermis. E-cadherin, a homophilic adhesion molecule, is synthesized and expressed by murine epidermal LC and found to mediate adhesion of LC to keratinocytes in vitro [17] and is presumably involved in the localization of LC in epidermis. Moreover, extracellular matrix proteins, such as fibronectin and laminin, which bind β1 integrins [18], can also regulate the direction of LC migration from the epidermis to the dermis by modulating their adhesion affinity. Thus, contact with dermal components could prevent LC from reentering the epidermis. Additionally, binding to laminin and fibronectin has been shown to reduce the expression of CD1a [19].

LC also elaborate important cytokines such as IL-1β, which is implicated as a critical molecule for initiation of primary immune responses in skin [20], and constitutively express IL-12, which initiates Th1-type immune responses. After maturation (incubation), LC IL-12 production spontaneously increases [21]. Furthermore, cytokines have an important impact on the development and movement of LC. For example, dendritic cells can be generated from bone marrow progenitors or blood mononuclear cells with the addition of GM-CSF, IL-4, and TNF-$\alpha$. TGF (transforming growth factor) $\beta$1, in the presence of GM-CSF and IL-4, has been reported to induce differentiation of blood monocytes into dendritic LC [22]. TNF-$\alpha$ is also known to induce dendritic cell migration and accumulation in draining lymph nodes, which optimizes contact sensitization [23–25].

Monocytes comprise around 10% of blood leukocytes and belong to the mononuclear phagocyte system. After entering tissues, they are stimulated, activated, and develop into macrophages, which are characterized by the presence of numerous lysosomes and, after phagocytosis, phagolysosomes. They are rich in cell surface receptors and exert functions involving almost all aspects of immunity (innate and specific) and tissue homeostasis. They express molecules shared with other cells such as HLA class I and class II (DR), CD11a-c/CD18, CD16, CD32, CD35, CD45, CD49d,e/CD29, CD64, CD87, and co-stimulatory molecules CD40, CD54, CD58, CD80(B7-1), CD86(B7-2). They also express distinguishing molecules such as CD14, CD36, and CD68. Their receptors for Fc$\gamma$ (CD64, CD32, CD16); C3b, C4b (CR1, CD35), iC3b (CR3, CD11b/CD18, $\beta$2 integrin); vascular cell adhesion molecule (VCAM)-1, fibronectin(CD49d/CD29, CD49e/CD29, $\beta$1 integrin); and co-stimulatory ligands are important and mostly involved in immune responses and cell migration. Monocytes/macrophages are capable of high levels of cytokine production, and their functions are also profoundly affected by both endogenous and exogenous cytokines. For example, superantigens can strongly induce IL-1 and TNF-$\alpha$ secretion from monocytes [26]. Although normally Fc$\epsilon$RIIb is undetectable in monocytes, it can be induced by IL-4, which is present in acute lesions of atopic dermatitis and thus could enhance IgE-mediated allergic response [27]. Moreover, IFN-$\gamma$ can induce a B7$^+$ CD16$^-$ macrophage phenotype and IL-10 can induce B7$^-$ CD16$^+$ phenotype on macrophages. Interaction with T cells results in an immune response or destruction of the targeted T cell, respectively, and these differential distinct pathways are mutually exclusive [28].

Keratinocytes, stimulated with IFN-$\gamma$, can express MHC class II molecule and CD40 [29] and act as APC, but unlike epidermal LC, they are unable to present conventional antigens to resting T cells. In murine studies, it has been shown that purified splenic T cells can be activated when they are incubated with keratinocytes bearing MHC class II molecules together with superantigens such as staphylococcal enterotoxin B or exfoliative toxin [30–32], and such T cells predominantly produce IL-4 [33]. In contrast, after incubation with professional APC and superantigens, T cells predominantly produce IFN-$\gamma$. The differential production of T-cell cytokines may result from the cytokines induced by stimulated keratinocytes such as TNF-$\alpha$, IL-10, and IL-12 [30,33].

## B. Immunocompetent Lymphoid Cells

T lymphocytes, B lymphocytes, and natural killer (NK) cells are the major component of immunocompetent lymphoid cells. T lymphocytes are the most important cells for the specific allergic immune responses. There are two broad groups of T lymphocytes: CD4$^+$ helper T lymphocytes (Th) recognizing antigens in association with MHC class II and CD8$^+$ cytotoxic T lymphocytes (Tc) recognizing antigens in association with MHC class I. CD4$^+$ T lymphocytes, according to their immunological function and pattern of cytokine production, have been further divided into subsets: Th1, which mediate delayed-type hypersensitivity and mainly produce IL-2, IFN-γ, and lymphotoxin and Th2, which provide B-cell help for antibody production, particularly IgE responses, and produce IL-4, IL-5, IL-6, IL-10, and IL-13 [34], which enhances eosinophil proliferation and function, commonly found in allergic responses. Moreover, a chemokine receptor CCR3 (eotaxin receptor) has been found predominantly on Th2-type lymphocytes, which co-localize with eosinophils [35], i.e., CCR3 T lymphocytes are recruited together with eosinophils. However, murine Th2 clones are different from those of humans, which are not highly restricted in cytokine production. Some clones produce IL-2 in addition to IL-4 and IL-5 [36]; IL-10 is produced by both Th1 and Th2 clones in humans [37]. The specific cell markers for Th1 and Th2 have recently been documented. Lymphocyte activation gene 3 (LAG-3, a member of the Ig superfamily) preferentially associates with Th1-like cells, which is upregulated by IFN-γ and downregulated by IL-4; CD30 (a member of the TNF receptor family) is mainly expressed in Th2-like cells, which is reciprocally dependent on IL-4 [38,39]. Th1 and Th2 differentiate from CD4$^+$ precursors and naive T0 cells under the influence of distinct cytokines: IL-12, IFN-γ, and TGF-β favor, but IL-4 hampers, Th1 development. Reciprocally, IL-4 favors but IFN-γ and TGF-β hamper Th2 development.

As with CD4$^+$ T cells, increasing evidence suggests that CD8$^+$ T cells can secrete either a Th1-like cytokine pattern or a Th2-like pattern in humans and mice. Similarly, IL-12 and IFN-γ promote the differentiation of precursors into Tc1 (cytotoxic type), as they do for Th1, and IL-4 induces the generation of both Th2 and Tc2. However, CD8$^+$ T cells require a higher dose of IL-4 than do CD4$^+$ cells in order to differentiate into IL-4–producing cells [39]. Thus, B-cell help by CD8$^+$ Tc2 cells may occur in vivo due to their secretion of type 2 cytokines (IL-4, IL-5, IL-6, and IL-10) and expression of CD40L, as CD4$^+$ Th2 cells for the activation of B cells [39]. CD8$^+$ T cells might also regulate IgE production by suppressing IgE synthesis via the inhibitory effect of IFN-γ on B cells and/or by affecting the differentiation and function of Th2-like CD4$^+$ T cells supporting IgE production [40]. Because cytokines play such a critical role in immunoregulation, rather than referring to Th1, Tc1$_{(cytotoxic)}$, and Th2, Tc2$_{(suppressor)}$ it is recommended that T cells be referred to as type 1 (IFN-γ, IL-2 predominant) and type 2 (IL-4, IL-5, IL-10 predominant), respectively [40–42], and also be termed as CD4 type 1, type 2 and CD8 type 1, type 2, correspondingly.

Histamine, an important inflammatory mediator in allergic diseases, has also been reported to have modulatory effects on T cells. Histamine inhibits IFN-γ production by type 1 cells but has no effect on IL-4 release and no effect on type 2 cells. However, histamine inhibits IL-4 but only slightly inhibits IFN-γ production by type 0 clones. The effect of histamine on T cells is via H2 receptors [43].

B-cell responses can be categorized as T-cell–dependent and T-cell–independent. After antigen is captured by B-cell membrane immunoglobulin, it is degraded, and certain of the resultant peptides are bound in the antigen-binding groove of class II MHC molecules, followed by translocation to the cell surface membrane of the B cell. The MHC/antigen structure, along with adhesive/aligning accessory/costimulatory molecules such as ICAM-1, B7 and LFA-3 then activate antigen-specific T cells, which express CD4, LFA-1, CD2 and the appropriate T-cell receptor (TCR).

CD40 is another co-stimulatory molecule on mature B cells. Upon binding to CD40L, which is expressed on activated CD4$^+$ T cells, B cells are triggered into an activation state. Thus, T and B cells mutually interact via costimulatory molecules. T-cell unresponsiveness can occur if activation of T cells occurs only through the TCR without engagement of other T-cell costimulatory molecules. Moreover, type 1 and type 2 pattern cytokines contribute to immunoglobulin isotype and class switching. For instance, in studies using lipopolysaccharide (LPS) as an independent activator, IL-4 mediates the switching of murine B cells to produce IgG1 and IgE. On the other hand, IFN-γ induces murine B cells to IgG2a and IgG3 [44]. In humans, upon T-cell–dependent activation IL-4 mediates the production of IgE and IgG4 by CD40–activated B cells [45]. In addition, IL-10 also regulates IgG by CD40-triggered B cells [46].

NK cells are non-T, non-B lymphocytes with the relatively distinct surface molecule, CD56, as well as CD16 (Fcγ RIII), CD2, and CD8, which they share with other cells. They produce certain important cytokines such as IFN-γ and TNF-α, which can activate dendritic APC and macrophages and can regulate T lymphocytes. NK cells and CD8$^+$ Tc are two major populations of cytotoxic lymphocytes that interact with each other. Regarding their cytotoxic effect, NK cells respond to offenders first as preactivated cytotoxic cells, which is then followed by specific T-cell responses. Then NK cells return to their preactivation state, implying that Tc may downregulate NK cell activity once specific immune responses are established. In addition, antigenic challenge of CD4$^+$T cells in association with NK cell activation and release of cytokines can lead to the development of a Th0/Th1 response or to a shift from a Th2 response toward a Th1/Th0 profile [47]. In severe atopic patients, the preferential Th2 pattern differentiation may be correlated with their defective NK cell function.

Interestingly, however, it recently has been reported that in mice, a minor population of CD1-specific CD4$^+$ NK1.1$^+$ T cells exists which can produce IL-4 promptly upon in vivo stimulation and can switch B cells to IgE production in response to injection of antibodies to IgD [48]. Therefore, CD4$^+$ NK1.1$^+$ T cells are important for the development of type 2/IgE immune responses in vivo. A comparable cell subset has also been recently defined in humans. It was shown that stimulation of naïve human CD4$^+$ T cells by anti-CD28 plus IL-2 induces expression of CD57 (an NK cell marker) and secretion of IL-4, which in turn induces IgE production by B cells independent of previous contact with IL-4. Thus, CD4$^+$CD57$^+$ T cells respond comparably to murine CD4$^+$ NK1.1$^+$ T cells. These T cells may produce early IL-4 and initiate Th2/IgE responses in allergy [49].

## C. Other Cells Important to Allergic Responses

Eosinophils, basophils, and mast cells are important to allergic responses derived from bone marrow granulocytic cells circulating in blood or found in tissues.

Eosinophils are present in normal peripheral blood. Major basic protein (MBP), eosinophil cationic protein (ECP), and eosinophil peroxidase (EPO) are major cationic granule proteins of eosinophils. These granules can induce histamine release from basophils and mast cells. There are a number of constitutively expressed receptors on normal blood eosinophils, such as IL-3R, IL-5R, IL-8R, CCR3 (eotaxin receptor), CR1, CR3, FcγRII, and RANTES, as well as inducible receptors, such as FcεRII (CD23), a low-affinity IgE receptor. Type 2 lymphocytes are the primary source for IL-3, IL-5, and GM-CSF, which are important to the survival, differentiation, and activation of eosinophils. Furthermore, activated T lymphocytes are also able to produce RANTES, a chemotactant for human eosinophils and memory T lymphocytes. This chemotactant from activated T cells may be responsible for the infiltration of eosinophils and memory T cells in the affected tissues of allergen-induced late-phase skin reactions in atopic subjects [50].

In allergy, it is believed that CCR3 is the principal chemokine receptor for the recruitment of eosinophils [51]. Eosinophils also express adhesion molecules such as CD11a, CD11b, CD11c/CD18, and VLA-4, which are probably responsible for the selective recruitment of eosinophils into tissues, especially when endothelial cells are activated during inflammation. In addition, β2 integrins play a crucial role in the activation of eosinophils stimulated by IgG [52]. Eosinophils also share surface molecule expression with other cells such as CD24, CD45, and the inducible molecules, HLA-DR, CD4, CD54. Activated eosinophils express HLA-DR and the adhesion molecule CD54 (ICAM-1), and participate in antigen uptake, processing, and presentation, thus they may serve as APCs for T lymphocytes. This eosinophil-mediated antigen presentation is inhibitable by treatment of eosinophils with chloroquine [53].

Basophils and mast cells contain similar basophilic-staining cytoplasmic granules but are distinct bone marrow–derived granulocytic cells. Basophils mature in the bone marrow, circulate in peripheral blood and can be recruited into tissues where allergic responses take place. IL-3, which may synergize with GM-CSF and IL-5, is the most important cytokine for basophil development and differentiation [54]. On the other hand, mast cells mature and develop in peripheral tissues with the crucial help of stem cell factor [55]. However, they share important common properties in allergic responses. They are the only cells that synthesize histamine and they express high-affinity IgE receptors. It seems that mast cells are well positioned in the skin to respond to locally invading allergens; by contrast, peripheral blood basophils have the potential to target distant sites of allergic inflammation. After activation by antigen-specific IgE interacting with receptor-bound IgE, basophils and mast cells degranulate, releasing preformed (e.g., histamine) and newly synthesized lipid (e.g., leukotrienes, LTC4) mediators. Basophils and mast cells and the different subsets of mast cells are characterized based on their content of tryptase and chymase (Tables 1 and 2). However, one should be aware that degranulation of mast cells and/or basophils may occur through non–IgE-dependent mechanisms and release the same mediators, causing clinical anaphylaxis syndrome such as urticaria, angioedema of the skin, asthma, cardiovascular collapse, etc. Neuropeptides are probably also major nonimmunological stimuli in the skin.

It has been documented that IL-4, an important type 2 cytokine, can be induced upon IgE receptor activation of mast cells [56] and basophils [57], which can enhance type 2 differentiation of T lymphocytes and sustain IgE production by B cells. In addition, IL-13 a newly defined cytokine, also contributes to IgE synthesis induced by all T-helper-cell subsets, including allergen-specific type 2 cells [34]. Furthermore, induction of human

**Table 1** Main Characteristics of Basophils and Mast Cells

|  | Basophils | Mast cells |
|---|---|---|
| In blood circulation | + | − |
| FcεR I | + | + |
| Histamine receptor 1 | + | + |
| Histamine receptor 2 | + | − |
| Lipid mediators | LTC4 | LTC4, PGD2 |
| Major basic protein | + | − |
| Inhibitory effect of corticosteroids | + | − |

LTC4 = leukotriene C4; PGD2 = prostaglandin $D_2$.

**Table 2** Characteristics of Human Mast Cell Subsets

|  | MCt | MCtc |
|---|---|---|
| Main distribution | Respiratory and intestinal mucosa | Skin |
| T-cell dependence | + | − |
| Inhibited by sodium cromoglycate | + | − |
| Involved in skin disorder | Atopic dermatitis | Urticaria |

MCt = mast cell containing tryptase only; MCtc = mast cell containing tryptase and chymase.

B-cell IgE synthesis by mast cells and basophils can also be independent of T cells. CD40L expression by freshly isolated mast cells and basophils, is able to provide signals in presence of IL-4 to induce IgE by B cells [58]. Integrins expressed on basophils may also play an important role during allergic inflammation. Cytokines such as IL-1 can induce expression of adhesion molecules on endothelial cells. It has been shown that vascular cell adhesion molecule-1 (VCAM-1) selectively binds and recruits eosinophils and basophils to sites of inflammation in vivo [59]. As with eosinophils, CCR3, an eotaxin receptor, is also expressed on basophils, thus eotaxin is likewise a potent chemotaxis of human basophils and plays a pathogenic role in allergic diseases by recruiting both basophils and eosinophils [60] to sites of inflammation.

## II. MAJOR PATHOLOGICAL MECHANISMS OF ALLERGIC SKIN RESPONSES

Atopic dermatitis, urticaria, and contact dermatitis are major allergic skin diseases and also represent the protypes of immunomechanisms of IgE-mediated and contact/delayed-type hypersensitivity. Our focus here is to delineate these two important immunopathological mechansims with particular respect to cell-mediated immunity.

### A. Ig-E Mediated Allergic Responses

The amount of IgE relative to other classes of immunoglobulin in serum and tissues is minimal; however, it plays a pivotal role particularly in immediate allergic responses. In the development of atopic (allergic) diseases [61], a genetic predisposition to develop allergen-specific IgE antibodies, such as for ragweed and grass pollen, exists. For the most part, no MHC-related genes causing allergic disease could be identified although there may still be a role for MHC in allergen-specific recognition [42].

The generation of allergen-specific IgE has been extensively studied with respect to the nature of the antigen, the antigen concentration, and the identity of antigen-presenting cells involved. In addition to natural allergens such as pollens, other proteins have been studied in mice or rats. Ovalbumin (OVA), *A. oryzae* lipase (AOL, an industrial enzyme), and bovine serum albumin (BSA) have been used as immunogens via mucosal tissue (intranasal) and a nonmucosal (intraperitoneal) route of exposure. OVA and AOL, but not BSA, stimulated strong IgE antibody responses. The quality of induced responses is not affected by the route of exposure [62]. In addition, OVA protein, through epicutaneous exposure in the absence of adjuvant, also induces a predominant type 2 response in mice. Mice receiving repeated protein antigen sustained elevated levels of specific IgE [63].

Chemical allergens, trimellitic anhydride (TMA, respiratory allergen), oxazolone (OX, contact allergen), and 2,4-dinitrochlorobenzene (DNCB, contact allergen), have also been studied. These chemicals were applied topically, and draining lymph node cells were derived for detection of IL-4 and hapten-specific and total IgE. Activation of mast cells was also determined. DNCB- and TMA-activated lymph node cells consistently expressed type 1 and type 2 cytokine patterns, respectively; i.e., TMA-treated lymph node cells express high levels of IL-4 and IL-10 but little IFN-$\gamma$. In contrast, DNCB-treated lymph node cells express the converse pattern of cytokine secretion [64,65]. In Brown Norway rats both chemicals, OX and TMA, stimulated hapten-specific IgG antibody responses, but only TMA induced specific IgE antibody, an increase in total serum IgE and active sensitization of mast cells. Furthermore, draining lymph node cells from TMA-treated rats express elevated IL-5 mRNA, and cells from TMA-treated rats, but not OX-treated rats cultured in the presence of Con A, secrete significantly higher levels of IL-4 than those from rats exposed to the controls (acetone/olive oil) [66]. Thus, the identity of the antigen is critical to the nature of the resulting immune response.

Antigen dose is another important component in generating optimal IgE responses. In general, low doses favor and large doses disfavor IgE production. An in vitro system that mimics responses generated in intact animals has been developed to examine the influence of antigen concentrations on the production of different classes and isotypes of immunoglobulin [67]. Lower concentrations of antigen favor maximal secretion of IgE, IgG1, and IgA, however, high antigen concentrations result in suppression of IgE, IgG1, and IgA synthesis [68]. Further studies show that this influence of antigen dose on IgE synthesis appears to be associated with the relative activation of type 1 (IFN-$\gamma$) and type 2 (IL-4) cells because IgE production is dependent upon the activation of IL 4-producing type 2, which could be detected in cultures having low, but not in those with high levels of antigen [69].

APC also participate in the induction of IgE production. In BALB/c mice application of DNCB, but not TMA, results in a 160% increase in Ia expression by LC, implying that TMA and DNCB exert differential effects on epidermal LC, possibly indicative of different antigen handling [70]. UVB irradiated LC from mice lose their ability to stimulate type 1 T-cell clones but retain their capacity to stimulate type 2 clones [71], and in chronic low-dose UVB irradiated mice the number of LC is markedly reduced with significant increase of IgE [72], suggesting that LC may be involved in TMA-induced IgE production together with accompanying release of relevant cytokines. In addition, it has been reported that sensitization with the hapten picryl chloride after barrier disruption of the skin down-regulated the expression of IFN-$\gamma$. The percent reduction in IFN-$\gamma$ expression correlated with the amount of stripping without changing the expression of IL-4. Furthermore, sensitization with house dust mite antigen on barrier-disrupted skin gives similar results. These results suggest that the percutaneous entry of environmental allergens through barrier-disrupted skin is associated with the induction of Th2-dominant allergic responses [73].

Once antigen-specific IgE is generated, IgE-mediated antigen presentation, by interaction with receptors for IgE of low affinity (CD23, Fc$\varepsilon$RII) on B cells, could lead to a continual activation of antigen-specific Th2 cells with very low concentrations of allergen. As the Th2 cell population expanded, which can induce more B cells to switch to IgE production, the presence of both Th2 cells specific for an allergen and high and persistent titers of allergen-specific IgE is the potent combination leading to expansion of allergic responses [74]. Thus the outcome of overproduction of IgE may explain the deterioration of the patients from being sensitive to a single group of allergens to being sensitive to multiple groups of allergens [75].

Based on immunomorphological and ultrastructural characterization, two distinct CD1a populations can be grouped, although they both are HLA-DR$^{bright}$/CD32$^{dim}$/CD23$^{dim/neg}$/CD1b$^{dim/neg}$: (1) classical LCs with CD1a$^{bright}$/FcεRI$^{dim}$/CD36$^{dim/neg}$ and (2) inflammatory dendritic epidermal cells with CD1a$^{dim}$/FcεRI$^{bright}$/CD36$^{bright}$ [76]. However, the functional effects of both populations have not been well defined yet [77]. As noted above, LC express FcεRI, which, interestingly, correlates with serum IgE levels in patients. However, unlike basophils, they are resistant to calcium flux following FcεRI engagement [15]. Furthermore, the location of FcεRI-bearing cells in skin is not random. In a patch test model, the presence of IgE in the epidermis, but not in the dermis, correlates well with the presence of (presumably IgE-bound) aeroallergens, such as host dust mites and grass pollen, suggesting that IgE-positive dermal cells might be related to food allergy as opposed to aeroallergens, which are more dependent on epidermal IgE-positive cells for induction of a cutaneous immune response. T-cell subsets have also been studied after patch testing. It has been shown that IgE-bearing LC are able to capture aeroallergens for antigen presentation, leading to activation of Th2 cells [78]. However, in the initiation phase of patch test with house dust mite allergen in patients with atopic dermatitis, IL-4 production by Th1 and Th0 cells is predominant over IFN-γ production by Th1 and Th0 cells. In the late and chronic phase the situation is reversed, i.e., IFN-γ production predominates over IL-4 production [79], suggesting that FcεRI$^+$ epidermal dendritic cells participate in the pathogenesis of atopic dermatitis. The presence of FcεRI$^+$ epidermal dendritic cells bearing IgE molecules seems to be a prerequisite to provoking eczematous skin lesions after application of aeroallergens to the skin of atopic patients [14].

The classical allergen-specific IgE-mediated clinical syndrome is anaphylaxis caused by specific allergen cross-linking two adjacent IgE molecules on mast cell surfaces, which initiates events leading to mediator (histamine) release. Anaphylaxis may occur locally or systemically and may be elicited by a variety of allergens, e.g., chemicals, drugs, foods aeroallergens, insect sting, etc. For example, in addition to the previously mentioned, latex could be a risk factor to atopic individuals [80], and various antigenic components of commercial latex have been identified. Drugs or their metabolites, such as the major determinant, benzylpenicilloyl, derived from penicillin, can bind as haptens to endogenous proteins. Nuts and shellfish are well-known food offenders. Pollen and house dust mites are common environmental allergens especially in atopic individuals. The basic immediate histamine-mediated response is characterized by constriction or dilation of smooth muscle resulting in vasodilation (erythema), increased vasopermeability between venular endothelial cells (raised wheal) seen in urticaria as cutaneous anaphylaxis, or cramps and diarrhea, or wheezing when gastrointestinal tract or pulmonary bronchi are targeted, respectively, which can be followed by cardiovascular collapse as systemic shock. The parenteral administration of an antigen is the route most associated with severe anaphylaxis. Any route, however, such as inhalational, oral, and topical administration, can be associated with the occurrence of anaphylactic reactions. Cutaneous anaphylaxis usually occurs within minutes once the sensitized individual encounters the specific allergen, peaks within 15–30 minutes, and fades within hours [81]. The cutaneous passive anaphylaxis (Prausnitz-Kustner reaction) is a helpful experimental model to elucidate the mechanism of IgE and its interaction with the mast cells. The reaction occurs after the injection into the dermis of antigen-specific IgE antibodies, which can then bind to FcεRI on the cell surface of tissue mast cells in the skin of normal recipients. After local challenge with antigen, which cross-links these IgE molecules, histamine and other mediators are released. This reaction has also been studied in oral allergy syndrome [82].

In many allergic individuals the immediate response to cutaneous antigenic challenge is followed 4–8 hours later by persistent swelling and leukocyte infiltration termed the late-phase response. The inflammatory infiltrate of the late-phase response is polymorphous, consisting of eosinophils, basophils, neutrophils, lymphocytes, and macrophages [83]. Relative to basophils, eosinophils are preferentially recruited to late-phase response. It has been documented that the central cause of the late-phase response is a result of mast cell degranulation. Histamine alone does not induce the late-phase response in the skin, rather products of the lipoxygenase pathway but not the cyclo-oxygenase pathway of arachiodonic acid metabolism are involved in cutaneous late-phase response [83]. It has been found that upon continuous antigen challenge, both histamine and mast cell tryptase are abruptly released, followed by a return to baseline tryptase content, but not histamine. It is postulated that basophils contribute histamine but basophils contains no tryptase. Again, using the skin chamber model to study the late-phase response for a 12-hour period shows that a difference between the early and late of this late-phase response is that prostaglandin $D_2$ (PGD2) production is absent late. It is likely that histamine originates from the basophil rather than mast cell, because, as with tryptase, basophils are not known to produce PGD2. In late phase, eosinophils are in an activated state and have enhanced production of LTC4 and release of eosinophil cationic proteins, particularly major basic protein. Furthermore, platelet-activating factor (PAF), one of the most potent chemotactic factors for eosinophils known, may also play an important role in the late-phase response. PAF is produced and released from eosinophils activated by their low-affinity receptors for IgE cross-linked by antigen, and in turn PAF can cause release of LTC4 from eosinophils. In addition, PAF also participates in increased vascular permeability, which leads to tissue edema.

In addition to soluble mediators, increasing data have shown that cytokines and chemokines may also play an important role in the late-phase response. Activated human basophils release IL-4 and IL-13 and human mast cells can produce IL-1, IL-4, IL-5, IL-6, IL-8, TNF-α, GM-CSF, and monocyte chemotactic protein-1 (MCP-1) [83–85]. It has been well documented that mediators and cytokines can induce vascular endothelial cells to express adhesion molecules. P-selectin is rapidly expressed on endothelial cells after exposure to histamine, PAF, LTB4, and LTD4. E-selectin, ICAM-1, and VCAM-1 can be induced by IL-1 and TNF-α [86]. Thus, neutrophils, eosinophils, basophils, monocytes, and lymphocytes can be recruited to the tissue sites of late-phase responses via vascular endothelial cells. Because of the high local concentration of IL-4, the development and expansion of type 2 lymphocytes may also be important [87]. Taken together, there are early- and late-phase responses. The late-phase response is initiated by IgE-mediated immediate, early-phase response followed by a complex recruitment of leukocytes and an interactive network of mediators, chemokines, and cytokines. Although accumulating evidence has provided better understanding of the basic aspects of allergic reactions, the mechanisms, especially of the late-phase response of the allergic reaction, have not been fully delineated. An outline of IgE-mediated allergic responses is shown in Figure 1.

## B. Contact and Delayed-Type Hypersensitivity

Allergic contact dermatitis is one of the most common skin diseases and represents the prototype of contact hypersensitivity (CHS). The skin is also an organ that demonstrates

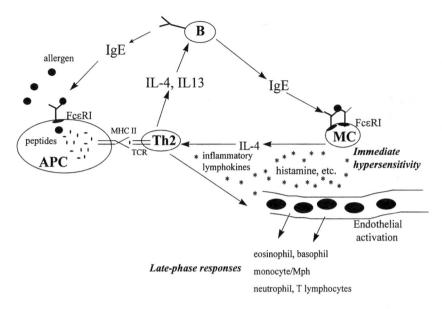

**Figure 1**   IgE-mediated allergic responses. APC = Antigen-presenting cell; B = B cell; MHC II = major histocompatibility complex class II; MC = mast cell; Mph = macrophage; TCR = T-cell receptor; Th2 = T-helper cell type 2.

delayed-type hypersensitivity (DTH): the tuberculin skin test is a classic example of DTH, which is elicited in sensitive individuals by intradermal injection of tuberculoprotein antigens. Although both CHS and DTH share certain common features, such as the delayed reaction in response to antigen by sensitized individuals, it appears that CHS-mediated effector T cells are of CD8+ phenotype, because depletion of CD4+ T cells enhances CHS, whereas depletion of CD8+ T cell suppresses CHS. By contrast, DTH responses are elicited by CD4+ T cells, because depletion of CD4+ T cells abrogates DTH [88]. In addition, it has been shown that CHS and DTH are different by the study of the in vivo effects of IL-10 on these reactions. IL-10 suppresses the induction of DTH but not CHS. However, IL-10 does block the elicitation of both CHS and DTH in mice. These data support the concept that CHS and DTH are related but their immunological reactions are different, particularly during initiation [89]. Although the differences between mechanisms of CHS and DTH have not been clearly defined, it is clear that the route of hapten administration, epicutaneous application versus intradermal injection, is highly relevant to the development of these reactions due to differential involvement of keratinocyte-, macrophage-, and LC (dendritic cell)–induced cytokines, which induce distinct microenvironments [88].

Two phases of CHS have been delineated. The sensitization phase of CHS is initiated by exposure to allergens on the skin surface. Elicitation occurs after subsequent reexposure to those specific allergens. Most environmental allergens are haptens, usually simple chemicals. Before acting as sensitizers they must first link covalently to carrier proteins to form a complete antigen.

Epidermal LC are the principal antigen-presenting cells involved in CHS. They are activated during capturing and processing of antigens. Subsequent secretion of IL-1β is essential for the development of epicutaneous sensitization [90–92]. Both IL-1β and TNF-α, which is induced by hapten from keratinocytes [23,90,92], are required for LC migration to the draining lymph nodes [25,93]. Other cytokines, such as IL-6, IL-12, IL-15, and GM-CSF [21,92,94] from either LC or keratinocytes or both, may also be involved in the process of primary sensitization. In addition, it has been defined in mice that the dermis contains potent MHC class II$^+$ CD11b$^-$ LC-like/indeterminant cells, which are distinct from dermal macrophages and from classical epidermal LC, positioned at the interface of the vasculature with the dermal interstitium. Therefore, they are important in the initial activation of T cells upon their entry into the skin from the blood and may be involved in trafficking of antigen between the skin and regional lymph nodes [11].

After LC are activated, they migrate to the draining lymph nodes where they present antigens and activate naïve T cells, resulting in generation of CHS effector cells. Recently, the in vivo function of CD4$^+$ and CD8$^+$ cells in CHS with the cytokines produced by each T-cell population has been extensively studied [95]. Depletion of CD8$^+$ T cells before sensitization of mice with dinitrofluorobenzene (DNFB) or oxazolone (OX) results in low or abrogated responses, in contrast, depletion of CD4$^+$ T cells results in increased and prolonged CHS responses. Determination of cytokine production in draining lymph nodes after sensitization with DNFB or OX shows that induced CD8$^+$ T cells produce IFN-$\gamma$ and no IL-4 and IL-10, and induced CD4$^+$ cells produce IL-4 and IL-10 and no or little detectable IFN-$\gamma$. Thus, these results provide interesting evidence that in CHS, two polarized and functionally opposing populations of T cells arise: IFN-$\gamma$–producing effector CD8$^+$ T cells and IL-4/IL-10–producing CD4$^+$ T cells that negatively regulate the response.

Because CD8$^+$ and CD4$^+$ T cells are restricted by MHC classes, studies on CHS responses to DNFB have been carried out on MHC class II (I$^+$ II$^-$)– and MHC class I (I$^-$II$^+$)–deficient mice [96,97]. Dendritic cell expression of MHC class I molecules is required for the induction of CHS and for the generation of hapten-specific CD8$^+$ T cells in lymphoid organs. MHC I$^+$II$^-$ DC are as potent as MHC I$^+$II$^+$ dendritic cells in inducing CHS, indicating that activation of effector CD8$^+$ T cells can occur independent of CD4$^+$ T-cell help. By contrast, I$^-$II$^+$dendritic cells can not induce CHS, as the presence of MHC I$^-$II$^+$ dendritic cells downregulate the inflammatory response. Thus, these results provide further evidence that CD8$^+$ T cells are effector cells and CD4$^+$ cells play a regulatory role and that their restriction to MHC class I and class II arise concurrently but independently in the sensitization of CHS.

The nature of sensitizers is also involved in cytokine profiles in CHS. In mice, both DNFB and fluorescein isothiocyanate (FITC) can induce CHS, but the expression of cytokine profiles is different. Studies on the cells from draining lymph nodes showed that in DNFB-sensitized mice IFN-$\gamma$–secreting cells are predominant, however, in FITC-sensitized mice IL-4–secreting cells are predominant. Thus, the DNFB response is associated with a type 1 immune response whereas the FITC response is associated with type 2 cytokines [98].

The importance of the dose of hapten in induction of CHS is also recognized [88,99]. Optimal doses of hapten may lead to the generation of CHS effector T cells by LC, and low doses of hapten (below threshold sensitivity) may induce tolerance. These subsensitizing doses of contact sensitizer on normal murine skin generate CD8$^+$ type 2 cells that give rise to hapten-specific tolerance. Studies have shown that the type 2 phenotype may be a consequence of clonal anergy [100].

It is well known that cell adhesion molecules (CAM) play an important role in cell-mediated immune responses. Mice sensitized with FITC have been used for the assessment of function of ICAM and LFA-1 in CHS sensitization. The combination of anti-ICAM-

1 and anti-LFA-1 monoclonal antibodies completely inhibited the induction of CHS to FITC. Dendritic lymph node cells from mice treated with anti-ICAM-1 or anti-LFA-1 monoclonal antibodies alone had significantly reduced numbers of brightly FITC-stained cells (LC) capable of stimulating a FITC-specific T-cell hybridoma indicating that the adhesion molecules, ICAM-1 and LFA-1, play a significant role in CHS sensitization, which may be in part due to their effect on APC migration [101].

It is also clear that co-stimulatory molecules, B7 [98,102,103] and CD40 [98,104], are involved in the sensitization phase of CHS. LC isolated from hapten-sensitized mice express high levels of B7-2 and low levels of B7-1. Anti-B7-2 antibody given during hapten sensitization inhibits outgrowth of effector CD8+ T cells and the magnitude of the CHS response. Anti-B7-1 antibody inhibits CHS but without inhibiting development of the IFN-γ–producing CD8+ cells; however, it increases the number of type 2 cells primed during hapten sensitization, implying that B7-2 plays a critical role on effector CD8+ T cells and B7-1 on regulatory CD4+ T cells to balance immune reaction during the sensitization of CHS [102,103]. Similarly, it has been shown that the blockade of B7-CD28 co-stimulatory pathway by CTLA-4-Ig (soluble form of CTLA-4) leads to tolerance in DNFB-induced type 1 CHS [98]. CD40-CD40L, like B7-CD28, is another pair of co-stimulatory molecules required in the sensitization, but not in elicitation phase of CHS. In DNFB-induced CHS, CD8+ T cells produce IFN-γ and exhibit effector function, while CD4+ T cells produce IL-4 and exhibit regulatory function. Anti-CD40L antibody decreases IFN-γ production and increases IL-4 production by draining lymph node cells from DNFB-sensitized mice, and it inhibits the elaboration of IL-12 in the regional lymph nodes. Because CD40L is expressed on CD4 cells, and CD40-CD40L interaction is critical for IL-12 production by APC such as macrophages and dendritic cells [105,106]. Thus, bidirectional CD40-CD40L signaling is required in the sensitization of CHS, and is associated with both APC IL-12 production and T-cell costimulation [104].

After primary sensitization, reexposure to specific allergens provokes the elicitation phase of CHS. T cells play a critical role in CHS; the skin-tropic subset of T cells is of memory/activated type and circulate in a tissue-selective manner [107]. Repeated activation in skin or skin-associated peripheral lymph nodes may reinforce cutaneous lymphocyte-associated antigen expression on T cells and thus enhance the functional efficiency of these cells by preferentially recirculating to the skin [108]. LC here are not necessary for presenting antigens to antigen-specific T cells. To the contrary, CHS responses in mice that were first sensitized with hapten and then challenged through skin that was previously treated by topical corticosteroid application to remove the majority of epidermal LC are markedly stronger when compared with vehicle-treated controls. These results indicate that depletion of most of the resident LC not only fails to impair but enhances the expression of CHS significantly [109]. It raises the possibility that other APC, such as LC-like interstitial dendritic APC [11], and nonprofessional APC may be involved in the elicitation phase of CHS. Epidermal keratinocytes normally do not express MHC class II antigens, although activation through IFN-γ can lead to their induction [1]. Activated T cells can also express MHC class II molecules as well as co-stimulatory molecules such as CD80, originally thought to be expressed only on classical APC [110]. The exact role of both professional and nonprofessional APC in the elicitation of CHS is still largely unclear.

Because haptens usually act not only as immunogens but as irritants as well, after local application of haptens to the skin, keratinocytes can be activated and a wide variety of cytokines induced [111]. Thus, locally applied specific haptens likely first induce the production of proinflammatory cytokines (such as IL-1, TNF-α) and chemokines (monocyte chemotactic protein-1, interferon-inducible protein-10, macrophage inflammatory protein 1α) mostly from activated keratinocytes during CHS elicitation, followed by upregulation of adhesion molecules and co-stimulatory molecules on APC, leukocytes and endothelial cells of post capillary venules, and recruitment of leukocytes. This process increases the likelihood that already sensitized T cells will encounter the specific allergens, and finally, elicited CHS occurs. Application of allergen and/or irritant to human subjects reveals that the response to both allergen and irritant was greater than to either alone. Doses of allergen, which did not produce a response when applied alone, produced a response when an irritant was added, indicating that irritants increase the allergic contact dermatitis response and may explain the presence of contact dermatitis in patients with negative patch tests [112]. Thus, nonspecific proinflammatory signals are important in elicitation of CHS (Fig. 2).

Interestingly, studies on CHS elicitation further showed that cytokine profiles of CHS are not invariable and can be shifted after repeated challenges of the same hapten. Mice sensitized with trinitrochlorobenzene (TNCB) have been employed for assessment of the temporal sequence of cytokine gene expression at various time points after elicitation with DNFB. In the acute lesions (day 0) increased mRNA levels for IFN-γ and IL-2 were rapidly detected and remained elevated, while mRNA expression for IL-4 and IL-10 was absent or minimally upregulated. In chronic lesions (day 24, applied at 2-day intervals), high levels of IL-4 mRNA were expressed and IL-10 mRNA was dramatically

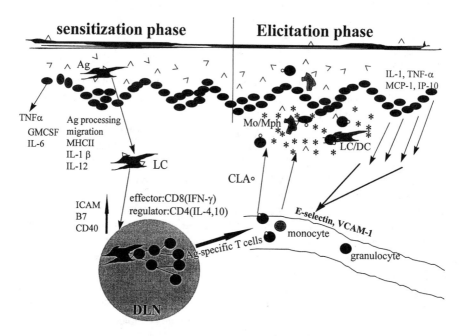

**Figure 2**   Contact hypersensitivity. Ag = Antigen; CLA = cutaneous lymphocyte-associated antigen; GMCSF = granulocyte macrophage colony stimulating factor; ICAM = intercellular adhesion molecule; IL = interleukin; DLN = draining lymph node; IFN = interferon; IP = inducible protein-10; LC/DC = Langerhans cell/dendritic cell; MCP-1 = macrophage chemotactic protein-1; MHC II = major histocompatibility complex class II; Mo/Mph = monocyte/macrophage; TNF = tumor necrosis factor; VCAM = vascular cell adhesion molecule.

upregulated. These transcripts correlated well with those of IL-4 and IL-10 protein produced locally, whereas the expression of type 1 cytokines was markedly reduced. This local cytokine pattern shifting from a type 1 to type 2 is site-restricted [113]. This shift toward type 2–dominated responses may explain clinically relevant events: that after repeated exposure to the same hapten, the deleterious type 1 response (dermatitis) diminishes.

Cell adhesion molecules not only are important in CHS sensitization, as mentioned above, but also are required for maximum CHS elicitation [114]. In a mouse study with DNFB sensitization, a specific anti-LFA-1 monoclonal antibody was injected into the ears of mice after sensitization but prior to challenge with DNFB. Twenty-four and 48 hours after challenge, ear swelling was dose-dependently suppressed and accompained a reduction of leukocyte infiltration into the dermis.

Co-stimulatory molecules are also required for CHS elicitation. After blockade of these molecules, tolerance occurs. However, the generation of tolerance is different in type 1 and type 2 CHS. In general, type 2 cells are more difficult to be anergized; for instance, such as FITC-induced (type 2) CHS elicitation is more difficult to be anergized than that DNFB-induced (type 1). It has been shown in mice that both anti-CD40L monoclonal antibody and CTLA 4-Ig treatment is effective in blocking the primary response to DNFB or FITC, but each alone is not effective in blocking the secondary response to FITC, although CTLA 4-Ig treatment is sufficient to suppress the ear-swelling response to DNFB. However, the combination of CTLA 4-Ig and anti-CD40L is able to induce long-lasting unresponsiveness to FITC. The results suggest that the cells mounting this type 2 response are capable of priming for a maximal response with receipt of signals through either CD28 or CD40L pathway [98]. An outline of contact hypersensitivity is shown in Figure 2.

## III. INTERVENTION: MECHANISMS OF CELL-MEDIATED IMMUNOSUPPRESSION

More than 20 years ago certain lymphoid cells, termed as suppressor cells, were noted to be capable of blocking the immune response, and later these cells were shown to be suppressor T cells. Animal studies, using synthetic polypeptide antigens along with natural protein antigens, showed that T-suppressor cells can block specific T-helper cells for B-cell help in the production of specific antibodies [115]. Moreover, the production of immunoglobulin is enhanced by treatment with anti-CD8 monoclonal antibody, further suggesting that CD8$^+$ cells play a downregulatory role in the production of immunoglobulins [116]. In cellular mediated responses, similarly, when antigen-specific CD4$^+$ T-cell clones are exposed to CD8$^+$ T-suppressor-cell clones and antigen, they become unresponsive to the specific antigen [117]. A series of studies since then revealed that macrophages are the most efficient APC in inducing T-suppressor cells [118]. Although the early study of T-suppressor cells focused on CD8$^+$ T suppressors, actually they are much more complicated. For example, CD4$^+$ suppressor-inducers are also involved in a cascade, which generates T suppressors [41], such as in humans, epidermal cells from ultraviolet light–exposed skin preferentially activate CD4$^+$ 2H4$^+$ lymphocytes (inducer of T-suppressor lymphocytes) and followed by the induction of CD8$^+$ suppressor cells [119,120]. However, with intensive study of cytokine function, accumulating evidence shows that the cell surface phenotype is not sufficient to represent the actual function of the cells and instead, the pattern of cytokines produced by the cells is more useful. Cytokines produced by type 1(IFN-$\gamma$, IL-2 predominant) and type 2 (IL-4, IL-5, IL-10 predominant) T cells are distinct and functionally reciprocal regardless of whether CD4 or CD8 cell surface molecules are present. If IgE production is used as a marker of cytokine activity, IL-4 is necessary for the production of IgE; by contrast, IFN-$\gamma$ inhibits the production of IgE. In general, mature, peripheral T cells are functionally inactivated through suppression, anergy, or apoptosis [121]. T-cell anergy is distinguished from suppression in that antigen-specific T-cell activation can be rescued by the addition of IL-2 in the presence of antigen. Suppression of T-cell responses can be mediated either by competition for antigen or by inhibitory cytokines. Apoptosis, such as induced by Fas/FasL interaction, can downmodulate lymphocyte-mediated immune responses [122]; in culture, mature LC spontaneously undergo apoptosis and can be accelerated by IL-10 [123]. Thus, cytokine suppression and apoptosis are pivotal factors, which have been studied along with immunocompetent cells to explore the mechanism of allergic responses and are potential tools for the intervention of allergic diseases.

As mentioned above, IgE-mediated hypersensitivity is a T-cell type 2 predominant cytokine–mediated allergic response. In the early stage of the response, histamine and other mediators are released, and correspondingly mast cell stabilizers (e.g., cromolyn), antihistamines, and other pharmaceutical interventions have been utilized to alleviate the responses and clinical symptoms. In terms of cell-mediated mechanisms, it has been proposed that alteration of cytokines such as inhibition of type-2 cytokines could be beneficial in the treatment of allergic diseases [42]. It has been known that antigen dose and APC can influence both cell-mediated and humoral immunity by T cells producing distinct sets of cytokines. In human studies [124,125], CD4$^+$ T cells from allergic donors produced high levels of IL-4 when stimulated in vitro with low concentrations of allergen, and more so when B-cell–enriched populations presented the antigen. In contrast, the same responding CD4$^+$ T-cell population produced little IL-4 when stimulated with high concentrations of antigen, especially when monocytes were used as antigen-presenting cells, implying that the cytokine profile of allergen-specific memory CD4$^+$ T cells can be modulated by the antigen dose and APC type and suggesting that methods that enhance allergen uptake by monocytes while inhibiting uptake by B cells will improve the clinical efficacy of immunotherapy in the treatment of allergic disease.

Allergen extracts had been utilized in the treatment of allergic disease, but IgE-mediated side effects have limited their utility in the clinic. Allergen-specific peptide-based therapy, thus, has been advocated for immunotherapy. Currently, individual allergen-specific peptides containing functional T-cell epitopes, but lacking IgE binding sites, have been recommended for effective immunotherapy. Such design allows administration of peptides at higher doses and for a shorter period of time than usual with full-length allergens with a lower risk of side effects [126,127]. The mechanism by which peptide treatment exerts its effect on allergic symptoms is not understood yet. The factors other than IgE antibody production such as cytokines must be studied on these anergized allergen-specific T cells [127].

IL-12, an IFN-$\gamma$ inducer, has also been proposed for the treatment of Th2-mediated allergic diseases. A study in a mouse model for asthma showed that antigen-induced airway hyperresponsiveness and type 2 cytokine expression are inhibited by administration of IL-12. Further studies showed that the response of memory T cells can also be altered, however, resting memory CD4$^+$ T cells are more sensitive than activated CD4$^+$ T cells to the effects of IL-12 [42,128]. The effect of IL-12 on human type 1, but not on type 2 cells is likely due to the IL-12 receptor $\beta$2 subunit, which is expressed on human type 1 but not type 2 clones and is induced during differentiation of human naïve cells along the type 1 but not type 2 pathway [129]. Importantly, IL-4 (type 2 cytokine) can also significantly inhibit IL-12R β2 expression after T-cell activation, leading to the loss of IL-12 signaling. Thus, administration of IL-12 followed by the induction of IFN-γ, inhibition of IL-4, preventing further loss of IL-12R β2 subunit, could be one potentially important treatment of ongoing allergic diseases [130].

Regulation of the human IL-2/IL-2 receptor system can also play a role in immuno-suppression in the treatment of allergic diseases. Expression of the high-affinity IL-2R (CD25) depends on the induction of IL-2Rα gene expression, which is low on normal resting T cells and upregulated by activation by antigen or mitogen. CD8 cells (including cytotoxic and mature suppressor T populations) actively suppress expression of the IL-2Rα in the non-CD8 cell population. Depletion of CD8 cells leads to superinduction of IL-2 activity and IL-2Rα, implying that in normal conditions CD8 plays an important role in the balance of cell-mediated immune responses [131]. In a study in adult hay fever patients, grass pollen immunotherapy was performed. Cellular infiltration and cytokine mRNA expression during allergen-induced late-phase cutaneous responses were observed. Clinical improvement was accompanied by a decrease in the size of the late-phase skin response. Analysis of skin biopsy specimens obtained 24 hours after intradermal introduction of allergen showed a significant reduction in the number of infiltrating CD3[+] and CD4[+] cells and a trend for a decrease in eosinophils but no influence of allergen-induced recruitment of CD8[+] cells and macrophages. Interestingly, the expression of CD25 was increased. Significant hybridization for IL-2 was also observed in the actively treated group. These findings indicate that immunotherapy is associated with suppression of allergen-induced CD4[+] T-lymphocyte infiltration and the upregulation of CD25 in the infiltrating cells [132]. The immunoregulation of these coupled genes is also involved in development of cell-mediated contact sensitivity. Altered regulation of these genes expression has been shown by our UV studies [133] and will be discussed below.

Contact and DTH is a T-cell type 1 predominant cytokine–mediated allergic response. Corticosteroids are the most common pharmacological intervention, administered locally or systemically, in the treatment of allergic contact dermatitis. It has been shown in an in vitro study that the production by T cells of both IFN-γ and IL-4 is inhibited in a dose-dependent manner, suggesting that the effect of corticosteroids on T-cell–mediated inflammation follows from inhibition of proliferation and cytokine production by T lymphocytes [134]. However, the production of IL-4 by T-cell clones is more sensitive to inhibition by corticosteroids in the treatment of type 2–mediated diseases such as asthma [135]. Thus, the sensitivity to inhibition by corticosteroids at the T-cell level may be influenced by its original immune status. Further insight is gained by observing the effects of corticosteroids on cytokine synthesis by cultures of human monocytes and T cells. Short incubation of monocytes with corticosteroids can have lasting effects on their ability to regulate cytokine synthesis by T cells. Corticosteroids significantly inhibit the production of monocyte IL-12, which results in a decreased capacity of the monocytes to induce IFN-γ and an increased ability to induce IL-4 in T cells [136]. Thus, it at least could be a part of mechanisms of the administration of corticorsteroids in the treatment of contact dermatitis.

The interaction of immune responses with environmental factors has always been recognized, and because the skin is the outermost part of the body, the interaction of environmental factors and the skin-associated immune system is important to health. Although overexposure to sunshine causes immunosuppression, induction of skin cancer, and infectious disease, it is also useful for the treatment of immunologically mediated skin diseases. Allergic and immunological skin disorders that improve by exposure to sunlight or phototherapy include atopic dermatitis, contact dermatitis, urticaria, and psoriasis [137]. The effects of ultraviolet light on skin have been studied for more than 30 years, and it was noticed that the elicitation of CHS reactions in guinea pigs is impaired by prior exposure of the test site to UVB radiation. Cell-mediated immunosuppressive mechanisms induced by UV radiation have been extensively studied since then.

UV comprises three distinct spectra: A (320–400 nm), B (290–320 nm), and C (200–290 nm). UVB is far more effective than UVA in inducing immunosuppression and skin tumors in human and experimental animals. UVB reaches terrestrial surface and human skin in significant doses. In contrast, UVC is absorbed by atmospheric ozone and is not present at the globe surface. Thus, UVB has been most intensively studied. Acute UV injury is a complex inflammatory and immunomodulatory process. Epidermal cells, mainly LC, keratinocytes, and melanocytes, are highly exposed to UV radiation. Initially, rapid membrane signal transduction events are triggered by UV, resulting in the triggering of cytokine [111] and mediator production and release [138], followed by the secondary activation of epidermal and dermal cells such as vascular cells, leukocytes, and extracellular matrix. DNA damage, photoisomerization of urocanic acid (UCA), and more recently α-melanocyte–stimulating hormone, Fas/Fas-ligand system and ligands for β1, β2 integrins are of special interest as contributors to the mechanisms of UV-induced cell-mediated immunosuppression. In addition to these events, there are a number of changes in the number and activation levels of immune cells, such as LC and monocyte/macrophages, present in the skin.

LC are intensely affected by UV exposure. UV injury depletes LC from the epidermis [139–147], causing LC to lose their dendritoxicity and downregulate some surface markers, such as MHC class II molecules [148]. UV also perturbs the functional expression of B7-1 and B7-2 co-stimulatory molecules on human LC [149], and prevents upregulation of ICAM-1 expression by LC in culture [150]. Although the hair follicle can be a critical reservoir of LC that repopulate the epidermis depleted of LC by UV, LC isolated from epidermis 72 hours after UVB do not upregulate B7-1 or B7-2 expression in culture compared with LC from unexposed control skin, suggesting that the phenotype of the hair follicle LC is different from normal interfollicular epidermal LC [151]. These alterations of LC after UV exposure may contribute to their inability to stimulate type 1, despite fully retaining their ability to stimulate type 2 lymphocytes [71,152], resulting in the conversion of LC from an immunogenic to a costimulatory signal-deficient state that induces T-cell anergy [153,154].

Immunocompetent cell populations are changed in the skin by UV exposure. UV injury induces inflammation with infiltration of neutrophils, differentiated macrophages, and monocyte/macrophagic APC in the dermis and epidermis [151,155–160]. Despite an overall expansion of HLA-DR$^+$ cells, the LC in epidermis and LC-like dendritic APC subsets of HLA-DR$^+$ cells in the dermis are depleted almost completely at 72 hours after UV. By contrast, UV exposure induces a selective expansion of the dermal macrophage subset, which is phenotypically identical to the monocytic/macrophagic APC that appear in the epidermis. These epidermal macrophages derive not only from transcapillary migration, but also from in situ proliferation of dermal precursors [158].

LC loss can occur without induction of tolerance to contact sensitizers (post-UVA exposure), and systemic suppression of CHS by UVB irradiation is not related to the numerical and morphological alterations in LC that occur locally at the site of irradiation

[161]. Thus, UV-induced unresponsiveness cannot be fully accounted for by alterations of LC. Furthermore, macrophages present in the skin after UV exposure are different from LC in their heightened responsiveness to FcIgG receptor-mediated signaling [162], high production of IL-10, and reduced production of IL-12 [21,159,160]. Therefore, different types of APC that are recruited to a site of antigen exposure, or the differentiation status of in situ APC, can dictate distinct outcomes of an immune response to that antigen.

As mentioned above, after UVB exposure, LC are replaced by infiltrating macrophages as the dominant APC in epidermis. We have named these cells UV macrophages (UV-Mph). Because UV-induced immunological tolerance is T-cell–mediated, we have reasoned that UV-Mph are critical to the induction of this tolerance. Several lines of evidence support this view. In mice, 3 days after in vivo UV exposure LC are depleted and macrophages appear in the epidermis. Intracutaneous injection of dinitrobenzenesulfonic acid-haptened UV-epidermal cell, but not normal controls, results in the induction of locally inducible antigen-specific tolerance to dinitrofluorobenzene. Removal of the CD11b$^+$ class II MHC$^+$ population (UV-Mph) shows that this population is indeed critical for tolerance induction [163]. Similarly, in vivo anti-CD11b treatment reduces the infiltration UV-Mph into UV-irradiated skin and blocks tolerance induction [164]. The time course after UV exposure of the induction of tolerance and the appearance of UV-Mph are the same. Partial tolerance is first detectable 6 hours and reaches its maximum 48 hours after UV exposure. Similarly, a small number of infiltrating UV-Mph are already apparent within the dermis at the 6-hour time point. Over the next few days the numbers of infiltrating UV-Mph parallel the intensity of the UV tolerance. By 48 hours post-UV exposure, when a state of maximum tolerance is obtained, both constitutive epidermal and dermal LC populations are at or near their nadir, in contrast, the infiltrating monocyte/macrophage population exhibits a dramatic increase in the epidermis at 48–72 hours, indicating that the induction of in vivo tolerance is closely associated with the expansion of monocytic/macrophagic cells in the dermis and epidermis. In humans, there is a also a concordant reduction in LC and increase in UV-Mph and UV-induced tolerance [156].

There are several features of UV-Mph that favor their ability to induce antigen-specific tolerance. First, IL-10 is dramatically induced and IL-12 is significantly reduced in UV-Mph, like other monocyte macrophages, both in vivo [159,160] and in vitro [166] after UV irradiation. Both IL-10 [167,168] and IL-12 [169,170] are critically involved in influencing the induction of UV-induced tolerance indicating that UV-Mph, as APC, other than LC, are well suited to play an important role in immunomodulation post UV injury.

The mechanisms of IL-10 induction and reduction of IL-12 by monocytes/macrophages after UV injury with the development of tolerance have been further explored. Monocytes/macrophages are rich in receptors for immunoglobulins, complement, and extracellular matrix components such fibronectin (Fn) and the third component of complement (C3). We found that monocytic β1 integrins, which bind to the UV-induced extracellular matrix ligand, Fn, and leukocyte β2 integrins binding to UV-induced C3 degradation product (iC3b) after extravasation of blood monocytes into the dermis is involved in the modulation of immunoregulatory monocytic cytokines. Immunostaining sections of human skin revealed that cellular Fn and iC3b are induced in the epidermis of UV-exposed skin relative to controls 24–72 hours after in vivo UV exposure and UV-Mph are found within the area enriched in Fn or iC3b. Stimulation of purified peripheral blood monocytes with iC3b-coated sheep RBC or Fn causes significantly enhanced IL-10 protein production [171]. To further model in vivo UV conditions in the skin, TNF-α was added, which further enhanced IL-10 production by these blood monocytes activated by iC3b [171].

Interestingly, Fn itself induces TNF-α release by monocytes as well and acts in an auto-crine manner to promote further IL-10 production. Furthermore, iC3b ligation also results in downregulation of IL-12 production [171]. Thus, UV-induced ligands for β1 and β2 integrins provide the stimuli for generating the IL-10$^{high}$ IL-12$^{lo}$ monocyte/macrophage phenotype in the micro-milieu of the skin after UV exposure (Fig. 3).

Because UV radiation activates C3 in the skin and its product, iC3b, can induce IL-10 and reduce IL-12 production by monocyte/macrophage, contact sensitizer applied through murine skin has been studied to explore whether iC3b plays a role in the immuno-suppressed state after UV exposure. Two different in vivo mouse model systems in which either C3 is deficient by C3 gene disruption or C3 is present and activation of C3 is inhibited by soluble CR1 were employed. Both C3-modulated systems totally reversed the failure to induce a contact sensitivity response to DNFB upon primary sensitization at the UV-exposed site as well as immunological tolerance to a secondary DNFB immuni-zation through normal skin. Treatment with soluble CR1 reduced the infiltration of monocytic/macrophagic cells into the epidermis and dermis of UV-irradiated skin but did not reverse the UV-induced depletion of epidermal LC. These results and the abrogation of locally induced UV immunosuppression by in vivo anti-CD11b treatment suggest a novel mechanism by which ligation of leukocyte β2 integrin, CD11b, by iC3b molecules derived from C$_3$ activation in UV-exposed skin, modifies cutaneous CD11b$^+$ cells such

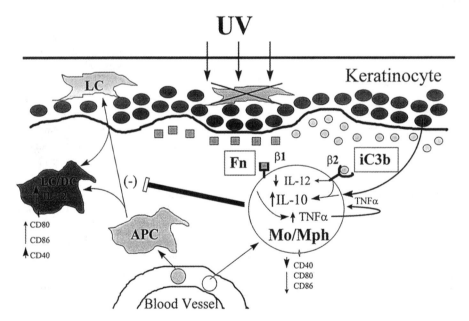

**Figure 3**  Integrin ligands are involved in induction of IL-10 and reduction of IL-12 by monocytes/macrophages after UV exposure of the skin. After UV exposure, Langerhans cells are depleted from epidermis, meanwhile, monocytes/macrophages migrate from the blood stream into dermis and epidermis. Cellular fibronectin, ligand for β1 integrin, and iC3b, ligand for β2 integrin, are newly formed in the dermis. Integrin-ligand interaction on monocytes/macrophages takes place and results in induction of IL-10 and reduction of IL-12 with or without TNF-α co-stimulation. Generation of IL-10$^{high}$ IL-12$^{low}$ micro-milieu in the skin by the infiltrating monocytes/macrophages suppresses normal function of Langerhans cells/dendritic antigen-presenting cells.

that skin APC are not only unable to sensitize in a primary immune response, but actively induce antigenic tolerance [172].

Because UV-induced tolerance is T-cell–mediated, one would expect that T-cell activation by UV-Mph and LC would be distinct. We have found in humans that allogeneic T cells stimulated in vitro by normal epidermal cells (LC as dominant APC) rapidly and markedly upregulate both IL-2 and IL-2Rα. In contrast, T cells stimulated with UV-exposed epidermal cells in which LC are depleted from the epidermis and UV-Mph are the dominant APC type were markedly deficient in their ability to express the IL-2Rα despite IL-2 expression and proliferation that were equal to that induced by APC in normal epidermis. Neutralizing the immunosuppressive cytokine TGF-β in cultures of UV-exposed epidermal cell–stimulated cultures restores CD4$^+$ cell surface IL-2Rα expression. Thus, LC upregulate allogeneic CD4$^+$ T cells IL-2 and IL-2Rα gene expression. By contrast, UV macrophage activation of these cells is characterized by TGF-β–dependent deficient IL-2Rα expression. The functional consequence of T-cell activation by UV-epidermal cells is that suppressor-inducer T lymphocytes are generated that activate CD8$^+$ cells [119,120], which in turn suppress lymphocyte responsiveness and possibly further enhance the function which induces deficiency of IL-2Rα on T cells [133]. As mentioned above CD8 cells actively suppress expression of the IL-2Rα in the non-CD8 cell population [131], thus, it is possible that in vivo these downregulatory T-cell responses are amplified.

Because the balance of IL-10 and IL-12 is important to the nature of immune responses and UV-Mph produce high levels of IL-10 and low levels of IL-12, one might expect that neutralizing IL-10 would restore IL-2Rα expression to UV-Mph–activated T cells. However, this is not the case. Studies are underway to determine whether deficient IL-12 production is more important to altered T-cell activation by UV-Mph. In addition to altered cytokine expression, UV-Mph are distinct from LC in their expression of important co-stimulatory molecules. As mentioned above, altered B7 and CD40 signals have been implicated in determining the function of activated T cells. Indeed, UV-Mph are deficient in their expression of B7-1, B7-2, and CD40. Of these, the CD40 deficiency was shown to be critical to altered (IL-2Rα$^-$) T-cell activation [165]. While the inability to respond to IL-2 inherent in the IL-2Rα$^-$ state is significant to the function of UV Mph-activated CD4$^+$ cells, a more direct issue is the cytokine profile of these T cells. A third issue is the growth factors that will expand these cells to a large enough population to have biological significance. Indeed, in human allogeneic primary cultures, UV-Mph but not LC induce IL-4–and IL-5–producing T cells. Upon secondary challenge with epidermal cells from the original skin donor, the percentage of these IL-4–and IL-5–producing cells preferentially expands [173]. Furthermore, T-cell growth induced by LC is dependent on IL-2, IL-7, and IL-15. In contrast, T-cell growth induced by UV-Mph is dependent on IL-4, but independent of IL-2 (as expected with deficient IL-2Rα expression), IL-7 and IL-15.

UV-Mph are thus well equipped to induce tolerance to otherwise sensitizing immunogens. They express high levels of IL-10 and low levels of IL-12. They are importantly deficient in their ability to express CD40. Lastly, the T cells secrete IL-4 and IL-5, type 2 cytokines associated with downregulation of cell mediated immune responses such as CHS and DTH. As such, UV-Mph are potentially important not only as a model system to understand the effects of UV on health and disease to give insight into the regulatory networks leading to sensitization and tolerance, but they also may prove useful as agents to downregulate allergic skin responses.

In addition to alterations in cytokine milieu and APC populations, photoproducts can also be involved in the induction of cell-mediated immunosuppression [174–179].

These photoproducts are derived from photoreceptors or chromophores, such as DNA and urocanic acid, which is present in high concentration in stratum corneum. UVB-induced DNA damage, in the form of cyclobutyl pyrimidine dimers, plays an important role in UV-induced suppression of cell-mediated immune responses. If the excision repair enzyme T4 endonuclease V is used to remove DNA damage from UV-irradiated mouse skin in vivo, UV-induced suppression of CHS and DTH responses to antigens applied or injected at a distant site is prevented [175]. The liposome-encapsulated HindIII added to cells causes double strand breaks in DNA and induces IL-10 and TNF-$\alpha$ production in a murine keratinocyte line in vitro [176]. However, the induction of tolerance and suppressor lymphocytes in response to contact sensitization are not mimicked by HindIII delivered by liposomes, suggesting that direct DNA damage alone may be insufficient for the generation of suppressor cells and tolerance. The administration of TNF-$\alpha$ plus hapten [180] or IL-10 plus antigen have likewise been unsuccessful to induce suppressor cells [174]. These imply that some additional, unidentified factors produced in response to the DNA damage–independent effects of UVB are required.

Urocanic acid (UCA) is produced by the deamination of histidine by histidase and is present in the stratum corneum of the skin as *trans*-UCA. After UVB or UVA irradiation, *trans*-UCA is converted to its photo-isomer, *cis*-UCA, which is more soluble and stable. Although the immunosuppressive properties of *cis*-UCA are well documented, the mechanisms of this suppression are still unclear because there is considerable variation in the experimental systems examined. The effects of UCA have mostly been studied during the induction phase. Although LC are the target and keratinocyte and/or LC TNF-$\alpha$ production is involved [181], pretreatment with the monoclonal antibody that reacts with *cis*-UCA abrogates the reduction in epidermal LC numbers but has no effect on the accumulation of dendritic cells in lymph nodes draining the site of UV exposure. This implies that UCA involvement in CHS is more complicated in terms of LC. Moreover, anti-*cis*-UCA antibodies do not prevent UV-induced suppression of CHS to sensitizer (e.g., oxazolone) but do restore UV-suppressed DTH to the clinically relevant herpes simplex virus [182]. Thus, it seems likely that UVB radiation–induced formation of *cis*-UCA in vivo is critical for systemically suppressing the DTH response but not CHS responses and its effect, perhaps indirectly is via IL-10 [177]. Another observation is that *cis*-UCA can synergize with histamine to increase prostaglandin E production by human keratinocytes [178] and peripheral blood monocytes. In turn, prostaglandin E activates suppressor T lymphocytes [183] and decreases IL-2 and IFN-$\gamma$ production by type 1 cells [184], thus, resulting in immunosuppression.

$\alpha$-Melanocyte–stimulating hormone is a neuroimmunomodulating peptide, recently shown to be synthesized and released by keratinocytes after UV, that significantly stimulates infiltrating monocytes of the skin to release IL-10 [85]. This result implies that there is another factor derived form keratinocytes that induces IL-10 by monocytes and contributes to immunosuppression.

In addition to positively regulating development, receptor-ligand interactions can also selectively initiate cell death and downregulate lymphocyte-mediated immune responses. FasL/Fas interaction is an example. Fas can be expressed on a variety of both lymphoid and nonlymphoid cells, such as T and B lymphocytes, NK cells, monocytes/macrophages, and fibroblasts. Not every cell that expresses Fas receptor is susceptible to Fas-induced apoptosis. Resting lymphocytes need to be stimulated to become sensitive to Fas-induced cell death. FasL can also be expressed on T cells, NK cells, and macrophages, but at lower levels than the expression of Fas. Resting human lymphocytes do not constitutively express FasL until they are stimulated by cytokine or through the T-cell receptor [122]. Recently, it has been found that Fas-deficient 1pr mice and FasL-deficient gld mice do not develop UV-induced tolerance. It has been shown that hapten-specific T-suppressor cells exist in the tolerance mice. T cells from UV-tolerized mice enhance Fas expression on dendritic cells and enhance dendritic cells death in a Fas/FasL-dependent manner, indicating that UV-induced T-suppressor cells may induce the death of APC via the Fas pathway [186]. The addition of IL-12, which can break established tolerance in vivo, prevents dendritic cell death, suggesting that IL-12 may break established tolerance via the prevention of dendritic cell death induced by T suppressor cells [186]. Summary of UV on cell-mediated immuno-alteration is shown in Figure 4.

In summary, allergic skin diseases such as urticaria, atopic dermatitis, and contact dermatitis are very common disorders in all human populations. The antigen-presenting cells and other immunocompetent cells, with the primary and secondary cytokines they produce, are integrated in a complex network that provides the mechanisms of allergic skin responses. The major professional antigen-presenting cells, such as dendritic Langerhans cells and monocytic/macrophagic cell–obtaining signals, direct and modulate T lymphocytes, which function as type 1 and type 2 subsets and reciprocally regulate as a Yin-Yang balance in the body (Fig. 5). Once imbalance of this system occurs, disorders correspondingly result as T-cell type 2–predominant, IgE-mediated atopic dermatitis and allergic urticaria and T cell type 1–predominant, allergic contact dermatitis. Current standards of therapy, such as corticosteroids, are aimed at blunting these undesirable responses. Future therapies more likely will be aimed at restoring appropriate balance through enhancing regulatory mechanisms.

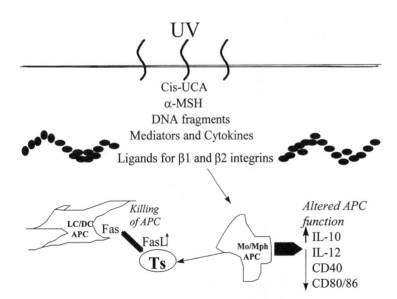

**Figure 4** Summary of UV on cell-mediated immuno-alteration. APC = Antigen-presenting cell; DC = dendritic cell; FasL = Fas ligand; LC = Langerhans cell; Mo/Mph = monocyte/macrophage; MSH = melanocyte-stimulating hormone; Ts = T-suppressor cell; UCA = urocanic acid.

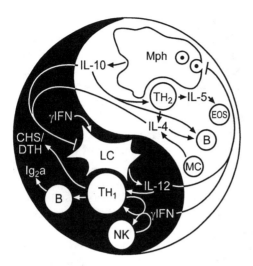

**Figure 5** Reciprocal regulation of antigen-presenting cells with T-cell subsets in a shape of Yin-Yang doctrine. (→) Stimulate; (⊣) inhibit. B = B cell; CHS = contact hypersensitivity; DTH = delayed-type hypersensitivity; eos = eosinophil; IFN = interferon; Ig = immunoglobulin; IL = interleukin; LC = Langerhans cell; MC = mast cell; Mph = macrophage; NK = natural killer cell; TH1 = T helper cell type 1; TH2 = T helper cell type 2.

## REFERENCES

1.  Nickoloff BJ, Turka LA. Immunological functions of non-professional antigen-presenting cells: new insights from studies of T-cell interactions with keratinocytes. Immunol Today 1994; 15:464–469.
2.  Takigawa MK, Iwatsuki M, Yamada H, Okamoto H, Imamura S. The Langerhans cell granule is an adsorptive endocytic organelle. J Invest Dermatol 1985; 85:12–15.
3.  Caux C, Liu Y-J, Banchereau J. Recent advances in the study of dendritic cells and follicular dendritic cells. Immunol Today 1995; 16:2–4.
4.  Bhardwaj N, Friedman SM, Cole BC, Nisanian AJ. Dendritic cells are potent antigen-presenting cells for microbial superantigens. J Exp Med 1992; 175:267–273.
5.  Streilein JW, Grammer S. In vitro evidence that antigen processing and presentation by Langerhans cells are spatially and temporally dissociated. FASEB J 1989; 312a.
6.  Romani N, Lenz A, Glassel H, Schuler G. Cultured human Langerhans cells resemble lymphoid dendritic cells in phenotype and function. J Invest Dermatol 1989; 93:600–609.
7.  Aiba S, Katz SI. Phenotypic and functional characteristics of in vivo-activated Langerhans cells. J Immunol 1990; 145:2791–2796.
8.  Schuler G, Steinman RM. Murine epidermal Langerhans cells mature into potent immunostimulatory dendritic cells in vitro. J Exp Med 1985; 161:526–546.
9.  Tse Y, Cooper KD. Cutaneous dermal Ia+ cells are capable of initiating delayed type hypersensitivity responses. J Invest Dermatol 1990; 94:267–272.
10. Meunier L, Gonzalez-Ramos A, Cooper KD. Heterogeneous populations of class II MHC+ cells in human dermal cell suspensions. Identification of a small subset responsible for potent dermal antigen-presenting cell activity with features analogous to Langerhans cells. J Immunol 1993; 151:4067–4080.

11. Duraiswamy N, Tse Y, Hammerberg C, Kang S, Cooper KD. Distinction of class II MHC+ Langerhans cell-like interstitial dendritic antigen-presenting cells in murine dermis from dermal macrophages. J Invest Dermatol 1994; 103:678–683.

12. Wang B, Rieger A, Kilgus O, Ochiai K, Maurer D, Fodinger D, Kinet JP, and Stingl G. Epidermal Langerhans cells from normal human skin bind monomeric IgE via Fc epsilon RI. J Exp Med 1992; 175:1353–1365.

13. Maurer D, Fiebiger E, Reininger B, Wolff-Winiski B, Jouvin M-H, Kilgus O, Kinet JP, Stingl G. Expression of functional high affinity immunoglobulin E receptors (Fc epsilon RI) on monocytes of atopic individuals. J Exp Med 1994; 179:745–750.

14. Bieber T. FcÎRI-expressing antigen-presenting cells: new players in the atopic game. J Immunol 1997; 159:599–605.

15. Shibaki A, Ohkawara A, Shimada S, Ra C, Aiba S, Cooper KD. Expression, but lack of calcium mobilization by high-affinity IgE Fc epsilon receptor I on human epidermal and dermal Langerhans cells. Exp Dermatol 1996; 5:272–278.

16. Bieber T, Delespesse G. Gamma-interferon promotes the release of IgE-binding factors (soluble CD23) by human epidermal Langerhans cells. J Invest Dermatol 1991; 97:600–603.

17. Tang A, Amagai M, Granger LG. Stanley JR, Udey MC. Adhesion of epidermal Langerhans cells to keratinocytes mediated by E-cadherin. Nature 1993; 361:82–85.

18. Le Varlet B, Dezutter-Dambuyant C, Staquet MJ, P. Delorme P, Schmitt D. Human epidermal Langerhans cells express integrins of the beta 1 subfamily. J Invest Dermatol 1991; 96:518–522.

19. Staquet M-J, Kobayashi Y, Dezutter-Dambuyant C, Schmitt D. Role of specific successive contact between extracellular matrix proteins and epidermal Langerhans cells in the control of their directed migration. Eur J Cell Biol 1995; 66:342–348.

20. Enk AH, Angeloni VL, Udey MC, Katz SI. An essential role for Langerhans cell-derived IL-1 beta in the initiation of primary immune responses in skin. J Immunol 1993; 150:3698–3704.

21. Kang K, Kubin M, Cooper KD, Lessin SR, Trinchieri G, Rook AH. IL-12 synthesis by human Langerhans cells. J Immunol 1996; 156:1402–1407.

22. Geissman F, Prost C, Monnet J-P, Dy M, Brousse N, Hermine D. Transforming growth factor b1, in the presence of granulocyte/macrophage colony-stimulating factor and interleukin 4, induces differentiation of human peripheral blood monocytes into dendritic Langerhans cells. J Exp Med 1998; 187:961–966.

23. Piguet PF, Grau GE, Hauser C, Vassalli P. Tumor necrosis factor is a critical mediator in hapten-induced irritant and contact hypersensitivity reactions. J Exp Med 1991; 173:673–679.

24. Cumberbatch M, Kimber I. Dermal tumor necrosis factor-alpha induces dendritic cell migration to draining lymph nodes, and possibly provides one stimulus for Langerhans' cell migration. Immunology 1992; 75:257–263.

25. Cumberbatch M, Kimber I. Tumour necrosis factor-alpha is required for accumulation of dendritic cells in draining lymph nodes and for optimal contact sensitization. Immunology 1995; 84:31.

26. Trede NS, Morio T, Scholl PR, Geha RS, Chatila T. Early activation events induced by the staphylococcal superantigen toxic shock syndrome toxin-1 in human peripheral blood monocytes. Clin Immunol Immunopathol 1994; 70:137–144.

27. Yokota A, Kikutani H, Tanaka T, Sato R, Barsumian EL, Suemura M, Kishimoto T. Two species of human FcÎ receptor II (FcÎRII/CD23): tissue specific and IL-4-specific regulation of gene expression. Cell 1988; 55:611–618.

28. Olikowsky T, Wang Z-Q, Dudhane A, Horowitz H, Conti B, Hoffmann MK. Two distinct pathways of human macrophage differentiation are mediated by interferon-gamma and interleukin-10. Immunology 1997; 91:104–108.

29. Gaspari AA, Sempowski GD, Chess P, Gish J, Phipps RP. Human epidermal keratinocytes

are induced to secrete interleukin-6 and co-stimulate T lymphocyte proliferation by a CD40-dependent mechanism. Eur J Immunol 1996; 26:1371–1377.

30.  Tokura Y, Yagi J, O'Malley M, Lewis JM, Takigawa M, Edelson RL, Tigelaar RE. Superantigenic staphylococcal exotoxins induce T-cell proliferation in the presence of Langerhans cells or class II-bearing keratinocytes and stimulate keratinocytes to produce T-cell-activating cytokines. J Invest Dermatol 1994; 102:31–38.

31.  Nickoloff BJ, Mitra RS, Green J, Zheng X-G, Shimizu Y, Thompson C, Turka LA. Accessory cell function of keratinocytes for superantigens. Dependence on lymphocyte function-associated antigen-1/intercellular adhesion molecule-1 interaction. J Immunol 1993; 150:2148–2159.

32.  Strange P, Skov L, Baadsgaard O. Interferon gamma-treated keratinocytes activate T cells in the presence of superantigens: involvement of major histocompatibility complex class II molecules. J Invest Dermatol 1994; 102:150–154.

33.  Goodman RE, Nestle F, Naidu YM, Green JM, Thompson CB, Nickoloff BJ, Turka LA. Keratinocyte-derived T cell costimulation induces preferential production of IL-2 and IL-4 but not IFN-gamma. J Immunol 1994; 152:5189–5198.

34.  Punnonen J, Yssel H, De Vries JE. The relative contribution of IL-4 and IL-13 to human IgE synthesis induced by activated CD4+ or CD8+ T cells. J Allergy Clin Immunol 1997; 100:792–801.

35.  Gerber BO, Zanni MP, Uguccioni M, Loetscher M, Mackay CR, Pichler WJ, Yawalkar N, Baggiolini M, Moser B. Functional expression of the eotaxin receptor CCR3 in T lymphocytes co-localizing with eosinophils. Curr Biol 1997; 7:836–843.

36.  Wierenga EA, Snoek M, De Groot C, Chretien I, Bos JD, Jansen HM, Kapsenberg L. Evidence for compartmentalization of functional subsets of CD4+ T lymphocytes in atopic patients. J Immunol 144:4651–4656.

37.  Moore KW, O'Garra A, de Waal Malefyt R, Vieira P, Mosmann TR. Interleukin-10. Annu Rev Immunol 1993; 11:165–190.

38.  Romagnani S. The Th1/Th2 paradigm. Immunol Today 1997; 18:263–266.

39.  Mosmann TR, Sad S. The expanding universe of T-cell subsets: Th1, Th2 and more. Immunol Today 1996; 17:138–146.

40.  Kemeny DM, Noble A, Holmes BJ, Diaz-Sanchez D. Immune regulation: a new role for the CD8+ T cell. Immunol Today 1994; 15:107–110.

41.  Bloom BR, Salgame P, Diamond B. Revisiting and revising suppressor T cells. Immunol Today 1992; 13:131–136.

42.  Umetsu DT, DeKruyff RH. Th1 and Th2 CD4+ cells in the pathogenesis of allergic diseases. Pathogen Allerg Dis 1997; 215:11–20.

43.  Lagier B, Lebel B, Bousquet J, Pene J. Different modulation by histamine of IL-4 and interferon-gamma (IFN-gamma) release according to the phenotype of human Th0, Th1 and Th2 clones. Clin Exp Immunol 1997; 108:545–551.

44.  Snapper CM, McIntyre TM, Mandler R, Pecanha LM, Finkelman FD, Lees A, Mond JJ. Induction of IgG3 secretion by interferon gamma: a model for T cell-independent class switching in response to T cell-independent type 2 antigens. J Exp Med 1992; 175:1367–1371.

45.  Jabara HH, Fu SM, Geha RS, Vercelli D. CD40 and IgE: synergism between anti-CD40 monoclonal antibody and Interleukin 4 in the induction of IgE synthesis by highly purified human B cells. J Exp Med 1990; 172:1861–1864.

46.  Defrance T, Vanbervliet B, Briere F, Durand I, Rousset F, Banchereau J. Interleukin 10 and transforming growth factor beta cooperate to induce anti-CD40-activated naive human B cells to secrete immunoglobulin A. J Exp Med 1992; 175:671–682.

47.  Kos FJ, Engleman EG. Immune regulation: a critical link between NK cells and CTLs. Immunol Today 1996; 17:174–176.

48.   Yoshimoto T, Bendelac A, Watson C, Hu-Li J, Paul WE. Role of NK1.1$^+$ T cells in a $T_H2$ response and in immunoglobulin E production. Science 1995; 270:1845–1847.
49.   Brinkmann V, Kristofic C. Massive production of Th2 cytokines by human CD4$^+$ effector T cells transiently expressing the natural killer cell marker CD57/HNK1. Immunology 1997; 91:541–547.
50.   Kameyoshi Y, Dorschner A, Mallet AI, Christophers E, Schroder JM. Cytokine RANTES released by thrombin-stimulated platelets is a potent attractant for human eosinophils. J Exp Med 1992; 176:587–592.
51.   Teixeira MM, Wells TN, Lukacs NW, Proudfoot AE, Kunkel SL, Williams TJ, Hellewell PG. Chemokine-induced eosinophil recruitment. Evidence of a role for endogenous eotaxin in an in vivo allergy model in mouse skin. J Clin Invest 1997; 100:1657–1666.
52.   Kaneko M, Horie S, Kato M, Gleich GJ, Kita H. A crucial role for beta2 integrin in the activation of eosinophils stimulated by IgG. J Immunol 1995; 155:2631–2641.
53.   Hansel TT, DeVries IJ, Carballido JM, Braun RK, Carballido-Perrig N, Rihs S, Blaser K, Walker C. Induction and function of eosinophil intercellular adhesion molecule-1 and HLA-DR. J Immunol 1992; 149:2130–2136.
54.   Valent P, Schmidt G, Besemer J, Mayer P, Zenke G, Liehl E, Hinterberger W, Lechner K, Mauer D, Bettelheim P. Interleukin-3 is a differentiation factor for human basophils. Blood 1989; 73:1763–1769.
55.   Valent P, Spanblochl E, Sperr WR, Sillaber C, Zsebo KM, Agis H, Strobl H, Geissler K, Bettelheim P, Lechner K. Induction of differentiation of human mast cells from bone marrow and peripheral blood mononuclear cells by recombinant human stem cell factor/kit-ligand in long-term culture. Blood 1992; 80:2237–2245.
56.   Bradding P, Feather IH, Howarth PH, Mueller R, Roberts JA, Britten K, Bews JP, Hunt TC, Okayama Y, Heusser CH, et al. Interleukin 4 is localized to and released by human mast cells. J Exp Med 1992; 176:1381–1386.
57.   Brunner T, Heusser CH, Dahinden CA. Human peripheral blood basophils primed by interleukin 3 (IL-3) produce IL-4 in response to immunoglobulin E receptor stimulation. J Exp Med 1993; 177:605–611.
58.   Gauchat J-F, Henchoz S, Mazzei G, Aubry J-P, Brunner T, Blasey H, Life P, Talabot D, Flores-Romo L, Thompson J, Kishi K, Butterfield J, Dahinden C, Bonnefoy J-Y. Induction of human IgE synthesis in B cells by mast cells and basophils. Nature 1998; 365: 340–343.
59.   Bochner BS, Luscinskas FW, Gimbrone MA, Jr., Newman W, Sterbinsky SA, Derse-Anthony CP, Klunk D, Schleimer RP. Adhesion of human basophils, eosinophils, and neutrophils to interleukin-1-activated human vascular endothelial cells: contributions of endothelial cell adhesion molecules. J Exp Med 1991; 173:1553–1557.
60.   Yamada H, Hirai K, Miyamasu M, Iikura M, Misaki Y, Shoji S, Takaishi T, Kasahara T, Morita Y, Ito K. Eotaxin is a potent chemotaxin for human basophils. Biochem Biophys Res Commun 1997; 231:365–368.
61.   Renz H. The central role of T-cells in allergic sensitization and IgE regulation. Exp Dermatol 1995; 4:173–182.
62.   Hilton J, Dearman RJ, Sattar N, Basketter DA, Kimber I. Characteristics of antibody responses induced in mice by protein allergens. Food Chem Toxicol 1997; 35:1209–1218.
63.   Wang L-F, Lin J-Y, Hsieh K-H, Lin R-H. Epicutaneous exposure of protein antigen induces a predominant Th2-like response with high IgE production in mice. J Immunol 1996; 156: 4079–4082.
64.   Dearman RJ, Smith S, Basketter DA, Kimber I. Classification of chemical allergens according to cytokine secretion profiles of murine lymph node cells. J Appl Toxicol 1997; 17:53–62.
65.   Ryan CA, Dearman RJ, Kimber I, Gerberick F. Inducible interleukin 4 (IL-4) production and mRNA expression following exposure of mice to chemical allergens. Toxicol Lett 1998; 94:1–11.

66. Vento KL, Dearman RJ, Kimber I, Basketter DA, Coleman JW. Selectivity of IgE responses, mast cell sensitization, and cytokine expression in the immune response of brown Norway rats to chemical allergens. Cell Immunol 1996; 172:246–253.

67. Kimber I, Hilton J, Dearman RJ, Gerberick GF, Ryan CA, Basketter DA, Lea L, House RV, Ladics GS, Loveless SE, Hastings KL. Assessment of the skin sensitization potential of topical medicaments using the local lymph node assay: an interlaboratory evaluation. J Toxicol Environ Health 1998; 53:563–579.

68. Marcelletti JF, Katz DH. Elicitation of antigen-induced primary and secondary murine Ige antibody responses in vitro. Cell Immunol 1991; 135:471–489.

69. Marcelletti JF, Katz DH. Antigen concentration determines helper T cell subset participation in IgE antibody responses. Cell Immunol 1992; 143:403–419.

70. Cumberbatch M, Gould SJ, Peters SW, Basketter DA, Dearman RJ, Kimber I. Langerhans cells, antigen presentation, and the diversity of responses to chemical allergens. J Invest Dermatol 1992; 99:107S–108S.

71. Simon JC, Cruz PD, Jr., Bergstresser PR, Tigelaar RE. Low dose ultraviolet B-irradiated Langerhans cells preferentially activate CD4+ cells of the T helper 2 subset. J Immunol 1990; 145:2087–2091.

72. El-Ghorr AA, Norval M, Lappin MB, Crosby JC. The effect of chronic low-dose UVB radiation on Langerhans cells, sunburn cells, urocanic acid isomers, contact hypersensitivity and serum immunoglobulins in mice. Photochem Photobiol 1995; 62:326–332.

73. Kondo H, Ichikawa Y, Imokawa G. Percutaneous sensitization with allergens through barrier-disrupted skin elicits a Th2-dominant cytokine response. Eur J Immunol 1998; 28:769–779.

74. Mudde GC, Reischl IG, Corvaia N, Hren A, Poellabauerk E-M. Antigen presentation in allergic sensitization. Immunol Cell Biol 1996; 74:167–173.

75. Guillet G, Guillet M-H. Natural history of sensitizations in atopic dermatitis. Arch Dermatol 1992; 128:187–192.

76. Wollenberg A, Kraft S, Hanau D, Bieber T. Immunomorphological and ultrastructural characterization of Langerhans cells and a novel, inflammatory dendritic epidermal cell (IDEC) population in lesional skin of atopic eczema. J Invest Dermatol 1996; 106:446–453.

77. Shibaki A, Meunier L, Ra C, Shimada S, Ohkawara A, Cooper KD. Differential responsiveness of Langerhans cell subsets of varying phenotypic states in normal human epidermis. J Invest Dermatol 1995; 104:42–46.

78. Mudde GG, Van Reijsen FC, Bruijnzeel-Koomen CAFM. IgE-positive Langerhans cells and TH2 allergen-specific T cells in atopic dermatitis. J Invest Dermatol 1992; 99:103S

79. Thepen T, Langeveld-Wildschut EG, Bihari IC, van Wichen DF, Van Reijsen FC, Mudde GC, Bruijnzeel-Koomen CA. Biphasic response against aeroallergen in atopic dermatis showing a switch from an initial TH2 response to a TH1 response in situ: an immunocytochemical study. J Allergy Clin Immunol 1996; 97:828–837.

80. Warpinski JR, Folgert J, Cohen M, Bush RK. Allergic reaction to latex: a risk factor for unsuspected anaphylaxis. Allergy Proc 1991; 12:95–102.

81. Atkinson TP, Kaliner MA. Anaphylaxis. Med Clin North Am 1992; 76:841–855.

82. Antico A. Oral allergy syndrome induced by chestnut. Ann Allergy Asthma Immunol 1996; 76:37–40.

83. Charlesworth EN. The role of basophils and mast cells in acute and late reactions in the skin. Allergy 1997; 52:31–43.

84. Marone G, Casolaro V, Patella V, Florio G, Triggiani M. Molecular and cellular biology of mast cells and basophils. Int. Arch. Allergy Immunol 1997; 114:207–217.

85. Metcalfe DD, Baram D, Mekori YA. Mast cells. Physiol Rev 1997; 77:1033–1079.

86. Carlos TM, Harlan JM. Leukocyte-endothelial adhesion molecules. Blood 1994; 84:2068–2101.

87. Muller KM, Jaunin F, Masouye I, Saurat JH, Hauser C. Th2 cells mediate IL-4-dependent local tissue inflammation. J Immunol 1993; 150:5576–5584.

88. Grabbe S, Schwarz T. Immunoregulatory mechanisms involved in elicitation of allergic contact hypersensitivity. Immunol Today 1998; 19:37–44.

89. Schwarz A, Grabbe S, Riemann H, Aragane Y, Simon M, Manon S, Andrade S, Luger TA, Zlotnik A, Schwarz T. In vivo effects of interleukin-10 on contact hypersensitivity and delayed-type hypersensitivity reactions. J Invest Dermatol 1994; 103:211–216.

90. Enk AH, Katz SI. Early molecular events in the induction phase of contact sensitivity. Proc Natl Acad Sci USA 1992; 89:1398–1402.

91. Muller G, Knop J, Enk AH. Is cytokine expression responsible for differences between allergens and irritants? Am J Contact Dermat 1996; 7:177–184.

92. Kimber I, Dearman J, Cumberbatch M. Epidermal cytokines and the induction of allergic and non-allergic contact dermatitis. Arch Toxicol Suppl 1997; 19:228–238.

93. Cuberbatch M, Dearman RJ, Kimber I. Langerhans cells require signals from both tumour necrosis factor-alpha and interleukin-1 beta for migration. Immunology 1997; 92:388–395.

94. Blauvelt A, Asada H, Klaus-Kovtun V, Altman DJ, Lucey DR, Katz SI. Interleukin-15 mRNA is expressed by human keratinocytes, Langerhans cells, and blood-derived dendritic cells and is downregulated by ultraviolet B radiation. J Invest Dermatol 1996; 22-202X:1047.

95. Xu H, DiIulio, NA, Fairchild RI. T cell populations primed by hapten sensitization in contact sensitivity are distinguished by polarized patterns of cytokine production: interferon gamma-producing (Tc1) effector CD8$^+$ T cells and interleukin (II) 4/Il-10-producing (Th2) negative regulatory CD4$^+$ T cells. J Exp Med 1996; 183:1001–1012.

96. Krasteva M, Kehren J, Horand F, Akiba H, Choquet G, Ducluzeau MT, Tedone R, Garrigue JL, Kaiserlian D, Nicolas JF. Dual role of dendritic cells in the induction and down-regulation of antigen-specific cutaneous inflammation. J Immunol 1998; 160:1181–1190.

97. Bouloc A, Cavani A, Katz SI. Contact hypersensitivity in MHC class II-deficient mice depends on CD8 T lymphocytes primed by immunostimulating Langerhans cells. J Invest Dermatol 1998; 111:44–49.

98. Tang A, Judge TA, Nickoloff BJ, Turka LA. Suppression of murine allergic contact dermatitis by CTLA41g. J Immunol 1996; 157:117–125.

99. Steinbrink K, Sorg C, Macher E. Low zone tolerance to contact allergens in mice. A functional role for CD8$^+$Tc2 responsible for DLN transfer of tolerance. J Exp Med 1996; 183:759–768.

100. Van Reijsen FC, Wijburg OLC, Gebhardt M, Van Ieperen-Van Dijk AG, Betz S, Poellabauer EM, Thepen T, Bruijnzeel-Koomen CAFM, Mudde GC. Different growth factor requirements for human Th2 cells may reflect in vivo induced anergy. Clin Exp Immunol 1994; 98:151–157.

101. Ma J, Wang J-H, Guo Y-J, Sy M-S, Bigby M. In vivo treatment with anti-ICAM-1 and anti-LFA-1 antibodies inhibits contact sensitization-induced migration of epidermal Langerhans cells to regional lymph nodes. Cell Immunol 1994; 158:389–399.

102. Xu H, Heeger PS, Fairchild RL. Distinct roles for B7-1 and B7-2 determinants during priming of effector CD8+ Tc1 and regulatory CD4+ Th2 cells for contact hypersensitivity. J Immunol 1997; 159:4217–4226.

103. Nuriya S, Yagita H, Okumura K, Azuma M. The differential role of CD86 and CD80 co-stimulatory molecules in the induction and the effector phases of contact hypersensitivity. Int Immunol 1996; 8:917–926.

104. Tang A, Judge TA, Turka LA. Blockade of CD40-CD40 ligand pathway induces tolerance in murine contact hypersensitivity. Eur J Immunol 1997; 27:3143–3150.

105. Kato T, Hakamada R, Yamane H, Nariuchi H. Induction of IL-12 p40 messenger RNA expression and IL-12 production of macrophages via CD40-CD40 ligand interaction. J Immunol 1996; 156:3932–3938.

106. Cella M, Scheidegger D, Palmer-Lehmann K, Lane P, Lanzavecchia A, Alber G. Ligation of CD40 on dendritic cells triggers production of high levels of interleukin-12 and enhances T cell stimulatory capacity: T-T help via APC activation. J Exp Med 1996; 184:747–752.

107. Mackay CR, Marston WL, Dudler L, Spertini O, Tedder TF, Hein WR. Tissue-specific migration pathways by phenotypically distinct subpopulations of memory T cells. Eur J Immunol 1992; 22:887–895.

108. Picker LJ, Treer JR, Ferguson-Darnell B, Collins PA, Bergstresser PR, Terstappen LWMM. Control of lymphocyte recirculation in man. II. Differential regulation of the cutaneous lymphocyte-associated antigen, a tissue-selective homing receptor for skin-homing T cells. J Immunol 1993; 150:1122–1136.

109. Grabbe S, Steinbrink K, Steinert M, Luger TA, Schwarz T. Removal of the majority of epidermal Langerhans cells by topical or systemic steroid application enhances the effector phase of murine contact hypersensitivity. J Immunol 1995; 155:4207–4217.

110. Pichler WJ, Wyss-Coray T. T cells as antigen-presenting cells. Immunol Today 1994; 15: 312–315.

111. Takashima A, Bergstresser PR. Impact of UVB radiation on the epidermal cytokine network. Photochem Photobiol 1996; 63:397–400.

112. McLelland J, Shuster S, Matthews JN. 'Irritants' increase the response to an allergen in allergic contact dermatitis. Arch Dermatol 1991; 127:1016–1019.

113. Kitigaki H, Ono N, Hayakawa K, Kitazawa T, Watanabe K, Shiohara T. Repeated elicitation of contact hypersensitivity induces a shift in cutaneous cytokine milieu from a T helper cell type 1 to a T helper cell type 2 profile. J Immunol 1997; 159:2484–2491.

114. Kondo S, Kono T, Brown WR, Pastore S, McKenzie RC, Sauder DN. Lymphocyte function-associated antigen-1 is required for maximum elicitation of allergic contact dermatitis. Br J Dermatol 1994; 131:354–359.

115. Webb DR, Kraig E, Derens BH. Suppressor cells and immunity. Chem Immunol 1994; 58: 146–192.

116. Coutelier JP. Enhancement of IgG production elicited in mice by treatment with anti-CD8 antibody. Eur J Immunol 1991; 21:2617–2620.

117. Salgame P, Modlin R, Bloom BR. On the mechanism of human T cell suppression. Int Immunol 1989; 1:121–129.

118. Dorf ME, Kuchroo VK, Collins M. Suppressor T cells: some answers but more questions. Immunol Today 1992; 13:241–243.

119. Baadsgaard O, Fox DA, Cooper KD. Human epidermal cells from ultraviolet light-exposed skin preferentially activate autoreactive CD4+2H4+ suppressor-inducer lymphocytes and CD8+ suppressor/cytotoxic lymphocytes. J Immunol 1988; 140:1738–1744.

120. Baadsgaard O, Salvo B, Mannie A, Dass B, Fox DA, Cooper KD. In vivo ultraviolet-exposed human epidermal cells activate T suppressor cell pathways that involve CD4+CD45RA+ suppressor-inducer T cells. J Immunol 1990; 145:2854–2861.

121. Schad VC. T cell tolerance; models for clinical application to allergy and autoimmunity. Chem Immunol 1994; 58:193–205.

122. Eischen CM, Leibson PJ. The Fas pathway in apoptosis. Adv Pharmacol 1997; 41:107–132.

123. Ludewig B, Graf D, Gelderblom HR, Becker Y, Kroczek RA, Pauli G. Spontaneous apoptosis of dendritic cells is efficiently inhibited by TRAP (CD40-ligand) and TNF-alpha, but strongly enhanced by interleukin-10. Eur J Immunol 1995; 25:1943–1950.

124. Secrist H, DeKruyff RH, Umetsu DT. Interleukin 4 production by CD4+ T cells from allergic individuals is modulated by antigen concentration and antigen-presenting cell type. J Exp Med 1995; 181:1081–1089.

125. Secrist H, Chelen CJ, Wen Y, Marshall JD, Umetsu DT. Allergen immunotherapy decreases interleukin 4 production in CD4+ T cells from allergic individuals. J Exp Med 1993; 178: 2123–2130.

126. Wallner BP, Gefter ML. Immunotherapy with T-cell-reactive peptides derived from allergens. Allergy 1994; 49:302–308.

127. Wallner BP, Gefter ML. Peptide therapy for treatment of allergic diseases. Clin Immunol Immunopathol 1996; 80:105–109.

128. Gavett SH, O'Hearn DJ, Li X, Huang SK, Finkelman FD, Wills-Karp M. Interleukin 12 inhibits antigen-indicued airway hyperresponsiveness, inflammation, and Th2 cytokine expression in mice. J Exp Med 1995; 182:1527–1536.

129. Rogge L, Barberis-Maino L, Biffi M, Passini N, Presky DH, Gubler U, Sinigaglia F. Selective expression of an interleukin-12 receptor component by human T helper 1 cells. J Exp Med 1997; 185:825–842.

130. Szabo SJ, Dighe AS, Gubler U, Murphy KM. Regulation of the interleukin (IL)-12Rb2 subunit expression in developing T helper 1 (Th1) and Th2 cells. J Exp Med 1997; 185:817–824.

131. Kaempfer R. Regulation of the human interleukin-2/interleukin-2 receptor system: a role for immunosuppression. Proc Soc Exp Biol Med 1994; 206:176–180.

132. Varney VA, Hamid QA, Gaga M, Jacobson SYM, Frew AJ, Kay AB, Durham SR. Influence of grass pollen immunotherapy on cellular infiltration and cytokine mRNA expression during allergen-induced late-phase cutaneous responses. J Clin Invest 1993; 92:644–651.

133. Stevens SR, Shibaki A, Meunier L, Cooper KD. Suppressor T cell-activating macrophages in UV-irradiated human skin induce a novel form of T cell activation characterized by reduced early activation gene IL-2R alpha expression. J Immunol 1995; 155:5601–5607.

134. Snijdewint FG, Kapsenberg ML, Wauben-Penris PJ, Bos JD. Corticosteroids class-dependently inhibit in vitro Th1- and Th2-type cytokine production. Immunopharmacology 1995; 29:93–101.

135. Krouwells FH, van der Heijden JF, Lutter R, van Neerven RJ, Jansen HM. Out TA. Glucocorticosteroids affect functions of airway- and blood-derived human T-cell clones, favoring the Th1 profile through two mechanisms. Am J Respir Cell Mol Biol 1996; 14:388–397.

136. Blotta MH, DeKruyff RH, Umetsu DT. Corticosteroids inhibit IL-12 production in human monocytes and enhance their capacity to induce IL-4 synthesis in CD4[+] lymphocytes. J Immunol 1997; 158:5589–5595.

137. Horio T. Skin disorders that improve by exposure to sunlight. Clin Dermatol 1998; 16:59–65.

138. Cooper KD. Cell-mediated immunosuppressive mechanisms induced by UV radiation. Photochem Photobiol 1996; 63:400–406.

139. Scheibner A, Hollis DE, Murray E, McCarthy WH, Milton GW. Effects of exposure to ultraviolet light on epidermal Langerhans cells and melanocytes in Australians of aboriginal, Asian and Celtic descent. Photodermatology 1987; 4:5–13.

140. Scheibner A, Hollis DE, McCarthy WH, Milton GW. Effects of sunlight exposure on Langerhans cells and melanocytes in human epidermis. Photodermatology 1986; 3:15–25.

141. Czernielewski JM, Masouye I, Pisani A, Ferracin J, Auvolat D, Ortonne JP. Effect of chronic sun exposure on human Langerhans cell densities. Photodermatology 1988; 5:116–120.

142. Noonan FP, Bucana C, Sauder DN, DeFabo EC. Mechanism of systemic immune suppression by UV irradiation in vivo. II. The UV effects on number and morphology of epidermal Langerhans cells and the UV-induced suppression of contact hypersensitivity have different wavelength dependencies. J Immunol 1984; 132:2408–2416.

143. Aberer G, Schuler G, Stingl G, Honigsmann H, Wolff K. Ultraviolet light depletes surface markers of Langerhans cells. J Invest Dermatol 1981; 76:202–210.

144. Aberer W, Schuler G, Stingl G, Honigsmann H, Wolff K. Effects of UV-light on epidermal Langerhans cells (abstr). J Invest Dermatol 1980; 74:458.

145. Krueger GG, Emam M. Biology of Langerhans cells: analysis by experiments to deplete Langerhans cells from human skin. J Invest Dermatol 1984; 82:613–617.

146. Cooper KD, Fox P, Neises G, Katz SI. Effects of ultraviolet radiation on human epidermal cell alloantigen presentation: Initial depression of Langerhans cell-dependent function is followed by the appearance of T6-Dr+ cells that enhance epidermal alloantigen presentation. J Immunol 1985; 134:129–137.

147. Alcalay J, Craig JN, Kripke ML. Alternations in Langerhans cells and Thy-1+ dendritic

epidermal cells in murine epidermis during the evolution of ultraviolet radiation-induced skin cancers. Cancer Res 1989; 49:4591–4596.

148. Toews GB, Bergstresser PR, Streilein JW, Sullivan S. Epidermal Langerhans cell density determines whether contact hypersensitivity or unresponsiveness follows skin painting with DNFB. J Immunol 1980; 124:445–453.

149. Weiss JM, Renkl AC, Denfeld RW, de Roche R, Spitzlei M, Schopf E, Simon JC. Low-dose UVB radiation perturbs the functional expression of B7-1 and B7-2 co-stimulatory molecules on human Langerhans cells. Eur J Immunol 1995; 25:2858–2862.

150. Tang A, Udey MC. Inhibition of epidermal Langerhans cell function by low dose ultraviolet B radiation. Ultraviolet B radiation selectively modulates ICAM-1 (CD54) expression by murine Langerhans cells. J Immunol 1991; 146:3347–3355.

151. Gilliam AC, Kremer IB, Yoshida Y, Stevens SR, Tootell E, Teunissen MBM, Hammerberg C, Cooper KD. The human hair follicle: a reservoir of CD40+ B7-deficient Langerhans cells that repopulate epidermis after UVB exposure. J Invest Dermatol 1998; 110:422–427.

152. Saijo S, Kodari E, Kripke ML, Strickland FM. UVB irradiation decreases the magnitude of the Th1 resonse to hapten but does not increase the Th2 response. Photodermatol Photoimmunol Photomed 1996; 12:145–153.

153. Bieber T, Dannenberg B, Ring J, Braun-Falco O. Keratinocytes in lesional skin of atopic eczema bear HLA-DR, CD1a and IgE molecules. Clin Exp Dermatol 1989; 14:35–39.

154. Hanifin JM. Atopic dermatitis in infants and children. Pediatr Clin North Am 1991; 38:763–789.

155. Cooper KD, Neises GR, Katz SI. Antigen-presenting OKM5+ melanophages appear in human epidermis after ultraviolet radiation. J Invest Dermatol 1986; 86:363–370.

156. Cooper KD, Oberhelman L, Hamilton TA, Baadsgaard O, Terhune M, LeVee G, Anderson T, Koren H. UV exposure reduces immunization rates and promotes tolerance to epicutaneous antigens in humans: relationship to dose, CD1a-DR+ epidermal macrophage induction, and Langerhans cell depletion. Proc Natl Acad Sci USA 1992; 89:8497–8501.

157. Cooper KD, Duraiswamy N, Hammerberg C, Allen E, Kimbrough-Green C, Dillon W, Thomas D. Neutrophils, differentiated macrophages, and monocyte/macrophage antigen presenting cells infiltrate murine epidermis after UV injury. J Invest Dermatol 1993; 101:155–163.

158. Meunier L, Bata-Csorgo Z, Cooper KD. In human dermis, UV induces expansion of a CD36+CD11b+CD1-macrophage subset by infiltration and proliferation; CD1+ Langerhans-like dendritic antigen-presenting cells are concomitantly depleted. J Invest Dermatol 1995; 105:782–788.

159. Kang K, Hammerberg C, Meunier L, Cooper KD. CD11b+macrophages that infiltrate human epidermis after in vivo ultraviolet exposure potently produce IL-10 and represent the major secretory source of epidermal IL-10 protein. J Immunol 1994; 153:5256–5264.

160. Kang K, Gilliam AC, Chen G, Tootell E, Cooper KD. In human skin, UVB initiates early induction of IL-10 over IL-12 preferentially in the expanding dermal monocytic/macrophagic population. J Invest Dermatol 1998; 111:31–38.

161. Morison WL, Bucana C, Kripke ML. Systemic suppression of contact hypersensitivity by UVB radiation is unrelated to the UVB-induced alterations in the morphology and number of Langerhans cells. Immunology 1984; 52:299–306.

162. Shibaki A, Ohkawara A, Cooper KD. Differential extracellular signalling via FcgammaR and FMLP in functionally distinct antigen presenting cell subsets: UV-induced epidermal macrophages vs. Langerhans cells. J Invest Dermatol 1995; 105:383–387.

163. Bhatti L, Sidell N. Transcriptional regulation by retinoic acid of interleukin-2alpha receptors in human B cells. Immunology 1994; 81:273–279.

164. Hammerberg C, Duraiswamy N, Cooper KD. Reversal of immunosuppression inducible through ultraviolet-exposed skin by in vivo anti-CD11b treatment. J Immunol 1996; 157:5254–5261.

165. Kremer IB, Cooper KD, Teunissen MBM, Stevens SR. Low expression of CD40 and B7 on macrophages infiltrating UV-exposed human skin; role in IL-2Rα⁻ T cell activation. Eur J Immunol 1998; 28:1–10.

166. Kremer IB, Hilkens CMU, Sylva-Steenland RMR, Koomen CW, Kapsenberg ML, Bos JD, Teunissen MBM. Reduced IL-12 production by monocytes upon ultraviolet-B irradiation selectively limits activation of T helper-1 cells. J Immunol 1996; 157:1913–1918.

167. Enk AH, Angeloni VL, Udey MC, Katz SI. Inhibition of Langerhans cell antigen-presenting function by IL-10. A role for IL-10 in induction of tolerance. J Immunol 1993; 151:2390–2398.

168. Enk AH, Saloga J, Becker D, Mohamadzadeh M, Knop J. Induction of hapten-specific tolerance by interleukin 10 in vivo. J Exp Med 1994; 179:1397–1402.

169. Schwarz A, Grabbe S, Aragane Y, Sandkuhl K, Riemann H, Luger TA, Kubin M, Trinchieri G, Schwarz T. Interleukin-12 prevents ultraviolet B-induced local immunosuppression and overcomes UVB-induced tolerance. J Invest Dermatol 1996; 106:1187–1191.

170. Riemann H, Schwarz A, Grabbe S, Aragane Y, Luger TA, Wysocka M, Kubin M, Trinchieri G, Schwarz T. Neutralization of IL-12 in vivo prevents induction of contact hypersensitivity and induces hapten-specific tolerance. J. Immunol. 156:1799–1803.

171. Kang K, Yoshida Y, Chen G, Gilliam AC, Hammerberg C, Cooper KD. Ligands for b1 and b2 integrins are induced in ultraviolet-exposed human skin and upregulate monocytic/macrophagic cell IL-10, but downregulate IL-12 production (abstr). J Invest Dermatol 1998; 110:490.

172. Hammerberg C, Katiyar SK, Carroll MC, Cooper KD. Activated complement component 3(C3) is required for UV induction of immunosuppression and antigenic tolerance. J Exp Med 1998; 187:1133–1138.

173. Stevens SR, Tarry-Lehmann M, Cooper KD. Distinct cytokine use and production by T cells after activation by Langerhans cells versus macrophages infiltrating UV-irradiated epidermis (abstr). J Invest Dermatol 1998; 110:490.

174. Vink M, Yarosh D, Kripke M. Chromophore for UV-induced immunosuppression. Photochem Photobiol 1996; 63:383–386.

175. Kripke ML, Cox PA, Alas LG, Yarosh DB. Pyrimidine dimers in DNA initiate systemic immunosuppression in UV-irradiated mice. Proc Natl Acad Sci USA 1992; 89:7516–7520.

176. O'Connor A, Nishigori C, Yarosh D, Alas L, Kibitel J, Burley L, Cox P, Bucana C, Ullrich S, Kripke M. DNA double strand breaks in epidermal cells cause immune suppression in vivo and cytokine production in vitro. J Immunol 1996; 157:271–278.

177. Moodycliffe AM, Bucana CD, Kripke ML, Norval M, Ullrich SE. Differential effects of a monoclonal antibody to *cis*-urocanic acid on the suppression of delayed and contact hypersensitivity following ultraviolet irradiation. J Immunol 1996; 157:2891–2899.

178. Jaksic A, Finlay-Jones JJ, Watson CJ, Spencer LK, Santucci I, Hart PH. Cis-urocanic acid synergizes with histamine for increased PGE(2) production immunosuppression. Photochem Photobiol 1995; 61:303–309.

179. Kurimoto I, Streilein JW. Deleterious effects of cis-urocanic acid and UVB radiation on Langerhans cells and on induction of contact hypersensitivity are mediated by tumor necrosis factor-alpha. J Invest Dermatol 1992; 99:69S–70S.

180. Vermeer M, Streilein JW. Ultraviolet B light-induced alterations in epidermal Langerhans cells are mediated in part by tumor necrosis factor-alpha. Photodermatol Photoimmunol Photomed 1990; 7:258–265.

181. Norval M. Chromophore for UV-induced immunosuppression: urocanic acid. Photochem Photobiol 1996; 63:386–390.

182. El-Ghorr AA, Norval M. A monoclonal antibody to cis-urocanic acid prevents the ultraviolet-induced changes in Langerhans cells and delayed hypersensitivity responses in mice, although not preventing dendritic cell accumulation in lymph nodes draining the site of irradiation and contact hypersensitivity responses. J Invest Dermatol 1995; 105:264–268.

183. Baadsgaard O. In vivo ultraviolet irradiation of human skin results in profound perturbation of the immune system. Relevance to ultraviolet-induced skin cancer. Arch Dermatol 1991; 127:99–109.

184. Phipps RP, Stein SH, Roper RL. A new view of prostaglandin E regulation of the immune response. Immunol Today 1991; 12:349–352.

185. Bhardwaj RS, Schwarz A, Becher E, Mahnke K, Aragane Y, Schwarz T, Luger TA. Pro-opiomelanocortin-derived peptides induce IL-10 production in human monocytes. Immunol 1996; 156:2517–2521.

186. Schwarz A, Grabbe S, Grosse-Heitmeyer K, Roters B, Riemann H, Luger TA, Trinchieri G, Schwarz T. Ultraviolet light-induced immune tolerance is mediated via the Fas/Fas-ligand system. J Immunol 1998; 160:4262–4270.

# 5

## Adhesion Molecules and Their Role in Allergic Skin Diseases

**Bruce S. Bochner and Lisa A. Beck**
*The Johns Hopkins University School of Medicine,*
*Baltimore, Maryland*

## I. INTRODUCTION

Localized inflammatory reactions are complex, highly regulated processes where different patterns of leukocytes accumulate within a tissue site. In the skin, for example, the preferential recruitment of neutrophils during wound healing, eosinophils during an experimental allergic late-phase reaction, or TH1 lymphocytes during classical delayed-type hypersensitivity responses are examples of how tissue-resident and circulating cells cooperate to generate characteristic inflammatory responses. While an extensive list of secreted and cell surface molecules contribute to these recruitment responses, this chapter will focus on those that permit cell-cell and cell-tissue matrix attachment: the cell adhesion molecules. For human cells, this family has now exceeded 35 members, which have been divided into subfamilies (selectins and their carbohydrate-containing counterligands, integrins, immunoglobulin-like structures, cadherins, and others) based on shared structural, molecular, functional, and biochemical characteristics. This chapter will briefly review the key structural and functional characteristics of each cell adhesion molecule subfamily, their respective ligands, and regulation of their surface expression and function. This is followed by a discussion emphasizing the roles played by adhesion molecules in allergic (IgE-dependent) inflammatory states in the skin, predominantly focusing on the endothelial contribution. Because of the extensive nature of the topic, the reader is referred to several recent comprehensive texts and reviews covering various aspects of the field of cell adhesion [1–6], as well as others reviewing the role of adhesion molecules on cells such as Langerhans cells, mast cells, and keratinocytes in skin biology [7–14].

## II. SELECTINS AND THEIR LIGANDS

The selectin gene family consists of three members: E-selectin, L-selectin, and P-selectin [6]. Each carries the designation CD62 followed by the respective first letters CD62E, CD62L, and CD62P. E-selectin (formerly endothelial-leukocyte adhesion molecule-1, or ELAM-1 [15]) is only expressed on activated endothelium. P-selectin (formerly GMP-

140 or PADGEM [16]) exhibits stimulus-dependent expression on platelets and two patterns of expression on endothelial cells, one of which is rapid and transient, while the other is slow and sustained (discussed below). L-selectin (formerly TQ1, LECCAM-1, LECAM-1, Leu-8, or LAM-1 [1,17]) is expressed on leukocytes. While selectins can mediate adhesion under static conditions [18–20], their primary function is that of leukocyte-endothelial tethering and rolling under the shear forces associated with blood flow [21–23]. They allow more rapidly moving cells to slow their velocity and initiate the subsequent steps of firm adhesion mediated via integrins. L-selectin has an additional set of unique functions: it facilitates lymphocyte trafficking to both peripheral and mesenteric lymph nodes [24,25].

Selectins share many structural characteristics (see Fig. 1) [6]. At their N-terminus, each possesses a calcium-dependent (C-type) lectin domain, attached to a smaller segment referred to as the EGF-like domain because of its high level of homology to a domain found in epidermal growth factor. This is the most important portion of the molecule for adhesion [26]. Next comes two to nine globular domains with homology to sequences found in complement regulatory proteins. Selectins attach to the cell surface via single spans of amino acids, and each has its own relatively distinct pattern of short intracellular sequences [27].

Regulation of surface expression of each of the selectins is quite different. E-selectin expression is not constitutive, but instead is induced in an mRNA synthesis and protein synthesis–dependent manner within several hours by stimuli such as IL-1, TNF, and bacterial endotoxin (LPS) [28]. This response can be potentiated by IFN-γ and inhibited by

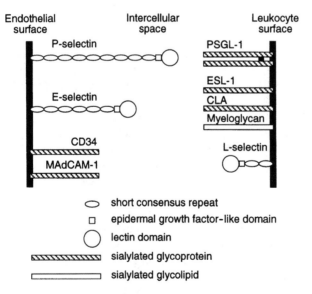

**Figure 1** Basic structures of selectins on leukocytes and endothelium. Examples of extensively glycosylated, mucin-like counterligands for each selectin are also displayed. The transmembrane and intracytoplasmic domains for each of these structures are not shown. Note that PSGL-1 is normally expressed as a homodimer. PSGL-1: P-selectin glycoprotein-1; ESL-1: E-selectin ligand-1; CLA: cutaneous lymphocyte antigen; MAdCAM-1: mucosal addressin cell adhesion molecule-1. (From Ref. 5.)

transforming growth factor β (TGF-β) [29,30]. Surface expression on cultured umbilical vein endothelium is transient, with levels declining towards baseline by 24 hours due to reinternalization and subsequent intracellular degradation [31–33]. E-selectin expression in vivo at sites of inflammation, however, may be more prolonged [34,35]. P-selectin is also not present on normal endothelium. It does, however, exist preformed within the Weibel-Palade bodies, where it can be transiently translocated to the cell surface within minutes in an mRNA synthesis and protein synthesis–independent manner after stimulation with a variety of agents including histamine, thrombin, leukotrienes, and complement fragments [36]. It also appears that other stimuli, such as IL-3 or IL-4, can induce a more gradual and sustained upregulation in surface expression in an mRNA synthesis and protein synthesis–dependent manner [37,38]. In contrast to both P-selectin and E-selectin, expression of L-selectin is constitutive and restricted to leukocytes. In further contrast to the requisite inducibility of these other two selectins, leukocyte activation leads to an irreversible downregulation of surface expression within minutes. This process is activated when leukocytes are exposed to chemotactic factors, cytokines, and other stimuli [39]. The mechanism involved in this process is not entirely understood, but it appears to be the result of activation of endogenous proteases that cleave the molecule at a site close to the cell surface [40,41]. Based on the ability of matrix metalloprotease inhibitors to prevent shedding of L-selectin and other lines of evidence [42–44], it is presumed that these enzymes (often referred to as shedases) are members of this family. Actually, it appears that control of expression of all three selectins is due, at least in part, to protease activity, because soluble forms of E-, L-, and P-selectin can be detected in various biological fluids [45,46].

Regarding the function of each of the selectins, there are many similarities, such as calcium dependence and function even at temperatures below 37°C [6,23,47,48]. Most important and unique to this family of adhesion molecules, however, is their function under conditions of shear forces. For each selectin, the lectin domain recognizes a variety of carbohydrate-containing mucin-like ligands [6,47,49] (see Fig. 1). Although the tetrasaccharide sialyl Lewis$^x$, which contains α2,3-linked terminal sialic acid residues and α1,3-linked fucose, can bind to all three selectins [50–52], differences exist among selectin ligands. For example, ligands for P-selectin are sialyl Lewis$^x$-containing glycoproteins, such as the homodimer PSGL-1 (P-selectin glycoprotein ligand-1) [53–55], while ligands for E-selectin may be a glycoprotein (ESL-1, E-selectin ligand-1 [56]) or instead an extended chain, sialyl Lewis$^x$-containing glycolipid termed myeloglycan [19,57–60]. For subsets of memory (CD45RO+) CD4+ skin-homing lymphocytes, another sialylated molecule termed CLA (cutaneous lymphocyte antigen) that resembles PSGL-1, mediates their binding to E-selectin but not to P-selectin [12,61,62]. In addition, differential expression of PSGL-1 itself on TH1 cells, but not on TH2 cells, has been reported as a possible mechanism responsible for recruitment of T-cell subsets [63]. L-selectin was originally discovered as a peripheral lymph node homing receptor responsible for lymphocyte attachment to high endothelial venules found in lymph nodes [64,65]. L-selectin has many other reported endothelial ligands, including CD34 [66] and mucosal addressin cell adhesion molecule-1 (MAdCAM-1) [22]. Along with PSGL-1, it may also participate in the phenomenon of leukocyte rolling on top of adherent leukocytes observed in in vitro models of shear [67]. Finally, adhesion via each of the selectins and their counterligands can result in alterations of cell function, and cell activation can alter selectin function [68–72]. Regardless of its form of display, biosynthesis of sialyl Lewis$^x$ results from the sequential activity of α1,3-fucosyltransferases (Fuc-T) on α2,3-sialylated lactosamine-type oligosaccharides [47,73]. Among the forms of α1,3-fucosyltransferases that have been cloned, Fuc-TVII appears to be critical for leukocyte synthesis of sialyl Lewis[x] [74–76].

## III.  INTEGRINS

Unlike the simple triumvirate of single-chain selectins, the integrin family is much larger and consists of structurally similar heterodimers with noncovalently associated α and β chains [77,78]. At least 23 different heterodimers, generated by the combination of 16 α subunits and eight β subunits, have been identified, because different α subunits can associate with more than one β subunit [78] (see Table 1). A schematic representation of an integrin is shown in Figure 2. In general, there is more homology among β subunits than among α subunits, and it is the α subunit that is felt to contribute more prominently to the ligand-binding specificity of the heterodimer [79,80]. Within the extracellular portions of α subunits are three or four domains resembling divalent cation-binding sites found in other proteins that contribute to the binding affinity of the heterodimer. Also found in many integrins (each of the β2 integrin α chains, as well as the α1 and α2 chains of β1 integrins) is an inserted, or I, domain, an important recognition site for integrin-binding activity [80,81]. A conserved feature of the β subunits is the presence of 56 cysteine

**Table 1**  Integrins and Their Ligands

| Subunit (CD, name) | Ligands |
|---|---|
| α1β1 (49a/29, VLA-1) | Laminin, collagen |
| α2β1 (49b/29, VLA-2) | Collagen, laminin, ECHO virus |
| α3β1 (49c/29, VLA-3) | Collagen, laminin, others |
| α4β1 (49d/29, VLA-4) | VCAM-1, fibronectin CS-1 domain, α4β1, α4β7 |
| α5β1 (49e/29, VLA-5) | Fibronectin |
| α6β1 (49f/29, VLA-6) | Laminin |
| α7β1 (α7/29) | Laminin |
| α8β1 (α8/29) | Fibronectin |
| α9β1 (α9/29) | Fibronectin, tenascin, VCAM-1 |
| αvβ1 (51/29) | Fibronectin, vitronectin |
| αLβ2 (11a/18, LFA-1) | ICAM-1, ICAM-2, ICAM-3 |
| αMβ2 (11b/18, Mac-1) | ICAM-1 and -2, C3bi, fibrinogen, heparin |
| αXβ2 (11c/18, p150,95) | C3bi, fibrinogen |
| αdβ2 (αd/18) | ICAM-3, VCAM-1 |
| αIIbβ3 (41/61, gpIIb/IIIa) | Fibrinogen, other RGD peptides |
| αvβ3 (51/61) | Vitronectin, PECAM-1, other RGD peptides |
| α6β4 (49f/104) | Laminin |
| αvβ5 (51/β5) | Vitronectin |
| αvβ6 (51/β6) | Fibronectin, tenascin |
| α4β7 (49d/β7, ACT-1) | MAdCAM-1, VCAM-1, fibronectin CS-1 domain |
| αEβ7 (103/β7, HML-1) | E-cadherin |
| α1β8 (49a/β8) | Laminin, collagen, fibronectin |
| αvβ8 (51/β8) | Laminin, collagen, fibronectin |

*Source*: Modified from Ref. 5.

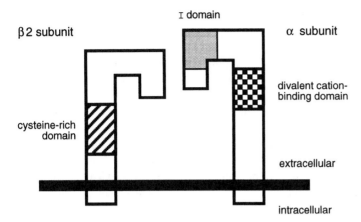

**Figure 2**  Schematic representation of a β2 integrin heterodimer. The I domain and divalent cation-binding domains on the α subunit that contribute to adhesive function are shown, as is the cysteine-rich repeat region of the β2 subunit that is conserved among integrin β subunits. (From Ref. 5.)

residues found in four tandem domains. Presumably, this structural feature keeps the entire molecule extended from the cell surface. Cell surface expression of integrins requires an intact β subunit. Genetic abnormalities involving mutations in the β2 subunit (especially near the N-terminal portion) have been identified in patients with leukocyte adhesion deficiency disease type I (LAD type I), where expression of β2 integrins is markedly impaired or totally absent on leukocytes [82].

Integrins have many ligands, including other adhesion molecules, complement protein fragments, and extracellular matrix proteins (Table 1). Expression of integrins varies widely among resident cutaneous cells [83,84], but there are several consistent characteristics. For example, the β1 integrin subfamily is primarily involved in matrix protein adhesion. Expression of the β2 integrin subfamily is restricted to leukocytes. Ligands for β2 integrins include ICAM-1, ICAM-2, and ICAM-3, as well as fibrinogen, the complement fragment C3bi, and other structures. These leukointegrins contribute to virtually all of the processes of firm adhesion, locomotion, and transendothelial migration involved during leukocyte extravasation into tissue sites. In yet another example, the β3 integrin subfamily, including the integrin αvβ3, is notable for important functions in platelet aggregation and angiogenesis [85,86]. Levels of surface expression vary, depending on cell type, stage of hematopoiesis, injury, or activation. For example, the expression of the very late activation antigen α1β1 (VLA-1) on lymphocytes is considered a marker of activation, because its de novo surface expression requires prolonged activation [87]. In another example, surface expression of integrins on epithelium and other cells in the skin becomes altered during the repair process of wound healing [88,89]. Other integrins, such as the β2 integrin αMβ2, exist both in an intracytoplasmic pool as well as on the cell surface; the intracellular pool is rapidly mobilized to the cell surface within minutes of activation [90].

Among the integrins, the α4β1 heterodimer (VLA-4) is of particular interest in allergic inflammation [5]. This is due in large part to its prominent expression on eosinophils and basophils and its lack of expression on neutrophils [91], although rat neutrophils [92,93] and even human neutrophils may be able, under certain conditions, to express α4 integrins [94]. VLA-4 binds to the alternatively spliced CS-1 (connecting segment-1) portion of the IIICS (type III connecting segment) region of fibronectin (containing the consensus amino acid sequence LDV [95]) and to regions within the first and fourth domains of VCAM-1 (vascular cell adhesion molecule-1), an immunoglobulin family adhesion molecule expressed on activated endothelial cells [4,96] (see below).

Integrins have other functions besides mediating adhesion. Integrins possess intracytoplasmic domains capable of interacting with cytoskeletal elements, where they influence shape change and contribute to migration responses [78,97,98]. Integrins also function in signal transduction via so-called outside-in signaling, whereby adhesion is translated into effects on cellular function [99–101]. Signaling via integrin clustering does not occur through the integrins themselves. Instead, outside-in signaling is felt to occur via interactions between integrins and other associated molecules, such as cytoskeletal proteins and members of the transmembrane 4 family of proteins that includes CD53, CD63, CD81, and CD82 [99,100,102–105]. Finally, in addition to the actual quantity of adhesion molecules expressed on the cell surface, the functional state of these structures also contributes to adhesion. It appears that rapid and reversible changes in tertiary conformation can occur, leading to dramatic changes in affinity of binding [78,106]. For example, activation by cytokines, chemokines, and other chemoattractants can rapidly alter integrin avidity [78,107–111]. These stimuli have also been shown to cause topographical redistribution of integrins in a way that facilitiates cell migration [112,113].

## IV. IMMUNOGLOBULIN SUPERFAMILY

Members of the immunoglobulin superfamily (IgSF) of adhesion molecules are type I transmembrane molecules that share the common structural characteristics of the globular domains found in immunoglobulins [114]. Like integrins, these molecules are responsible for adhesion to other cell-surface ligands and have important signaling functions. Examples of ligand pairs for IgSF family members involved in endothelial cell–endothelial cell, endothelial cell–leukocyte, and leukocyte-leukocyte adhesion are shown in Figure 3. Family members include the intercellular adhesion molecules (ICAM-1 (CD54), ICAM-2 (CD102), ICAM-3 (CD50), and others [115]), vascular cell adhesion molecule-1 (VCAM-1, CD106 [116]), and platelet-endothelial cell adhesion molecule-1 (PECAM-1, CD31 [117]). Other IgSF members, which will not be discussed here in detail, include MAdCAM-1 found in Peyer's patches and gut lamina propria [118], CD2, CD3, CD4, CD8, CD56 (an isoform of neural cell adhesion molecule), CD58, MHC class I and II, and the T-cell receptor, along with a subfamily, called the I-type lectins or sialoadhesins, that include CD22 and CD33 [114,119,120].

Expression of ICAM molecules can be constitutive, inducible, or both. For example, ICAM-1 is constitutively expressed on the luminal, intercellular, and subluminal surfaces of endothelial cells [121], as well as on many leukocytes [122] and respiratory epithelium [123]. Various stimuli, including IL-1, TNF, LPS, and IFN-γ, are capable of inducing or enhancing its expression [124–127]. ICAM-1 expression can also be induced on eosinophils [128,129]. In contrast, ICAM-2 is constitutively expressed on endothelial cells, mononuclear cells, basophils, mast cells, and platelets [122], and expression is unaffected by cytokines. ICAM-3 is constitutively and exclusively expressed on all leukocytes and on mast cells [122], where it also acts as a signaling molecule [130–132]. Ligands for these structures have both overlapping and unique specificities. The integrin CD11a/CD18 binds to all three ICAMs, but additional ligands for ICAM-1 include CD11b/CD18, fibrinogen,

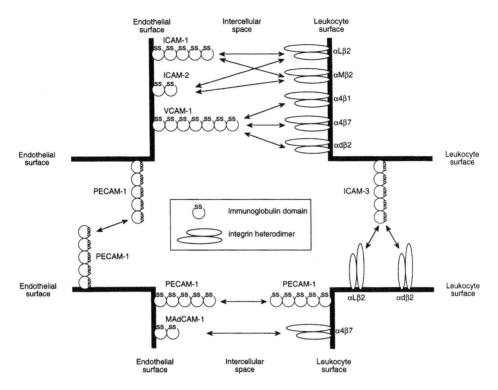

**Figure 3** Schematic representation of several immunoglobulin gene superfamily molecules expressed on endothelial cells and leukocytes. Counterligands, most of which are integrins, are also shown. Arrows denote ligand-counterligand interactions but do not indicate domains used for binding. Note that MAdCAM-1 expression appears to be limited to endothelium in the lamina propria of the gut and to Peyer's patches, while others, such as VCAM-1, require specific stimuli to induce expression. (From Ref. 5, modified to include new data regarding αdβ2 function from Ref. 140.)

and most serotypes of rhinovirus [133–138], while the integrin αd/CD18 binds to ICAM-3 and VCAM-1 [139–141].

VCAM-1, another IgSF structure, was initially identified as a cytokine-inducible endothelial cell structure, as it is not constituively expressed [116,142,143]. On endothelium, expression of VCAM-1 is located primarily on the luminal surface [121] and can be induced de novo within several hours after exposure to IL-1, TNF, or LPS; expression reaches maximal levels by 24–48 hours [116,143–145]. These treatment conditions lead to increased expression of other endothelial adhesion molecules as well [5]. In contrast, treatment of endothelial cells with IL-4 or IL-13 [146–149] leads to selective induction of VCAM-1 expression, and the combination of IL-4 with TNF is synergistic [150–152]. However, this pattern of cytokine responsiveness differs among endothelial cell types. For example, human dermal microvascular endothelial cells express VCAM-1 after stimulation with TNF but not with IL-1 or IL-4 [153]. VCAM-1 can also be found on other cells, including macrophages, dendritic cells, astrocytes, and bone marrow stromal cells [154,155], and exists in two alternatively spliced versions, a predominant seven-domain form and a more rare six-domain form missing domain 4 [156]. There is extensive homology between the three N-terminal domains and the fourth through sixth domains, probably a result of gene duplication [157–159]. Within the extracellular portions of VCAM-1, domains 1 and 4 are most homologous to each other; these are the domains that carry the IDSPL (isoleucine-aspartic acid-serine-proline-leucine) binding site for integrin VLA-4 ($\alpha 4\beta 1$) and probably for $\alpha d\beta 2$ as well [141,160].

PECAM-1 is constitutively expressed on endothelial cells, platelets, and most leukocytes [122]. It is found at particularly high concentrations at interendothelial cell interfaces, and studies suggest a critical role for this molecule during transendothelial migration in vitro and in vivo [161–163]. Both homotypic and heterotypic adhesion, the latter via the integrin $\alpha v\beta 3$, have been reported [117,164].

## V.  OTHER ADHESION MOLECULES

Several other adhesion molecules have been identified, including those that may function during leukocyte recruitment responses into the skin. For example, vascular adhesion protein-1 (VAP-1) is a sialylated homodimeric protein ligand for lymphocytes identified on high endothelial venules of peripheral lymph nodes, smooth muscle, and at sites of cutaneous inflammatory disorders, although its exact counterligand is not yet known [165–170]. It has no known homology with other adhesion molecules and instead bears some resemblance to proteins belonging to an ectoenzyme family with amine oxidase activity [170]. Another molecule is L-VAP-2 (lymphocyte-vascular adhesion protein-2, or CD73), which is expressed on endothelial cells and B- and T-lymphocyte subsets; on endothelium, it can function as a lymphocyte ligand [171–173]. It too has ectoenzyme activity, originally having been described as an ecto-5′-nucleotidase [174]. Yet another adhesion molecule, CD44, is found at high levels on most leukocytes, endothelial cells, dermal and respiratory epithelial cells, keratinocytes, and other cell types, where a number of splice variants have been identified [175]. CD44 functions as a ligand for hyaluronic acid and has been implicated as an important adhesion molecule for peripheral lymph node homing, endothelial-leukocyte rolling, tumor metastasis, and extravasation of cells into inflamed peritoneum and skin [175–178]. One final superfamily is the cadherins. One subset in this family are the classical cadherins, consisting of E-cadherin of endothelial and epithelial origin, P-cadherin of placental origin, and N-cadherin of neural origin. They mediate homotypic interactions at adherens junctions and interact with actin, catenins, and other cytoskeletal proteins, while the other subset, containing the desmocollins and desmogleins, or so-called desmosomal cadherins, are found at desmosomes, where interactions with keratin filaments contribute to barrier tissue integrity and cellular transmigration [10,179–181]. In the skin, for example, it has been proposed that interactions of Langerhans cells with keratinocytes via surface E-cadherin on the Langerhans cells may contribute to their localization and persistence within the epidermis [182].

## VI.  CONTRIBUTIONS OF ENDOTHELIAL ADHESION
## MOLECULE TOPOGRAPHY AND PHYSIOLOGY
## DURING THE PROCESS OF CELL
## RECRUITMENT INTO THE SKIN

During the migration of leukocytes out of the vasculature into tissues, different adhesion molecules contribute within different anatomical locations and at different stages of the process [7,13,183,184]. An excellent example of this is inflammation in the skin, where endothelial adhesion molecule expression is compartmentalized within the vascular beds of the subepidermal capillary loops versus the superficial and deep vascular plexes. While the deep vascular plexus is capable of expressing both E-selectin and VCAM-1 on microvessels, arteries, and veins, VCAM-1 expression is not usually found on either the subepidermal capillary loops or the superficial vascular plexus. Under some conditions, such as in skin explants from dermatitic patients exposed in vitro to the combination of TNF and IL-4, more superficial vascular VCAM-1 expression can be detected [185]. This contrasts with E-selectin expression in these zones, where it is detectable only at the level of the postcapillary venules [186]. Given the topography of endothelial adhesion molecule expression, it is not surprising that cell recruitment, dependent on specific endothelial adhesion molecule expression, influences the routing of extravasating cells to different regions of the skin [187–189].

Differences between the vasculature of the skin and other organs are further highlighted by additional in vitro studies, in which the adhesion molecule phenotype of dermal microvascular endothelial cells has been compared to that of larger vessels, typically from umbilical veins (Table 2) [125,186,190–196]. For example, dermal endothelial cells express higher basal levels of ICAM-1 than umbilical vein endothelial cells and, unlike umbilical vein endothelial cells, do not respond to IL-4 or IL-13 by expressing VCAM-1, even though both will express VCAM-1 in response to TNF [153,197–199]. These differences appear to be due to differences in cell-surface cytokine receptors as well as differences in intracellular signaling pathways [199,200]. Cytokine-induced expression of E-selectin on umbilical vein endothelial cells is transient, while on dermal endothelial cells it is prolonged, apparently due to differences in shedding, reinternalization, or mRNA stability [31,32,35,201,202]. It has also been shown that a variety of treatments used for dermatological diseases, including ultraviolet A and B radiation, can activate endothelial adhesion molecule expression [203,204], while others, such as retinoic acid, have inhibitory effects [205].

Before firm conclusions can be made regarding possible heterogeneity seen among endothelial types based on in vitro studies, these findings need to be compared and sometimes reconciled with results from in vivo studies, where some discrepancies have been observed. For example, regarding effects of IL-4 on VCAM-1 expression, intradermal injection with IL-4 of mice [206], but not humans [195], causes an eosinophil-rich infiltrate, a characteristic of particular relevance to cutaneous allergic inflammatory responses. In other mouse models, IL-4 transgenic mice developed tissue eosinophilia and an allergic-like syndrome [207], and mice inoculated with an IL-4–transfected tumor cell line developed local tissue eosinophilia [208]. In rat models of eosinophil recruitment induced by intracutaneous injection of TNF, IL-4, eotaxin, or other chemoattractants, consistent roles for $\alpha 4$ integrins have been observed when blocking antibodies have been used [209–212]. This suggests that the induction of VCAM-1 expression on dermal microvascular endothelium in vitro may not be entirely predictive of that seen in vivo with the same stimuli.

With respect to the physiology of cell recruitment, it is now well established that a series of adhesion-dependent events are involved in cellular emigration into tissue sites during inflammation [213]. One of the earliest detectable events is the beginning of leukocyte "rolling" on the endothelium under the influence of shear forces caused by blood flow. These interactions are mediated primarily by carbohydrates and their selectin counterligands, although under certain conditions the integrins VLA-4 and $\alpha d \beta 2$ may also partici-

**Table 2** Stimuli That Induce Expression of Adhesion Molecules on Endothelium In Vitro and In Vivo

| Stimulus | HUVEC | DMVEC | Skin explants | Dermal injection |
|---|---|---|---|---|
| E-Selectin | | | | |
| IL-1 | + | + | + | + |
| TNF-α | + | + | + | + |
| IL-4 | − | − | ND | − |
| TNF + IL-4 | − | ND | ND | − |
| IL-13 | − | − | ND | ND |
| IFN-γ | − | ND | ND | − |
| LPS | + | ND | + | + |
| ICAM-1 | | | | |
| IL-1 | + | + | ND | − |
| TNF-α | + | + | ND | + |
| IL-4 | − | − | ND | − |
| TNF + IL-4 | − | ND | ND | − |
| IL-13 | − | − | ND | ND |
| IFN-γ | + | + | ND | + |
| LPS | + | + | ND | + |
| VCAM-1 | | | | |
| IL-1 | + | − | + | + |
| TNF-α | + | + | + | + |
| IL-4 | + | − | + | − |
| TNF + IL-4 | + | ND | ND | + |
| IL-13 | + | ND | ND | ND |
| IFN-γ | − | ND | ND | + |
| TNF + IFN-γ | + | ND | ND | ND |
| LPS | + | ND | ND | + |

HUVEC = human umbilical vein endothelial; DMVEC = dermal microvascular endothelial cells; ND = not determined.
*Source*: Refs. 125, 184, 190–196.

pate [21,141,214–216]. This can be visualized microscopically in vitro using flow chambers or in vivo animal models in tissues such as the skin or exteriorized mesentery, where endothelial-activating cytokines and others, such as vascular endothelial growth factor, can alter these events [217,218].

The subsequent process of firm adhesion, during which rolling cells attach more strongly to the luminal endothelial surface, appears to require leukocyte activation. Currently it is believed that this activation step involves primarily the integrins and occurs as a result of leukocyte seven-spanner chemoattractant receptor interactions with endothelial-displayed stimuli such as platelet-activating factor or chemokines [2,108,111,219–222]. During transendothelial migration, leukocytes travel between endothelial cells, events primarily involving PECAM-1 [117,161], although cadherins, integrins, selectins, and selectin ligands may also participate [152,223–226]. Finally, the burrowing cell must penetrate the basement membrane, composed of extracellular matrix proteins, a process in which enzymes such as matrix metalloproteases play important roles [44,227]. Once inside the extravascular space, adhesion molecules, via interactions with additional matrix proteins, ultimately influence cell localization and function [78]. These events appear to apply to skin mast cells and Langerhans cells as well with respect to their localization and migration within cutaneous tissues [228,229]. Thus, patterns of leukocyte infiltration and localization are the net result of recruitment and migration events involving adhesion mechanisms and activating factors. Disease phenotypes in humans support this stepwise recruitment paradigm. In patients with genetic defects in human leukocyte β2 integrins (LAD type 1) or defects in human leukocyte β2 integrin activation (LAD type 1 variant), impaired neu-trophil adhesion and bacterial immunity are observed [82,230]. Similarly, in LAD type II, in which abnormal GDP-fucose synthesis is associated with abnormalities in the genera-tion of many carbohydrate antigens, including sialyl Lewis[x], impaired leukocyte rolling and mild reductions in bacterial immunity, manifesting as periodontal disease, are seen [231–235]. The disease phenotype of a variety of single and dual adhesion molecule knockout mice has also been explored (reviewed in Ref. 5). While some have relatively subtle deficits (e.g., E- or P-selectin knockouts), others, such as β2 integrin, L-selectin, and dual adhesion molecule knockouts, display more profound impairment of inflamma-tory and immune responses in tissues including the skin [5,236–238].

## VI. EXPRESSION AND FUNCTION OF ADHESION MOLECULES IN VIVO IN ALLERGIC AND OTHER CUTANEOUS DISORDERS IN HUMANS

The potential role of adhesion molecules in cutaneous diseases has been studied using a number of different approaches, and in certain diseases associations between aberrant adhesion molecule expression or function and disease have emerged. In psoriasis, for example, altered levels, function, and locations of β1 integrin expression on keratinocytes, with loss of polarized surface expression, have been strongly implicated in the pathogene-sis of this disorder [88,185,239,240]. These conclusions are supported by findings in a transgenic model in which altered topography of integrin expression within the epidermis results in psoriatic skin changes [241]. In several bullous diseases, cutaneous abnormalities have been traced to abnormalities in adhesion molecules. Junctional epidermolysis bullosa with pyloric atresia is associated with genetic defects in the expression of the integrin α6β4, a receptor for laminin-5 (formerly called epiligrin, nicein, or kalinin) [242–244]. Infusion of anti-laminin-5 antibodies into mice results in blistering that mimics this disease [245]. An autoimmune response directed against desmosomal cadherins is now felt to be responsible for the development of both pemphigus vulgaris and pemphigus foliaceus [10], and soluble forms of E-cadherin correlate with disease severity [246].

The exact role of adhesion molecules in allergic cutaneous disease is less certain. Several strategies have been employed to study these molecules in these disorders. One approach has been to detect the expression of endothelial adhesion molecules immunohis-tochemically in the skin following experimental allergen challenge, as well as in atopic dermatitis and other eosinophilic skin diseases. In challenge studies, within 6–12 hours of intradermal injection of allergic subjects with allergen, induction of endothelial expres-sion of E-selectin and VCAM-1 and increases in constitutive expression of ICAM-1 are typically observed [247,248]. In one study, VCAM-1 expression correlated with the num-bers of infiltrating eosinophils [249]. E-selectin expression induced in this situation was inhibited when the site was immediately biopsied and placed into culture with a mixture of antibodies that neutralized IL-1 and TNF [248]. Cutaneous allergen challenge is also associated with the recruitment of eosinophils, memory (CD45RO+) CLA+ T cells and CD68+ macrophages [250–254]. In another study, allergen challenge was associated with the appearance of increased numbers of mRNA+ cells for IL-4 and IL-13 [255], both of which are capable of selectively activating endothelial expression of VCAM-1 [147,149]. In this study, correlations were observed between IL-13 (but not IL-4) and infiltrating cells as well as endothelial VCAM-1 expression [255].

Along with experimental allergen challenge studies, cell adhesion molecules have been implicated in the pathophysiology of atopic dermatitis. Endothelial activation occurs in this disease, as documented histologically by altered endothelial adhesion molecule expression [256,257]. Whether VCAM-1 expression persists in more chronic lesions is more controversial, with both positive [199] and negative [257] findings having been reported. Increased serum levels of soluble E-selectin, ICAM-1, and/or VCAM-1 have also been observed [258–261]. In another study, elevated levels of these serum markers in severe atopic dermatitis patients treated with ultraviolet A radiation failed to decrease after successful therapy [262]. However, further support for the role of VCAM-1 in eosinophilic inflammation was provided by the demonstration of VCAM-1 staining of blood vessels, without E-selectin staining, in the skin of patients with eosinophilic vasculitis [263]. Direct proof of adhesion molecule involvement in allergic diseases will, by necessity, require the use of specific adhesion molecule antagonists [264,265]. Although no data exists for allergic skin diseases in humans, antibodies to adhesion molecules have been used in some clinical trials [4]. Ultimately, information on the role of adhesion molecules in cutaneous inflammatory diseases in vivo must await studies with novel antagonists currently under development.

## REFERENCES

1. Carlos TM, Harlan JM. Leukocyte-endothelial adhesion molecules. Blood 1994; 84:2068–2101.
2. Springer TA. Traffic signals on endothelium for lymphocyte recirculation and leukocyte emigration. Annu Rev Physiol 1995; 57:827–872.
3. Gumbiner BM. Cell adhesion: the molecular basis of tissue architecture and morphogenesis. Cell 1996; 84:345–357.
4. Kavanaugh A. Overview of cell adhesion molecules and their antagonism. In: Bochner BS, ed. Cell Adhesion Molecules in Allergic Disease. New York: Marcel Dekker, 1997: 1–24.
5. Bochner BS. Cellular adhesion in inflammation. In: Middleton J, Reed C, Ellis E, Adkinson J, Yunginger J, Busse W, eds. Allergy Principles and Practice. 5th ed. St. Louis: Mosby, 1998:94–107.
6. Tedder TF, Steeber DA, Chen A, Engel P. The selectins: vascular adhesion molecules. FASEB J 1995; 9:866–873.
7. Nickoloff BJ, Griffiths CEM, Barker JNWN. The role of adhesion molecules, chemotactic factors, and cytokines in inflammatory and neoplastic skin disease. J Invest Dermatol 1990; 94:S151–S157.
8. Kupper T. Immune and inflammatory processes in cutaneous tissues. Mechanisms and speculations. J Clin Invest 1990; 86:1783–1789.
9. Lawley TJ, Caughman SW, Swerlick RA, Xu Y. The role of adhesion molecules in cutaneous inflammation. J Dermatol 1994; 21:790–794.
10. Amagai M. Adhesion molecules. I: Keratinocyte-keratinocyte interactions; cadherins and pemphigus. J Invest Dermatol 1995; 104:146–152.

11. Yancey KB. Adhesion molecules. II: Interactions of keratinocytes with epidermal basement membrane. J Invest Dermatol 1995; 104:1008–1014.

12. Leung DYM, Picker LJ. Adhesion pathways controlling recruitment responses of lymphocytes during allergic inflammatory reactions in vivo. In: Bochner BS, ed. Adhesion Molecules in Allergic Diseases. New York: Marcel Dekker, 1997:297–314.

13. Beck LA, Georas SN. Expression of cell adhesion molecules in eosinophilic disorders of the skin and nose. In: Bochner BS, ed. Adhesion Molecules in Allergic Diseases. New York: Marcel Dekker, Inc., 1997:339–366.

14. Ioffreda MD, Murphy GF. Mast cell activation and leukocyte recruitment responses into skin sites: role of cell adhesion molecules. In: Bochner BS, ed. Adhesion Molecules in Allergic Diseases. New York: Marcel Dekker, Inc., 1997:257–278.

15. Bevilacqua MP, Stengelin S, Gimbrone MA Jr., Seed B. Endothelial leukocyte adhesion molecule 1: an inducible receptor for neutrophils related to complement regulatory proteins and lectins. Science 1989; 243:1160–1165.

16. Johnston GI, Cook RG, McEver RP. Cloning of GMP-140, a granule membrane protein of platelets and endothelium: sequence similarity to proteins involved in cell adhesion and inflammation. Cell 1989; 56:1033–1044.

17. Tedder TF, Isaacs CM, Ernst TJ, Demetri GD, Adler DA, Disteche CM. Isolation and chromosomal localization of cDNAs encoding a novel human lymphocyte cell surface molecule, LAM-1. J Exp Med 1989; 170:123–133.

18. Patel KD, Moore KL, Nollert MU, McEver RP. Neutrophils use both shared and distinct mechanisms to adhere to selectins under static and flow conditions. J Clin Invest 1995; 96: 1887–1896.

19. Bochner BS, Sterbinsky SA, Bickel CA, Werfel S, Wein M, Newman W. Differences between human eosinophils and neutrophils in the function and expression of sialic acid-containing counterligands for E-selectin. J Immunol 1994; 152:774–782.

20. Bochner BS, Sterbinsky SA, Saini SS, Briskin M, MacGlashan DW Jr. Counter-receptors on human basophils for endothelial cell adhesion molecules. J Immunol 1996; 157:844–850.

21. Lawrence MB, Springer TA. Leukocytes roll on a selectin at physiologic flow rates: distinction from and prerequisite for adhesion through integrins. Cell 1991; 65:859–873.

22. Berg EL, McEvoy LM, Berlin C, Bargatze RF, Butcher EC. L-selectin-mediated lymphocyte rolling on MAdCAM-1. Nature 1993; 366:695–698.

23. Finger EB, Puri KD, Alon R, Lawrence MB, von Andrian UH, Springer TA. Adhesion through L-selectin requires a threshold hydrodynamic shear. Nature 1996; 379:266–269.

24. Watson SR, Imai Y, Fennie C, Geoffroy J, Rosen SD, Lasky LA. A homing receptor-IgG chimera as a probe for adhesive ligands of lymph node high endothelial venules. J Cell Biol 1990; 110:2221–2229.

25. Briskin M. Pathways of cell recruitment to mucosal surfaces. In: Bochner BS, ed. Adhesion Molecules in Allergic Diseases. New York: Marcel Dekker, 1997:105–128.

26. Spertini O, Kansas GS, Reimann KA, Mackay CR, Tedder TF. Function and evolutionary conservation of distinct epitopes on the leukocyte adhesion molecule-1 (TQ-1, Leu-8) that regulate leukocyte migration. J Immunol 1991; 147:942–949.

27. Lasky LA. Selectins—interpreters of cell-specific carbohydrate information during inflammation. Science 1992; 258:964–969.

28. Bevilacqua MP, Nelson RM. Selectins. J Clin Invest 1993; 91:379–387.

29. Leeuwenberg JFM, von Asmuth EJU, Jeunhomme TMAA, Buurman WA. IFN-γ regulates the expression of the adhesion molecule ELAM-1 and IL-6 production by human endothelial cells in vitro. J Immunol 1990; 145:2110–2114.

30. Gamble JR, Khew-Goodall Y, Vadas MA. Transforming growth factor-β inhibits E-selectin expression on human endothelial cells. J Immunol 1993; 150:4494–4503.

31. Bevilacqua MP, Pober JS, Mendrick DL, Cotran RS, Gimbrone MA Jr. Identification of an inducible endothelial-leukocyte adhesion molecule. Proc Natl Acad Sci USA 1987; 84:9238–9242.

32. Kuijpers TW, Raleigh M, Kavanagh T, Janssen H, Calafat J, Roos D, Harlan JM. Cytokine-activated endothelial cells internalize E-selectin into a lysosomal compartment of vesiculotubular shape. J Immunol 1994; 152:5060–5069.

33. Newman W, Beall LD, Carson CW, Hunder GG, Graben N, Randhawa ZI, Gopal TV, Wienerkronish J, Matthay MA. Soluble E-selectin is found in supernatants of activated endothelial cells and is elevated in the serum of patients with septic shock. J Immunol 1993; 150:644–654.

34. Cotran RS, Gimbrone MA Jr., Bevilacqua MP, Mendrick DL, Pober JS. Induction and detection of a human endothelial activation antigen in vivo. J Exp Med 1986; 164:661–666.

35. Chu W, Presky DH, Swerlick RA, Burns DK. Alternatively processed human E-selectin transcripts linked to chronic expression of E-selectin in vivo. J Immunol 1994; 153:4179–4189.

36. Lorant DE, Topham MK, Whatley RE, McEver RP, McIntyre TM, Prescott SM, Zimmerman GA. Inflammatory roles of P-selectin. J Clin Invest 1993; 92:559–570.

37. Khew-Goodall Y, Butcher CM, Litwin MS, Newlands S, Korpelainen EI, Noack LM, Berndt MC, Lopez AF, Gamble JR, Vadas MA. Chronic expression of P-selectin on endothelial cells stimulated by the T-cell cytokine, interleukin-3. Blood 1996; 84:1432–1438.

38. Yao LB, Pan JL, Setiadi H, Patel KD, McEver RP. Interleukin 4 or oncostatin m induces a prolonged increase in P-selectin mRNA and protein in human endothelial cells. J Exp Med 1996; 184:81–92.

39. Kishimoto TK, Jutila MA, Berg EL, Butcher EC. Neutrophil Mac-1 and MEL-14 adhesion proteins inversely regulated by chemotactic factors. Science 1989; 245:1238–1241.

40. Migaki GI, Kahn J, Kishimoto TK. Mutational analysis of the membrane-proximal cleavage site of L-selectin: relaxed sequence specificity surrounding the cleavage site. J Exp Med 1995; 182:549–557.

41. Chen AJ, Engel P, Tedder TF. Structural requirements regulate endoproteolytic release of the L-selectin (CD62L) adhesion receptor from the cell surface of leukocytes. J Exp Med 1995; 182:519–530.

42. Bennett TA, Lynam EB, Sklar LA, Rogelj S. Hydroxamate-based metalloprotease inhibitor blocks shedding of L-selectin adhesion molecule from leukocytes—functional consequences for neutrophil aggregation. J Immunol 1996; 156:3093–3097.

43. Mullberg J, Rauch CT, Wolfson MF, Castner B, Fitzner JN, Otten-Evans C, Mohler KM, Cosman D, Black RA. Further evidence for a common mechanism for shedding of cell surface proteins. FEBS Lett 1997; 401:235–238.

44. Massova I, Kotra LP, Fridman R, Mobashery S. Matrix metalloproteinases: structures, evolution, and diversification. FASEB J 1998; 12:1075–1095.

45. Gearing AJH, Newman W. Circulating adhesion molecules in disease. Immunol Today 1993; 14:506–512.

46. Koch AE, Halloran MM, Haskell CJ, Shah MR, Polverini PJ. Angiogenesis mediated by soluble forms of E-selectin and vascular cell adhesion molecule-1. Nature 1995; 376:517–519.

47. Lowe JB. Specificity and expression of carbohydrate ligands. In: Wegner CD, ed. Adhesion Molecules. London: Academic Press, 1994:113–140.

48. Ley K, Tedder TF. Leukocyte interactions with vascular endothelium—new insights into selectin-mediated attachment and rolling—commentary. J Immunol 1995; 155:525–528.

49. Varki A. Selectin ligands: Will the real ones please stand up? J Clin Invest 1997; 99:158–162.

50. Walz G, Aruffo A, Kolanus W, Bevilacqua M, Seed B. Recognition by ELAM-1 of the sialyl-Le$^x$ determinant on myeloid and tumor cells. Science 1990; 250:1132–1135.

51. Phillips ML, Nudelman E, Gaeta FCA, Perez M, Singhal AK, Hakomori S-I, Paulson JC. ELAM-1 mediates cell adhesion by recognition of a carbohydrate ligand, sialyl-Le$^x$. Science 1990; 250:1130–1132.

52. Foxall C, Watson SR, Dowbenko D, Fennie C, Lasky LA, Kiso M, Hasegawa A, Asa D, Brandley BK. The three members of the selectin receptor family recognize a common carbohydrate epitope, the Sialyl Lewis X oligosaccharide. J Cell Biol 1992; 117:895–902.

53. Sako D, Chang X-J, Barone KM, Vachino G, White HM, Shaw G, Veldman GM, Bean KM, Ahern TJ, Furie B, Cumming DA, Larsen GR. Expression cloning of a functional glycoprotein ligand for P-selectin. Cell 1993; 75:1179–1186.

54. McEver RP, Cummings RD. Role of PSGL-1 binding to selectins in leukocyte recruitment. J Clin Invest 1997; 100:485–492.

55. Snapp KR, Craig R, Herron M, Nelson RD, Stoolman LM, Kansas GS. Dimerization of P-selectin glycoprotein ligand-1 (PSGL-1) required for optimal recognition of P-selectin. J Cell Biol 1998; 142:263–270.

56. Steegmaier M, Levinovitz A, Isenmann S, Borges E, Lenter M, Kocher HP, Kleuser B, Vestweber D. The E-selectin ligand ESL-1 is a variant of a receptor for fibroblast growth factor. Nature 1995; 373:615–620.

57. Larsen GR, Sako D, Ahern TJ, Shaffer M, Erban J, Sajer SA, Gibson RM, Wagner DD, Furie BC, Furie B. P-selectin and E-selectin. Distinct but overlapping leukocyte ligand specificities. J Biol Chem 1992; 267:11104–11110.

58. Wein M, Sterbinsky SA, Bickel CA, Schleimer RP, Bochner BS. Comparison of eosinophil and neutrophil ligands for P-selectin: ligands for P-selectin differ from those for E-selectin. Am J Respir Cell Mol Biol 1995; 12:315–319.

59. Stroud MR, Handa K, Ito K, Salyan MEK, Fang H, Levery SB, Hakomori S, Reinhold BB, Reinhold VN. Myeloglycan, a series of E-selectin-binding polylactosaminolipids found in normal human leukocytes and myelocytic leukemia HL60 cells. Biochem Biophys Res Commun 1995; 209:777–787.

60. Collins BE, Bochner BS, Schnaar RL. Glycolipids may be endogenous neutrophil E-selectin ligands (abstr). Glycoconjugate J 1995; 12:535.

61. Fuhlbrigge RC, Kieffer JD, Armerding D, Kupper TS. Cutaneous lymphocyte antigen is a specialized form of PSGL-1 expressed on skin-homing T cells. Nature 1997; 389:978–981.

62. Tietz W, Allemand Y, Borges E, vonLaer D, Hallmann R, Vestweber D, Hamann A. CD4(+) T cells migrate into inflamed skin only if they express ligands for E- and P-selectin. J Immunol 1998; 161:963–970.

63. Borges E, Tietz W, Steegmaier M, Moll T, Hallmann R, Hamann A, Vestweber D. P-selectin glycoprotein ligand-1 (PSGL-1) on T helper 1 but not on T helper 2 cells binds to P-selectin and supports migration into inflamed skin. J Exp Med 1997; 185:573–578.

64. Butcher EC, Picker LJ. Lymphocyte homing and homeostasis. Science 1996; 272:60–66.

65. Girard JP, Springer TA. High endothelial venules (HEVs): specialized endothelium for lymphocyte migration. Immunol Today 1995; 16:449–457.

66. Baumhueter S, Singer MS, Henzel W, Hemmerich S, Renz M, Rosen SD, Lasky LA. Binding of L-selectin to the vascular sialomucin CD34. Science 1993; 262:436–438.

67. Walcheck B, Moore KL, McEver RP, Kishimoto TK. Neutrophil-neutrophil interactions under hydrodynamic shear stress involve L-selectin and PSGL-1-a mechanism that amplifies initial leukocyte accumulation on P-selectin in vitro. J Clin Invest 1996; 98:1081–1087.

68. Wong CS, Gamble JR, Skinner MP, Lucas CM, Berndt MC, Vadas MA. Adhesion protein GMP-140 inhibits superoxide release by human neutrophils. Proc Natl Acad Sci USA 1991; 88:2397.

69. Cooper D, Butcher CM, Berndt MC, Vadas MA. P-selectin interacts with a β2-integrin to enhance phagocytosis. J Immunol 1994; 153:3199–3209.

70. Weyrich AS, McIntyre TM, McEver RP, Prescott SM, Zimmerman GA. Monocyte tethering by P-selectin regulates monocyte chemotactic protein-1 and tumor necrosis factor-α secretion. J Clin Invest 1995; 95:2297–2303.

71. Lorant DE, McEver RP, Mcintyre TM, Moore KL, Prescott SM, Zimmerman GA. Activation

of polymorphonuclear leukocytes reduces their adhesion to P-selectin and causes redistribution of ligands for P-selectin on their surfaces. J Clin Invest 1995; 96:171–182.

72. Giblin PA, Hwang ST, Katsumoto TR, Rosen SD. Ligation of L-selectin on T lymphocytes activates β1 integrins and promotes adhesion to fibronectin. J Immunol 1997; 159:3498–3507.

73. Kuijpers TW. Terminal glycosyltransferase activity—a selective role in cell adhesion. Blood 1993; 81:873–882.

74. Knibbs RN, Craig RA, Natsuka S, Chang A, Cameron M, Lowe JB, Stoolman LM. The fucosyltransferase FucT-VII regulates E-selectin ligand synthesis in human T cells. J Cell Biol 1996; 133:911–920.

75. Lowe JB, Ward PA. Therapeutic inhibition of carbohydrate-protein interactions in vivo. J Clin Invest 1997; 99:822–826.

76. Maly P, Thall AD, Petryniak B, Rogers GE, Smith PL, Marks RM, Kelly RJ, Gersten KM, Cheng GY, Saunders TL, Camper SA, Camphausen RT, Sullivan FX, Isogai Y, Hindsgaul O, von Andrian UH, Lowe JB. The α(1,3) fucosyltransferase Fuc-TVII controls leukocyte trafficking through an essential role in L-, E-, and P-selectin ligand biosynthesis. Cell 1996; 86:643–653.

77. Hynes RO. Integrins: versatility, modulation, and signaling in cell adhesion. Cell 1992; 69:11–25.

78. Hunt SW III, Kellermann S-A, Shimizu Y. Integrins, integrin regulators and the extracellular matrix: the role of signal transduction and leukocyte migration. In: Bochner BS, ed. Cell Adhesion Molecules in Allergic Disease. New York: Marcel Dekker, 1997:73–104.

79. Ruoslahti E, Engvall E. Integrins and vascular extracellular matrix assembly. J Clin Invest 1997; 99:1149–1152.

80. Loftus JC, Liddington RC. New insights into integrin-ligand interaction. J Clin Invest 1997; 99:2302–2306.

81. Balsam LB, Liang TW, Parkos CA. Functional mapping of CD11b/CD18 epitopes important in neutrophil-epithelial interactions: A central role of the I domain. J Immunol 1998; 160:5058–5065.

82. Anderson DC, Springer TA. Leukocyte adhesion deficiency: an inherited defect in the Mac-1, LFA-1, and p150,95 glycoproteins. Annu Rev Med 1987; 38:175–194.

83. Adams JC, Watt FM. Expression of β1-integrin, β3-integrin, β4-integrin and β5-integrin by human epidermal keratinocytes and non-differentiating keratinocytes. J Cell Biol 1991; 115:829–841.

84. Zambruno G, Manca V, Santantonio ML, Soligo D, Giannetti A. VLA protein expression on epidermal cells (keratinocytes, Langerhans cells, melanocytes)—a light and electron microscopic immunohistochemical study. Br J Dermatol 1991; 124:135–145.

85. Swerlick RA, Brown EJ, Xu Y, Lee K, Manos S, Lawley TJ. Expression and modulation of the vitronectin receptor on human dermal microvascular endothelial cells. J Invest Dermatol 1992; 99:715–722.

86. Brooks PC, Clark RAF, Cheresh DA. Requirement of vascular integrin αvβ3 for angiogenesis. Science 1994; 264:569–571.

87. Hemler ME. VLA proteins in the integrin family: structures, functions, and their role on leukocytes. Annu Rev Immunol 1990; 8:365–400.

88. Hertle MD, Kubler MD, Leigh IM, Watt FM. Aberrant integrin expression during epidermal wound healing and in psoriatic epidermis. J Clin Invest 1992; 89:1892–1901.

89. Juhasz I, Murphy GF, Yan HC, Herlyn M, Albelda SM. Regulation of extracellular matrix proteins and integrin cell substratum adhesion receptors on epithelium during cutaneous human wound healing in vivo. Am J Pathol 1993; 143:1458–1469.

90. Bainton DF, Miller LJ, Kishimoto TK, Springer TA. Leukocyte adhesion receptors are stored in peroxidase-negative granules of human neutrophils. J Exp Med 1987; 166:1641–1653.

91. Bochner BS, Luscinskas FW, Gimbrone MA Jr., Newman W, Sterbinsky SA, Derse-Anthony

C, Klunk D, Schleimer RP. Adhesion of human basophils, eosinophils, and neutrophils to IL-1-activated human vascular endothelial cells: contributions of endothelial cell adhesion molecules. J Exp Med 1991; 173:1553–1557.

92. Issekutz TB, Miyasaka M, Issekutz AC. Rat blood neutrophils express very late antigen 4 and it mediates migration to arthritic joint and dermal inflammation. J Exp Med 1996; 183: 2175–2184.

93. Davenpeck KL, Sterbinsky SA, Bochner BS. Rat neutrophils express $\alpha 4$ and $\beta 1$ integrins and bind to vascular cell adhesion molecule-1 (VCAM-1) and mucosal addressin cell adhesion molecule-1 (MAdCAM-1). Blood 1998; 91:2341–2346.

94. Kubes P, Niu XF, Smith CW, Kehrli ME, Reinhardt PH, Woodman RC. A novel $\beta 1$ integrin-dependent adhesion pathway on neutrophils: a mechanism invoked by dihydrocytochalasin b or endothelial transmigration. FASEB J 1995; 9:1103–1111.

95. Wayner EA, Garcia-Pardo A, Humphries MJ, McDonald JA, Carter WG. Identification and characterization of the T lymphocyte adhesion receptor for an alternative cell attachment domain (CS-1) in plasma fibronectin. J Cell Biol 1989; 109:1321–1330.

96. Elices MJ, Osborn L, Takada Y, Crouse C, Luhowskyj S, Hemler ME, Lobb RR. VCAM-1 on activated endothelium interacts with the leukocyte integrin VLA-4 at a site distinct from the VLA-4/fibronectin binding site. Cell 1990; 60:577–584.

97. Simon KO, Burridge K. Interactions between integrins and the cytoskeleton: structure and regulation. In: Cheresh DA, Mecham RP, eds. Integrins:Molecular and Biological Responses to the Extracellular Matrix. San Diego: Academic Press, 1994:49–78.

98. Clark EA, Brugge JS. Integrins and signal transduction pathways: the road taken. Science 1995; 268:233–239.

99. Yamada KM, Miyamoto S. Integrin transmembrane signaling and cytoskeletal control. Curr Opin Cell Biol 1995; 7:681–686.

100. Wahl SM, Feldman GM, McCarthy JB. Regulation of leukocyte adhesion and signaling in inflammation and disease. J Leukoc Biol 1996; 59:789–796.

101. Petty HR, Todd RF. Integrins as promiscuous signal transduction devices. Immunol Today 1996; 7:209–212.

102. Rubinstein E, Lenaour F, Billard M, Prenant M, Boucheix C. CD9 antigen is an accessory subunit of the VLA integrin complexes. Eur J Immunol 1994; 24:3005–3013.

103. Berditchevski F, Bazzoni G, Hemler ME. Specific association of CD63 with the VLA-3 and VLA-6 integrins. J Biol Chem 1995; 270: 17784–17790.

104. Mannion BA, Berditchevski F, Kraeft S-K, Chen LB, Hemler ME. Transmembrane-4 super-family proteins CD81 (TAPA-1), CD82, CD63, and CD53 specifically associate with integrin $\alpha 4\beta 1$ (CD49d/CD29). J Immunol 1996; 157:2039–2047.

105. Berditchevsky F, Tolias KF, Wong K, Carpenter CL, Hemler ME. A novel link between integrins, transmembrane-4 superfamily proteins (CD63 and CD81), and phosphatidylinositol 4-kinase. J Biol Chem 1997; 272:2595–2598.

106. Diamond MS, Springer TA. The dynamic regulation of integrin adhesiveness. Curr Biol 1994; 4:506–517.

107. Honda S, Campbell JJ, Andrew DP, Engelhardt B, Butcher BA, Warnock RA, Ye RD, Butcher EC. Ligand-induced adhesion to activated endothelium and to vascular cell adhesion molecule-1 in lymphocytes transfected with the N-formyl peptide receptor. J Immunol 1994; 152:4026–4035.

108. Campbell JJ, Qin S, Bacon KB, Mackay CR, Butcher EC. Biology of chemokine and classical chemoattractant receptors: differential requirements for adhesion-triggering versus chemotactic responses in lymphoid cells. J Cell Biol 1996; 134:255–266.

109. Weber C, Alon R, Moser B, Springer TA. Sequential regulation of $\alpha 4\beta 1$ and $\alpha 5\beta 1$ integrin avidity by CC chemokines in monocytes: implications for transendothelial chemotaxis. J Cell Biol 1996; 134:1063–1073.

110. Werfel S, Yednock T, Matsumoto K, Sterbinsky SA, Schleimer RP, Bochner BS. Functional

regulation of β1 integrins and human eosinophils by divalent cations and cytokines. Am J Respir Cell Mol Biol 1996; 14:45–52.

111. Kitayama J, Mackay CR, Ponath PD, Springer TA. The C-C chemokine receptor CCR3 participates in stimulation of eosinophil arrest on inflammatory endothelium in shear flow. J Clin Invest 1998; 101:2017–2024.

112. Lawson MA, Maxfield FR. $Ca^{2+}$ and calcineurin-dependent recycling of an integrin to the front of migrating neutrophils. Nature 1995; 377:75–79.

113. Delpozo MA, Sanchez-Mateos P, Sanchez-Madrid F. Cellular polarization induced by chemokines: a mechanism for leukocyte recruitment? Immunol Today 1996; 17:127–131.

114. Springer TA. Adhesion receptors of the immune system. Nature 1990; 346:425–434.

115. Hayflick J, Kilgannon P, Gallatin W. The intercellular adhesion molecule (ICAM) family of proteins. New members and novel functions. Immunol Res 1998; 17:313–327.

116. Osborn L, Hession C, Tizard R, Vassallo C, Luhowskyj S, Chi-Rosso G, Lobb R. Direct expression cloning of vascular cell adhesion molecule 1, a cytokine-induced endothelial protein that binds to lymphocytes. Cell 1989; 59:1203–1211.

117. DeLisser HM, Newman PJ, Albelda SM. Molecular and functional aspects of PECAM-1/CD31. Immunol Today 1994; 15:490–495.

118. Briskin MJ, McEvoy LM, Butcher EC. MAdCAM-1 has homology to immunoglobulin and mucin-like adhesion receptors and to IgA1. Nature 1993; 363:461–464.

119. Kelm S, Pelz A, Schauer R, Filbin MT, Tang S, de Bellard M-E, Schnaar RL, Mahoney JA, Hartnell A, Bradfield P, Crocker PR. Sialoadhesin, myelin-associated glycoprotein and CD22 define a new family of sialic acid-dependent adhesion molecules of the immunoglobulin superfamily. Curr Biol 1994; 4:965–972.

120. Powell LD, Varki A. I-type lectins. J Biol Chem 1995; 270:14243–14246.

121. Oppenheimer-Marks N, Davis LS, Bogue DT, Ramberg J, Lipsky PE. Differential utilization of ICAM-1 and VCAM-1 during the adhesion and transendothelial migration of human T lymphocytes. J Immunol 1991; 147:2913–2921.

122. Shaw S, Luce GG, Gilks WR, Anderson K, Ault K, Bochner BS, Boumsell L, Denning SM, Engleman EG, Fleisher T, Freedman AS, Fox DA, Gailit J, Carlos Gutierrez-Ramos J, Hurtubise PE, Lansdorp P, Lotze MT, Mawhorter S, Marti G, Matsuo Y, Minowada J, Michelson A, Picker L, Ritz J, Roos E, Van der Schoot CE, Springer TA, Tedder TF, Telen MJ, Thompson JS, Valent P. Leukocyte differentiation antigen database. In:Schlossman S, Boumsell L, Gilks W, Harlan J, Kishimoto T, Morimoto C, Ritz J, Shaw S, Silverstein R, Springer T, Tedder T, Todd R, eds. Leukocyte Typing V: White Cell Differentiation Antigens. New York: Oxford University Press, 1995:16–198.

123. Polito AJ, Proud D. Epithelial cells: phenotype, substratum and mediator production. In: Bochner BS, ed. Cell Adhesion Molecules in Allergic Disease. New York: Marcel Dekker, 1997:43–72.

124. Dustin ML, Rothlein R, Bhan AK, Dinarello CA, Springer TA. Induction by IL 1 and interferon-γ: tissue distribution, biochemistry, and function of a natural adherence molecule (ICAM-1). J Immunol 1986; 137:245–254.

125. Pober JS, Gimbrone MA Jr., Lapierre LA, Mendrick DL, Fiers W, Rothlein R, Springer TA. Overlapping patterns of activation of human endothelial cells by interleukin 1, tumor necrosis factor, and immune interferon. J Immunol 1986; 137:1893–1896.

126. Tosi MF, Stark JM, Smith CW, Hamedani A, Gruenert DC, Infeld MD. Induction of ICAM-1 expression on human airway epithelial cells by inflammatory cytokines—effects on neutrophil-epithelial cell adhesion. Am J Respir Cell Mol Biol 1992; 7:214–221.

127. Bloemen PG, van den Tweel MC, Henricks PAJ, Engels F, Wagenaar SS, Rutten AAJJL, Nijkamp FP. Expression and modulation of adhesion molecules on human bronchial epithelial cells. Am J Respir Cell Mol Biol 1993; 9:586–593.

128. Hansel TT, Braunstein JB, Walker C, Blaser K, Bruijnzeel PLB, Virchow JC, Virchow C.

Sputum eosinophils from asthmatics express ICAM-1 and HLA-DR. Clin Exp Immunol 1991; 86:271–277.

129. Czech W, Krutmann J, Budnik A, Schopf E, Kapp A. Induction of ICAM-1 expression on normal human eosinophils by inflammatory cytokines. J Invest Derm 1993; 100:417–423.
130. Juan M, Vinas O, Pinootin MR, Places L, Martinezcaceres E, Barcelo JJ, Miralles A, Vilella R, Delafuente MA, Vives J, Yague J, Gaya A. CD50 (intercellular adhesion molecule 3) stimulation induces calcium mobilization and tyrosine phosphorylation through p59(fyn) and p56(lck) in Jurkat T cell line. J Exp Med 1994; 179:1747–1756.
131. Cid MC, Esparza J, Juan M, Miralles A, Ordi J, Vilella R, Urbano-Marquez A, Gaya A, Vives J, Yague J. Signaling through CD50 (ICAM-3) stimulates T lymphocyte binding to human umbilical vein endothelial cells and extracellular matrix proteins via an increase in β1 and β2 integrin function. Eur J Immunol 1994; 24:1377–1382.
132. Saini S, White J, Gallatin WM, Hoffman PA, Lichtenstein LM, Bochner BS. Potentiation of basophil function by antibodies to ICAM-3 (abstr). J Allergy Clin Immunol 1996; 97: 264.
133. Marlin SD, Springer TA. Purified intercellular adhesion molecule-1 (ICAM-1) is a ligand for lymphocyte function-associated antigen-1 (LFA-1). Cell 1987; 51:813–819.
134. Languino LR, Plescia J, Duperray A, Brian AA, Plow EF, Geltosky JE, Altieri DC. Fibrinogen mediates leukocyte adhesion to vascular endothelium through an ICAM-1-dependent pathway. Cell 1993; 73:1423–1434.
135. Greve JM, Davis G, Meyer AM, Forte CP, Yost SC, Marlor CW, Kamarck ME, McClelland A. The major human rhinovirus receptor is ICAM-1. Cell 1989; 56:839–847.
136. Staunton DE, Dustin ML, Erickson HP, Springer TA. The arrangement of the immunoglobulin-like domains of ICAM-1 and the binding sites for LFA-1 and rhinovirus. Cell 1990; 61: 243–254.
137. Diamond MS, Staunton DE, de Fougerolles AR, Stacker SA, Garcia-Aguilar J, Hibbs ML, Springer TA. ICAM-1 (CD54): a counter-receptor for Mac-1 (CD11b/CD18). J Cell Biol 1990;111:3129–3139.
138. Wang JH, Springer TA. Structural specializations of immunoglobulin superfamily members for adhesion to integrins and viruses. Immunol Rev 1998; 163:197–215.
139. Van der Vieren M, Letrong H, Wood CL, Moore PF, St. John T, Staunton DE, Gallatin WM. A novel leukointegrin, αdβ2, binds preferentially to ICAM-3. Immunity 1995; 3:683–690.
140. Grayson MH, Van der Vieren M, Sterbinsky SA, Gallatin WM, Hoffman PA, Staunton DE, Bochner BS. αdβ2 integrin is expressed on human eosinophils and functions as an alternative ligand for VCAM-1. J Exp Med 1998; 2187–2191.
141. Van der Vieren M, Crowe DT, Hoekstra D, Adams L, Vazeux R, Grayson MH, Bochner BS, Staunton DE. The leukocyte integrin αdβ2 binds VCAM-1. J Immunol 1999 (in press).
142. Rice GE, Bevilacqua MP. An inducible endothelial surface glycoprotein mediates melanoma adhesion. Science 1989; 246:1303–1306.
143. Graber N, Gopal TV, Wilson D, Beall LD, Polte T, Newman W. T cells bind to cytokine-activated endothelial cells via a novel, inducible sialoglycoprotein and endothelial leukocyte adhesion molecule-1. J Immunol 1990; 145:819–830.
144. Wellicome SM, Thornhill MH, Pitzalis C, Thomas DS, Lanchbury JSS, Panayi GS, Haskard DO. A monoclonal antibody that detects a novel antigen on endothelial cells that is induced by tumor necrosis factor, IL-1, or lipopolysaccharide. J Immunol 1990; 144:2558–2565.
145. Rice GE, Munro JM, Bevilacqua MP. Inducible cell adhesion molecule 110 (INCAM-110) is an endothelial receptor for lymphocytes. A CD11/CD18-independent adhesion mechanism. J Exp Med 1990; 171:1369–1374.
146. Thornhill MH, Kyan-Aung U, Haskard DO. IL-4 increases human endothelial cell adhesiveness for T cells but not for neutrophils. J Immunol 1990; 144:3060–3065.
147. Schleimer RP, Sterbinsky SA, Kaiser J, Bickel CA, Klunk DA, Tomioka K, Newman W,

Luscinskas FW, Gimbrone MA Jr., McIntyre BW, Bochner BS. Interleukin-4 induces adherence of human eosinophils and basophils but not neutrophils to endothelium: association with expression of VCAM-1. J Immunol 1992; 148:1086–1092.

148. Sironi M, Sciacca FL, Matteucci C, Conni M, Vecchi A, Bernasconi S, Minty A, Caput D, Ferrara P, Colotta F, Mantovani A. Regulation of endothelial and mesothelial cell function by interleukin-13: Selective induction of vascular cell adhesion molecule-1 and amplification of interleukin-6 production. Blood 1994; 84:1913–1921.

149. Bochner BS, Klunk DA, Sterbinsky SA, Coffman RL, Schleimer RP. Interleukin-13 selectively induces vascular cell adhesion molecule-1 (VCAM-1) expression in human endothelial cells. J Immunol 1995; 154:799–803.

150. Thornhill MH, Haskard DO. IL-4 regulates endothelial cell activation by IL-1, tumor necrosis factor, or IFN-γ. J Immunol 1990; 145:865–872.

151. Masinovsky B, Urdal D, Gallatin WM. IL-4 acts synergistically with IL-1β to promote lymphocyte adhesion to microvascular endothelium by induction of vascular cell adhesion molecule-1. J Immunol 1990; 145:2886–2895.

152. Ebisawa M, Bochner BS, Schleimer RP. Eosinophil-endothelial interactions and transendothelial migration. In: Bochner BS, ed. Adhesion Molecules in Allergic Diseases. New York: Marcel Dekker, Inc., 1997:173–186.

153. Swerlick RA, Lee KH, Li L, Sepp NT, Caughman SW, Lawley TJ. Regulation of vascular cell adhesion molecule 1 on human dermal microvascular endothelial cells. J Immunol 1992; 149:698–705.

154. Rice GE, Munro JM, Corless C, Bevilacqua MP. Vascular and nonvascular expression of INCAM-110. Am J Pathol 1991; 138:385–393.

155. Rosenman SJ, Shrikant P, Dubb L, Benveniste EN, Ransohoff RM. Cytokine-induced expression of vascular cell adhesion molecule-1 (VCAM-1) by astrocytes and astrocytoma cell lines. J Immunol 1995; 154:1888–1899.

156. Pepinsky B, Hession C, Chen LL, Moy P, Burkly L, Jakubowski A, Chow EP, Benjamin C, Chirosso G, Luhowskyj S, Lobb R. Structure/function studies on vascular cell adhesion molecule-1. J Biol Chem 1992; 267:17820–17826.

157. Polte T, Newman W, Raghunathan G, Gopal TV. Structural and functional studies of full length vascular cell adhesion molecule-1: internal duplication and homology to several adhesion proteins. DNA Cell Biol 1991; 10:349–357.

158. Cybulsky MI, Fries JWU, Williams AJ, Sultan P, Eddy R, Byers M, Shows T, Gimbrone MA Jr., Collins T. Gene structure, chromosomal location, and basis for alternative messenger RNA splicing of the human VCAM-1 gene. Proc Natl Acad Sci USA 1991; 88:7859–7863.

159. Hession C, Tizard R, Vassallo C, Schiffer SB, Goff D, Moy P, Chi-Rosso G, Luhowskyj S, Lobb R, Osborn L. Cloning of an alternative form of vascular cell adhesion molecule-1 (VCAM-1). J Biol Chem 1991; 266:6682–6685.

160. Lobb RR, Hemler ME. The pathophysiologic role of α4 integrins in vivo. J Clin Invest 1994; 94:1722–1728.

161. Muller WA. The role of PECAM-1 (CD31) in leukocyte emigration: studies in vitro and in vivo. J Leukoc Biol 1995; 57:523–528.

162. Vaporciyan AA, DeLisser HM, Yan H-C, Mendiguren II, Thom SR, Jones ML, Ward PA, Albelda SM. Involvement of platelet-endothelial cell adhesion molecule-1 in neutrophil recruitment in vivo. Science 1993; 262:1580–1582.

163. Zocchi MR, Ferrero E, Leone BE, Rovere P, Bianchi E, Toninelli E, Pardi R. CD31/PECAM-1-driven chemokine-independent transmigration of human T lymphocytes. Eur J Immunol 1996; 26:759–767.

164. Piali L, Hammel P, Uherek C, Bachmann F, Gisler RH, Dunon D, Imhof BA. CD31/PECAM-1 is a ligand for αvβ3 integrin involved in adhesion of leukocytes to endothelium. J Cell Biol 1995; 130:451–460.

165. Salmi M, Jalkanen S. A 90-kilodalton endothelial cell molecule mediating lymphocyte binding in humans. Science 1992; 257:1407–1409.

166. Salmi M, Kalimo K, Jalkanen S. Induction and function of vascular adhesion protein-1 at sites of inflammation. J Exp Med 1993; 178:2255–2260.

167. Salmi M, Jalkanen S. Human vascular adhesion protein 1 (VAP-1) is a unique sialoglycoprotein that mediates carbohydrate-dependent binding of lymphocytes to endothelial cells. J Exp Med 1996; 183:569–579.

168. Arvilommi AM, Salmi M, Kalimo K, Jalkanen S. Lymphocyte binding to vascular endothelium in inflamed skin revisited: a central role for vascular adhesion protein-1 (VAP-1). Eur J Immunol 1996; 26:825–833.

169. Arvilommi AM, Salmi M, Airas L, Kalimo K, Jalkanen S. CD73 mediates lymphocyte binding to vascular endothelium in inflamed human skin. Eur J Immunol 1997; 27:248–254.

170. Smith DJ, Salmi M, Bono P, Hellman J, Leu T, Jalkanen S. Cloning of vascular adhesion protein 1 reveals a novel multifunctional adhesion molecule. J Exp Med 1998; 188:17–27.

171. Airas L, Salmi M, Jalkanen S. Lymphocyte-vascular adhesion protein-2 is a novel 70-kDa molecule involved in lymphocyte adhesion to vascular endothelium. J Immunol 1993; 151:4228–4238.

172. Airas L, Hellman J, Salmi M, Bono P, Puurunen T, Smith DJ, Jalkanen S. CD73 is involved in lymphocyte binding to the endothelium: characterization of lymphocyte vascular adhesion protein 2 identifies it as CD73. J Exp Med 1995; 182:1603–1608.

173. Airas L, Niemela J, Salmi M, Puurunen T, Smith DJ, Jalkanen S. Differential regulation and function of CD73, a glycosyl-phosphatidylinositol-linked 70-kD adhesion molecule, on lymphocytes and endothelial cells. J Cell Biol 1997; 136:421–431.

174. Zimmermann H. 5′-Nucleotidase: molecular structure and functional aspects. Biochem J 1992; 285:345–365.

175. Lesley JR, Hyman R, Kincade PW. CD44 and its interaction with extracellular matrix. Adv Immunol 1993; 54:271–298.

176. Degrendele HC, Estess P, Picker LJ, Siegelman MH. CD44 and its ligand hyaluronate mediate rolling under physiologic flow: a novel lymphocyte-endothelial cell primary adhesion pathway. J Exp Med 1996; 183:1119–1130.

177. DeGrendele HC, Estess P, Siegelman MH. Requirement for CD44 in activated T cell extravasation into an inflammatory site. Science 1997; 278:672–675.

178. Seiter S, Schadendorf D, Tilgen W, Zoller M. CD44 variant isoform expression in a variety of skin-associated autoimmune diseases. Clin Immunol Immunopathol 1998; 89:79–93.

179. Shapiro L, Fannon AM, Kwong PD, Thompson A, Lehmann MS, Grubel G, Legrand JF, Alsnielsen J, Colman DR, Hendrickson WA. Structural basis of cell-cell adhesion by cadherins. Nature 1995; 374:327–337.

180. Cowin P. Unraveling the cytoplasmic interactions of the cadherin superfamily. Proc Natl Acad Sci USA 1994; 91:10759–10761.

181. Luscinskas FW. The endothelium in leukocyte recruitment. In: Bochner BS, ed. Adhesion Molecules in Allergic Diseases. New York: Marcel Dekker, Inc., 1997:25–41.

182. Tang AM, Amagai M, Granger LG, Stanley JR, Udey MC. Adhesion of epidermal Langerhans cells to keratinocytes mediated by E-cadherin. Nature 1993; 361:82–85.

183. Butcher EC. Leukocyte-endothelial cell recognition: Three (or more) steps to specificity and diversity. Cell 1991; 67:1033–1036.

184. Swerlick RA, Lawley TJ. Role of microvascular endothelial cells in inflammation. J Invest Dermatol 1993; 100:111S–115S.

185. Petzelbauer P, Pober JS, Keh A, Braverman IM. Inducibility and expression of microvascular endothelial adhesion molecules in lesional, perilesional, and uninvolved skin of psoriatic patients. J Invest Dermatol 1994; 103:300–305.

186. Petzelbauer P, Bender JR, Wilson J, Pober JS. Heterogeneity of dermal microvascular endo-

thelial cell antigen expression and cytokine responsiveness in situ and in cell culture. J Immunol 1993; 151:5062–5072.

187. Kunstfeld R, Lechleitner S, Groger M, Wolff K, Petzelbauer P. HECA-452+ T cells migrate through superficial vascular plexus but not through deep vascular plexus endothelium. J Invest Dermatol 1997; 108:343–348.

188. Yan H-C, Juhasz I, Pilewsi J, Murphy GF, Herlyn M, Albelda SM. Human/severe combined immunodeficient mouse chimeras. An experimental in vivo model system to study the regulation of human endothelial cell-leukocyte adhesion molecules. J Clin Invest 1993; 91:986–996.

189. Yan HC, Delisser HM, Pilewski JM, Barone KM, Szklut PJ, Chang XJ, Ahern TJ, Langersafer P, Albelda SM. Leukocyte recruitment into human skin transplanted onto severe combined immunodeficient mice induced by TNFα is dependent on E-selectin. J Immunol 1994; 152:3053–3063.

190. Kaiser J, Bickel C, Bochner BS, Schleimer RP. The effects of the potent glucocorticoid budesonide on adhesion of eosinophils to human vascular endothelium and on endothelial expression of adhesion molecules. J Pharmacol Exp Therap 1993; 267:245–249.

191. Messadi DV, Pober JS, Fiers W, Gimbrone MA Jr., Murphy GF. Induction of an activation antigen on postcapillary venular endothelium in human skin organ culture. J Immunol 1987; 139:1557–1562.

192. Groves RW, Allen MH, Barker JNWN, Haskard DO, MacDonald DM. Endothelial leucocyte adhesion molecule-1 (ELAM-1) expression in cutaneous inflammation. Br J Dermatol 1991; 124:117–123.

193. Groves RW, Ross E, Barker JNWN, Ross JS, Camp RDR, MacDonald DM. Effect of in vivo interleukin-1 on adhesion molecule expression in normal human skin. J Invest Dermatol 1992; 98:384–387.

194. Groves RW, Allen MH, Ross EL, Barker JNWN, MacDonald DM. Tumour necrosis factor alpha is pro-inflammatory in normal human skin and modulates cutaneous adhesion molecule expression. Br J Dermatol 1995; 132:345–352.

195. Briscoe D, Cotran R, Pober J. Effects of TNF, LPS, and IL-4 on the expression of VCAM-1 in vivo: correlation with CD3+ T cell infiltration. J Immunol 1992; 149:2954–2960.

196. Lechleitner S, Gille J, Johnson DR, Petzelbauer P. Interferon enhances tumor necrosis factor-induced vascular cell adhesion molecule 1 (CD106) expression in human endothelial cells by an interferon-related factor 1-dependent pathway. J Exp Med 1998; 187:2023–2030.

197. Detmar M, Imcke E, Ruszczak Z, Orfanos CE. Effects of recombinant tumor necrosis factor-alpha on cultured microvascular endothelial cells derived from human dermis. J Invest Dermatol 1990; 95:S219–S222.

198. Swerlick RA, Garcia-Gonzalez E, Kubota Y, Xu YL, Lawley TJ. Studies of the modulation of MHC antigen and cell adhesion molecule expression on human dermal microvascular endothelial cells. J Invest Dermatol 1991; 97:190–196.

199. de Vries IJM, Langeveld-Wildschut EG, van Reijsen FC, Dubois GR, van den Hoek JA, Bihari IC, van Wichen D, de Weger RA, Knol EF, Thepen T, Bruijnzeel-Koomen CAFM. Adhesion molecule expression on skin endothelia in atopic dermatitis: effects of TNFα and IL-4. J Allergy Clin Immunol 1998; 102:461–468.

200. Gille J, Swerlick R, Lawley T, Caughman S. Differential regulation of vascular cell adhesion molecule-1 gene transcription by tumor necrosis factor alpha and interleukin-1 alpha in dermal microvascular endothelial cells. Blood 1996; 87:211–217.

201. Kluger MS, Johnson DR, Pober JS. Mechanism of sustained E-selectin expression in cultured human dermal microvascular endothelial cells. J Immunol 1997; 158:887–896.

202. Sepp NT, Gille J, Li LJ, Caughman SW, Lawley TJ, Swerlick RA. A factor in human plasma permits persistent expression of E-selectin by human endothelial cells. J Invest Dermatol 1994; 102:445–450.

203. Cornelius LA, Sepp N, Li LJ, Degitz K, Swerlick RA, Lawley TJ, Caughman SW. Selective

upregulation of intercellular adhesion molecule (ICAM-1) by ultraviolet b in human dermal microvascular endothelial cells. J Invest Dermatol 1994; 103:23–28.

204. Heckmann M, Eberlein-Konig B, Wollenberg A, Przybilla B, Plewig G. Ultraviolet-A radiation induces adhesion molecule expression on human dermal microvascular endothelial cells. Br J Dermatol 1994; 131:311–318.

205. Gille J, Paxton LLL, Lawley TJ, Caughman SW, Swerlick RA. Retinoic acid inhibits the regulated expression of vascular cell adhesion molecule-1 by cultured dermal microvascular endothelial cells. J Clin Invest 1997; 99:492–500.

206. Moser R, Groscurth P, Carballido JM, Bruijnzeel PLB, Blaser K, Heusser CH, Fehr J. Interleukin-4 induces tissue eosinophilia in mice: Correlation with its in vitro capacity to stimulate the endothelial cell-dependent selective transmigration of human eosinophils. J Lab Clin Med 1993; 122:567–575.

207. Tepper RI, Levinson DA, Stanger BZ, Campos-Torres J, Abbas AK, Leder P. IL-4 induces allergic-like inflammatory disease and alters T cell development in transgenic mice. Cell 1990; 62:457–467.

208. Tepper RI, Pattengale PK, Leder P. Murine interleukin-4 displays potent anti-tumor activity in vivo. Cell 1989; 57:503–512.

209. Weg VB, Williams TJ, Lobb RR, Nourshargh S. A monoclonal antibody recognizing very late activation antigen-4 inhibits eosinophil accumulation in vivo. J Exp Med 1993; 177: 561–566.

210. Sanz MJ, Hartnell A, Chisholm P, Williams C, Davies D, Weg VB, Feldmann M, Bolanowski MA, Lobb RR, Nourshargh S. Tumor necrosis factor $\alpha$-induced eosinophil accumulation in rat skin is dependent on $\alpha 4$ integrin/vascular cell adhesion molecule-1 adhesion pathways. Blood 1997; 90:4144–4152.

211. Sanz MJ, Marinova-Mutafchieva L, Green P, Lobb RR, Feldmann M, Nourshargh S. IL-4-induced eosinophil accumulation in rat skin is dependent on endogenous TNF-$\alpha$ and $\alpha 4$ integrin/VCAM-1 adhesion pathways. J Immunol 1998; 160:5637–5645.

212. Sanz MJ, Ponath PD, Mackay CR, Newman W, Miyasaka M, Tamatani T, Flanagan BF, Lobb RR, Williams TJ, Nourshargh S, Jose PJ. Human eotaxin induces $\alpha 4$ and $\beta 2$ integrin-dependent eosinophil accumulation in rat skin in vivo: Delayed generation of eotaxin in response to IL-4. J Immunol 1998; 160:3569–3576.

213. Springer TA. Traffic signals for lymphocyte recirculation and leukocyte emigration: the multistep paradigm. Cell 1994; 76:301–314.

214. Lawrence MB, Springer TA. Neutrophils roll on E-selectin. J Immunol 1993; 151:6338–6346.

215. Sriramarao P, von Andrian UH, Butcher EC, Bourdon MA, Broide DH. L-selectin and very late antigen-4 integrin promote eosinophil rolling at physiological shear rates in vivo. J Immunol 1994; 153:4238–4246.

216. Johnston B, Issekutz TB, Kubes P. The $\alpha 4$-integrin supports leukocyte rolling and adhesion in chronically inflamed postcapillary venules in vivo. J Exp Med 1996; 183:1995–2006.

217. Granger DN, Kubes P. The microcirculation and inflammation: modulation of leukocyte-endothelial adhesion. J Leukoc Biol 1994; 55:662–675.

218. Detmar M, Brown LF, Schon MP, Elicker BM, Velasco P, Richard L, Fukumura D, Monsky W, Claffey KP, Jain RK. Increased microvascular density and enhanced leukocyte rolling and adhesion in the skin of VEGF transgenic mice. J Invest Dermatol 1998; 111:1–6.

219. Lorant DE, Patel KD, Mcintyre TM, McEver RP, Prescott SM, Zimmerman GA. Coexpression of GMP-140 and PAF by endothelium stimulated by histamine or thrombin—a juxtacrine system for adhesion and activation of neutrophils. J Cell Biol 1991; 115:223–234.

220. Tanaka Y, Adams DH, Hubscher S, Hirano H, Siebenlist U, Shaw S. T-cell adhesion induced by proteoglycan-immobilized cytokine MIP-1$\beta$. Nature 1993; 361:79–82.

221. Schall TJ, Bacon KB. Chemokines, leukocyte trafficking, and inflammation. Curr Opin Immunol 1994; 6:865–873.

222. Schall T. Fractalkine—a strange attractor in the chemokine landscape. Immunol Today 1997; 18:147–147.

223. Hakkert BC, Kuijpers TW, Leeuwenberg JFM, van Mourik JA, Roos D. Neutrophil and monocyte adherence to and migration across monolayers of cytokine-activated endothelial cells: the contribution of CD18, ELAM-1, and VLA-4. Blood 1991; 78:2721–2726.

224. Luscinskas FW, Cybulsky MI, Kiely J-M, Peckins CS, Davis VM, Gimbrone MA Jr. Cytokine-activated human endothelial monolayers support enhanced neutrophil transmigration via a mechanism involving both endothelial-leukocyte adhesion molecule-1 and intracellular adhesion molecule-1. J Immunol 1991; 146:1617–1625.

225. Babi LFS, Moser R, Soler MTP, Picker LJ, Blaser K, Hauser C. Migration of skin-homing T cells across cytokine-activated human endothelial cell layers involves interaction of the cutaneous lymphocyte-associated antigen (CLA), the very late antigen-4 (VLA-4), and the lymphocyte function-associated antigen-1 (LFA-1). J Immunol 1995; 154:1543–1550.

226. Allport JR, Ding H, Collins T, Gerritsen ME, Luscinskas FW. Endothelial-dependent mechanisms regulate leukocyte transmigration: A process involving the proteasome and disruption of the vascular endothelial-cadherin complex at endothelial cell-to-cell junctions. J Exp Med 1997; 186:517–527.

227. Okada S, Kita H, George TJ, Gleich GJ, Leiferman KM. Migration of eosinophils through basement membrane components in vitro: Role of matrix metalloproteinase-9. Am J Respir Cell Molec Biol 1997; 17:519–528.

228. Vliagoftis H, Metcalfe DD. Cell adhesion molecules in mast cell adhesion and migration. In: Bochner BS, ed. Adhesion Molecules in Allergic Diseases. New York: Marcel Dekker, Inc., 1997:151–172.

229. Price AA, Cumberbatch M, Kimber I, Ager A. α6 integrins are required for Langerhans cell migration from the epidermis. J Exp Med 1997; 186:1725–1735.

230. Kuijpers TW, vanLier RAW, Hamann D, de Boer M, Thung LY, Weening RS, Verhoeven AJ, Roos D. Leukocyte adhesion deficiency type 1 (LAD-1)/variant—a novel immunodeficiency syndrome characterized by dysfunctional β2 integrins. J Clin Invest 1997; 100:1725–1733.

231. Etzioni A, Frydman M, Pollack S, Avidor I, Phillips ML, Paulson JC, Gershoni-Baruch R. Brief report—recurrent severe infections caused by a novel leukocyte adhesion deficiency. N Engl J Med 1992; 327:1789–1792.

232. von Andrian UH, Berger EM, Ramezani L, Chambers JD, Ochs HD, Harlan JM, Paulson JC, Etzioni A, Arfors KE. In vivo behavior of neutrophils from 2 patients with distinct inherited leukocyte adhesion deficiency syndromes. J Clin Invest 1993; 91:2893–2897.

233. Karsan A, Cornejo CJ, Winn RK, Schwartz BR, Way W, Lannir N, Gershoni-Baruch R, Etzioni A, Ochs HD, Harlan JM. Leukocyte Adhesion Deficiency Type II is a generalized defect of de novo GDP-fucose biosynthesis—endothelial cell fucosylation is not required for neutrophil rolling on human nonlymphoid endothelium. J Clin Invest 1998; 101:2438–2445.

234. Sturla L, Etzioni A, Bisso A, Zanardi D, DeFlora G, Silengo L, DeFlora A, Tonetti M. Defective intracellular activity of GDP-D-mannose-4,6-dehydratase in leukocyte adhesion deficiency type II syndrome. FEBS Lett 1998; 429:274–278.

235. Etzioni A, Gershoni-Baruch R, Pollack S, Shehadeh N. Leukocyte adhesion deficiency type II: long term follow-up. J Allergy Clin Immunol 1998; 102:323–324.

236. Scharffetter-Kochanek K, Lu HF, Norman K, van Nood N, Munoz F, Grabbe S, McArthur M, Lorenzo I, Kaplan S, Ley K, Smith CW, Montgomery CA, Rich S, Beaudet AL. Spontaneous skin ulceration and defective T cell function in CD18 null mice. J Exp Med 1998; 188:119–131.

237. Mizgerd JP, Kubo H, Kutkoski GJ, Bhagwan SD, Scharffetter-Kochanek K, Beaudet AL, Doerschuk CM. Neutrophil emigration in the skin, lungs, and peritoneum: different requirements for CD11/CD18 revealed by CD18-deficient mice. J Exp Med 1997; 186:1357–1364.

238. Tang MLK, Hale LP, Steeber DA, Tedder TF. L-selectin is involved in lymphocyte migration to sites of inflammation in the skin—delayed rejection of allografts in L-selectin-deficient mice. J Immunol 1997; 158:5191–5199.

239. Pellegrini G, Deluca M, Orecchia G, Balzac F, Cremona O, Savoia P, Cancedda R, Marchisio PC. Expression, topography, and function of integrin receptors are severely altered in keratinocytes from involved and uninvolved psoriatic skin. J Clin Invest 1992; 89:1783–1795.

240. Penas PF, Gomez M, Buezo GF, Rios L, Yanez-Mo M, Cabanas C, Sanchez-Madrid F, Garcia-Diez A. Differential expression of activation epitopes of β1 integrins in psoriasis and normal skin. J Invest Dermatol 1998; 111:19–24.

241. Carroll JM, Romero MR, Watt FM. Suprabasal integrin expression in the epidermis of transgenic mice results in developmental defects and a phenotype resembling psoriasis. Cell 1995; 83:957–968.

242. Brown TA, Gil SG, Sybert VP, Lestringant GG, Tadini G, Caputo R, Carter WG. Defective integrin α6β4 expression in the skin of patients with junctional epidermolysis bullosa and pyloric atresia. J Invest Dermatol 1996; 107:384–391.

243. Pulkkinen L, Bruckner-Tuderman L, August C, Uitto J. Compound heterozygosity for missense (L156P) and nonsense (R554X) mutations in the β4 integrin gene (ITGB4) underlies mild, nonlethal phenotype of epidermolysis bullosa with pyloric atresia. Am J Pathol 1998; 152:935–941.

244. Ruzzi L, Gagnoux-Palacios L, Pinola M, Belli S, Meneguzzi G, D'Alessio M, Zambruno G. A homozygous mutation in the integrin α6 gene in junctional epidermolysis bullosa with pyloric atresia. J Clin Invest 1997; 99:2826–2831.

245. Lazarova Z, Yee C, Darling T, Briggaman RA, Yancey KB. Passive transfer of anti-laminin 5 antibodies induces subepidermal blisters in neonatal mice. J Clin Invest 1996; 98:1509–1518.

246. Matsuyoshi N, Tanaka T, Toda K, Okamoto H, Furukawa F, Imamura S. Soluble E-cadherin: a novel cutaneous disease marker. Br J Dermatol 1995; 132:745–749.

247. Kyan-Aung U, Haskard DO, Poston RN, Thornhill MH, Lee TH. Endothelial leukocyte adhesion molecule-1 and intercellular adhesion molecule-1 mediate the adhesion of eosinophils to endothelial cells in vitro and are expressed by endothelium in allergic cutaneous inflammation in vivo. J Immunol 1991; 146:521–528.

248. Leung DYM, Pober JS, Cotran RS. Expression of endothelial-leukocyte adhesion molecule-1 in elicited late phase allergic reactions. J Clin Invest 1991; 87:1805–1809.

249. Schleimer RP, Bochner BS. Letter to the editor. J Immunol 1991; 147:380–381.

250. Frew AJ, Kay AB. UCHL1+ (CD45RO+) memory T-cells predominate in the CD4+ cellular infiltrate associated with allergen-induced late-phase skin reactions in atopic subjects. Clin Exp Immunol 1991; 84:270–274.

251. Gaga M, Frew AJ, Varney VA, Kay AB. Eosinophil activation and T lymphocyte infiltration in allergen-induced late phase skin reactions and classical delayed-type hypersensitivity. J Immunol 1991; 147:816–822.

252. Babi LFS, Picker LJ, Soler MTP, Drzimalla K, Flohr P, Blaser K, Hauser C. Circulating allergen-reactive T cells from patients with atopic dermatitis and allergic contact dermatitis express the skin-selective homing receptor, the cutaneous lymphocyte-associated antigen. J Exp Med 1995; 181:1935–1940.

253. Werfel S, Massey W, Lichtenstein LM, Bochner BS. Preferential recruitment of activated, memory T-lymphocytes into skin chamber fluids during human cutaneous late phase allergic reactions. J Allergy Clin Immunol 1995; 96:57–65.

254. de Vries IJM, Langeveld-Wildschut EG, van Reijsen FC, Bihari IC, Bruijnzeel-Koomen CAFM, Thepen T. Nonspecific T-cell homing during inflammation in atopic dermatitis: expression of cutaneous lymphocyte-associated antigen and integrin alpha E beta 7 on skin-infiltrating T cells. J Allergy Clin Immunol 1997; 100:694–701.

255. Ying S, Meng Q, Barata LT, Robinson DS, Durham SR, Kay AB. Associations between IL-

13 and IL-4 (mRNA and protein), vascular cell adhesion molecule-1 expression, and the infiltration of eosinophils, macrophages, and T cells in allergen-induced late-phase cutaneous reactions in atopic subjects. J Immunol 1997; 158:5050–5057.

256. Jung K, Linse F, Heller R, Moths C, Goebel R, Neumann C. Adhesion molecules in atopic dermatitis: VCAM-1 and ICAM-1 expression is increased in healthy-appearing skin. Allergy 1996; 51:452–460.

257. Wakita H, Sakamoto T, Tokura Y, Takigawa M. E-selectin and vascular cell adhesion molecule-1 as critical adhesion molecules for infiltration of T lymphocytes and eosinophils in atopic dermatitis. J Cutan Pathol 1994; 21:33–39.

258. Groves RW, Kapahi P, Barker JNWN, Haskard DO, MacDonald DM. Detection of circulating adhesion molecules in erythrodermic skin disease. J Am Acad Dermatol 1995; 33:32–36.

259. Czech W, Schopf E, Kapp A. Soluble E-selectin in sera of patients with atopic dermatitis and psoriasis—correlation with disease activity. Br J Dermatol 1996; 134:17–21.

260. Wolkerstorfer A, Laan MP, Savelkoul HFJ, Neijens HJ, Mulder PGH, Oudesluys-Murphy AM, Sukhai RN, Oranje AP. Soluble E-selectin, other markers of inflammation and disease severity in children with atopic dermatitis. Br J Dermatol 1998; 138:431–435.

261. Yamashita N, Kaneko S, Kouro O, Furue M, Yamamoto S, Sakane T. Soluble E-selectin as a marker of disease activity in atopic dermatitis. J Allergy Clin Immunol 1997; 99:410–416.

262. Kowalzick L, Kleinheinz A, Weichenthal M, Neuber K, Kohler I, Grosch J, Ring J. Effects of medium-dose UV-A1 on clinical course and serum levels of sICAM-1, sE-selection, sIL-2R and ECP in severe atopic eczema. J Invest Dermatol 1995; 105:82A.

263. Chen K-R, Pittelkow MR, Su WPD, Gleich GJ, Newman W, Leiferman KM. Recurrent cutaneous necrotizing eosinophilic vasculitis: a novel eosinophil mediated syndrome. Arch Dermatol 1994; 130:1159–1166.

264. Bochner BS. Cellular adhesion and its antagonism. J Allergy Clin Immunol 1997; 100:581–585.

265. Bochner BS. Targeting VLA-4 integrin function: potential therapeutic implications. In: Mousa SA, ed. Cell Adhesion Molecules and Matrix Proteins in Health and Disease. Georgetown, TX: Landes Bioscience, 1998:113–131.

# 6

## Pathophysiology of Pruritus

**Malcoln W. Greaves**

*United Medical and Dental School of Guy's and St. Thomas' Hospitals, King's College, London, England*

## I. INTRODUCTION

Itching is the dominant symptom of skin diseases. Almost all skin lesions, whether inflammatory neoplastic, proliferative, or degenerative, can and do itch. Since, by definition, itching leads to rubbing or scratching, this intervention can modify the clinical appearances of the skin, making diagnosis more difficult. Itching is also a common and important manifestation of systemic disease and may be associated with a skin that looks healthy apart from the consequences of rubbing or scratching including excoriations, nodules, papules, lichenification (superficial thickening and coarsening of the skin), and bruising. Itching in the presence of a normal-looking skin should prompt thorough clinical laboratory and radiological assessment. However, all too frequently itching, either localized or generalized, is a presenting complaint in an otherwise apparently healthy individual. Patients with "idiopathic" pruritus constitute about 40% of the patients attending my regular itch clinic. Their management is a major problem, but recent better understanding of the molecular and neurophysiological basis of itching could shortly lead to a better success rate in treatment.

It is important to appreciate that, at the time of writing, there are no selective "anti-itch" drugs. Antihistamines relieve the itching of urticaria and some other inflammatory skin disorders, but they are not intrinsically antipruritic; they simply relieve itching when it is caused by histamine but are otherwise ineffective. Likewise corticosteroids only relieve itching associated with inflammation; they are not true antipruritics. Some newer agents including opioid peptide antagonists and capsaicin seem promising but have yet to achieve the status of antipruritic drugs.

Itching is evolutionarily venerable. Feathered dinosaurs have been shown by paleontologists to have had ectoparasites on their feathers. It is suggested that the purpose of itching was originally to enable these to be detached by scratching. Scratching an itch can be quite pleasurable, but for many it causes acute distress, depression, and even suicidal inclination.

## II. MEASUREMENT OF ITCH

One of the problems that has retarded research on itch and its treatment is the lack of direct objective measurements of itch. There is no satisfactory animal model for itch. The recent report [1] of an "itchy" gene mutation in a18H mice that leads to scratching is misleading. This mutation actually leads to multisystem inflammatory disease including the skin, a consequence of which is scratching. In fact, there is no means of knowing whether an animal that scratches actually perceives itching; other noxious sensations could well lead to scratching.

In humans there is no such problem; everyone can recognize itching when it occurs. Thus, the most widely used measure of itching in humans has been the visual analog scale for intensity of itching and its recent refinement, the microcomputer-based self-data-logging portable system [2]. However, this method is indirect, subjective, and does not lend itself to statistical analysis. Scratching can be measured fairly easily; it is an objective measurement but indirect, since it depends on the assumption of a linear quantitative relationship between itch and scratch. Numerous ingenious methods have been devised including using self-winding watches to measure scratching instead of recording the time and placing of transducers on the nail plates of both middle fingers (since scratching or rubbing is normally executed with the middle finger) [3]. Perhaps the recent identification, by functional positron emission topography, of an "itch center" in the brain (see below) may lead to a direct objective measure of itch.

## III. PATHOPHYSIOLOGY OF ITCH AND MOLECULAR MECHANISMS

### A. Receptors and Mediators

There are no specialized receptors for itch in the skin. Thus, itch appears to cause responses in unspecialized free nerve endings in the epidermis and around the dermo-epidermal junction. These "itch points" were originally identified by using the ultrafine spicules of cowhage. These spicules, when inserted into the skin at an "itch point" (i.e., at the site of an unspecialized nerve ending) could cause intense itching due to release of proteolytic enzymes. In inflamed skin, including urticaria, atopic eczema, contact allergic dermatitis, it is assumed that pharmacological mediators (histamine, interleukin-2, proteases, neuro-peptides) released from the inflamed skin, evoke itching by a direct action on these receptors. Some of these pruritogenic mediators, their sources, and receptors are listed in Table 1.

Prostaglandins, although not intrinsically pruritogenic, enhance itching due to other pruritic mediators such as histamine [4]. Histamine generates itch through $H_1$ but not $H_2$ receptors [5]. It also causes itching in two distinct ways. Intradermal injection of histamine causes itch directly by its action on receptive nerve endings through an $H_1$ action as outlined above. It also renders a zone of surrounding skin abnormally sensitive to other stimuli normally perceived as causing tactile, pressure, or temperature-change sensations. Instead

**Table 1**  Candidate Mediators of Itch

| Mediator | Source | Receptor |
|---|---|---|
| Histamine | Mast cells, basophils | $H_1$ |
| Interleukin-2 | TH1 lymphocytes | IL-2r |
| Opioid peptides | Neurones | $\mu, \delta$ |
| Subst. P. | Neurones | SPr |
| Proteases | Granulocytes, macrophages | ? |

of these stimuli being perceived as the corresponding sensation, they are instead perceived as itch—a phenomenon described years ago as "itchy skin" by Bickford and more recently termed "alloknesis." It may explain the intense pruritus experienced by atopic eczema patients in response to sudden changes in temperature and contact of skin with clothing.

Interleukin 2 (IL-2) has only recently been recognized as an important mediator of itching in inflammatory skin disease. It causes intense itching when injected intradermally and following systemic administration [7,8]. Reduction in IL-2 tissue levels may also be the explanation for the rapid suppression of itching caused by cyclosporine in patients with atopic dermatitis. Evidence for the importance of substance P in itching is mainly indirect and is based upon immunocytochemical evidence of co-localization of unmyelinated nerve endings and substance P in epidermis and the association of depletion of this neuropeptide by topical capsaicin with amelioration of itching.

## B.  Neuronal Pathways

For many years the standard teaching was that pain and itch utilized identical neural pathways, itching being no more than a mild form of pain. However, this view was clearly inconsistent with a number of simple observational data including the fact that itch and pain can be perceived simultaneously at the same site, that itch and pain elicit different reflex responses, and that morphine relieves pain but exacerbates itch. Itch is never felt in deeper organs such as joints, muscle, and intestines, which can be the source of exquisite pain. Recently evidence has emerged to strengthen a long-held suspicion that there may be itch-dedicated unmyelinated nociceptor C fibers. These so-called silent fibers, each of which enjoys an unusually large receptive field, were identified in humans by microneurography and proved insensitive to mechanical and heat stimulation but highly sensitive to histamine iontophoresis-induced itch. However, they only represent a small (5–10%) proportion of the total C fibers [9]. One other remarkable fact about these seemingly dedicated itch nerve fibers is that they show a uniquely slow conduction velocity, explaining the clinical observation that there is a delay of a few seconds before itch is perceived after an itch stimulus is applied to the skin.

Secondary transmission neurones conduct the itch signal across the spinal cord to the opposite side and ascend in the contra-lateral spinothalamic tract to the thalamus. From the thalamus a final neural pathway is presumed to relay the signal to the cerebral cortex, thus enabling conscious perception of itch. However, this part of the itch neural pathway has not been fully anatomically characterized.

Is there an "itch center" in the brain? Recent studies using functional positron emission tomography suggest there may be. Induction of itch in the leg by histamine iontophoresis leads to focal increase in metabolic activity in the contra-lateral anterior cingulate gyrus region (Brodman area 24). In contrast the intention to scratch is associated with focal increase in blood flow in the premotor area on the opposite side [10]. These data need to be reproduced using other nonhistaminic pruritic stimuli. The pathways outlined above are illustrated in Figure 1.

## C.  Modulation of Perception of Itch

Why does scratching or rubbing relieve itch, albeit temporarily? The explanation lies in the phenomenon of "surround inhibition" [11]. Pinpoint activation of itching, e.g., by

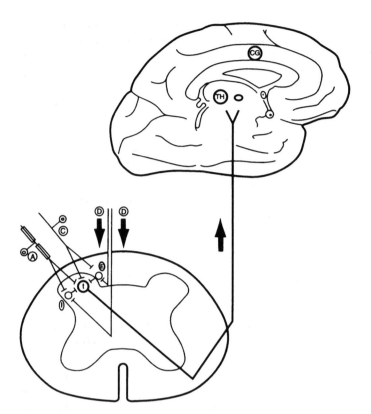

**Figure 1**  Pathways for itch in cord and brain. A = Fast-conducting myelinated A neurones; C = slow conducting unmyelinated C neurones; I = inhibitory neuronal circuits; E = excitatory neuronal circuits; t = transmission neurone; D = descending pathways from peri-aqueductal region; TH = thalamus; CG = cingulate gyrus (Brodman area 24).

applying the end of a stiff hair to the skin, causes a signal to be transmitted through a nociceptor C fiber. Concurrent activation of amplifying neuronal circuits in the substantia gelatinosa of the grey matter of the cord (E in Fig. 1) leads to augmentation of the signal, a state of local excitation perceived by the subject as an almost intolerable itch. Rubbing or scratching activates fast-conducting myelinated A fibers, which in turn activate inhibitory neuronal circuits in the grey matter of the dorsal horn (I in Fig. 1), leading to downregulation of the itch signal or ''surround inhibition'' and a temporarily suppressed state of itching. Probably application of local vibratory stimuli and transepidermal electrical nerve stimulation (TENS) act similarly. These excitatory and inhibitory neuronal circuits, which help modulate itch, are also influenced by signals descending from higher centers in the periaqueductal region of the brain (marked D in Fig. 1).

Perception of itch can be modulated by skin temperature changes. Cooling (10°C) usually reduces or abolishes itch, whereas warming the skin (45°C) greatly aggravates itching in one third of subjects but reduces or abolishes it in one third [12]. These responses, which are probably due to a direct action of temperature on itch-sensitive nerve endings, may go some way towards explaining the common observation of pruritic patients that the symptom seems to be worse when warm and mitigated when cool.

## D. Opioid Peptides

That intraspinal morphine analgesia frequently causes troublesome localized or more widespread pruritus has been recognized for many years and is explained by the existence of $\mu$ or $\delta$ opioid receptors in the central nervous system. A similar response is recognized to occur following intravenous morphine. These responses are inhibited by the opioid $\mu$ receptor antagonist naloxone. Interestingly, use of this antagonist is not necessarily associated with loss of analgesia [13]. Opioids cause itching not only in the central nervous system but also peripherally. Morphine and opioid peptides cause itching upon intradermal injection and also enhance the itching actions of other pruritogenic mediators [14]. At least part of their peripheral actions may also be explained by the release of histamine (and probably other mediators) from cutaneous mast cells [15]. The importance of the opioid peptides as mediators of pruritus remains to be established, but persuasive data (see below) suggest their importance in the pruritus of cholestasis. Interpretation of findings using selective antagonists such as naloxone will have to take into account both peripheral and central actions of opioid peptides.

## IV. ITCH AS A SYMPTOM OF SYSTEMIC DISEASE

Itch occurring in the skin looks clinically normal (apart from the effects of rubbing or scratching) must always be looked upon as a manifestation of underlying systemic disease until proved otherwise.

## A. Diabetes Mellitus

Generalized itching is a very rare manifestation of diabetes mellitus despite statements in reviews and textbooks to the contrary. This piece of medical apocrypha originated in a 1927 paper reporting findings in the skin in 500 cases of diabetes. Only 16 had generalized pruritus (3%) [16] This percentage, which has been confirmed by more recent studies, is not significantly different than in the nondiabetic general population [17]. However, localized anogenital pruritus, often associated with candidosis, is quite common in diabetics, who may also suffer from a peculiar localized scalp pruritus.

## B. Itch and Malignant Disease

Should patients with generalized pruritus be evaluated for underlying malignancy? There is very little hard evidence, but it is prudent to look for lympho-reticular malignancy including Hodgkin's lymphoma and non-Hodgkin's lymphoma in patients with onset of generalized pruritus. An association with solid tumors is doubtful except for gall bladder, liver or pancreatic tumors causing cholestasis. This subject has been usefully reviewed [18].

## C. Cholestatic Itching

Traditionally, cholestatic itching due to biliary obstruction has been attributed to elevated plasma bile salt levels, on the basis that cholestyramine, an oral exchange resin that lowers plasma levels of bile salts, causes some relief of pruritus and the pruritic action of bile salts when applied to a raw blister base in skin. However, the correlation between bile salt levels and pruritus is poor and recently opioid peptides have been implicated. Almost 20 years ago intravenous naloxone was demonstrated on a double-blind placebo-controlled basis to relieve the pruritus of obstructive jaundice [19]. This finding has been subsequently confirmed independently. It is of interest that administration of naloxone to patients with cholestasis may lead to symptoms resembling those typical of opiate withdrawal [20]. Other treatments proposed to relieve the itching of cholestasis include phenobarbitone, charcoal, and ursodeoxycholic acid.

Besides the well-known causes of cholestasis (gallstones, carcinoma of the bile ducts or head of pancreas, viral hepatitis, sclerosing cholangitis, drug hepatotoxicity), less well-recognized causes need to be considered. These include cholestasis of pregnancy [21] and the Alagille syndrome (congenital hypoplasia of intrahepatic bile ducts, pruritus, jaundice, xanthomata, and vascular anomalies) as a cause of pruritus in infancy [22].

## D.  Renal Itching

A number of factors are believed to contribute to the pruritus of renal failure. These include an excessively dry skin, secondary hyperparathyroidism, increased numbers of cutaneous mast cells and polyneuropathy. Undoubtedly use of emollients helps some patients, but dryness is not a major cause. Secondary hyperparathyroidism occurs as a specific clinical problem in only a small number of renal failure patients, and parathormone itself is not pruritogenic. The increased numbers of mast cells and nerve fibers in the skin in renal failure are probably reactive. Recently a placebo-controlled trial has yielded data suggesting that naltrexone, an oral μ receptor opioid antagonist, may be helpful in these patients [23]. Other treatments proposed include cholestyramine, ultraviolet B phototherapy, parenteral lignocaine, and heparin.

## V.  SOME IMPORTANT ITCHES

A number of important causes of itch can easily be missed.

## A.  Itching in the Elderly

Itching in old people is an increasingly common problem given the increasing proportion of the elderly in our populations. In every elderly patient with an itch, great care must be taken to exclude cutaneous and systemic causes, especially renal and hepatic disease. In many patients the itch can be attributed to excessive drying of the skin (xerosis). One interesting type of itching in the elderly with a dry skin is the condition Kligman and I termed ''water-induced itching of the elderly'' [24]. It, like other types of itch due to xerosis, responds well to emollient treatment, which distinguishes it from ordinary aquagenic pruritus (see below), in which the skin is normally hydrated and which does not respond to emollients. Dry skin in the elderly is due to a combination of deterioration of the hygroscopic qualities and barrier function of the epidermis, together with environmental factors, especially prolonged institutional exposure to high-temperature, low-humidity environments.

## B. Hydroxyethyl Starch–Induced Pruritus

This plasma substitute is used to improve arterial perfusion in a range of disorders including peripheral vascular disease and neurological and otological disorders. It is also used to help maintain plasma volume in patients during cardiopulmonary bypass surgery. The pruritus usually persists for around a year after the administration of the plasma expander and is both widespread and severe. Examination of skin biopsy material reveals vacuolated macrophages and Schwann cells in which electron-dense material can be found, presumably due to phagocytosis of the starch material by these cells [25]. Pruritus in the patients is highly resistant to treatment, but topical capsaicin or ultraviolet B phototherapy may help.

## C. Pemphigoid Nodularis

This is a mainly nonbullous variant of the autoimmune blistering disorder bullous pemphigoid, which presents with extensive prurigo nodularis. The presenting complaint is of widespread pruritus evoking scratching, rubbing, and the development of multiple firm, pigmented papules and nodules. Blistering may occur later on in the course of the disease, but initially it is not conspicuous. A skin biopsy shows epidermal acanthosis characteristic of nodular prurigo. However, direct immuno-fluorescence examination reveals deposition of immuno-reactants (IgG and C'3) at the dermoepidermal junction. The sodium chloride split skin technique reveals that these immuno-reactants map to the roof of the blister, and immuno-blotting shows that the antibodies are reacting with 180 and 230 KDa epitopes related to the hemidesmosomal and desmoplakin proteins [26]. The pruritus responds to systemic steroids with or without oral azathioprine.

## D. Onchocerciasis

This diagnosis should be considered in anyone with widespread pruritus and unremarkable skin changes who has spent some time (resident) in Africa or Central or South America. A mild papular or slightly lichenified eruption on the affected skin may be all that is visible. The disease is due to infestation by a filarial worm *Onchocerca volvulus*. The microfilaria migrate to the skin and eye, causing pruritus and blindness. A skin snip examined microscopically reveals the causative microfilaria. Ivermectin is a highly effective treatment in a single-dose regime [27].

## E. Aquagenic Pruritus

Although first described by W. B. Shelley, this pruritus was originally established as a distinct clinical and pathological entity by the author [28]. The condition is not rare and still causes diagnostic confusion. Patients, usually adults, give a protracted history of intense, distressing, widespread pruritus occurring after contact with water at any temperature and without visible signs in the skin. Lack of visible changes in the skin frequently results in patients being labeled as psychoneurotic. However, elevated skin histamine levels and increased mast cell population density in skin are demonstrable. The importance of recognizing the condition is substantiated by its good response to PUVA (photochemotherapy with 8-methoxy psoralen and UVA) [29] as is the importance of follow-up because some of these patients go on subsequently to develop polycythemia vera or other bone-marrow–derived disorders. This condition is described in greater detail in Chapter 8, p. 181.

## F.  Brachioradial Pruritus

As the western world becomes populated by an increasing proportion of leisured, well-to-do elderly, problems relating to chronic sun damage become increasingly prevalent. One such problem is brachioradial pruritus, a chronic pruritic condition mainly affecting the outer surfaces of the upper arm, elbow, and forearm. It is due to chronic sun damage and occurs in golfers, sailing enthusiasts, tennis players, and other exponents of outdoor leisure activities in sunny climes. It occurs particularly in those who habitually wear short-sleeved shirts and can be more than simply a nuisance, but it does respond to topical capsaicin [30].

## G.  The Itch of HIV

Pruritus is a common complaint in HIV-infected patients. However, it is important to exclude primary skin disease (seborrhoeic eczema, psoriasis, adverse drug reactions, urticaria) and systemic causes (chronic renal or hepatobiliary disease, thyroid disease, lymphoma). Characteristically pruritus of HIV disease presents as scattered excoriated pink or pigmented papules and scars. Lichenification may also be present. The pruritus may respond to oral metronidazole, phototherapy (UVB or PUVA), or topical 5% doxepin. HIV pruritus needs to be distinguished from eosinophilic folliculitis, which may also be pruritic and which may also respond to PUVA [31].

## VI.  INVESTIGATION OF PRURITUS

This section focuses on the problem of the patient with generalized pruritus but without a visible rash. It is worthwhile pointing out that some physical urticarias (dermographism, cholinergic urticaria) not uncommonly present with pruritus without a rash at the time of examination, although the typical urticarial eruption is easily provoked by appropriate physical urticaria challenge testing.

## A.  History

Few appreciate the importance of obtaining a detailed history of the character of the pruritus. Pruritus evoked by contact with clothes, change of temperature, or bathing suggests an underlying cutaneously derived itch (dryness, low-grade eczema causing alloknesis, or dermographism). The itch of inflammatory skin disease is usually burning or pricking in nature, but patients with an itch of a psychoneurotic type frequently mention a sensation of insects crawling on the skin. However, this symptom may also be described by patients who actually do have insects crawling over the skin (pediculosis). The regional distribution is also important. Aquagenic pruritus frequently affects the legs with or without spread to other areas of the body.

## B.  Examination and Review of Systems

A careful examination of the skin can yield dividends (xerosis, warm sweaty skin of thyrotoxicosis, jaundice, minimal atopic eczema, mastocytosis, micropapular lichen planus, cholinergic urticaria are a few examples easily missed). The routine screening labora-

**Table 2**  Recommended Screening Laboratory Tests for the Itchy Patient

1. Full blood count, with differential white blood cell count and erythrocyte sedimentation rate
2. Renal function tests including blood urea and serum creatinine
3. Liver function tests including alkaline phosphatase, serum bilirubin, and hepatitis B/C serology
4. Thyroid function tests including T4 and thyroid-stimulating hormone (TSH) plasma level
5. Sugar in urine and blood
6. Stool[a] for occult blood
7. Chest x-ray
8. Plasma FSH and LH in postmenopausal females

[a] Also stool examination for parasites if there is a blood eosinophilia.

tory tests that should be carried out in all patients without an evident cutaneous cause for the itch are listed in Table 2.

The localized nature of some types of pruritus is well recognized. These include pruritus of the scalp in diabetics, itching of the center of the back in notalgia paraesthetica, and brachioradial pruritus (see above). A careful drug history is important since drugs can cause intense pruritus in the absence of a rash. Examples include hydroxyethyl starch (see above) and IgE-mediated (type I) hypersensitivity reactions to drugs. The occupation of the patient may also be important. Pruritus can be caused by occupational contact with glass fiber and by chronic sun exposure.

Establishing the diurnal periodicity of itching is especially important when considering a treatment regime. Many patients itch principally in the evening and at night when their attention is less distracted and the ambient temperature may be warm. Clearly antihistamines and other antipruritic measures should be focused appropriately in such a case. Other important factors to be elicited from the history include bathing habits (I have seen generalised pruritus as a consequence of overzealous, three-times-daily bathing in a foam bath in a cleanliness-obsessed individual), contact with domestic pets (papular urticaria), a history of previous foreign residence (onchocerciasis), and a history of atopy. I do not believe the literature supports a role for reduced serum or tissue iron levels as a cause for pruritus, so I do not advocate routine serum iron or ferritin examination. In the presence of localizing pointers in the history or clinical examination, further endoscopic or radiological studies may be indicated.

## VII.  TREATMENT OF THE ITCHY PATIENT

Obviously, making a diagnosis of the cause, be it in the skin or systemic, is the first step in treatment, although unfortunately, even when identified, a cause may not be easily corrected.

There are a number of common-sense measures that are appropriate for most cases. The skin is almost invariably less itchy when cool. An air-conditioned environment, light clothing and bedclothes, and a tepid shower or bath are often very helpful. Avoidance of woollen clothing next to the skin should be advised. I also advise patients to eschew alcoholic drinks and temperature-hot and spicy-hot foods and drinks and strong soaps, bath salts, and detergents.

There are no specifically antipruritic drugs of proven value. Clearly antihistamines orally or topically (e.g., 5% doxepin cream) may relieve itching when it is due to histamine release. Likewise topical steroids, though not antipruritic, may suppress itching when it is associated with inflammatory skin disease. There is no case for use of steroids topically or systemically in patients who do not suffer from itching due to inflammatory skin disease. Although oral doxepin (an $H_1$- plus $H_2$-antihistamine) should normally be prescribed for patients with histamine-mediated itchy disorders, it can, exceptionally, be used for other causes of itching due to its additional anxiolytic and antidepressant properties. When antihistamines are employed, it is reasonable to use a low-sedation antihistamine in the morning and a sedative antihistamine at night. Combined $H_1$- and $H_2$-antihistamines may be useful in physical urticaria such as dermographism.

Other measures to combat itching include 1% menthol cream, 10% crotamiton cream, and capsaicin 0.025–0.075% cream. Capsaicin is derived from hot chili pepper and is a vanillyl derivative. It causes depletion of substance P from nociceptor nerve endings via VR1 protein ion channels, preventing an influx of calcium ions. When applied to the skin repeatedly for several days it causes abolition of pruritus. It has therefore been used to treat localized skin conditions such as notalgia paraesthetica and brachioradial pruritus, as well as atopic eczema. The problem is that it causes considerable burning, redness, and irritation of the skin, so compliance is poor [32].

Physical methods of treating chronic pruritus are nonspecific but nevertheless of value. These include phototherapy (UVB, suberythema dosage 3 times weekly), transepidermal electrical nerve stimulation (TENS), and application of vibratory stimuli.

## REFERENCES

1. Perry WL, Hustad CM, Swing DA, O'Sullivan N, Jenkins NA, Copeland NG. The itching focus encodes a novel ubiquitin protein ligase that is disrupted in a18H mice. Nature Genetics 1998; 18:143–148.
2. Hagermark O, Wahlgren C-F. Some methods for evaluating clinical itch and their applications for studying pathophysiological mechanisms. J Dermatol Sci 1992; 4:55–62.
3. Talbot TL, Schmitt JM, Bergasa NV, Jones EA, Walker EC. Application of piezo film technology for quantitative assessment of pruritus. Biomed Instrum Technol 1991; 25:400–403.
4. Greaves MW, McDonald-Gibson W. Itch: role of prostaglandins. Br Med J 1973; 3:608–609.
5. Davies MG, Greaves MW. Sensory responses of human skin to synthetic histamine analogues and histamine. Br J Clin Pharmacol 1980; 9:461–465 (1980).
6. Bickford RG. Experiments relating to the itch sensation: its peripheral mechanism and central pathways. Clin Sci 1938; 3:377–386.
7. Wahlgren C-F, Linder MT, Hagermark O, Sibeynices A. Itch and inflammation induced by intradermally injected interleukin-2 in atopic patients and healthy subjects. Arch Dermatol Res 1995; 287:572–580.
8. Gaspari AA, Lotze MT, Rossenberg SA, Stern JB, Katz SI. Dermatological changes associated with interleukin-2 administration. J Am Med Assoc 1987; 258:1624–1629.
9. Schmelz M, Schmidt R, Bickel A, Handwerker HO, Torebjork H. Specific C receptors for itch in human skin. J Neurophysiol 1997; 17:8003–8008.
10. Hsieh J-C, Hagermark O, Stahle-Backdahl M, Ericson K, Eriksson L, Stone-Elander S, Ingvar M. Urge to scratch represented in the human cerebral cortex during itch. J Neurophysiol 1994; 72:3004–3008.
11. Greaves MW, Wall PD. Pathophysiology of itching. Lancet 1996; 348:938–940.
12. Fruhstorfer H, Hermanns M, Latzke L. The effects of thermal stimulation on clinical and experimental itch. Pain 1986; 24:259–269.

13. Bromage PR. The price of intraspinal narcotics: basic constraints. Anaesth Analg 1981; 60: 461–463.

14. Fjellner B, Hagermark O. Potentiation of histamine-induced itch and flare responses in human skin by the enkephalin analogue FK33-824 B-endorphin and morphine. Arch Dermatol Res 1982; 274:29–37.

15. Khalifa N, Greaves MW, Wall P, McMahon SB. Opioid peptides and itch. J Acad Dermatol 1998; 11 (supp 2): S67.

16. Greenwood AM. A study of the skin in five hundred cases of diabetes. J Am Med Assoc 1927; 89:774–776.

17. Neilly JB, Martin A, Simpson N, MacCuish AC. Pruritus in diabetes mellitus: Investigation of prevalence and correlation with disease control. Diabetes Care 1986; 9:273–275.

18. Lober CW. Should the patient with generalised pruritus be evaluated for malignancy? J Am Acad Dermatol 1988; 19:350–352.

19. Summerfield JA. Naloxone modulates the perception of itch in man. Br J Clin Pharmacol 1980; 10: 180–183 (1980).

20. Bergasa NV, Alling DW, Talbot TL, Swain MG, Yurdaydin C, Turner ML, Schmitt JM, Walker EC, Jones EA. Effects of naloxone infusions in patients with pruritus of cholestasis. Ann Int Med 1995; 123:161–167.

21. Fagan EA. Intrahepatic cholestasis of pregnancy. Br Med J 1994; 309:1243–1244.

22. Alagille D, Estrada A, Hadchouel M, Gautier M. Syndromic paucity of interlobular bile ducts (Alagille syndrome or arterio hepatic dysplasia): review of 80 cases. J Paediatr 1987; 110: 195–200 (1987).

23. Peer G, Kivity S, Agami O, Fireman E, Silverbert D, Bleum M, Iaina A. Randomised crossover trial of naltretone in uraemic pruritus. Lancet 1996; 348:1552–1554.

24. Kligman AM, Greaves MW, Steinman H. Water induced itching without cutaneous signs: aquagenic pruritus. Arch Dermatol 1986; 122:183–186.

25. Speight EL, MacSween RM, Stevens A. Persistent itching due to etherified starch plasma expander. Br Med J 1997; 314:1460–1467.

26. Ross JS, McKee PH, Smith NP, Shimizu H, Griffiths WAD, Bhogal BS, Black MM. Unusual variants of pemphigoid from pruritus to pemphigoid nodularis. J Cutan Pathol 1992; 19:212–216.

27. Murdoch ME, Hay RJ, MacKinzie CD. A clinical classification and grading system of the cutaneous changes in onchocerciasis. Br J Dermatol 1993; 129:260–269.

28. Greaves MW, Black AK, Eady RAJ. Aquagenic pruritus. Brit Med J 1981; 282:2008–2010.

29. Menage H du P, Norris P, Hawk J, Greaves MW. The efficacy of psoralen photochemotherapy in the treatment of aquagenic pruritus. Br J Dermatol 1993; 129:163–165.

30. Wallengren J. Brachioradial pruritus, a recurrent solar dermopathy. J Am Acad Dermatol, 1998; 39:803–806.

31. Bason MM, Berger TG, Nesbitt LT. Pruritic papular eruption of HIV disease. Int J Dermatol 1993; 32:784–789.

32. Holst-Folster R, Brasch J. Effect of topically applied capsaicin treatment on pruritus of atopic dermatitis. J Dermatol 1996; 7:13–15.

# 7
## Atopic Dermatitis

**Mark Boguniewicz**
*National Jewish Medical and Research Center, Denver, Colorado*

**Donald Y. M. Leung**
*National Jewish Center for Immunology and Respiratory Medicine, Denver, Colorado*

## I. INTRODUCTION

Atopic dermatitis (AD) is a chronically relapsing inflammatory skin disease commonly associated with respiratory allergy [1,2]. It is the most common chronic skin disease of young children, and its prevalence has continued to rise in western countries, similar to what has been observed in asthma. Poorly controlled AD may be associated with school absenteeism, occupational disability, and emotional stress. AD may also be associated with significant morbidity, especially when complicated by erythroderma or concomitant infection. Like asthma and allergic rhinitis, acute AD is associated with the local infiltration of T cells with a T helper-2 (Th2) cytokine profile [3]. Over 50% of patients with AD will develop asthma and allergic rhinitis [4]. In addition, data suggest that the eosinophil is a key effector cell in chronic AD similar to the allergic respiratory diseases [5]. Furthermore, like patients with asthma and allergic rhinitis, patients with AD can have nonspecific as well as specific triggers.

## II. HISTORICAL OVERVIEW

At the end of the last century, Besnier described the prurigo group of diseases, characterized by pruritus and a familial predisposition that included asthma and hay fever along with skin rash [6]. Subsequently, Coca and Cooke introduced the term ''atopy,'' derived from the Greek *atopos* or strangeness, to describe a familial altered end-organ hypersensitivity to environmental proteins in hay fever and asthma [7]. This definition was broadened to include the propensity to produce heat-labile reaginic antibody, later identified as IgE, to common allergens and to include atopic eczema [8]. In the 1930s, Hill and Sulzberger [9] suggested the term ''atopic dermatitis'' to describe both the weeping eczema of infancy and childhood and the chronic xerosis and lichenified lesions more typical of older patients. This term also recognized the close relationship between AD, asthma, and allergic rhinitis.

## III.  EPIDEMIOLOGY

Recent studies suggest an increasing prevalence of AD. Schultz Larsen [10] in Denmark demonstrated a cumulative incidence rate up to 7 years of 12% for twins born between 1975 and 1979 compared with a rate of 3% for twins born between 1960 and 1964. A cross-sectional questionnaire study conducted in 1992 confirmed this increased prevalence [11]. In this study of 3000 7-year-olds from Denmark, Germany, and Sweden, the frequency of AD was 15.6%. Similarly, questionnaire studies of Swedish schoolchildren in 1979 and 1991 showed an increase in prevalence of AD from 7% in 1979 to 18% in 1991 [12]. The point prevalence of AD in a study of schoolchildren living in northern Norway was found to be 23% [13].

In a recently published study, the authors performed skin examinations rather than relying on questionnaires to ascertain the prevalence of childhood and adolescent AD in a Japanese population [14]. They examined 994 5- to 6-year-olds, 1240 7- to 9-year-olds, 1152 10- to 12-year-olds, 1670 13- to 15-year-olds, and 2159 16- to 18-year olds. The examination was performed in the spring of 1994–96, when exacerbations of childhood and adolescent AD occur most frequently in Japan. AD was observed in 24% of the 5- to 6-year-old group, in 19% of the 7- to 9-year-old group, in 15% of the 10- to 12-year-old group, in 14% of the 13- to 15-year-old group, and in 11% of the 16- to 18-year-old group. Of note, the prevalence of AD in 9- to 12-year-old children was two times, and in 18-year-old adolescents five times as high as in similar age groups examined 20 years ago.

Increased exposure to pollutants, indoor allergens, especially house dust mites and a decline in breast-feeding, along with increased awareness of AD have been suggested as reasons for the increased frequency of AD [15]. In a prospective study, Zieger et al. [16] found that restricting the mother's diet during the third trimester of pregnancy and lactation as well as the child's diet during the first 2 years of life resulted in decreased prevalence in AD of the prophylactic group as compared to a control group that followed standard feeding practices at 12 months of age, but not at 24 months. Follow-up through 7 years of age showed no difference between the prophylactic and control groups for AD or respiratory allergy [17]. In a large study of an ethnically and socially diverse group of children in suburban Birmingham, England, Kay et al. [18] also found that breast-feeding did not affect the lifetime prevalence of 20%. A study of prevalence of childhood eczema found a correlation with increased socioeconomic class that was not due to heightened parental awareness [19].

The effects of genetic and environmental factors on allergic diseases were studied in two Japanese cities with differing climates [20]. The prevalence of allergic diseases and AD in the city with a temperature climate was significantly higher than in the one with a subtropical climate even after controlling for genetic and environmental factors. In both cities, children from atopic families had a significantly higher risk of contracting respiratory allergies and AD.

## IV.  GENETICS

Although genetic susceptibility to respiratory allergy has been suggested by localization of a locus for atopy on chromosome 11q13 [21], linkage to this gene has not been demonstrated in patients with AD [22]. Other studies have found linkage of serum IgE levels to an extended region on chromosome 5q containing genes that code for several interleukins and growth factors, including IL-4 [23]. Chan et al. [24] found that abnormal IL-4 gene expression in AD may be linked to alterations in nuclear protein interactions with IL-4 promoter elements. More recently, Kawashima et al. examined linkage between markers at and near the IL-4 gene and AD in 88 Japanese nuclear families [25]. A case-control comparison suggested a genotypic association between the T allele of the −590C/T polymorphism of the IL-4 gene with AD. Since the T allele was reported to be associated with increased IL-4 gene promoter activity compared with the C allele, the data indicate that genetic differences in transcriptional activity of the IL-4 gene may influence predisposition for AD, particularly in a Japanese population, because of the high frequency of the T allele. In addition, Hershey et al. [26] studied a small group of AD patients and reported an association of atopy with a gain-of-function mutation in the alpha subunit of the IL-4 receptor. The authors speculate that the R576 allele may predispose persons to allergic diseases by altering the signaling function of the receptor [26]. Linkage of both AD and asthma to polymorphisms within the gene for the β subunit of the high-affinity IgE receptor on chromosome 11q12-13 has recently been reported but has yet to be substantiated [27].

Of potential interest, Mao et al. [28] demonstrated a significant association between a specific polymorphism in the mast cell chymase gene and AD, but no association with asthma or allergic rhinitis. This finding, which requires confirmation, suggests that a genetic variant of mast cell chymase, which is a serine protease secreted by skin mast cells, may have an organ-specific effect and contribute to the genetic risk for AD.

Although the mode of transmission remains uncertain, some studies support an autosomal dominant inheritance pattern. Uehara and Kimura [29] found that 60% of adults with AD had children with AD. The prevalence of AD in children was 81% when both parents had AD, 59% when one parent had AD and the other had respiratory allergy, and 56% when one parent had AD and the other had neither AD nor respiratory allergy.

Diepgen and Fartasch [30] showed that 42% of first-degree relatives of patients with AD also had AD, while 28% had respiratory allergy. In contrast, only 12% of first-degree relatives of persons with respiratory allergy without skin disease had AD, while 43% had respiratory allergy. A follow-up study from this group investigated the familial aggregation of AD, allergic rhinitis, and allergic asthma in the relatives of 426 patients with AD and 628 subjects with no history of AD [31]. The odds ratio of familial aggregation for AD was 2.16 if no distinction was made between the degree of relationship. Further analyses within the members of the family showed a high odds ratio of 3.86 among siblings, while the odds ratio between parents and siblings was only 1.90. For AD the odds ratio differed between mother-sibling pairs (2.66) and father-sibling pairs (1.29), possibly because of environmental events that affect the fetus in utero or the shared physical environment of mother and child. However, since all of the atopic diseases demonstrated a stronger correlation between siblings than between siblings and parents, this supports the hypothesis that exposure to environmental factors during childhood is responsible for the recently observed increased prevalence of atopic diseases.

## V. NATURAL HISTORY

AD typically presents in early childhood with onset before 5 years of age in approximately 90% of patients [1]. In adults with new onset dermatitis, especially without a history of childhood eczema, asthma or allergic rhinitis, other diseases need to be considered.

Although Vickers' 20-year follow-up suggests that approximately 84% of children outgrow their AD by adolescence [32], more recent studies present less optimistic outcomes. AD had disappeared in only 18% of children followed from infancy until 11–13 years of age, although it became less severe in 65% [4]. Another study [33] found that 72% of patients diagnosed in the first 2 years of life continued to have AD 20 years later. In a prospective study from Finland, between 77 and 91% of adolescent patients treated for moderate or severe AD had persistent or frequently relapsing dermatitis as adults, although only 6% had severe disease [34]. In addition, more than half of the adolescents treated for mild dermatitis experienced a relapse of disease as adults. Finally, adults with childhood AD in remission for a number of years may present with hand dermatitis, especially if daily activities require repeated hand wetting [35].

## VI. ATOPIC DERMATITIS, ASTHMA, AND ALLERGIES

AD, asthma, and allergic rhinitis are classified as atopic diseases, i.e., diseases occurring in individuals with the genetic predisposition to develop an IgE response to common environmental allergens. This abnormal IgE response, however, is dependent on T-cell dysfunction with the overproduction of Th2 cytokines likely accounting for the elevated IgE levels and eosinophilia seen in these diseases. Of interest, a recent study found a linkage of both AD and asthma to polymorphisms within the gene for the β subunit of the high affinity IgE receptor on chromosome 11q12-13 [27].

Early onset of AD has been found to be associated with an increased risk for respiratory allergy. Pasternack first observed that the highest incidence of asthma at a given age occurred in children with onset of AD before 3 months of age, in those with severe AD, and with a family history of asthma [36]. A more recent study confirmed the association of increased risk for respiratory allergy (asthma and/or rhinoconjunctivitis) with early onset of AD [37]. Respiratory allergy occurred in 50% of children with onset of AD in the first 3 months of life and with two or more atopic family members compared to 12% of those with onset of AD after 3 months of age and with no atopic family members.

Like patients with asthma and allergic rhinitis, patients with AD can react to both allergic and nonspecific triggers. Skin reactivity to irritants such as sodium lauryl sulfate (SLS) has been shown in patients with both active and inactive AD as well as in patients with allergic respiratory disease with no dermatitis compared to normal nonatopic subjects [38]. The authors hypothesized that an abnormal intrinsic hyperreactivity in inflammatory cells in atopic individuals predisposes to a lowered threshold of irritant responsiveness. Importantly, in patients with AD, no constitutionally impaired stratum corneum barrier has been definitively proven [39]. Rather, atopy has been shown to be transferred through bone marrow transplantation [40], suggesting that the cutaneous abnormality results from inflammation stemming from a complex interaction of resident and infiltrating cells. In a recent study of bronchial and skin reactivity in asthmatic patients with and without AD [41], the authors found a latent predisposition for bronchial asthma in AD patients and implicated activated eosinophils as the common effector cells.

Of note, a global survey of the prevalence of asthma, allergic rhinoconjunctivitis, and AD studied 463,801 children aged 13–14 years in 155 collaborating centers in 56 countries [42]. For AD, the highest prevalences were reported from scattered centers, including Scandinavia and Africa, that were not among centers with the highest asthma prevalences; however, the lowest prevalence rates for AD were similar to centers with the lowest prevalence of asthma and allergic rhinoconjunctivitis. Thus, the ultimate presentation of an atopic disease may depend on a complex interaction of environmental exposures with end-organ response in a genetically prediposed individual.

## VII. CLINICAL FEATURES

AD has no pathognomonic skin lesion(s) or unique laboratory parameters. Thus, diagnosis is based on the presence of major and associated clinical features (Table 1). The principal features include severe pruritus, a chronically relapsing course, typical morphology, and distribution of the skin lesions and a history of atopic disease [1]. The presence of pruritus is critical to the diagnosis of AD and patients with AD have been shown to have a reduced threshold for pruritus.

Acute AD is characterized by intensely pruritic, erythematous papules associated with excoriations, vesiculations, and serious exudate (Fig. 1). Subacute AD is characterized by erythematous, excoriated, scaling papules, while chronic AD is characterized by thickened skin with accentuated markings (lichenification) and fibrotic papules (Fig. 2). Patients with chronic AD may have all three types of lesions present concurrently. In addition, patients usually have dry skin (Fig. 3). Significant differences can be observed between the pH, capacitance, and transepidermal water loss of AD lesions compared with uninvolved skin in the same patients and with the skin of normal controls [43].

**Table 1**  Clinical Features of Atopic Dermatitis

Major features
   Pruritus
   Facial and extensor involvement in infants and
      children
   Flexural lichenification in adults
   Chronic or relapsing dermatitis
   Personal or family history of atopic disease
Minor features
   Xerosis
   Cutaneous infections
   Nonspecific dermatitis of the hands or feet
   Ichthyosis, palmar hyperlinearity, keratosis pilaris
   Pityriasis alba
   Nipple eczema
   White dermatographism and delayed blanch
      response
   Anterior subcapsular cataracts
   Elevated serum IgE levels
   Positive immediate-type allergy skin tests

*Source*: Adapted from Ref. 1.

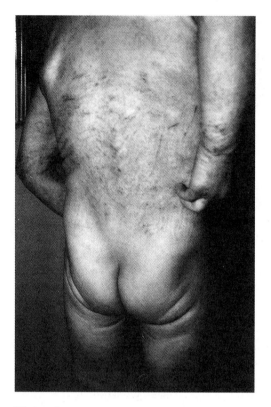

**Figure 1**  Acute AD with excoritated lesions associated with pruritus with sparing of the diaper area.

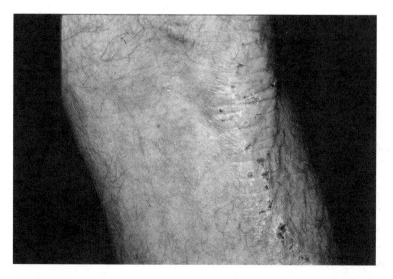

**Figure 2**  Chronic AD with significant lichenification of popliteal fossa.

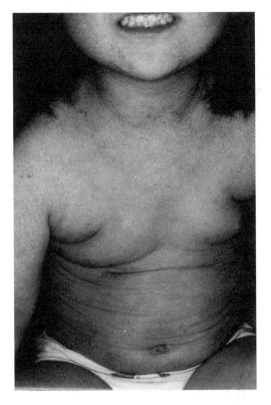

**Figure 3**   Generalized xerosis in AD.

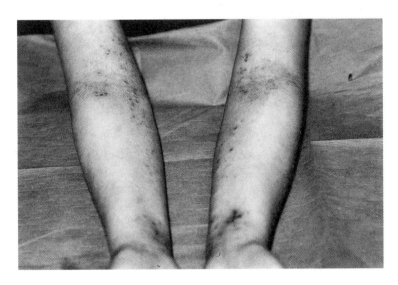

**Figure 4**   Flexural distribution in chronic AD.

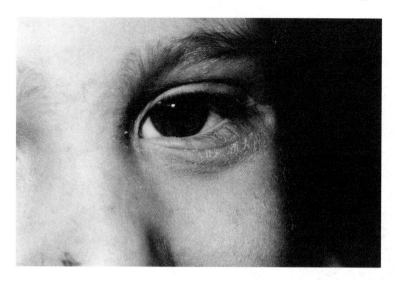

**Figure 5**  Periorbital dermatitis in AD with Dennie-Morgan line.

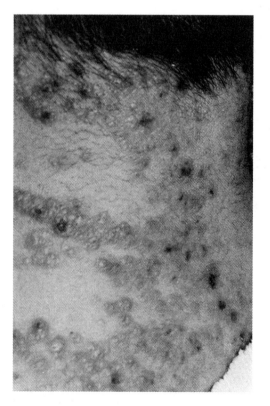

**Figure 6**  Prurigo nodules on neck and upper back of adolescent with chronic AD.

During infancy, AD involves primarily the face, scalp, and extensor surfaces of the extremities. The diaper area is usually spared (Fig. 1). When involved, it may be secondarily infected with *Candida*, in which case the dermatitis does not spare the inguinal folds. In contrast, infragluteal involvement is a common distribution in children. In older patients with long-standing disease, the flexural folds of the extremities are the predominant location of lesions (Fig. 4). Localization of AD to the eyelids may be an isolated manifestation but should be differentiated from an allergic contact dermatitis (Fig. 5). Chronic traumatization of the skin due to pruritus can at times result in prurigo nodules (Fig. 6).

Recently, the United Kingdom's Working Party proposed a set of diagnostic criteria for AD with a sensitivity of 85% and specificity of 96% [44]. These included itchy skin plus three or more of the following: history of flexural involvement, a history of asthma/hay fever, generalized dry skin, onset of rash under the age of 2 years, or flexural dermatitis. This group also found that certain signs including keratosis pilaris, xerosis, orbital pigmentation, fine hair, and extensor dermatitis showed poor between-observer agreement [45]. Subsequently, Nagaraja et al. [46] reported ichthyosis, nipple eczema, cheilitis, keratoconus, anterior subcapsular cataracts, hypopigmented patches, anterior neck folds, and food intolerance to be nonspecific findings in children with AD. In addition, associated features varied according to age group. These studies highlight the need for a laboratory test that could definitively establish the diagnosis.

## VIII. COMPLICATING FEATURES

### A. Ocular Problems

Ocular complications associated with AD can lead to significant morbidity. Of interest, increased numbers of IgE-bearing Langerhans cells have been found in the conjunctival epithelium in patients with AD [47]. These cells may capture aeroallergens and present them to infiltrating T cells, thus contributing to ocular inflammation. Atopic keratoconjunctivitis is always bilateral, and symptoms include itching, burning, tearing, and copious mucoid discharge [48]. It is frequently associated with eyelid dermatitis and chronic blepharitis and may result in visual impairment from corneal scarring. Vernal conjunctivitis is a severe bilateral recurrent chronic inflammatory process of the upper eyelid conjunctiva usually occurring primarily in younger patients. It has a marked seasonal incidence often in the spring. The associated intense pruritus is exacerbated by exposure to irritants, light, or sweating. Examination of the eye reveals a papillary hypertrophy or "cobblestoning" of the upper inner eyelid surface. Keratoconus is a conical deformity of the cornea believed to result from persistent rubbing of the eyes in patients with AD and allergic rhinitis. Anterior subcapsular cataracts may develop during adolescence or early adult life

### B. Hand Dermatitis

Patients with AD often have a nonspecific hand dermatitis. This is frequently irritant in nature and aggravated by repeated wetting, especially in the occupational setting (Fig. 7) [49]. The authors of a recent study suggest that a history of past or present AD at least doubles the effects of irritant exposure and, thus, doubles the risk in occupations where hand eczema is a common problem [50].

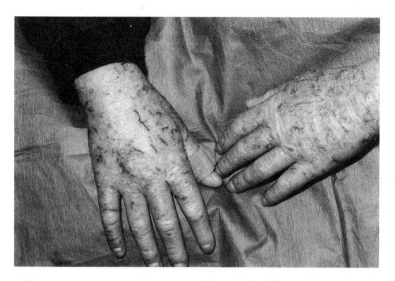

**Figure 7**  Severe chronic hand dermatitis in patient with AD.


## C.  Infections

Patients with AD have an increased susceptibility to infection or colonization with a variety of organisms [51] (see also Chapter XX). These include viral infections with *Herpes simplex* [52], *Molluscum contagiosum* [53], and human papillomavirus [54]. Raychaudhuri and Raychaudhuri [55] demonstrated a direct relationship between IFN-γ concentrations and the cytopathic effect of *Herpes simplex* and an inverse relationship between IL-4 and the cytopathic effect of *Herpes simplex*. This suggests that the T-cell–associated cytokine abnormalities seen in AD can enhance viral infections.

Superimposed dermatophytosis may cause AD to flare [56]. Patients with AD appear to have a threefold increase of *Trichophyton rubrum* infections compared to controls [57]. *Pityrosporum ovale* has also been associated with a predominantly head and neck distribution of AD [58].

A number of studies have elucidated the importance of *Staphylococcus aureus* in AD. *S. aureus* can be cultured from the skin of more than 90% of patients with AD compared to only 5% of normal subjects [59]. *S. aureus* colonization occurs even in infants with AD [60]. A recent study confirms the higher rate of *S. aureus* colonization in atopic dermatitis lesions compared to lesions from other skin disorders [61]. The authors further show that this finding may be associated with colonization of the nares. In addition, this study points to the importance of *S. aureus* carriage on the hand, suggesting that this may be the vector for transmitting these bacteria from the nasal reservoir to lesional skin and to close contacts of these patients. Of interest, treatment for nasal carriage with an intranasal antibiotic showed a trend for reduction in *S. aureus* carriage, although this did not reach significance [62]. However, hand carriage was significantly reduced in the treated group compared with controls. In another study looking at reservoirs, the prevalence of *S. aureus* in the anterior nares of patients with AD was more than five times higher than in the anterior nares of patients with other skin diseases or in healthy adult controls and the prevalence of *S. aureus* in the subungual spaces was 10 times higher in the AD patients compared to the other groups studied [63]. The phage type of *S. aureus* strains isolated from the anterior nares was similar to that of the strains isolated from the subungual spaces. Patients without obvious superinfection may show a better response to combined antistaphylococcal and topical corticosteroid therapy than to corticosteroids alone [64]. Although recurrent staphylococcal pustulosis can be a significant problem in AD, invasive *S. aureus* infections occur rarely and should raise the possibility of an immunodeficiency such as hyper-IgE syndrome [65].

## IX.  DIFFERENTIAL DIAGNOSIS

A number of diseases may be confused with AD (see Chapter 18). Scabies can present as a pruritic skin disease. However, distribution in the genital and axillary areas, presence of linear lesions as well as skin scrapings may help to distinguish it from AD. It is especially important to recognize that an adult who presents with an eczematous dermatitis with no history of childhood eczema and without other atopic features may have a contact dermatitis, but more importantly cutaneous T-cell lymphoma needs to be ruled out. Ideally, biopsies should be sent from three separate sites, since histology may show spongiosis and cellular infiltrate similar to AD. In addition, eczematous rash suggestive of AD has been reported with HIV [66].

A contactant should be considered in those patients whose AD does not respond to appropriate therapy. Typical distribution for a suspected contactant may be suggestive. However, allergic contact dermatitis complicating AD may appear as an acute flare of the underlying disease, rather than the more typical vesiculobullous eruption. Proper diagnosis depends on confirmation of a suspected allergen with patch testing. Standardized testing with the T.R.U.E. Test® is available for 24 of the most common contact allergens (discussed in Chapter 20). More extensive testing by an occupational dermatologist may be appropriate in selective cases.

## X.  PSYCHOLOGICAL IMPLICATIONS

Patients with AD have been characterized as having high levels of anxiety and problems in dealing with anger and hostility [67]. While these do not cause AD, they can exacerbate the illness. Patients often respond to stress or frustration with itching and scratching. Stimulation of the central nervous system may intensify cutaneous vasomotor and sweat responses and contribute to the itch-scratch cycle. In some instances, scratching is associated with significant secondary gain or with a strong component of habit. Finally, severe disease may have a significant impact on patients leading to problems with social interactions and self-esteem.

## XI.  THE ROLE OF ALLERGENS

Although elevated serum IgE levels can be demonstrated in 80–85% of patients with AD [68] and a similar number have immediate skin tests or in vitro tests to food and inhalant allergens [69], the relationship between the course of AD and implicated allergens has been difficult to establish. Nevertheless, a number of well-controlled studies suggest that various allergens can impact the course of this disease.

## A.  Foods

May [70] first recognized that patients with AD and positive food allergen tests often had negative food challenges to the implicated allergen, distinguishing between symptomatic and asymptomatic hypersensitivity. Thus, triggers for clinical disease cannot be predicted simply by performing allergy testing. However, double-blinded, placebo-controlled food challenges (DBPCFC) have demonstrated that food allergens can cause exacerbations in a subset of patients with AD [71]. A recent study confirmed that seven foods (milk, egg, peanut, soy, wheat, fish, and nuts) account for nearly 90% of the positive challenges [72]. In addition, a study of patients referred to a university dermatology practice for evaluation of their eczema, rather than for suspected food allergy, showed that approximately one third had IgE-mediated food hypersensitivity [73]. The study reaffirms the need to consider the role of food allergens in children with atopic dermatitis who do not respond readily to conventional therapy. Although lesions induced by single positive challenges are usually transient, repeated challenges, more typical of real-life exposure, can result in eczematous lesions. Furthermore, elimination of food allergens results in amelioration of skin disease and a decrease in spontaneous basophil histamine release [74].

## B.  Aeroallergens

The evidence supporting a role for aeroallergens in AD includes the finding of both allergen-specific IgE antibodies [75] and allergen-specific T cells [76]. Exacerbation of AD can occur with exposure to allergens such as house dust mites, animal danders, and pollens. In the 1940s, Tuft demonstrated that introduction of aerollergens intranasally could exacerbate AD [77]. More recently, 9 of 20 patients with AD who underwent bronchial provocation with a standardized house dust mite extract in a double-blind, randomized, placebo-controlled fashion developed unequivocal cutaneous lesions after inhalation of dust mite [78]. All of the patients with dust mite–induced dermatitis had a history of asthma, and in eight of these nine patients skin reaction was preceded by an early bronchial reaction. Brinkman et al. also showed that allergen inhalation challenge causes a flare-up of skin lesions 24 hours after the challenge in atopic dermatitis patients with or without asthma, but more pronounced in the former group [79]. Thus, the respiratory route may be important in the induction and exacerbation of AD. In addition, studies with patch testing have shown that direct contact with inhalant allergens can also result in eczematous skin eruptions [80–82]. A recent study suggests that the presence of antigen-specific Th2 cells found in acute allergen patch test reactions indicates that the Th2 differentiation pathway is seen preferentially in allergen-exposed skin [83]. In addition, the cytokine profile of T-cell clones obtained from naturally occurring skin lesions in this study was similar to those from the patch test lesions, suggesting that the patch test represents a model to investigate the pathogenesis of AD. However, the authors of a recently published study suggest that allergic patch test to Der p1 and Der p2 are rare and that irritant reactions from *Dermatophagoides pteronyssinus* proteolytic activity may be a more common phenomenon when patch testing atopic dermatitis patients with house dust mite antigen extract [84]. Nevertheless, environmental control measures have been shown to result in clinical improvement of AD [85]. These studies suggest that inhalation or contact with aeroaller-gens may be involved in the pathogenesis of AD.

## C. Microbial Agents and Toxins

In addition to their role as infectious agents, both the lipophilic yeast *Pityrosporum ovale (orbiculare)* [86] and the superficial dermatophyte *Trichophyton rubrum* [87] have been associated with elevated specific IgE in patients with AD. Patients with AD predominantly of the head and neck compared to a group without this distribution and normal individuals more often demonstrate positive skin tests, RAST, and specific histamine release to *P. ovale* [58]. In one study, the majority of T-cell clones derived from lesional skin of such patients showed a Th2-like cytokine profile, suggesting that *P. ovale* may play a role in maintaining IgE-mediated skin inflammation in AD [88]. The clinical significance of these findings is suggested by clinical improvement of such patients following treatment with antifungal therapy [56]. However, it is worth noting that a recent study found that a number of AD patients produced IgE to fungal glycoproteins without a significant histamine re-lease or skin test reactivity possibly because of nonspecific interaction with carbohydrate moieties on IgE and poor biological activity of IgE directed to cross-reactive carbohydrate determinants of fungal glycoproteins [89]. Thus, the clinical relevance of antifungal IgE in patients with AD remains to be fully elucidated.

Exotoxins secreted by *S. aureus* have been shown to act as superantigens, which could contribute to persistent inflammation or exacerbations of AD [90]. Over half of the AD patients studied had *S. aureus* cultured from their skin that secreted primarily enterotoxins A and B and toxic shock syndrome toxin-1. In addition, almost half of the patients made specific IgE antibodies directed against the staphylococcal toxins found on their skin. Basophils from patients with antitoxin IgE released histamine on exposure to the relevant toxin, but not in response to toxins to which they had no specific IgE. These observations have been confirmed in subsequent studies with up to 80% of pa-tients showing specific IgE antibodies against SEA and/or SEB [91]. In addition, SEB applied to the skin can induce skin changes of erythema and induration [92]. In a study utilizing a humanized murine model of skin inflammation, *S. aureus* toxin plus allergen was shown to have an additive effect in inducing cutaneous inflammation [93]. In a dif-ferent study, PBMC from children with AD showed significantly higher proliferative responses to both *S. aureus* and SEB and diminished production of IFN-γ in response to *S. aureus* and SEB [94]. In contrast, PBMC from children with AD were more likely to produce IL-4 in response to *S. aureus*. These investigators suggested that impaired IFN-γ production to *S. aureus* in vivo may result in failure to eradicate this organism from the skin. Persistence on the skin could contribute to inflammation by causing con-tinued T-cell activation and release of pro-inflammatory mediators. Furthermore, by eliciting an IgE response, staphylococcal toxins could exacerbate AD by activating mast cells, basophils, or other Fcε receptor–bearing cells. Other staphylococcal proteins such as protein A and α-toxin could also participate in the induction of local inflamma-tion in AD by releasing TNF-α from epidermal keratinocytes [95]. In contrast to the superantigenic toxins, staphylococcal α-toxin can also induce profound cytotoxicity in these cells.

## XII.  IMMUNE RESPONSES IN AD

The finding of elevated serum IgE levels and the occurrence of eczematous lesions indistinguishable from AD in patients with primary T-cell immunodeficiency disorders suggest an immunological basis for AD [96]. In Wiskott-Aldrich syndrome, bone marrow transplantation results in correction of the immunological defect and resolution of the dermatitis. In addition, nonatopic recipients of bone marrow transplants from atopic donors have been shown to develop atopic symptoms and positive skin tests following successful engraftment [40]. These data suggest that AD results from a bone marrow–derived cell dysfunction rather than from a constitutive skin defect.

## A.  Immunoregulatory Dysfunction

A number of immunoregulatory abnormalities have been described in AD (Table 2). B cells from patients with AD synthesize high levels of IgE [97]. Lymphocytes from these patients produce increased amounts of IL-4 and express abnormally high levels of IL-4 receptor [97,98]. In addition, the spontaneous production of IgE can be inhibited in vitro by addition of anti-IL-4 [99]. Peripheral blood mononuclear cells isolated from AD patients have a decreased capacity to make IFN-$\gamma$, and this is inversely correlated with serum IgE levels [100].

   A number of studies have also shown an increased frequency of both circulating and cutaneous allergen-specific IL-4 and IL-5 secreting T-helper cells in AD patients [76,101]. Recently, Nakazawa et al. used flow cytometry to demonstrate at the single cell level that the frequency of Th2 cytokine–secreting cells was significantly higher in AD patients compared to normal controls [102]. In addition, CD30, an activation marker of T-cell clones thought to show a Th2 cytokine profile has been found to be significantly elevated in soluble form in children with AD [103].

   In addition to acting as an IgE isotype–specific switch, IL-4 also inhibits production of IFN-$\gamma$ and downregulates the differentiation of Th1 cells [104]. IFN-$\gamma$ production is

**Table 2**  Immunoregulatory Abnormalities in Atopic Dermatitis

| |
|---|
| Increased number of activated CLA+ T cells |
| Increased secretion of IL-4, IL-5, and IL-13 by Th2-type cells |
| Decreased secretion of IFN-$\gamma$ by Th1-type cells |
| Increased soluble E-selectin levels |
| Increased serum eosinophil cationic protein levels |
| Increased synthesis of IgE |
| Increased specific IgE to multiple allergens including foods, aeroallergens, microorganisms, enterotoxins |
| Increased expression of CD23 on B cells and monocytes |
| Increased basophil histamine release |
| Impaired delayed-type hypersensitivity response |
| Decreased CD8 suppressor/cytotoxic T-cell number and function |
| Increased soluble IL-2 receptor levels |
| Elevated levels of monocyte cAMP-phosphodiesterase with increased IL-10 and PGE$_2$ |

also inhibited by prostaglandin (PG) $E_2$ and IL-10, both of which are secreted in increased amounts by monocytes from AD patients [105,106]. A recent study found no defect in the capacity of cells from AD patients to produce IL-12, an important inducer of IFN-$\gamma$ [107]. However, neutralization of IL-10 and IL-4 was able to correct production IFN-$\gamma$. Thus, the activation of Th2-like cells and monocytes may be central to the immune dysregulation in AD.

More recently, a role for the co-stimulatory molecules CD80/CD86 has been investigated in AD. Using immunohistochemical analysis, Ohki et al. showed predominantly CD86 on Langerhans cells in both the epidermis and the dermis in AD [108]. They also demonstrated almost complete inhibition of antigen specific T-cell proliferation with an anti-CD86 monoclonal antibody. Studies have also suggested that these accessory molecules differ in their capacity to generate Th1-versus Th2-type T-cell responses. A recent study found that the expression of CD86 on B cells of AD patients was significantly higher than on B cells from normals and psoriasis patients [109]. In contrast, there was no significant difference in CD80 expression among the three subject groups. Interestingly, total serum IgE from AD patients and normal subjects correlated significantly with CD86 expression on B cells, suggesting a role for CD86+ B cells in IgE synthesis. Purified CD86+ B cells produced significantly more IgE than CD86− B cells in vitro and anti-CD86, but not CD80, mAb significantly decreased IgE production by PBMC stimulated with IL-4 and anti-CD40 mAb. Furthermore, CD86+ B cells had a significantly higher level of IL-4R and CD23 expression than CD80+ B cells. These data demonstrate the predominant expression of CD86 in AD and suggest a role in IgE synthesis.

## B. Immunopathological Features

Routine histology of clinically normal-appearing skin in AD reveals mild epidermal hyperplasia and a sparse, predominantly lymphocytic infiltrate in the dermis [110]. Acute eczematous lesions are characterized by both intercellular edema of the epidermis (spongiosis) and intracellular edema. A sparse lymphocytic infiltrate may be observed in the epidermis, while a marked perivenular infiltrate consisting of lymphocytes and some monocytes with rare eosinophils, basophils, and neutrophils is seen in the dermis. Mast cells are found in normal numbers in different stages of degranulation. In chronic lichenified lesions, the epidermis shows prominent hyperkeratosis with increased numbers of epidermal Langerhans cells and predominantly monocytes/macrophages in the dermal infiltrate. Mast cells are usually increased in number but are not degranulated.

Immunohistochemical staining of acute and chronic skin lesions in AD shows that the lymphocytes are predominantly CD3, CD4, and CD45RO memory T cells, i.e., they have previously encountered antigen [65,111]. These cells also express CD25 and HLA-DR on their surface, indicative of intralesional activation [65]. In addition, almost all of the T cells infiltrating into atopic skin lesions express high levels of the skin lymphocyte homing receptor, cutaneous lymphocyte antigen (CLA), a ligand for the vascular adhesion molecule, E-selectin [112].

Vascular endothelial cells from atopic skin lesions express abnormally high levels of E-selectin as well as vascular cell adhesion molecule-1 (VCAM-1) and CD54 [113]. Mast cells, monocytes, Langerhans cells, and keratinocytes are all potential sources of IL-1 and TNF-$\alpha$, which induce E-selectin, a molecule critical to targeting of CLA expressing T cells to sites of cutaneous inflammation [114]. Furthermore, migration of skin-homing T cells into atopic skin lesions also involves interaction between VCAM-1 and very late antigen-4 as well as CD54 and leukocyte function–associated antigen-1 [115]. In addition, VCAM-1, which can be induced by IL-4 and IL-13, is involved in eosinophil and mononuclear cell movement into sites of allergic inflammation [116].

In contrast to epidermal Langerhans cells from normal subjects, Langerhans cells found in the epidermis and dermis of chronic AD express CD1b, CD36, and HLA-DR surface antigens and are potent activators of autologous resting CD4 T cells [117]. Furthermore, both Langerhans cells and macrophages infiltrating into the AD skin lesion have been shown to have surface-bound IgE [118,119]. Interestingly, a recent study found a distinct population of CD1a inflammatory dendritic epidermal cells in cutaneous lesions in AD [120]. Exposure of these cells to specific signals results in upregulation of FcεRI in AD skin.

Activated eosinophils are present in significantly greater numbers in chronic as compared to acute lesions [3]. In addition, deposition of eosinophil major basic protein (MBP) can be detected throughout the upper dermis and to a lesser extent deeper in the dermis [121]. MBP deposition is more prominent in involved areas as compared to uninvolved skin. MBP may contribute to the pathogenesis of AD through its cytotoxic properties and its capacity to induce basophil and mast cell degranulation [122]. Furthermore, serum levels of eosinophil cationic protein are elevated in AD and correlate with disease severity [123].

## C.  Cytokine and Chemokine Expression

Cytokine expression in AD lesions reflects the nature of the underlying inflammation. In this respect, Hamid et al. [3] used in situ hybridization to study IL-4, IL-5, and IFN-γ mRNA expression in acute and chronic skin lesions as well as uninvolved skin in AD. Biopsies from uninvolved atopic skin showed a significant increase in the number of cells expressing IL-4, but not IL-5 or IFN-γ mRNA. Both acute and chronic lesions had significantly greater numbers of cells that were positive for IL-4 and IL-5, compared to uninvolved or normal skin. Neither acutely involved or uninvolved atopic skin showed significant numbers of IFN-γ mRNA–expressing cells. In contrast, chronic AD skin lesions, when compared with acute AD skin lesions, had significantly fewer IL-4 mRNA–expressing cells and significantly more IL-5 mRNA–expressing cells. T cells comprised the majority of IL-5–expressing cells in both the acute and chronic lesions. Activated eosinophils were found in significantly greater numbers in the chronic, as compared to acute lesions. These data suggest that while both acute and chronic lesions in AD are associated with increased IL-4 and IL-5 gene activation, acute skin inflammation is associated with predominantly IL-4 expression, whereas chronic inflammation is associated with IL-5 expression and eosinophil infiltration. Consistent with the relative importance of these cytokines, further studies revealed that acute AD is associated with a high expression of IL-4 receptor α, whereas IL-5 receptor α is predominantly increased in chronic AD [124]. These investigators also found that IL-13 expression was higher in acute compared with chronic atopic lesions or psoriatic lesions [125]. These data suggest that IL-13 may be involved in the pathogenesis of AD and further support the hypothesis that acute inflammation in AD is mediated by Th2-type cytokines. Chronic lesions had increased numbers of IL-12 mRNA–positive cells compared with acute and uninvolved skin. IL-12 is known to be a potent inducer of IFN-γ synthesis; therefore, it is of interest that increased IFN-γ expression has been reported in chronic AD lesions [126,127]. Although the clinical significance of this biphasic response needs to be further elucidated [since some AD patients respond to treatment with recombinant human IFN-γ (rhIFN-γ)], these findings support the biphasic role of cytokines in the pathophysiology of AD. Most recently, IL-16, a potent chemoattractant for CD4$^+$ T cells, was shown to be significantly increased in acute AD lesions compared to chronic and uninvolved or normal skin [128]. The source of the IL-16 in the epidermis appears to be keratinocytes, which have recently been recognized as important sources of cytokines, including IL-1, IL-8, IL-10, IL-12, GM-CSF, and RANTES. Thus, by mediating infiltration of CD4 cells, IL-16 may play a role in the pathogenesis of AD.

The C—C chemokines RANTES and monocyte chemotactic protein-3 (MCP-3) are potent chemoattractants in vitro for eosinophils and other cell types associated with allergic inflammation. Allergen-induced infiltration of eosinophils, T cells, and macrophages in the skin of atopic subjects is accompanied by the appearance of mRNA+ cells for RANTES and MCP-3 [129]. Kinetic studies support the view that MCP-3 is involved in the regulation of the early eosinophil response to specific allergen, whereas RANTES may have more relevance to the later accumulation of T cells and macrophages. In a recent study of acute versus chronic AD lesions, both keratinocytes and infiltrating cells were found to express mRNA for chemokines with a significantly higher number of cells positive for eotaxin and MCP-4 in chronic lesions [130].

## D.  Immunopharmacological Abnormalities

Leukocytes from patients with AD have been found to have genetically determined increased cAMP-phosphodiesterase (PDE) enzyme activity [131]. Cellular abnormalities associated with this finding include increased IgE synthesis by B cells, increased IL-4 production by T cells, and increased histamine releasability in basophils [132]. The greatest PDE abnormality is seen in AD monocytes, which have been shown to have a unique, highly active isoenzyme [133]. However, in a mixed cell system, PDE inhibitors have been shown to downregulate antigen-driven proliferation and gene expression of proinflammatory cytokines predominantly through their effects on lymphocytes rather than monocytes [134].

Monocytes from patients with AD can modulate T-cell dysfunction through inhibition of IFN-γ production. This is mediated in part by increased monocyte PGE$_2$ production associated with elevated PDE activity [105] and by monocyte-associated IL-10 [106]. In addition, enhanced survival or decreased apoptosis of circulating and infiltrating monocytes in association with increased production of GM-CSF in AD may play an important role in the establishment of chronic inflammation [135].

## E.  The Role of IgE in Cutaneous Inflammation

In AD, IgE may play an important role in allergen-induced cell-mediated reactions involving Th2-like cells that are distinct from conventional delayed-type hypersensitivity reactions mediated by Th1-like cells [136]. IgE-dependent biphasic reactions are frequently associated with clinically significant allergic reactions and may contribute to the inflammatory process of AD [137]. Immediate-type reactions due to mediator release by mast cells bearing allergen-specific IgE may result in the pruritus and erythema that occurs after exposure to relevant allergens. IgE-dependent late-phase reactions (LPR) can then lead to more persistent symptoms. The T-cell infiltrate in cutaneous allergen-induced LPR has been shown to have increased mRNA for IL-3, IL-4, IL-5, and granulocyte/macrophage colony-stimulating factor, but not for IFN-$\gamma$ [138]. These cells are therefore similar to the Th2-like cells found in AD lesions. In addition, the cutaneous LPR is associated with a similar pattern of adhesion molecule expression as AD [139]. Thus, a sustained IgE-dependent LPR may be part of the chronic inflammatory process in AD.

Furthermore, epidermal Langerhans cells in AD skin have been shown to express IgE on their cell surface and to be significantly more efficient than IgE-negative Langerhans cells at presenting allergen to T cells [140]. A study by Jürgens et al. [141] extends these observations by demonstrating that Langerhans cells from atopic individuals have a much higher level of Fc$\epsilon$RI expression. Furthermore, Klubal et al. propose that the high-affinity IgE receptor is the only biologically relevant IgE-binding receptor on a heterogeneous group of cells found in the skin in atopic dermatitis [142]. This underscores the importance of IgE antibodies in capturing and focusing allergens on antigen-presenting cells, thus contributing to the pathogenesis of this disease. Presentation to Th2 cells in atopic skin may be an important mechanism for sustaining local T-cell activation.

## F.   Skin-Directed Th2-Like Cell Response

A number of studies in recent years have demonstrated important similarities in the allergic inflammation of asthma and AD. Common features include local infiltration of Th2-like cells in response to allergens, development of specific IgE to allergens, a chronic inflammatory process, and organ-specific hyperreactivity. In both diseases, IL-4–and IL-5–secreting memory Th2-like cells have a central role in the induction of local IgE responses and recruitment of eosinophils [3,143]. The recognition of T-cell heterogeneity based on expression of tissue-selective homing receptors [144] suggests that an individual's propensity for specific allergic disease may be a function of end-organ targeting by their effector T cells. In this respect, T cells migrating to the skin express CLA, whereas most memory/effector T cells isolated from asthmatic airways do not [145].

In a study of patients with milk-induced AD, casein-reactive T cells expressed significantly higher levels of CLA than did *Candida albicans*–reactive T cells from these patients or casein-reactive T cells from patients with milk-induced enterocolitis or eosinophilic gasteroenteritis [146]. Additional evidence for selective end-organ targeting by T-cell subsets in allergic inflammation includes recent data showing that dust mite–specific T-cell proliferation in mite-sensitized patients with AD was localized to the CLA-expressing fraction of T cells [147]. In contrast, T cells isolated from mite allergic asthmatics that proliferated on exposure to the relevant allergen were CLA-negative. Furthermore, CLA-expressing T cells isolated from patients with AD, but not from normal controls, showed evidence of activation (HLA-DR expression) and also spontaneously produced IL-4, but not IFN-$\gamma$. This suggests that T-cell effector function in AD is closely linked to CLA expression.

## G. Immunological Basis for Chronic Allergic Skin Inflammation

The mechanisms responsible for chronic inflammation in AD have not been fully elucidated but likely involve a number of interdependent factors. This includes repeated or chronic exposure to allergens such as foods, aeroallergens, and micro-organisms leading to chronic allergic responses and Th2-like cell expansion. Consistent with this concept, specific allergen avoidance can result in clinical improvement or clearing of AD [85,148]. In addition, clinical improvement after treatment with antistaphylococcal antibiotics may be related to the reduction of *S. aureus* exotoxin levels on the skin.

Toxins acting as superantigens are capable of inducing CLA expression by stimulating IL-12 production [149]. In addition, by stimulating epidermal Langerhans cells and macrophages to secrete IL-1 and TNF-$\alpha$, staphylococcal exotoxins can induce vascular endothelial E-selectin expression. This in turn would facilitate migration of CLA-positive T cells to the area. Furthermore, toxin-stimulated Langerhans cells migrating to regional skin-associated lymph nodes act as antigen-presenting cells and could produce IL-12 locally, thus influencing the skin-homing capability of antigen-stimulated T cells. Toxins also stimulate a high proportion of T cells via the variable domain of the T-cell receptor $\beta$ chain to proliferate and secrete cytokines implicated in tissue inflammation. A recent study found that children with active AD had an increased percentage of circulating CLA+ T cells expressing V$\beta$ elements specific for *S. aureus* superantigens [150]. By eliciting an IgE response, staphylococcal toxins could exacerbate AD by activating mast cells, basophils, or other Fc$\epsilon$ receptor–bearing cells. In addition, other staphylococcal proteins such as protein A and $\alpha$-toxin can participate in the induction of local inflammation in AD by releasing TNF-$\alpha$ from epidermal keratinocytes [95]. Such amplifying pathways could then lead to persistent cutaneous inflammation.

Furthermore, cytokines secreted by Th2-like cells after exposure to allergen inhibit IFN-$\gamma$ production by Th1-like cells, increase IgE synthesis and promote migration, differentiation, and proliferation of eosinophils [151]. Mast cells can also produce IL-4 after allergen stimulation [152]. Monocytes from AD patients express high levels of IL-10 and PGE$_2$, which antagonize Th1-like cells [106]. Thus, conditions favoring a persistent Th2-like cell response may be established in AD. Monocytes from AD patients also have a lower incidence of spontaneous apoptosis associated with increased production of GM-CSF [135]. Together with IL-5, GM-CSF contributes to increased survival and infiltration of eosinophils in chronic AD. Finally, allergen-induced inflammation can alter corticosteroid receptor binding affinity, thus blunting the anti-inflammatory effects of corticosteroids [153].

The itch-scratch cycle likely contributes to skin inflammation in AD as well. Recent studies demonstrating that keratinocytes are an important source of cytokines have provided new insights into the mechanisms by which scratching could promote inflammation. In this regard, scratching can injure or stimulate keratinocytes, leading to the release of cytokines such as IL-1 [154] and TNF-$\alpha$ [95] necessary for the induction of adhesion molecules that attract cells into cutaneous sites of inflammation. Both resident and infiltrating cells could then perpetuate the inflammatory process by secreting cytokines and mediators.

In summary, antigen or superantigen exposure, allergen-induced IgE synthesis and Th2-like cell expansion, mast cell degranulation, and keratinocyte injury may all contribute to chronic AD skin inflammation and possibly to nonspecific cutaneous hyperresponsiveness as well.

## XIII.  MANAGEMENT

### A.  Conventional Therapy

Our current understanding of the pathophysiology of AD supports the concept that assessing the role of allergens, infectious agents, irritants, physical environment, and emotional stressors is equal in importance to initiating therapy with first-line agents. The acute and chronic aspects of AD need to be considered when designing an individual treatment plan. Patients should understand that therapy is not curative, but that avoidance of exacerbating factors together with proper daily skin care can result in the control of symptoms and improve long-term outcome.

### B.  Identification and Elimination of Exacerbating Factors

#### 1.  Irritants

Patients with AD have a lowered threshold of irritant responsiveness [38]. Thus, recognition and avoidance of irritants is integral to successful management of this disease. These include detergents, soaps, chemicals, pollutants, and abrasive materials as well as extremes of temperature and humidity. Cleansers with minimal defatting activity and a neutral pH should be used rather than soaps. Gentle cleansers include Dove®, Oil of Olay®, Basis®, Aveeno®, and Cetaphil®. New clothes should be laundered before wearing to remove formaldehyde and other chemicals. Residual laundry detergent in clothing may be irritating, and using a liquid rather than powder detergent and adding a second rinse cycle may be beneficial. Occlusive clothing should be avoided and cotton or cotton blends used. Ideally, temperature in the home and work environments should be temperate to minimize sweating. Chemicals such as chlorine or bromine in a pool can be irritating if allowed to dry on the skin. Rather than instructing patients to avoid swimming, they should be given appropriate skin care instructions. Usually, showering with the use of a cleanser and moisturizer after swimming allows the patient to enjoy this activity without irritating their skin. While sunlight may be beneficial to some patients with AD, nonsensitizing sunscreens should be used to avoid sunburn. Products developed for use on the face are often best tolerated by patients with AD. Prolonged sun exposure can cause evaporative losses, overheating, and sweating, which can be irritating.

#### 2.  Allergens

Identification of allergens involves taking a careful history and doing selective immediate hypersensitivity skin tests or in vitro tests when appropriate. Negative skin tests with proper controls have a high predictive value for ruling out a suspected allergen. Positive skin tests have a lower correlation with clinical symptoms in suspected food allergen–induced AD and should be confirmed with DBPCFC, unless there is a coincidental history of anaphylaxis to the suspected food. In children who have undergone DBPCFC, milk, egg, peanut, soy, wheat, and fish account for approximately 90% of the food allergens found to exacerbate AD [155]. More importantly, avoidance of foods implicated in controlled challenges results in clinical improvement [71,74]. Extensive elimination diets, which may be both extremely burdensome and at times nutritionally unsound, are almost never warranted since even patients with multiple positive skin tests are rarely clinically sensitive to more than three foods on DBPCFC [155].

Sampson subsequently showed that for selected foods (i.e., egg, milk, peanut, and fish), allergen-specific IgE levels could be measured in an in vitro system that could identify clinically allergic patients [156]. It is important not to extrapolate these results to other food allergens, such as wheat and soy, where antibody levels did not provide positive predictive values. Nevertheless, since egg, milk, peanut, and fish account for approximately 80% of documented food allergy in children, the CAP System FEIA can identify many at-risk patients when doing blinded, placebo-controlled challenges is not feasible. Characterization of relevant allergens in other foods should lead to additional predictive in vitro assays. Meanwhile, the CAP System FEIA may also prove to be a useful tool in monitoring the natural history of food allergy and help to determine when a food could be reintroduced.

In dust mite–allegic individuals, environmental control measures aimed at reducing dust mite load have been shown to improve AD in patients who demonstrate specific IgE to dust mite allergen [85]. These include use of dust mite–proof casings on pillows, mattresses, and boxsprings; washing linens in hot water weekly; removal of bedroom carpeting; and decreasing indoor humidity levels.

## C. Psychosocial Factors

Counseling is often helpful in dealing with the frustrations associated with AD. Relaxation, behavioral modification, or biofeedback may all be of benefit, especially in those patients with habitual scratching [157,158]. A recent review describes potentially long-lasting benefits of insight-oriented psychotherapy for selected patients [159].

## D. Patient Education

Learning about the chronic nature of AD, exacerbating factors, and appropriate treatment options is important for both patients and family members [160]. Clinicians should provide patients or their families with both general disease information and detailed written skin care recommendations. The treatment plan should be reviewed, and the patient or family member should demonstrate an appropriate level of understanding to help ensure a good outcome. Educational pamphlets and video may be obtained from the Eczema Association for Science and Education (1221 SW Yamhill, Suite 303, Portland, OR 97205; (503)228-4430), a national nonprofit, patient-oriented organization. In addition, patients and their families should be counseled with regard to the natural history and prognosis of the disease with appropriate vocational counseling.

## E. Hydration

Atopic dry skin shows enhanced transepidermal water loss [161] and reduced water-binding capacity [162]. Therefore, skin hydration is an essential component of therapy. The best way to reestablish the skin's barrier function is to soak the affected area or bathe for 15–20 minutes in warm water, then apply an occlusive agent to retain the absorbed water.

Addition of substances such as oatmeal or baking soda to the bath water may feel soothing to some patients but does not effect water absorption. Hydration of the face or neck can be achieved by applying a wet facecloth or towel to the involved area for 15–20 minutes. A wet washcloth may be more readily accepted if holes are cut out for eyes and mouth, allowing the patient to remain functional. Hand or foot dermatitis can be treated by soaking the affected part in a basin. Daily baths may need to be taken on a chronic basis and even increased to several times daily during flares of AD, while showers may be adequate for patients with mild disease. It is essential to use an occlusive preparation within a few minutes after hydrating the skin to prevent evaporation, which can be both drying and irritating. Patients and their families need to be properly educated about hydration of the skin.

## F.   Moisturizers and Occlusives

Use of an effective emollient, especially when combined with hydration therapy, will help restore and preserve the stratum corneum barrier and can result in a decreased need for topical corticosteroids. Moisturizers are available as lotions, creams, and ointments. Lotions contain more water than creams and may be more drying due to an evaporative effect. Both lotions and creams may cause skin irritation secondary to added preservatives and fragrances. Since moisturizers usually need to be applied several times daily on a long-term basis, they should be obtained in one pound jars if available. Effective moisturizers include Aquaphor® Ointment, Eucerin® Creme, Vanicream®, Cetaphil® Cream, and Moisturel® Cream. Crisco® shortening can be used if an inexpensive moisturizer is needed. Petroleum jelly (Vaseline®) is an effective occlusive when used to seal in water after bathing.

## G.   Corticosteroids

Corticosteroids reduce inflammation and pruritus in AD. Topical corticosteroids are available in a wide variety of formulations, ranging from extremely high to low-potency preparations (see Chapter 27). Choice of a particular product depends on the severity and distribution of skin lesions. Patients need to be informed of the potency of their corticosteroid and the potential side effects. In general, the topical corticosteroid of lowest potency that is effective should be used. However, choosing a preparation that is too weak may result in persistent or worsening AD. Resistant lesions occasionally may respond to a potent topical corticosteroid under occlusion [163].

With appropriately used low to medium-potency topical corticosteroids, side effects are infrequent [164]. Thinning of the skin with telangiectasias, bruising, hypopigmentation, acne, striae, and secondary infections may occur. The face, especially the eyelids and the intertriginous areas, are especially sensitive to these adverse effects, and only low-potency preparations should be used routinely on these areas. Use of high-potency topical corticosteriods, especially under occlusion, may result in significant atrophic changes as well as systemic side effects and needs to be done cautiously.

Topical corticosteriods are available in a variety of bases including ointments, creams, lotions, solutions, gels, sprays, and even tapes. There is, therefore, no need to compound these medications. Ointments are most occlusive and as a rule provide better delivery of the medication while preventing evaporative losses. In a humid environment, creams may be better tolerated than ointments since the increased occlusion may cause itching or even folliculitis. In general, however, creams and lotions, while easier to spread, are less effective and can contribute to skin dryness and irritation. Solutions can be used on the scalp and hirsute areas, although their alcohol content can be quite irritating, especially if used on inflamed or open lesions. In addition to their irritant potential, additives used to formulate the different bases may cause sensitization. Furthermore, allergic contact dermatitis to corticosteroid compounds is being recognized with increasing frequency [165]. Thus, contact allergy to topical corticosteroids can complicate treatment of inflammatory skin diseases, often in an insidious manner. A recent study highlights the difficulty in testing for this problem [166].

Patients should be instructed in the proper use of topical corticosteroids. Application of an emollient immediately prior to or over a topical corticosteiod preparation may decrease the effectiveness of the corticosteriod. With clinical improvement, a less potent corticosteroid should be prescribed and the frequency of use decreased. Topical corticosteroids can be discontinued when the inflammation resolves, but hydration and moisturizers need to be continued.

In addition to their anti-inflammatory properties, topical corticosteroids can decrease *S. aureus* colonization in AD [167]. In a double-blind, randomized one-week trial of desonide compared with vehicle in children with AD, clinical scores improved and *S. aureus* density significantly decreased in the desonide, but not in the vehicle group [168].

Systemic corticosteroids, including oral prednisone, should be avoided in the management of a chronic, relapsing disorder such as AD. Often patients or parents demand immediate improvement of their disease and find systemic corticosteroids more convenient to use than topical therapy. However, the dramatic improvement observed with systemic corticosteroids may be associated with an equally dramatic flaring of AD following their discontinuation. If a short course of oral corticosteroids is given, it is usually best to prescribe a tapering dose. Topical skin care, particularly with topical corticosteroids, should be intensified during the taper to suppress rebound flaring of AD.

## H.  Tar Preparations

Crude coal tar extracts have anti-inflammatory properties that are not as pronounced as those of topical corticosteroids. Tar preparations used in conjunction with topical corticosteroids in chronic AD may reduce the need for more potent corticosteroid preparations. Tar shampoos are often beneficial for scalp involvement. Moisturizer applied over tar products can decrease their drying effects on the skin. To avoid the inconvenience of multiple layers, a compounded product such as 5% LCD (Liquor Carbonis detergents) in Aquaphor® ointment can be used. Use at bedtime helps to increase compliance. This allows the patient to remove any residual tar and associated odor by washing in the morning and limits staining to pajamas and bed sheets. Use of tar preparations on acutely inflamed skin should be avoided, since this may result in skin irritation. Other than dryness or irritation, side effects associated with tar products are rare but include photosensitivity reactions and folliculitis.

## I.  Anti-Infective Therapy

Systemic antibiotic therapy may be necessary to treat AD secondarily infected with *S. aureus*. Erythromycin or a semisynthetic penicillin is usually the first choice of therapy, although erythromycin-resistant organisms are fairly common. First- or second-generation cephalosporins are an effective and convenient alternative. Maintenance antibiotic therapy is rarely indicated and may result in colonization by methicillin-resistant organisms. The topical antistaphylococcal antibiotic mupirocin (Bactroban®) applied three times daily to affected areas for 7–10 days may be effective for treating localized areas of involvement [169]. Although antibacterial cleansers have been shown to be effective in reducing bacterial skin flora [170], they can cause significant skin irritation.

Patients with disseminated eczema herpeticum, also referred to as Kaposi's varicelliform eruption, usually require treatment with systemic acyclovir [171]. Recurrent cutaneous herpetic infections can be controlled with daily prophylactic oral acyclovir. Superficial dermatophytosis and *P. ovale* can be treated with topical or rarely systemic antifungal drugs [56].

## J.  Antihistamines

Pruritus is the most common and usually least tolerated symptom of AD. Even partial reduction of pruritus can result in significant improvement in quality of life for patients with severe AD [172]. Systemic antihistamines and anxiolytics may be most useful through their tranquilizing and sedative effects and can be used primarily in the evening to avoid daytime drowsiness [173]. The tricyclic antidepressant doxepin, which has both histamine $H_1$- and $H_2$-receptor binding affinity as well as a long half-life, may be given as a single 10–50 mg dose in the evening. If nocturnal pruritus remains severe, short-term use of a sedative to allow adequate rest may be appropriate.

Nonsedating antihistamines may be ineffective in treating the pruritus associated with AD [174]. However, a recent study of loratadine 10 mg daily showed it to be significantly better than placebo in a double-blind, multicrossover study [175]. A beneficial effect has also been reported in a double-blind study in children with AD treated with cetirizine 5–10 mg daily for 8 weeks [176]. Of potential interest, cetirizine 10 mg twice daily has also been shown in a placebo-controlled, double-blind study in allergen-specific challenge to reduce both eosinophils and neutrophils in early and late phase reactions, suggesting anti-inflammatory, along with antihistamine effects [177].

Treatment of AD with topical antihistamines and local anesthetics should be used cautiously because of potential sensitization. A multicenter, double-blind, vehicle-controlled study of topical 5% doxepin cream resulted in significant reduction of pruritus [178]. In this one-week study, sensitization was not reported, although rechallenge with the drug after the 7-day course of therapy was not evaluated. Since then, several case reports have documented reactions to topical doxepin [179].

## XIV.  RECALCITRANT DISEASE

### A.  Wet Dressings

Wet dressings can be used together with hydration and topical therapy in severe AD or to potentiate therapy with less potent corticosteroids [180]. The prolonged hydration and occlusion provided by these wraps increases the absorption of topical medications and promotes healing. They can also serve as an effective barrier against the persistent scratching that often undermines therapy. Total body dressings can be achieved by using wet pajamas or long underwear with dry pajamas or sweatsuit on top. Hands and feet can be covered by wet tube socks under dry tube socks. Alternatively, the face, trunk, or extremities can be covered by wet gauze with dry gauze over it and secured in place with an elastic bandage or by pieces of tube socks. Dressings may be removed when they dry out or they may be remoistened. They are often best tolerated at bedtime. Overuse of wet dressings, however, can result in chilling, maceration of the skin, or secondary infection.

## B. Hospitalization

AD patients who are erythrodermic or who appear toxic may need to hospitalized. Hospitalization may also be appropriate for patients with severe disseminated disease resistant to first-line therapy. Often removing the patient from environmental allergens or stressors, together with intense education and assurance of compliance with therapy, results in marked clinical improvement. In this setting, the patient can also undergo appropriately controlled provocative challenges to help identify potential triggering factors.

## C. Phototherapy and Photochemotherapy

Ultraviolet (UV) light therapy can be a useful treatment modality for chronic recalcitrant AD. A recent study showed that treatment with UVA and UVB was associated with clinical improvement and a decrease in the expression of activation markers such as HLA-DR, interleukin-2 receptor, and CD30 on CLA-positive T cells [181]. Patients who do not experience photoexacerbations of their AD and who are not fair complexioned may benefit from moderate amounts of natural sunlight. However, they should be cautioned not to sunburn and to avoid perspiring, which can induce pruritus. Sunlamp treatment at home is usually not recommended because of the danger of overexposure. Under medical supervision, UVB has been shown to be effective in the treatment of AD [182], although narrow-band UVB may be a safer alternative [183]. Addition of UVA to UVB can increase the therapeutic response [184]. Alternatively, high-dose UVA1 has been found to be a fast-acting and effective phototherapeutic approach in patients with acute exacerbations of AD [185]. Unlike traditional UVA-UVB phototherapy, which appears less effective for acute exacerbations and acts primarily in the epidermis, high-dose UVA1 therapy significantly decreases dermal IgE-binding cells, including mast cells and dendritic cells [186]. UVA1 may exert anti-inflammatory effects indirectly by downregulating pro-inflammatory cytokines or directly by inducing apoptosis in skin-infiltrating CD4$^+$ T cells [187].

Photochemotherapy with oral methoxypsoralen therapy followed by UVA (PUVA) may be indicated in patients with severe AD, especially with failure of topical therapy in patients with significant corticosteroid side effects [188]. Short-term adverse effects may include erythema, pruritus, and pigmentation, while long-term adverse effects include premature skin aging and cutaneous malignancies [189]. Topical psoralens combined with UVA may be equally effective [190]. Topical PUVA has no risk of systemic side effects and may be especially useful for patients with chronic hand eczema who are resistant to other topical medications [191].

PUVA therapy in children with severe AD and growth suppression has resulted in accelerated growth [192]. In a follow-up study [193], children with severe AD unresponsive to other therapy were treated with twice-weekly PUVA with significant improvement observed in 74% after a mean of 9 weeks. Forty-two percent had sustained remission a year after discontinuing treatment. However, long-term risk of cutaneous malignancies has usually precluded treatment of children with PUVA.

## XV.  IMMUNOMODULATORY THERAPY

Since AD is associated with a number of immunoregulatory abnormalities, therapy directed toward correction of the immune dysfunction represents a rational alternative for those patients unresponsive to conventional therapies. Alternative treatment modalities may be especially useful for patients in whom corticosteroid resistance could be contributing to treatment failure [153].

### A.  Thymopentin

Thymopentin, a synthetic pentapeptide corresponding to amino acid residues 32–36 of the linear 48-amino-acid sequence of human thymopoietin, promotes differentiation of thymocytes and T-cell function [194]. Several blinded, placebo-controlled studies with subcutaneous thymopentin 50 mg given either once daily for 6 weeks or three times weekly for 12 weeks have shown it to be safe and effective in reducing pruritus and erythema [195,196].

### B.  Interferons

IFN-γ suppresses IgE synthesis [197] and inhibits Th2 cell function [198]. Treatment with subcutaneous rhIFN-γ has been shown to result in reduced clinical severity and decreased total circulating eosinophil counts in patients with AD [199,200]. In addition, treatment with rhIFN-γ has been shown to significantly decrease the number of circulating CD25+ lymphocytes [201]. Some patients may show persistent improvement several months after discontinuing therapy [202]. Thus, the in vivo effects of rhIFN-γ therapy are likely to be complex with modulation of Th2-cell–directed allergic inflammation the primary action. Recently, two open long-term studies have shown clinical efficacy in AD patients treated for a minimum of 22 months with 50 μg/m$^2$ rhIFN-γ given daily or every other day [203,204]. Importantly, the authors have shown that patients with AD can be treated chronically with rhIFN-γ without deterioration in their disease or significant adverse effects. This is noteworthy since IFN-γ has been shown to have pro-inflammatory effects in some clinical settings. Importantly, effective dosing with rhIFN-γ is associated with a decrease in eosinophil counts, suggesting that rhIFN-γ acts primarily on the allergic inflammatory response as opposed to IgE synthesis. Thus, it is likely that some patients treated with rhIFN-γ would respond better to individualized titration of their treatment dose. An increased understanding of the immunopathogenesis of AD could possibly help identify those patients who would respond to this treatment modality [205].

Recombinant IFN-α has also been used to treat patients with AD in several small, uncontrolled trials. Although a few reports suggest some clinical benefit using this immunomodulator [206], other studies have not confirmed this finding, although a significant decrease in circulating eosinophils has been observed [207]. In one report, after six weeks of therapy, epidermal inflammation was reduced with a corresponding decrease in infiltrating CD4 and CD8 cells [208]. In another study, although total serum IgE and eosinophil-derived proteins were not reduced, a significant reduction in IgE-receptor–mediated basophil histamine release was observed in six of nine patients [209]. A study of two patients with AD suggests improvement in their AD when rIFN-γ and rIFN-α were used sequentially [210].

## C. Cyclosporin A

Cyclosporin A (CsA) is an immunosuppressive drug that acts primarily on T cells, interfering with cytokine transcription [211]. The drug binds to an intracellular protein, cyclophilin, and this complex in turn inhibits calcineurin, a $Ca^{2+}$-calmodulin–dependent protein phosphatase involved in signal transduction [212]. Activation of calcineurin is necessary for cytokine gene transcription to be initiated. Maintenance of chronic inflammation in AD appears to be associated with increased IL-5 gene expression and eosinophil infiltration [3], and preliminary in vitro data with mononuclear cells from atopic patients demonstrate suppression of IL-5 production by CsA [213]. A significant decrease in the number of circulating eosinophils has also been observed with CsA therapy. These studies provide a rationale for the use of CsA in AD.

Van Joost et al. [214] first reported the benefit of oral CsA in severe AD. This was subsequently confirmed in both open trials and in an 8-week double-blind, placebo-controlled, crossover study with 5 mg/kg per day [215]. In addition, health-related quality of life showed significant improvement after treatment with CsA [216]. Short-term, blinded, placebo-controlled studies confirm the clinical benefit of oral CsA in severe re-fractory AD in adults [217,218]. These data have been substantiated in long-term trials, although patients relapse even after 48 months of therapy [219].

Two recent open studies demonstrate that children with AD treated with CsA tolerated the treatment well and showed significant improvement in both clinical signs and quality of life [220,221]. Unfortunately, discontinuation of treatment resulted in relapse, although the rate of relapse was variable.

Short-term oral CsA therapy can result in increased serum urea, creatinine, and bilirubin concentrations, but these have been shown to normalize after treatment is discontinued [215,222]. Although short-term therapy is well tolerated, most patients relapse soon after discontinuation of the drug [216]. Because of the concern for progressive or irreversible nephrotoxicity with extended treatment [223], few patients have been evaluated on maintenance therapy. In a recently published study [224], patients with severe AD treated with oral CsA 5 mg/kg per day for 6 weeks were followed until relapse, then treated with a second 6-week course. After both treatment periods, approximately half of the patients relapsed after 2 weeks, and the relapse rate after 6 weeks was 71 and 90%, respectively. However, a few patients did not relapse after the first or second treatment courses. All of these patients were still in remission after one year, suggesting that although this treatment regimen did not result in lasting remission for the majority of patients, a subset of patients may get extended clinical benefit. Because of concerns for systemic toxicity, topical administration of CsA has been tried. A 3-week, double-blind, vehicle-controlled study with 10% CsA gel and 10% CsA ointment failed to show significant improvement [225].

## D. Tacrolimus Ointment

Tacrolimus (FK506), a macrolide lactone isolated from a soil mold by Japanese researchers, is an immunosuppressive agent with a spectrum of activity similar to CsA, although it is structurally unrelated to CsA [226]. Tacrolimus also interacts with a cyclophilin-like cytoplasmic protein, FK506 binding protein, and this complex in turn inhibits calcineurin, interfering with gene transcription [212]. Preliminary data with tacrolimus in ointment form suggest clinical benefit in AD, with markedly diminished pruritus within 3 days of initiating therapy [227]. Biopsy results from days 3 and 7 of treatment revealed markedly diminished T-cell and eosinophilic infiltrates. No systemic side effects were noted over the 21 days of treatment. Further studies have shown that, unlike topical corticostroids, tacrolimus ointment does not cause cutaneous atrophy [228]. A study by Ruzicka et al. was conducted in a randomized, double-blind fashion with three concentrations of tacrolimus ointment in adults with atopic dermatitis [229]. In this 3-week trial, tacrolimus was applied on up to 1000 $cm^2$ BSA, and all three tacrolimus preparations were found to be significantly better than the vehicle alone. Burning at the application site was the only adverse event seen with active drug. Importantly, blood tacrolimus levels were not elevated during this study. A similar study was also done in children with AD, and the results showed that all three concentrations of tacrolimus ointment were superior to vehicle alone [230]. Again, no serious adverse events were noted. Since skin inflammation in AD is associated with increased permeability, an interesting aspect of therapy with tacrolimus ointment that may contribute to its safety profile is its self-regulatory activity, i.e., as it heals inflamed skin, tacrolimus absorption is decreased [231]. Of note, multicentered, blinded, vehicle-controlled phase 3 trials with tacrolimus in both adults and children with AD have been completed, and importantly, since AD is a chronic disease, long-term studies with tacrolimus ointment applied on up to 100% body surface area are in progress. The optimal treatment regimen using this agent remains to be defined.

The mechanism by which tacrolimus exerts its beneficial effects remains to be elucidated, although it likely involves the inhibition of IL-4 and IL-5 gene transcription. Tacrolimus also inhibits the transcription and release of other T-cell–derived cytokines such as IL-3, IFN-$\gamma$, TNF-$\alpha$, and GM-CSF, which can also contribute to allergic inflammation [211,232]. Of note, other cell types important in allergic skin inflammation including mast cells, basophils, eosinophils, keratinocytes, and Langerhans cells have tacrolimus (FK506)–binding proteins and downregulate their mediator or cytokine expression following treatment with tacrolimus [233–235]. Since recent studies suggest that the T-cell activation in AD is biphasic with activation of the Th2-like cytokines, IL-4, IL-5, and IL-13, during the acute phase with increased expression of the Th1 cytokines, IFN-$\gamma$ and IL-12, present in chronic lesions [3,76,106,126,236], the capacity of tacrolimus to inhibit the activation of multiple cell types and different cytokines may account for its ability to effectively reduce skin inflammation in AD.

## XVI.  EXPERIMENTAL AND UNPROVEN THERAPIES

### A.  Allergen Desensitization

A number of uncontrolled trials have suggested that desensitization to specific allergens may improve AD [237,238]. In a controlled study, patients with AD were treated with either allergen extract or placebo in a blinded fashion for over 24 months [239]. Eighty-one percent of patients in the active treatment group improved compared to 40% in the placebo group. However, patients were not treated with the same extract, and standardized allergens were not available. In a more recent double-blind, controlled trial of desensitization to house dust mite with tyrosine-adsorbed *D. pteronyssinus* extract, children with AD and immediate hypersensitivity to *D. pteronyssinus* failed to demonstrate any clinical benefit compared to placebo after an 8-month course of treatment [240]. In a second phase, children initially administered *D. pteronyssinus* extract were randomly assigned to continue on active treatment or placebo for an additional 6 months. The clinical scores suggested that extended desensitization may be more effective than placebo, but the numbers were too small to permit confident conclusions. A high placebo effect may have served to conceal any additional therapeutic effect from active treatment. Further controlled trials with standardized extracts of relevant allergens in AD are needed before this form of therapy can be recommended.

A different approach to allergen desensitization in AD has been attempted with allergen-antibody complexes. In a single-center study, adults with AD and hypersensitivity to *D. pteronyssinus* treated in a double-blind, placebo-controlled trial with intradermal injections of complexes containing *D. pteronyssinus* and autologous *D. pteronyssinus* specific antibodies showed significant clinical improvement, which was maintained for several months after discontinuing the injections [241]. These results need to be confirmed in multicenter trials.

## B. Traditional Chinese Herbal Therapy

Traditional Chinese herbal therapy (TCHT) in the form of decoctions (boiled, then strained extracts) has been proposed as a therapy for AD. A placebo-controlled, double-blind crossover trial with a standardized formulation of TCHT was carried out in children with widespread nonexudative AD [242]. Thirty-seven of 47 children enrolled completed the study. Response to active treatment was superior to placebo and was clinically significant with no evidence of systemic toxicity. All of the children were then enrolled in a long-term study [243]. At the end of the year, 18 children showed ≥90% reduction in eczema activity score. Seven children were able to discontinue treatment without relapse and while 16 required maintenance therapy, only 4 required daily treatment. Fourteen children withdrew from the study-10 due to lack of response and 4 because of unpalatability or difficulty in preparation of the decoction. Asymptomatic elevation of liver function tests was noted on one occasion in two children, but liver function normalized after discontinuation of TCHT.

This therapy was also tested in a double-blind, placebo-controlled study in 40 adult patients with long-standing refractory AD [244]. They were randomized to receive either TCHT or placebo herbs for 2 months followed by a crossover to the other treatment after a 4-week washout period. The mean scores for erythema and surface damage showed significant improvement at the end of active treatment. There was subjective improvement in itching and sleep during the active treatment phase. No side effects were reported by the patients. In a 12-month open-label extension of this study, patients who chose to continue on the herbal therapy had a 60–90% reduction in their clinical scores compared with baseline values, while clinical scores of patients who discontinued the herbal treatments gradually deteriorated [245]. No patient in the TCHT group felt able to discontinue treatment permanently, but some tolerated an alternate-day or every third-day regimen. Toxicology screening revealed no abnormalities in blood counts or biochemical parameters in any of the patients on continued treatment. Improvement in disease was not associated with any significant change in serum IgE level or peripheral blood lymphocyte subsets.

TCHT used in these studies is comprised of 10 herbs, some with known pharmacological properties [246]. These may include antimicrobial, sedative, anti-inflammatory, and corticosteroid-like activities. Recent data suggest that TCHT can inhibit the low-affinity receptor for IgE on peripheral blood monocytes in a dose-dependent manner that was not due to a toxic effect [247]. A more recent study suggests that changes in clinical severity are more closely related to the expression of CD23 on mature antigen-presenting cells in lesional skin rather than to differentiating peripheral blood monocyte CD23 expression [248]. The specific ingredients of TCHT that may be responsible for clinical improvement in AD remain to be elucidated. The clinical benefits of TCHT may be short-lived, and effectiveness may diminish despite continued treatment [249]. In addition, the possibility of toxicity associated with long-term use or idiosyncratic reactions remains a concern [250,251]. At present, TCHT for AD remains investigational.

## C. Essential Fatty Acids

A number of disturbances in the metabolism of essential fatty acids (EFAs) have been reported in patients with AD [252]. Consequently, clinical trials with either fish oil as a source of n-3 series EFAs [253] or oil extracted from the seeds of *Oenothera biennis* (evening primrose) as a source of n-6 series EFA [254] have been conducted with conflicting results. A double-blind, placebo-controlled, parallel-group randomized study that avoided the methodological and analytical problems of a number of previous studies found no clinical benefit of either evening primrose oil or fish oil in AD [255].

## D. Intravenous Gammaglobulin

Since chronic inflammation and T-cell activation appear to play a critical role in the pathogenesis of AD, intravenous gammaglobulin (IVGG) could have immunomodulatory effects in this disease. IVGG could also interact directly with antigens, such as infectious agents or toxins involved in the pathogenesis of AD. IVGG has been shown to contain high concentrations of staphylococcal toxin–specific antibodies, which inhibit the in vitro activation of T cells by staphylococcal toxins [256]. In this study, two different pooled IVGG preparations both contained high titers of antibodies to eight staphylococcal toxins, and binding by the pooled IVGG was toxin specific. Importantly, the mechanism of inhibition by IVGG was shown to be direct blocking of toxin binding to, or presentation by, antigen-presenting cells.

Treatment of severe refractory AD with IVGG has yielded conflicting results. Studies have not been controlled and have involved small numbers of patients. Kimata reported dramatic improvement of AD with this treatment modality [257]. However, in a more recent open label study, nine patients with severe AD were treated with high-dose (2 g/kg) IVGG (Venoglobulin I-Alpha Therapeutic Corporation) monthly for seven infusions [258]. Skin disease improved slightly in six patients, while their average daily prednisone dosage did not change significantly. Mean serum IgE levels did not decrease significantly during IVGG therapy, and in vitro IgE production by PBMC following IL-4 and anti-CD40 stimulation was not significantly reduced. The authors concluded that IVGG was of no clear clinical benefit in this small group of patients. In a novel approach, IVGG was applied topically to AD lesions on one extremity and a halogenated corticosteroid to a corresponding control area on the opposite extremity in six patients [259]. Treated areas were covered by nonocclusive dressings. After once-daily treatment for 9 days, the IVGG treated areas showed significant improvement in five of six patients and was superior to topical corticosteroids in two of these patients and equivalent in three. Controlled studies are needed before this treatment modality can be recommended.

## E. Leukotriene Modifiers

The role of cysteinyl leukotrienes has not been defined in AD, and no controlled studies have been reported to date with this group of drugs. Case reports with the LTD 4 receptor antagonist zafirlukast suggest possible benefit in some patient with AD [260].

## XVII. FUTURE DIRECTIONS

### A. Anticytokine/Cytokine Receptor Therapy

Targeting specific cytokines or their receptors represents a potentially unique and specific treatment modality for AD. Anti-IL-5 antibody has been shown to completely block eosinophil infiltration in sensitized animals whether administered before or after allergen challenge [261]. Preliminary data with a humanized monoclonal antibody against IL-5 in a monkey model suggest that a single dose can inhibit eosinophilia for an extended period of time [262]. These results suggest that anti-IL-5 therapy could be of benefit in AD since chronic inflammation in AD has been shown to be associated with increased IL-5 expression and eosinophil infiltration [3].

Soluble IL-4 receptor (sIL-4R) molecules can effectively bind IL-4 and suppress IL-4–mediated T- and B-cell functions [263]. In patients with AD, sIL-4R has been shown to downregulate allergen-specific lymphocyte function in vitro and may prove to be an effective therapeutic agent [264].

### B. Phosphodiesterase Inhibitors

Since monocytes from AD patients have an abnormal increase in PDE enzyme activity, PDE inhibitors such as Ro 20-1724 have been shown to decrease IgE synthesis [265] and basophil histamine release in vitro [266]. Culture of AD monocytes with Ro 20-1724 also resulted in significant reduction of abnormal levels of IL-4, IL-10, and $PGE_2$ [132]. Recently, patients with AD treated with CP80,633, a potent inhibitor of PDE type IV, applied topically in a blinded, placebo-controlled paired-lesion study, showed significant clinical improvement with the active drug [132].

### C. SDZ ASM 981 (Ascomycin Derivative)

Topical 1% SDZ ASM 981 was recently studied in a randomized, double-blind, placebo-controlled, right- and-left comparison trial [267]. Thirty-four adult patients with moderate AD were treated with topical 1% SDZ ASM 981 cream applied either once or twice daily and compared with a corresponding placebo cream base. Twice-daily application of 1% SDZ ASM 981 cream was significantly more effective than use of the corresponding placebo and more effective than once-daily treatment over a 21-day period. No clinically relevant drug-related adverse effects were noted. Phase 2 and 3 trials are in progress.

## XVIII. CONCLUSIONS

AD is a common inflammatory skin disease whose prevalence has increased similarly to asthma and allergic rhinitis. Recent studies have elucidated how allergens, IgE, T cells with skin homing capability, Langerhans cells, keratinocytes, eosinophils, and mast cells may all contribute to the inflammatory process in AD. These studies have also pointed out immune abnormalities shared by patients with AD and respiratory allergies. Thus, further investigations of AD may provide a ''window'' to gain new insights into the immunopathogenesis of the other atopic diseases as well. Although most patients respond to conventional therapy, novel treatment modalities based on a better understanding of the complex nature of the inflammatory process in AD may lead to improved outcomes, especially in recalcitrant disease, and possibly point the way toward even more specific, rather than symptomatic therapy. However, much remains to be learned about the complex inter-relationship of genetic, environmental, immunological and pharmacological factors in this disease before the ultimate goal of prevention can become a reality.

## REFERENCES

1.  Hanifin JM, Raika G. Diagnostic features of atopic dermatitis. Acta Dermatol Venereol (Stockh) 1980; 92:44–47.
2.  Boguniewicz M, Leung D. Atopic dermatitis. In: Middleton Jr E, Reed C, Ellis E, Adkinson Jr N, Yunginger J, Busse W, eds. Allergy: Principles and Practice. St. Louis: Mosby; 1998: 1123–1134.
3.  Hamid Q, Boguniewicz M, Leung DYM. Differential in situ cytokine gene expression in acute versus chronic atopic dermatitis. J Clin Invest 1994; 94(2):870–876.
4.  Linna O, Kokkonen J, Lahtela P, Tammela O. Ten-year prognosis for generalized infantile eczema. Acta Paediatr 1992; 81(12):1013–1016.
5.  Schauer U, Trube M, Jager R, Gieler U, Rieger CH. Blood eosinophils, eosinophil-derived proteins, and leukotriene C4 generation in relation to bronchial hyperreactivity in children with atopic dermatitis. Allergy 1995; 50(2):126–132.
6.  Besnier E. Première note et observations préliminaires pour servir d'introduction à l'étude diathesiques. Ann Dermatol Syphiligr (Paris) 1892; 23:634–648.
7.  Coca AF, Cooke RA. On the classification of the phenomena of hypersensitiveness. J Immunol 1923; 8:163–182.
8.  Pepys J. Atopy. In: Gill PGH, Coombs RRA, Lachmann PJ, eds. Clinical Aspects of Immunology. 3d ed. Malden: Blackwell Scientific, 1975:877–902.
9.  Hill LW, Sulzberger MB. Evolution of atopic dermatitis. Arch Dermatol Syph 1935; 32: 451–463.
10. Schultz Larsen F. Atopic dermatitis: a genetic-epidemiologic study in a population-based twin sample. J Am Acad Dermatol 1993; 28(5 Pt 1):719–723.
11. Schultz Larsen F, Diepgen T, Svensson A. The occurrence of atopic dermatitis in north Europe: an international questionnaire study. J Am Acad Dermatol 1996; 34(5 Pt 1): 760–764.
12. Aberg N, Hesselmar B, Aberg B, Eriksson B. Increase of asthma, allergic rhinitis and eczema in Swedish schoolchildren between 1979 and 1991. Clin Exp Allergy 1995; 25(9):815–819.
13. Dotterud LK, Kvammen B, Lund E, Falk ES. Prevalence and some clinical aspects of atopic dermatitis in the community of Sor-Varanger. Acta Derm Venereol 1995; 75(1):50–53.
14. Sugiura H, Umemoto N, Deguchi H, Murata Y, Tanaka K, Sawai T, Omoto M, Uchiyama M, Kiriyama T, Uehara M. Prevalence of childhood and adolescent atopic dermatitis in a Japanese population: comparison with the disease frequency examined 20 years ago. Acta Derm Venereol 1998; 78(4):293–294.
15. Williams HC. Is the prevalence of atopic dermatitis increasing? Clin Exp Dermatol 1992; 17:385–391.
16. Zeiger R, Heller S, Mellon M, et al. Genetic and environmental factors affecting the development of atopy through age 4 in children of atopic parents: a prospective randomized study of food allergen avoidance. Pediatr Allergy Immunol 1992; 3:110–127.
17. Zeiger RS, Heller S. The development and prediction of atopy in high-risk children: follow-up at age seven years in a prospective randomized study of combined maternal and infant food allergen avoidance. J Allergy Clin Immunol 1995; 95(6):1179–1190.
18. Kay J, Gawkrodger DJ, Mortimer MJ, Jaron AG. The prevalence of childhood atopic eczema in a general population. J Am Acad Dermatol 1994; 30(1):35–39.

19. Williams HC, Strachan DP, Hay RJ. Childhood eczema: disease of the advantaged? Br Med J 1994; 308:1132–1135.

20. Hayashi T, Kawakami N, Kondo N, Agata H, Fukutomi O, Shimizu H, Orii T. Prevalence of and risk factors for allergic diseases: comparison of two cities in Japan. Ann Allergy Asthma Immunol 1995; 75(6 Pt 1):525–529.

21. Cookson WOCM, Sharp PA, Faux JA, Hopkin JM. Linkage between Immunoglobulin E responses underlying asthma and rhinitis and chromosome 11q. Lancet 1989; 1:1292–1295.

22. Coleman R, Trembath RC, Harper JI. Chromosome 11q13 and atopy underlying atopic eczema. Lancet 1993; 341(8853):1121–1122.

23. Marsh DG, Neely JD, Breazeale DR, Ghosh B, Friedhoff LR, Ehrlich-Kautzky E, Schou C, Krishnaswamy G, Beaty TH. Linkage analysis of IL4 and other chromosome 5q31.1 markers and total serum immunoglobulin E concentrations. Science 1994; 264:1152–1156.

24. Chan SC, Brown MA, Willcox TM, Li SH, Stevens SR, Tara D, Hanifin JM. Abnormal IL-4 gene expression by atopic dermatitis T lymphocytes is reflected in altered nuclear protein interactions with IL-4 transcriptional regulatory element. J Invest Dermatol 1996; 106(5): 1131–1136.

25. Kawashima T, Noguchi E, Arinami T, Yamakawa-Kobayashi K, Nakagawa H, Otsuka F, Hamaguchi H. Linkage and association of an interleukin 4 gene polymorphism with atopic dermatitis in Japanese families. J Med Genet 1998; 35(6):502–504.

26. Hershey GK, Friedrich MF, Esswein LA, Thomas ML, Chatila TA. The association of atopy with a gain-of-function mutation in the alpha subunit of the interleukin-4 receptor. N Engl J Med 1997; 337(24):1720–1725.

27. Cox HE, Moffatt MF, Faux JA, Walley AJ, Coleman R, Trembath RC, Cookson WO, Harper JI. Association of atopic dermatitis to the beta subunit of the high affinity immunoglobulin E receptor. Br J Dermatol 1998; 138(1):182–187.

28. Mao XQ, Shirakawa T, Yoshikawa T, et al. Association between genetic variants of mast-cell chymase and eczema. Lancet 1996; 348:581–583.

29. Uehara M, Kimura C. Descendant family history of atopic dermatitis. Acta Derm Venereol 1993; 73:62–63.

30. Diepgen TL, Fartasch M. Recent epidemiological and genetic studies in atopic dermatitis. Acta Derm Venereol Suppl (Stockh) 1992; 176:13–18.

31. Diepgen TL, Blettner M. Analysis of familial aggregation of atopic eczema and other atopic diseases by odds ratio regression models. J Invest Dermatol 1996; 106(5):977–981.

32. Vickers CFH. The natural history of atopic eczema. Acta Derm Venerol 1980; 92:113–115.

33. Kissling S, Wuthrich B. Sites, types of manifestations and micromanifestations of atopic dermatitis in young adults. A personal follow-up 20 years after diagnosis in childhood. Hautarzt 1994; 45(6):368–371.

34. Lammintausta K, Kalimo K, Raitala R, Forsten Y. Prognosis of atopic dermatitis. A prospective study in early adulthood. Int J Dermatol 1991; 30(8):563–568.

35. Shmunes E, Keil J. Occupational dermatoses in South Carolina: a descriptive analysis of cost variables. J Am Acad Dermatol 1983; 9:861–866.

36. Pasternack D. The prediction of asthma in infantile eczema: a statistical approach. J Pediatr 1965; 66:164–165.

37. Bergmann RL, Edenharter G, Bergmann KE, Forster J, Bauer CP, Wahn V, Zepp F, Wahn U. Atopic dermatitis in early infancy predicts allergic airway disease at 5 years. Clin Exp Allergy 1998; 28:965–970.

38. Nassif A, Chan SC, Storrs FJ, Hanifin JM. Abnormal skin irritancy in atopic dermatitis and in atopy without dermatitis. Arch Dermatol 1994; 130(11):1402–1407.

39. Hanifin JM, Storrs FJ, Chan SC, Nassif A. Irritant reactivity in noncutaneous atopy [letter]. J Am Acad Dermatol 1997; 37(1):139.

40. Agosti JM, Sprenger JD, Lum LG, Witherspoon RP, Fisher LD, Storb R, Henderson WR.

Transfer of allergen-specific IgE-mediated hypersensitivity with allogeneic bone marrow transplantation. N Engl J Med 1988; 319:1623–1628.

41. Brinkman L, Raajimakers JAM, Bruijnzeel-Koomen C, Koenderman L, Lammers JW. Bronchial and skin reactivity in asthmatic patients with and without atopic dermatitis. Eur Respir J 1997; 10(5):1033–1040.

42. Worldwide variation in prevalence of symptoms of asthma, allergic rhinoconjunctivitis, and atopic eczema: ISAAC. The International Study of Asthma and Allergies in Childhood (ISAAC) Steering Committee. Lancet 1998; 351(9111):1225–1232.

43. Seidenari S, Giusti G. Objective assessment of the skin of children affected by atopic dermatitis: a study of pH, capacitance and TEWL in eczematous and clinically uninvolved skin. Acta Derm Venereol 1995; 75(6):429–433.

44. Williams HC, Burney PG, Pembroke AC, Hay RJ. The U.K. Working Party's diagnostic criteria for atopic dermatitis. III. Independent hospital validation. Br J Dermatol 1994; 131(3): 406–416.

45. Williams HC, Burney PG, Strachan D, Hay RJ. The U.K. Working Party's diagnostic criteria for atopic dermatitis. II. Observer variation of clinical diagnosis and signs of atopic dermatitis. Br J Dermatol 1994; 131(3):397–405.

46. Nagaraja, Kanwar AM, Dhar S, Singh S. Frequency and significance of minor clinical features in various age-related subgroups of atopic dermatitis in children. Pediatr Dermatol 1996; 13:10–13.

47. Yoshida A, Imayama S, Sugai S, Kawano Y, Ishibashi T. Increased number of IgE positive Langerhans cells in the conjunctiva of patients with atopic dermatitis. Br J Ophthalmol 1997; 81(5):402–406.

48. Tuft SJ, Kemeny DM, Dart JK, Buckley RJ. Clinical features of atopic keratoconjunctivitis. Ophthalmology 1991; 98(2):150–158.

49. Rystedt I. Work-related hand eczema in atopics. Contact Dermatitis 1985; 12:164–171.

50. Coenraads PJ, Diepgen TL. Risk for hand eczema in employees with past or present atopic dermatitis. Int Arch Occup Environ Health 1998; 71(1):7–13.

51. Ring J, Abeck D, Neuber K. Atopic eczema: role of microorganisms on the skin surface. Allergy 1992; 47:265–269.

52. Rystedt I, Strannegard IL, Strannegard O. Recurrent viral infections in patients with past or present atopic dermatitis. Br J Dermatol 1986; 114(5):575–582.

53. Pauly CR, Artis WM, Jones HE. Atopic dermatitis, impaired cellular immunity, and molluscum contagiosum. Arch Dermatol 1978; 114:391–393.

54. Currie JM, Wright RC, Miller OW. The frequency of warts in atopic patients. Cutis 1971; 8:244–245.

55. Raychaudhuri SP, Raychaudhuri SK. Revisit to Kaposi's varicelliform eruption: role of IL-4. Int J Dermatol 1995; 34(12):854–856.

56. Kolmer HL, Taketomi EA, Hazen KC, Hughs E, Wilson BB, Platts-Mills TA. Effect of combined antibacterial and antifungal treatment in severe atopic dermatitis. J Allergy Clin Immunol 1996; 98(3):702–707.

57. Jones HE, Reinhardt JH, Rinaldi MG. A clinical, mycological and immunological survey for dermatophytosis. Arch Dermatol 1973; 108:61–65.

58. Svejgaard E, Faergeman J, Jemec G, Kieffer M, Ottevanger V. Recent investigations on the relationship between fungal skin diseases and atopic dermatitis. Acta Derm Venereol Suppl (Stockh) 1989; 144:140–142.

59. Leyden JE, Marples RR, Kligman AM. *Staphylococcus aureus* in the lesions of atopic dermatitis. Br J Dermatol 1974; 90:525–530.

60. Higaki S, Morimatsu S, Morohashi M, Yamagishi T, Hasegawa Y. *Staphylococcus* species on the skin surface of infant atopic dermatitis patients. J Int Med Res 1998; 26(2):98–101.

61. Williams J, Vowels B, Honig P, Leyden J. *S. aureus* isolation from the lesions, the hands,

and the anterior nares of patients with atopic dermatitis. Pediatr Dermatol 1998; 15:194–198.

62. Doebbeling B, Reagan D, Pfaller M, Houston A, Hollis R, Wenzel R. Long-term efficacy of intranasal mupirocin ointment. A prospective cohort study of *Staphylococcus aureus* carriage. Arch Intern Med 1994; 154:1505–1508.

63. Nishijima S, Namura S, Higashida T, Kawai S. *Staphylococcus aureus* in the anterior nares and subungual spaces of the hands in atopic dermatitis. J Int Med Res 1997; 25(3): 155–158.

64. Leyden J, Kligman A. The case for steroid-antibiotic combinations. Br J Dermatol 1997; 96: 179–187.

65. Leung DYM, Bhan AK, Schneeberger EE, Geha RS. Characterization of the mononuclear cell infiltrate in atopic dermatitis using monoclonal antibodies. J Allergy Clin Immunol 1983; 71:47–56.

66. Cockerell CJ. Seborrheic dermatitis-like and atopic dermatitis-like eruptions in HIV-infected patients. Clin Dermatol 1991; 9(1):49–51.

67. White A, Horne DJ, Varigos GA. Psychological profile of the atopic eczema patient. Australas J Dermatol 1990; 31(1):13–16.

68. Jones HE, Inouye JC, McGerity JL, Lewis CW. Atopic disease and serum immunoglobulin E. Br J Dermatol 1975; 92:17–25.

69. Rajka G. Prurigo Besnier (atopic dermatitis) with special reference to the role of allergic factors. II. The evaluation of the results of skin reactions. Acta Derm Venereol 1961; 41: 1–39.

70. May CE. Objective clinical laboratory studies of immediate hypersensitivity reactions to foods in asthmatic children. J Allergy Clin Immunol 1976; 58:500–515.

71. Sampson HA, McCaskill CC. Food hypersensitivity and atopic dermatitis: evaluation of 113 patients. J Pediatr 1985; 107:669–675.

72. Burks AW, James JM, Hiegel A, Wilson G, Wheeler JG, Jones SM, Zuerlein N. Atopic dermatitis and food hypersensitivity reactions. J Pediatr 1998; 132(1):132–136.

73. Eigenmann P, Sicherer S, Borkowski T, Cohen B, Sampson H. Prevalence of IgE-mediated food allergy among children with atopic dermatitis. Pediatrics 1998; 101:E8.

74. Sampson HA, Broadbent K, Bernhisel-Broadbent J. Spontaneous basophil histamine release and histamine-releasing factor in patients with atopic dermatitis and food hypersensitivity. N Engl J Med 1989; 321:228–232.

75. Hoffman DR, Yamamoto FY, Geller B, Haddad Z. Specific IgE antibodies in atopic eczema. J Allergy Clin Immunol 1975; 55:256–267.

76. Van der Heijden F, Wierenga EA, Bos JD, Kapsenberg JL. High frequency of IL-4 producting CD4 + allergen-specific T lymphocytes in atopic dermatitis lesional skin. J Invest Dermatol 1991; 97:389–394.

77. Tuft L. Importance of inhalant allergens in atopic dermatitis. J Invest Dermatol 1949; 12: 211–219.

78. Tupker RA, De Monchy JG, Coenraads PJ, Homan A, van der Meer JB. Induction of atopic dermatitis by inhalation of house dust mite. J Allergy Clin Immunol 1996; 97(5):1064–1070.

79. Brinkman L, Aslander MM, Raaijmakers JA, Lammers JW, Koenderman L, Bruijnzeel-Koomen CA. Bronchial and cutaneous responses in atopic dermatitis patients after allergen inhalation challenge. Clin Exp Allergy 1997; 27(9):1043–1051.

80. Mitchell EB, Crow J, Chapman MD, Jouhal SS, Pope FM, Platts-Mills TAE. Basophils in allergen-induced patch test sites in atopic dermatitis. Lancet 1982; 1:127–130.

81. Clark RA, Adinoff AD. The relationship between positive aeroallergen patch test reactions and aeroallergen exacerbations of atopic dermatitis. Clin Immunol Immunopathol 1989; 53: S132–140.

82. Ring J, Darsow U, Gfesser M, Vieluf D. The atopy patch test in evaluating the role of aeroallergens in atopic eczema. Int Arch Allergy Immunol 1997; 113(1-3):379–383.

83. Neumann C, Gutgesell C, Fliegert F, Bonifer R, Hermann F. Comparative analysis of the frequency of house dust mite specific and nonspecific Th1 and Th2 cells in skin lesions and peripheral blood of patients with atopic dermatitis. J Mol Med 1996; 74(7):401–406.

84. Deleuran M, Ellingsen AR, Paludan K, Schou C, Thestrup-Pedersen K. Purified Der p1 and p2 patch tests in patients with atopic dermatitis: evidence for both allergenicity and proteolytic irritancy. Acta Dermato Venereol 1998; 78(4):241–243.

85. Tan BB, Weald D, Strickland I, Friedmann PS. Double-blind controlled trial of effect of housedust-mite allergen avoidance on atopic dermatitis. Lancet 1996; 347(8993):15–18.

86. Nordvall SL, Johansson S. IgE antibodies to *Pityrosporum orbiculare* in children with atopic diseases. Acta Paediatr Scand 1990; 79:343–348.

87. Wilson BB, Deuell B, Mills TA. Atopic dermatitis associated with dermatophyte infection and *Trichophyton* hypersensitivity. Cutis 1993; 51:191–192.

88. Tengvall Linder M, Johansson C, Zargari A, Bengtsson A, van der Ploeg I, Jones I, Harfast B, Scheynius A. Detection of *Pityrosporum orbiculare* reactive T cells from skin and blood in atopic dermatitis and characterization of their cytokine profiles. Clin Exp Allergy 1996; 26(11):1286–1297.

89. Nissen D, Petersen LJ, Esch R, Svejgaard E, Skov PS, Poulsen LK, Nolte H. IgE-sensitization to cellular and culture filtrates of fungal extracts in patients with atopic dermatitis. Ann Allergy Asthma Immunol 1998; 81(3):247–255.

90. Leung DYM, Harbeck R, Bina P, Hanifin JM, Reiser RF, Sampson HA. Presence of IgE antibodies to staphylococcal exotoxins on the skin of patients with atopic dermatitis: evidence for a new group of allergens. J Clin Invest 1993; 92:1374–1380.

91. Tada J, Toi Y, Akiyama H, Arata J, Kato H. Presence of specific IgE antibodies to staphylococcal enterotoxins in patients with atopic dermatitis. Eur J Dermatol 1996; 6(8):552–554.

92. Strange P, Skov L, Lisby S, Nielsen PL, Baadsgaard O. Staphylococcal enterotoxin B applied on intact normal and intact atopic skin induces dermatitis. Arch Dermatol 1996; 132(1):27–33.

93. Herz U, Schnoy N, Borelli S, Weigl L, Kasbohrer U, Daser A, Wahn U, Kottgen E, Renz H. A human-SCID mouse model for allergic immune response bacterial superantigen enhances skin inflammation and suppresses IgE production. J Invest Dermatol 1998; 110(3):224–231.

94. Campbell DE, Kemp AS. Proliferation and production of interferon-gamma (IFN-gamma) and IL-4 in response to *Staphylococcus aureus* and staphylococcal superantigen in childhood atopic dermatitis. Clin Exp Immunol 1997; 107(2):392–397.

95. Ezepchuk YV, Leung DYM, Middleton MH, Bina P, Reiser R, Norris DA. Staphylococcal toxins and protein A differentially induce cytotoxicity and release of tumor necrosis factor-alpha from human keratinocytes. J Invest Dermatol 1996; 107(4)603–609.

96. Saurat JH. Eczema in primary immune-deficiencies: clues to the pathogenesis of atopic dermatitis with special reference to the Wiskott-Aldrich syndrome. Acta Derm Venereol 1985; 114:125–128.

97. Rousset F, Robert J, Andary M, Bonnin J-P, Souillet G, Chrétien I, Brière F, Pène J, de Vries JE. Shifts in interleukin-4 and interferon-γ production by T cells of patients with elevated serum IgE levels and the modulatory effects of these lymphokines on spontaneous IgE synthesis. J Allergy Clin Immunol 1991; 87:58–69.

98. Renz H, Jujo K, Bradley KL, Domenico J, Gelfand EW, Leung DYM. Enhanced IL-4 production and IL-4 receptor expression in atopic dermatitis and their modulation by interferon-gamma. J Invest Dermatol 1992; 99:403–408.

99. Vollenweider S, Saurat J-H, Röcken M, Hauser C. Evidence suggesting involvement of interleukin-4 (IL-4) production in spontaneous in vitro IgE synthesis in patients with atopic dermatitis. J Allergy Clin Immunol 1991; 87:1088–1095.

100. Reinhold U, Pawelec G, Wehrmann W, Herold M, Wernet P, Kreysel HW. Immunoglobulin E and immunoglobulin G subclass distribution in vivo and relationship to in vitro generation

of interferon-gamma and neopterin in patients with severe atopic dermatitis. Int Arch Allergy Appl Immunol 1988; 87:120–126.

101. Van Reijsen FC, Bruijnzeel-Koomen CA, Kalthoff FS, Maggi E, Romagnani S, Westland JK, Mudde GC. Skin-derived aeroallergen-specific T-cell clones of Th2 phenotype in patients with atopic dermatitis. J Allergy Clin Immunol 1992; 90:184–193.

102. Nakazawa M, Sugi N, Kawaguchi H, Ishii N, Nakajima H, Minami M. Predominance of type 2 cytokine-producing CD4+ and CD8+ cells in patients with atopic dermatitis. J Allergy Clin Immunol 1997; 99(5):673–682.

103. Frezzolini A, Paradisi M, Ruffelli M, Cadoni S, De Pita O. Soluble CD30 in pediatric patients with atopic dermatitis. Allergy 1997; 52(1):106–109.

104. Vercelli D, Jabara HH, Lauener RP, Geha RS. IL-4 inhibits the synthesis of IFN-$\gamma$ and induces the synthesis of IgE in human mixed lymphocyte cultures. J Immunol 1990; 144:570–573.

105. Chan SC, Kim JW, Henderson WR, Hanifin JM. Altered prostaglandin $E_2$ regulation of cytokine production in atopic dermatitis. J Immunol 1993; 151:3345–3352.

106. Ohmen JD, Hanifin JM, Nickoloff BJ, Rea TH, Wyzykowski R, Kim J, Jullien D, McHugh T, Nassif AS, Chan SC, Modlin RL. Overexpression of IL-10 in atopic dermatitis. Contrasting cytokine patterns with delayed-type hypersensitivity reactions. J Immunol 1995; 154(4):1956–1963.

107. Lester MR, Hofer MF, Gately M, Trumble A, Leung DYM. Down-regulating effects of IL-4 and IL-10 on the IFN-gamma response in atopic dermatitis. J Immunol 1995; 154(11): 6174–6181.

108. Ohki O, Yokozeki H, Katayama I, Umeda T, Azuma M, Okumura K, Nishioka K. Functional CD86 (B7-2/B70) is predominantly expressed on Langerhans cells in atopic dermatitis. Br J Dermatol 1997; 136(6):838–845.

109. Jirapongsananuruk O, Hofer MF, Trumble AE, Norris DA, Leung DYM. Enhanced expression of B7.2 (CD86) in patients with atopic dermatitis: a potential role in the modulation of IgE synthesis. J Immunol 1998; 160(9):4622–4627.

110. Mihm MC, Soter NA, Dvorak HF, Austen KJ. The structure of normal skin and the morphology of atopic eczema. J Invest Dermatol 1976; 67:305–312.

111. Bos JD, Hagenara C, Das PK, Krieg SR, Voorn WJ, Kapsenberg ML. Predominance of "memory" T cells (CD4+, CDw29+) over "naive" T cells (CD4+, CD45R+) in both normal and diseased human skin. Arch Dermatol Res 1989; 81:24–30.

112. Picker LJ, Butcher EC. Physiogical and molecular mechanisms of lymphocyte homing. Annu Rev Immunol 1992; 10:561–591.

113. Wakita H, Sakamoto T, Tokura Y, Takigawa M. E-selectin and vascular cell adhesion molecule-1 as critical adhesion molecules for infiltration of T lymphocytes and eosinophils in atopic dermatitis. J Cutan Pathol 1994; 21(1):33–39.

114. Rossiter H, van Reijsen F, Mudde G. Skin disease-related T cells bind to endothelial selectins: expression of cutaneous lymphocyte antigen (CLA) predicts E-selectin but not P-selectin binding. Eur J Immunol 1994; 24:205–210.

115. Babi LFS, Moser R, Soler MTP, Picker LJ, Blaser K, Hauser C. Migration of skin-homing T cells across cytokine-activated human endothelial cell layers involves interaction of the cutaneous lymphocyte-associated antigen (CLA), the very late antigen-4 (VLA-4), and the cutaneous lymphocyte-associated antigen-1 (LFA-1). J Immunol 1995; 154:1543–1550.

116. Bochner BS, Klunk DA, Sterbinsky SA, Coffman RL, Schleimer RP. IL-13 selectively induces vascular cell adhesion molecule-1 expression in human endothelial cells. J Immunol 1995; 154(2):799–803.

117. Taylor RS, Baadsgaard O, Hammerberg C, Cooper KD. Hyperstimulatory CD1a+ CD1b+CD36+ Langerhans cells are responsible for increased autologous T lymphocyte reactivity to lesional epidermal cells of patients with atopic dermatitis. J Immunol 1991; 147: 3794–3802.

118. Bruijnzeel-Koomen C, van Wichen DF, Toonstra J, Berrens L, Bruijnzeel PLB. The presence of IgE molecules on epidermal Langerhans cells in patients with atopic dermatitis. Arch Derm Res 1986; 278:199–205.

119. Leung DYM, Schneeberger EE, Siraganian RP, Geha RS, Bhan AK. The presence of IgE on monocytes/macrophages infiltrating into the skin lesion of atopic dermatitis. Clin Immunol Immunopathol 1987; 42:328–337.

120. Wollenberg A, Kraft S, Hanau D, Bieber T. Immunomorphological and ultrastructural characterization of Langerhans cells and a novel, inflammatory dendritic epidermal cell (IDEC) population in lesional skin of atopic eczema. J Invest Dermatol 1996; 106(3):446–453.

121. Leiferman KM, Ackerman SJ, Sampson HA, Haugen HS, Venecie PY, Gleich GJ. Dermal deposition of eosinophil granule major basic protein in atopic dermatitis: Comparison with onchocerciasis. N Engl J Med 1985; 313:282–285.

122. Gleich GJ, Leiferman KM. Eosinophils and hypersensitivity disease. In: Read CE, ed. Proc XII Int Congress Allergol Clin Immunol. St. Louis: C.V. Mosby Co., 1986:124–130.

123. Kagi MK, Joller-Jemelka H, Wuthrich B. Correlation of eosinophils, eosinophil cationic protein, soluble interleukin-2 receptor with the clinical activity of atopic dermatitis. Dermatology 1992; 185:88–92.

124. Taha RA, Leung DYM, Ghaffar O, Boguniewicz M, Hamid Q. In vivo expression of cytokine receptor mRNA in atopic dermatitis. J Allergy Clin Immunol 1998; 102(2):245–250.

125. Hamid Q, Naseer T, Minshall EM, Song YL, Boguniewicz M, Leung DY. In vivo expression of IL-12 and IL-13 in atopic dermatitis. J Allergy Clin Immunol 1996; 98:225–231.

126. Grewe M, Gyufko K, Schopf E, Krutmann J. Lesional expression of interferon-gamma in atopic eczema. Lancet 1994; 343(8888):25–26.

127. Thepen T, Langeveld-Wildschut EG, Bihari IC, van Wichen DF, van Reijsen FC, Mudde GC, Bruijnzeel-Koomen CAFM. Biphasic response against aeroallergen in atopic dermatitis showing a switch from an initial TH2 response to a TH1 response in situ: an immunocytochemical study. J Allergy Clin Immunol 1996; 97(3):828–837.

128. Laberge S, Ghaffar O, Boguniewicz M, Center D, Leung D, Q H. Association of increased CD4+ T-cell infiltration with increased IL-16 gene expression in atopic dermatitis. J Allergy Clin Immunol 1998; 102:645–650.

129. Ying S, Taborda-Barata L, Meng Q, Humbert M, Kay AB. The kinetics of allergen-induced transcription of messenger RNA for monocyte chemotactic protein-3 and RANTES in the skin of human atopic subjects: relationship to eosinophil, T cell, and macrophage recruitment. J Exp Med 1995; 181(6):2153–2159.

130. Taha RA, Leung DYM, Minshall E, Boguniewicz M, Luster A, Hamid Q. Eotaxin and monocyte chemoattractant protein (MCP)-4 mRNA expression in acute versus chronic atopic dermatitis. J Allergy Clin Immunol 1998; 101:S228.

131. Sawai T, Ikai K, Uehara M. Elevated cyclic adenosine monophosphate phosphodiesterase activity in peripheral blood mononuclear leucocytes from children with atopic dermatitis. Br J Dermatol 1995; 132(1):22–24.

132. Hanifin JM, Chan SC, Cheng JB, Tofte SJ, Henderson WR, Jr., Kirby DS, Weiner ES. Type 4 phosphodiesterase inhibitors have clinical and in vitro anti-inflammatory effects in atopic dermatitis. J Invest Dermatol 1996; 107(1):51–56.

133. Chan SC, Hanifin JM. Differential inhibitor effects on cyclic adenosine monophosph-phosphodiesterase isoforms in atopic and normal leukocytes. J Lab Clin Med 1993; 121:44–51.

134. Essayan DM, Huang SK, Kageysobotka A, Lichtenstein LM. Differential efficacy of lymphocyte- and monocyte-selective pretreatment with a type 4 phosphodiesterase inhibitor on antigen-driven proliferation and cytokine gene expression. J Allergy Clin Immunol 1997; 99(1 Part 1):28–37.

135. Bratton DL, Hamid Q, Boguniewicz M, Doherty DE, Kailey JM, Leung DYM. Granulocyte macrophage colony-stimulating factor contributes to enhanced monocyte survival in chronic atopic dermatitis. J Clin Invest 1995; 95(1): 211–218.

136. Muller KM, Jaunin F, Masouye I, Saurat JH, Hauser C. Th2 cells mediate IL-4-dependent local tissue inflammation. J Immunol 1993; 150:5576–5584.

137. Solley GO, Gleich GJ, Jordan RE, Schroeter AL. The late phase of the immediate wheal and flare skin reaction: its dependence upon IgE antibodies. J Clin Invest 1976; 58:408–420.

138. Kay AM, Ying S, Varney V, Gaga M, Durham SR, Moqbel R, Wardlaw AJ, Hamid Q. Messenger RNA expression of cytokine gene cluster, interleukin 3 (IL-3), IL-5, and granulocyte/macrophage colony-stimulating factor in allergen-induced late-phase cutaneous reactions in atopic subjects. J Exp Med 1991; 173:775–778.

139. Leung DYM, Cotran RS, Pober JS. Expression of an endothelial leukocyte adhesion molecule (ELAM-1) in elicited late phase allergic skin reactions. J Clin Invest 1991; 87:1805–1810.

140. Mudde GC, Van Reijsen FC, Boland GJ, DeGast GC, Bruijnzeel PLB, Bruijnzeel-Koomen CAFM. Allergen presentation by epidermal Langerhans cells from patients with atopic dermatitis is mediated by IgE. Immunology 1990; 69:335–341.

141. Jürgens M, Wollenberg A, Hanau D, de la Salle H, Bieber T. Activation of human epidermal Langerhans cells by engagement of the high affinity receptor for IgE, Fc epsilon RI. J Immunol 1995; 155(11):5184–5189.

142. Klubal R, Osterhoff B, Wang B, Kinet JP, Maurer D, Stingl G. The high-affinity receptor for IgE is the predominant IgE-binding structure in lesional skin of atopic dermatitis patients. J Invest Dermatol 1997; 108(3):336–342.

143. Robinson DS, Hamid Q, Ying S, Tsicopoulos A, Barkans J, Bentley AM, Corrigan C, Durham SR, Kay AB. Predominant $T_{H2}$-like bronchoalveolar T-lymphocyte population in atopic asthma. N Engl J Med 1992; 326:298–304.

144. Picker LJ, Treer JR, Ferguson-Darnell B, Collins PA, Bergstresser PR, Terstappen LW. Control of lymphocyte recirculation in man: II. differential regulation of the cutaneous lymphocyte-associated antigen, a tissue-selective homing receptor for skin-homing T cells. J Immunol 1993; 150:1122–1136.

145. Picker LJ, Martin RJ, Trumble AE, Newman L, Collins PA, Bergstresser PR, Leung DYM. Control of lymphocyte recirculation in man: Differential expression of homing-associated adhesion molecules by memory/effector T cells in pulmonary vs. cutaneous effector sites. Eur J Immunol 1994; 24:1269–1277.

146. Abernathy-Carver KJ, Sampson HA, Picker LJ, Leung DYM. Milk-induced eczema is associated with the expansion of T cells expressing cutaneous lymphocyte antigen. J Clin Invest 1995; 95(2):913–918.

147. Babi LFS, Picker LJ, Soler MTP, Drzimalla K, Flohr P, Blaser K, Hauser C. Circulating allergen-reactive T cells from patients with atopic dermatitis and allergic contact dermatitis express the skin-selective homing receptor, the cutaneous lymphocyte-associated antigen. J Exp Med 1995; 181:1935–1940.

148. Jones S, Sampson H. The role of allergens in atopic dermatitis. In: Leung DYM, ed. Atopic Dermatitis: From Pathogenesis to Treatment. Austin: RG Landes, 1996:41–65.

149. Leung DYM, Gately M, Trumble A, Ferguson-Darnell B, Schlievert PM, Picker LJ. Bacterial superantigens induce T cell expression of the skin-selective homing receptor, the cutaneous lymphocyte-associated antigen, via stimulation of interleukin 12 production. J Exp Med 1995; 181(2):747–753.

150. Torres MJ, Gonzalez FJ, Corzo JL, Giron MD, Carvajal MJ, Garcia V, Pinedo A, Martinez-Valverde A, Blanca M, Santamaria LF. Circulating CLA+ lymphocytes from children with atopic dermatitis contain an increased percentage of cells bearing staphylococcal-related T-cell receptor variable segments. Clin Exp Allergy 1998; 28:1264–1272.

151. Leung DYM. Atopic dermatitis: the skin as a window into the pathogenesis of chronic allergic diseases. J Allergy Clin Immunol 1995; 96(3):302–318.

152. Plaut M, Pierce JH, Watson CJ, Hanley-Hyde J, Nordan RP, Paul WE. Mast cell lines produce lymphokines in response to cross-linkage of FcεRI to calcium ionophores. Nature 1989; 229:64–67.

153. Clayton MH, Leung DYM, Surs W, Szefler SJ. Altered glucocorticoid receptor binding in atopic dermatitis. J Allergy Clin Immunol 1995; 96(3):421–423.

154. Kupper TS. Interleukin-1 and other human keratinocyte cytokines: molecular and functional characterization. Adv Dermatol 1988:293–307.

155. Sampson HA. The role of food allergy and mediator release in atopic dermatitis. J Allergy Clin Immunol 1988; 81:635–645.

156. Sampson HA, Ho DG. Relationship between food-specific IgE concentrations and the risk of positive food challenges in children and adolescents. J Allergy Clin Immunol 1997; 100(4): 444–451.

157. Noren P, Melin L. The effect of combined topical steroids and habit-reversal treatment in patients with atopic dermatitis. Br J Dermatol 1989; 121(3):359–366.

158. Horne DJ, White AE, Varigos GA. A preliminary study of psychological therapy in the management of atopic eczema. Br J Med Psychol 1989; 62(Pt3):241–248.

159. Koblenzer CS. Psychotherapy for intractable inflammatory dermatoses. J Am Acad Dermatol 1995; 32(4):609–612.

160. Broberg A, Kalimo K, Lindblad B, Swanbeck G. Parental education in the treatment of childhood atopic eczema. Acta Derm Venereol 1990; 70(6):495–499.

161. Werner Y, Lindberg M. Transepidermal water loss in dry and clinically normal skin in patients with atopic dermatitis. Acta Derm Venereol (Stockh) 1985; 65:102–105.

162. Linde Y. Dry skin in atopic dermatitis. Acta Derm Venereol Suppl (Stockh) 1992; 77: 9–13.

163. Volden G. Successful treatment of therapy-resistant atopic dermatitis with clobetasol propionate and a hydrocolloid occlusive dressing. Acta Derm Venereol Suppl (Stockh) 1992; 176: 126–128.

164. Vernon HJ, Lane AT, Weston W. Comparison of mometasone furoate 0.1% cream and hydrocortisone 1.0% cream in treatment of childhood atopic dermatitis. J Am Acad Dermatol 1991; 24:603–607.

165. Dooms-Goossens A, Morren M. Results of routine patch testing with corticosteroid series in 2073 patients. Contact Dermatitis 1992; 26:182–191.

166. Seukeran D, Wilkinson S, Beck M. Patch testing to detect corticosteroid allergy: Is it adequate? Contact Dermatitis 1997; 36:127–130.

167. Nilsson EJ, Henning CG, Magnusson J. Topical corticosteroids and *Staphylococcus aureus* in atopic dermatitis. J Am Acad Dermatol 1992; 27:29–34.

168. Stalder JF, Fleury M, Sourisse M, Rostin M, Pheline F, Litoux P. Local steroid therapy and bacterial skin flora in atopic dermatitis. Br J Dermatol 1994; 131(4):536–540.

169. Luber H, Amornsiripanitch S, Lucky AW. Mupirocin and the eradication of *Staphylococcus aureus* in atopic dermatitis. Arch Dermatol 1988; 124:853–854.

170. Stalder JF, Fleury M, Sourisse M, Allavoine T, Chalamet C, Brosset P, Litoux P. Comparative effects of two topical antiseptics (chlorhexidine vs KMnO4) on bacterial skin flora in atopic dermatitis. Acta Derm Venereol Suppl (Stockh) 1992; 176:132–134.

171. Bork K, Brauninger W. Increasing incidence of eczema herpeticum: analysis of seventy-five cases. J Am Acad Dermatol 1988; 19(6):1024–1029.

172. Doherty V, Sylvester DGH, Kennedy CTC, Harvey SG, Calthrop JG, Gibsom JR. Treatment of itching in atopic eczema with antihistamines with a low sedative profile. BMJ 1989; 298: 96.

173. Kraus L, Shuster S. Mechanism of action of antipruritic drugs. BMJ 1983; 287:1199–1200.

174. Berth-Jones J, Graham-Brown RAC. Failure of terfenadine in relieving the pruritus of atopic dermatitis. Br J Dermatol 1989; 121:635–637.

175. Langeland T, Fagertun HE, Larsen S. Therapeutic effect of loratadine on pruritus in patients with atopic dermatitis. A multi-crossover-designed study. Allergy 1994; 49(1):22–26.

176. La Rosa M, Ranno C, Musarra I, Guglielmo F, Corrias A, Bellanti JA. Double-blind study of cetirizine in atopic eczema in children. Ann Allergy 1994; 73(2):117–122.

177. Ciprandi G, Buscaglia S, Pesce G, Passalacqua G, Rihoux JP, Bagnasco M, Canonica GW. Cetirizine reduces inflammatory cell recruitment and ICAM-1 (or CD54) expression on conjunctival epithelium in both early-and late-phase reactions after allergen-specific challenge. J Allergy Clin Immunol 1995; 95:612–621.

178. Drake LA, Fallon JD, Sober A, Group DS. Relief of pruritus in patients with atopic dermatitis after treatment with topical doxepin cream. J Am Acad Dermatol 1994; 31(4):613–616.

179. Shelley WB, Shelley ED, Talanin NY. Self-potentiating allergic contact dermatitis caused by doxepin hydrochloride cream. J Am Acad Dermatol 1996; 34(1):143–144.

180. Nicol NH. Atopic dermatitis: the (wet) wrap-up. Am J Nurs 1987; 87(12):1560–1563.

181. Piletta PA, Wirth S, Hommel L, Saurat JH, Hauser C. Circulating skin-homing T cells in atopic dermatitis. Selective up-regulation of HLA-DR, interleukin-2R, and CD30 and decrease after combined UV-A and UV-B phototherapy. Arch Dermatol 1996; 132(10):1171–1176.

182. Jekler J, Larko O. UVB phototherapy for atopic dermatitis. Br J Dermatol 1988; 119:697–705.

183. George SA, Bilsland DJ, Johnson BE, Ferguson J. Narrow band (TL-01) UVB air conditioned phototherapy for chronic severe adult atopic dermatitis. Br J Dermatol 1993; 128:49–56.

184. Midelfart K, Stenvold SE, Voloden G. Combined UVB and UVA phototherapy of atopic eczema. Dermatologica 1985; 171:95–98.

185. Krutmann J, Czech W, Diepgen T, Niedner R, Kapp A, Schopf E. High-dose UVA1 therapy in the treatment of patients with atopic dermatitis. J Am Acad Dermatol 1992; 26:225–230.

186. Krutmann J, Diepgen TL, Luger TA, Grabbe S, Meffert H, Sonnichsen N, Czech W, Kapp A, Stege H, Grewe M, Schopf E. High-dose UVA1 therapy for atopic dermatitis: results of a multicenter trial. J Am Acad Dermatol 1998; 38(4):589–593.

187. Morita A, Werfel T, Stege H, Ahrens C, Karmann K, Grewe M, Grether-Beck S, Ruzicka T, Kapp A, Klotz LO, Sies H, Krutmann J. Evidence that singlet oxygen-induced human T helper cell apoptosis is the basic mechanism of ultraviolet-A radiation phototherapy. J Exp Med 1997; 186(10):1763–1768.

188. Morison WL, Parrish JA, Fitzpatrick TB. Oral psoralen photochemotherapy of atopic eczema. Br J Dermatol 1978; 98:25–30.

189. Honig B, Morison WL, Karp D. Photochemotherapy beyond psoriasis. J Am Acad Dermatol 1994; 31:775–790.

190. Yoshiike T, Sindhvananda J, Aikawa Y, Nakajima S, Ogawa H. Topical psoralen photochemotherapy for atopic dermatitis: evaluation of two therapeutic regimens for inpatients and outpatients. J Dermatol 1991; 18:201–205.

191. Gritiyarangsan P, Sukhum A, Tresukosol P, Kullavanijaya P. Topical PUVA therapy for chronic hand eczema. J Dermatol 1998; 25(5):299–301.

192. Atherton DJ, Carabott F, Glover MT, Hawk JLM. The role of psoralen chemotherapy (PUVA) in the treatment of severe atopic eczema in adolescents. Br J Dermatol 1988; 118:791–795.

193. Sheehan MP, Atherton DJ, Norris P, Hawk J. Oral psoralen photochemotherapy in severe childhood atopic eczema: an update. Br J Dermatol 1993; 129(4):431–436.

194. Meroni PL, Barcellini W, Frasca D, Sguotti C, Borghi MO, De Bartolo G, Doria G, Zanussi C. In vivo immunopotentiating activity of thymopentin in aging humans: increase of IL-2 production. Clin Immunol Immunopathol 1987; 42(2):151–159.

195. Leung DYM, Hirsch RL, Schneider L, Moody C, Takaoka R, Li SH, Meyerson LA, Mariam SG, Goldstein G, Hanifin JM. Thymopentin therapy reduces the clinical severity of atopic dermatitis. J Allergy Clin Immunol 1990; 85:927–933.

196. Stiller MJ, Shupack JL, Kenny C, Jondreau L, Cohen DE, Soter NA. A double-blind, placebo-controlled clinical trial to evaluate the safety and efficacy of thymopentin as an adjunctive treatment in atopic dermatitis. J Am Acad Dermatol 1994; 30(4):597–602.

197. Pène J, Rousset F, Brière F, Chrétien I, Bonnefoy JY, Spits H, Yokota T, Arai N, Arai K, Banchereau J, et al. IgE production by normal human lymphocytes is induced by interleukin 4 and suppressed by interferons gamma and alpha and prostaglandin E2. Proc Natl Acad Sci USA 1988; 85(18):6880–6884.

198. Gajewski TF, Fitch FW. Anti-proliferative effect of IFN-γ in immune regulation. I. IFN-γ inhibits the proliferation of Th2 but not Th1 murine helper T lymphocyte clones. J Immunol 1988; 140:4245–4252.

199. Boguniewicz M, Jaffe HS, Izu A, Sullivan MJ, York D, Geha RS, Leung DYM. Recombinant gamma interferon in treatment of patients with atopic dermatitis and elevated IgE levels. Am J Med 1990; 88(4):365–370.

200. Hanifin JM, Schneider LC, Leung DYM, Ellis CN, Jaffe HS, Izu AE, Bucalo LR, Hirabayashi SE, Tofte SJ, Cantu-Gonzales G, Milgrom H, Boguniewicz M, Cooper KD. Recombinant interferon gamma therapy for atopic dermatitis. J Am Acad Dermatol 1993; 28(2 Pt 1):189–197.

201. Musial J, Milewski M, Undas A, Kopinski P, Duplaga M, Szczeklik A. Interferon-gamma in the treatment of atopic dermatitis: influence on T-cell activation. Allergy 1995; 50(6):520–523.

202. Reinhold U, Kukel S, Brzoska J, Kreysel HW. Systemic interferon gamma treatment in severe atopic dermatitis. J Am Acad Dermatol 1993; 29(1):58–63.

203. Schneider LC, Baz Z, Zarcone C, Zurakowski D. Long-term therapy with recombinant interferon-gamma (rIFN-gamma) for atopic dermatitis. Ann Allergy Asthma Immunol 1998; 80(3):263–268.

204. Stevens SR, Hanifin JM, Hamilton T, Tofte SJ, Cooper KD. Long-term effectiveness and safety of recombinant human interferon gamma therapy for atopic dermatitis despite unchanged serum IgE levels. Arch Dermatol 1998; 134(7):799–804.

205. Boguniewicz M, Leung DYM. Atopic dermatitis: a question of balance. Arch Dermatol 1998; 134(7):870–871.

206. Torrelo A, Harto A, Sendagorta E, Czarnetzki BM, Ledo A. Interferon-alpha therapy in atopic dermatitis. Acta Derm Venereol 1992; 72(5):370–372.

207. Paukkonen K, Fraki J, Horsmanheimo M. Interferon-alpha treatment decreases the number of blood eosinophils in patients with severe atopic dermatitis. Acta Derm Venereol 1993; 73(2):141–142.

208. Gruschwitz MS, Peters KP, Heese A, Stosiek N, Koch HU, Hornstein OP. Effects of interferon-alpha-2b on the clinical course, inflammatory skin infiltrates and peripheral blood lymphocytes in patients with severe atopic eczema. Int Arch Allergy Immunol 1993; 101(1):20–30.

209. Nielsen BW, Reimert CM, Hammer R, Schiotz PO, Thestrup-Pedersen K. Interferon therapy for atopic dermatitis reduces basophil histamine release, but does not reduce serum IgE or eosinophilic proteins. Allergy 1994; 49(2):120–128.

210. Pung YH, Vetro SW, Bellanti JA. Use of interferons in atopic (IgE-mediated) diseases. Ann Allergy 1993; 71(3):234–238.

211. Schreiber SL, Crabtree GR. The mechanism of action of cyclosporin A and FK506. Immunol Today 1992; 13:136–142.

212. Liu J, Farmer JD, Lane WS, Friedman J, Weissman I, Schreiber SL. Calcineurin is a common target of cyclophilin-cyclosporin A and FKBP-FK506 complexes. Cell 1991; 66:807–815.

213. Mori A, Suko M, Nishizaki Y, Kaminuma O, Matsuzaki G, Ito K, Etoh T, Nakagawa H, Tsuruoka N, Okudaira H. Regulation of interleukin-5 production by peripheral blood mononuclear cells from atopic patients with FK506, cyclosporin A and glucocorticoid. Int Arch Allergy Immunol 1994; 104(1):32–35.

214. van Joost T, Stolz E, Heule F. Efficacy of low-dose cyclosporine in severe atopic skin disease. Arch Dermatol 1987; 123(2):166–167.

215. Sowden JM, Berth-Jones J, Ross JS, Motley RJ, Marks R, Finlay AY, Salek MS, Graham-

Brown RA, Allen BR, Camp RD. Double-blind, controlled, crossover study of cyclosporin in adults with severe refractory atopic dermatitis. Lancet 1991; 338(8760):137–140.

216. Salek MS, Finlay AY, Luscombe DK, Allen BR, Berth-Jones J, Camp RD, Graham-Brown RA, Khan GK, Marks R, Motley RJ, et al. Cyclosporin greatly improves the quality of life of adults with severe atopic dermatitis. A randomized, double-blind, placebo-controlled trial. Br J Dermatol 1993; 129(4):422–430.

217. Wahlgren CF, Scheynius A, Hagermark O. Antipruritic effect of oral cyclosporin A in atopic dermatitis. Acta Derm Venereol 1990; 70:323–329.

218. van Joost T, Heule F, Korstanje M, van den Broek MJ, Stenveld HJ, van Vloten WA. Cyclosporin in atopic dermatitis: a multicentre placebo-controlled study. Br J Dermatol 1994; 130: 634–640.

219. Berth-Jones J, Graham-Brown RA, Marks R, Camp RD, English JS, Freeman K, Holden CA, Rogers SC, Oliwiecki S, Friedmann PS, Lewis-Jones MS, Archer CB, Adriaans B, Douglas WS, Allen BR. Long-term efficacy and safety of cyclosporin in severe adult atopic dermatitis. Br J Dermatol 1997; 136(1):76–81.

220. Berth-Jones J, Finlay AY, Zaki I, Tan B, Goodyear H, Lewis-Jones S, Cork MJ, Bleehen SS, Salek MS, Allen BR, Smith S, Graham-Brown RA. Cyclosporine in severe childhood atopic dermatitis: a multicenter study. J Am Acad Dermatol 1996; 34(6):1016–1021.

221. Zaki I, Emerson R, Allen BR. Treatment of severe atopic dermatitis in childhood with cyclosporin. Br J Dermatol 1996; 135 (suppl 48):21–24.

222. van Joost T, Heule F, Korstanje M, van den Broek MJ, Stenveld HJ, van Vloten WA. Cyclosporin in atopic dermatitis: a multicentre placebo-controlled study. Br J Dermatol 1994; 130(5):634–640.

223. Zachariae H, Kragballe K, Hansen HE, Marcussen N, Olsen S. Renal biopsy findings in long-term cyclosporin treatment of psoriasis. Br J Dermatol 1997; 136:531–535.

224. Granlund H, Erkko P, Sinisalo M, Reitamo S. Cyclosporin in atopic dermatitis: time to relapse and effect of intermittent therapy. Br J Dermatol 1995; 132(1):106–112.

225. De Rie MA, Meinardi MHM, Bos JD. Lack of efficacy of topical cyclosporin A in atopic dermatitis and allergic contact dermatitis. Acta Derm Venereol 1991; 71(5):452–454.

226. Kino T, Hatanaka H, Hashimoto M, Nishiyama M, Goto T, Okuhara M, Kohsaka M, Aoki H, Imanaka H. FK-506, a novel immunosuppressant isolated from a Streptomyces. I. Fermentation, isolation, physico-chemical and biological characteristics. J Antibiot 1987; 40:1249–1255.

227. Nakagawa H, Etoh T, Ishibashi Y, Higaki Y, Kawashima M, Torii H, Harada S. Tacrolimus ointment for atopic dermatitis. Lancet 1994; 344(8926):24.

228. Reitamo S, Rissanen J, Remitz A, Granlund H, Erkko P, Elg P, Autio P, Lauerma AI. Tacrolimus ointment does not affect collagen synthesis: results of a single-center randomized trial. J Invest Dermatol 1998; 111(3):396–398.

229. Ruzicka T, Bieber T, Schopf E, Rubins A, Dobozy A, Bos JD, Jablonska S, Ahmed I, Thestrup-Pedersen K, Daniel F, Finzi A, Reitamo S, European Tacrolimus Multicenter Atopic Dermatitis Study Group. A short-term trial of tacrolimus ointment for atopic dermatitis. N Engl J Med 1997; 337(12):816–821.

230. Boguniewicz M, Fiedler VC, Raimer S, Lawrence ID, Leung DYM, Hanifin JM. A randomized, vehicle-controlled trial of tacrolimus ointment for treatment of atopic dermatitis in children. Pediatric Tacrolimus Study Group. J Allergy Clin Immunol 1998; 102:637–644.

231. Bieber T. Topical tacrolimus (FK506): a new milestone in the management of atopic dermatitis. J Allergy Clin Immunol 1998; 102:555–557.

232. Yoshimura N, Matsui S, Hamashima T, Oka T. Effect of a new immunosuppressive agent, FK506, on human lymphocyte responses in vitro. II. Inhibition of the production of IL-2 and gamma-IFN, but not B cell-stimulating factor 2. Transplantation 1989; 47:356–359.

233. de Paulis A, Stellato C, Cirillo R, Ciccarelli A, Oriente A, Marone G. Anti-inflammatory effect of FK-506 on human skin mast cells. J Invest Dermatol 1992; 99:723–728.

234. Kaplan A, Matsue H, Shibaki A, Kawashima T, Kobayashi H, Ohkawara A. The effect of cyclosporin A and FK506 on human skin mast cells. J Dermatol Sci 1995; 10:130–138.

235. Thomson A, Nalesnik M, Abu-Elmagd K, Starzl T. Influence of FK 506 on T lymphocytes, Langerhans' cells and the expression of cytokine receptors and adhesion molecules in psoriatic skin lesions: a preliminary study. Transplant Proc 1991; 23:3330–3331.

236. Hamid Q, Naseer T, Minshall EM, Song YL, Boguniewicz M, Leung DYM. In vivo expression of IL-12 and IL-13 in atopic dermatitis. J Allergy Clin Immunol 1996; 98(1):225–231.

237. Zachariae H, Cramers M, Herlin T, Jensen J, Kragballe K, Ternowitz T, Thestrup-Pedersen K. Non-specific immunotherapy and specific hyposensitization in severe atopic dermatitis. Acta Derm Venereol Suppl (Stockh) 1985; 114:48–54.

238. Heijer A. Hyposensitization with aeroallergens in atopic eczema. Allergo J 1993; 2:3–7.

239. Kaufman HS, Roth HL. Hyposensitization with alum precipitated extracts in atopic dermatitis: a placebo-controlled study. Ann Allergy 1974; 32(6):321–330.

240. Glover MT, Atherton DJ. A double-blind controlled trial of hyposensitization to *Dermatophagoides pteronyssinus* in children with atopic eczema. Clin Exp Allergy 1992; 22(4):440–446.

241. Leroy BP, Boden G, Lachapelle JM, Jacquemin MG, Saint-Remy JM. A novel therapy for atopic dermatitis with allergen-antibody complexes: a double-blind, placebo-controlled study. J Am Acad Dermatol 1993; 28(2 Pt 1):232–239.

242. Sheehan MP, Atherton DJ. A controlled trial of traditional Chinese medicinal plants in widespread non-exudative atopic eczema. Br J Dermatol 1992; 126(2):179–184.

243. Sheehan MP, Atherton DJ. One-year follow up of children treated with Chinese medicinal herbs for atopic eczema. Br J Dermatol 1994; 130(4):488–493.

244. Sheehan MP, Rustin MH, Atherton DJ, Buckley C, Harris DJ, Brostoff J, Ostlere L, Dawson A, Harris DJ. Efficacy of traditional Chinese herbal therapy in adult atopic dermatitis. Lancet 1992; 340(8810):13–17.

245. Sheehan MP, Stevens H, Ostlere LS, Atherton DJ, Brostoff J, Rustin MH. Follow-up of adult patients with atopic eczema treated with Chinese herbal therapy for 1 year. Clin Exp Dermatol 1995; 20(2):136–140.

246. Latchman Y, Whittle B, Rustin M, Atherton DJ, Brostoff J. The efficacy of traditional Chinese herbal therapy in atopic eczema. Int Arch Allergy Immunol 1994; 104(3):222–226.

247. Latchman Y, Bungy GA, Atherton DJ, Rustin MHA, Brostoff J. Efficacy of traditional Chinese herbal therapy in vitro. A model system for atopic eczema: inhibition of CD23 expression on blood monocytes. Br J Dermatol 1995; 132:592–598.

248. Banerjee P, Xu XJ, Poulter LW, Rustin MH. Changes in CD23 expression of blood and skin in atopic eczema after Chinese herbal therapy. Clin Exp Allergy 1998; 28(3):306–314.

249. Harper J. Traditional Chinese medicine for eczema. BMJ 1994; 308(6927):489–490.

250. Davis EG, Pollock I, Steel HM. Chinese herbs for eczema. Lancet 1990; 336:177.

251. Ferguson JE, Chalmers RJG, Rowlands DJ. Reversible dilated cardiomyopathy following treatment of atopic eczema with Chinese herbal medicine. Br J Dermatol 1997; 136(4):592–593.

252. Melnik B, Plewig G. Are disturbances of ω-6-fatty acid metabolism involved in the pathogenesis of atopic dermatitis? Acta Derm Venereol (Stockh) 1992; 176:77–85.

253. Bjorneboe A, Soyland E, Bjorneboe GE, Rajka G, Drevon CA. Effect of dietary supplementation with eicosapentaenoic acid in the treatment of atopic dermatitis. Br J Dermatol 1987; 117(4):463–469.

254. Sharpe GR, Farr PM. Evening primrose oil and eczema. Lancet 1990; 335:667–668.

255. Berth-Jones J, Graham-Brown RA. Placebo-controlled trial of essential fatty acid supplementation in atopic dermatitis. Lancet 1993; 341(8860):1557–1560.

256. Takei S, Arora YK, Walker SM. Intravenous immunoglobulin contains specific antibodies inhibitory to activation of T cells by Staphylococcal toxin superantigens. J Clin Invest 1993; 91:602–607.

257. Kimata H. High-dose intravenous gamma-globulin treatment for hyperimmunoglobulinemia E syndrome. J Allergy Clin Immunol 1995; 95(3):771–774.
258. Wakim M, Alazard M, Yajima A, Speights D, Saxon A, Stiehm E. High dose intravenous immunoglobulin in atopic dermatitis and hyper-IgE syndrome. Ann Allergy Asthma Immunol 1998; 81:153–158.
259. Burek-Kozlowska A, Morell A, Hunziker T. Topical immunoglobulin G in atopic dermatitis. Int Arch Allergy Immunol 1994; 104(1):104–106.
260. Carucci JA, Washenik K, Weinstein A, Shupack J, Cohen DE. The leukotriene antagonist zafirlukast as a therapeutic agent for atopic dermatitis. Arch Dermatol 1998; 134(7):785–786.
261. Mauser PJ, Pitman A, Witt A, Fernandez X, Zurcher J, Kung T, Jones H, Watnick AS, Egan RW, Kreutner W, et al. Inhibitory effect of the TRFK-5 anti-IL-5 antibody in a guinea pig model of asthma. Am Rev Respir Dis 1993; 148(6 Pt 1):1623–1627.
262. Egan RW, Athwahl D, Chou CC, Emtage S, Jehn CH, Kung TT, Mauser PJ, Murgolo NJ, Bodmer MW. Inhibition of pulmonary eosinophilia and hyperreactivity by antibodies to interleukin-5. Int Arch Allergy Immunol 1995; 107:321–322.
263. Garrone P, Djossou O, Galizzi J-P, Banchereau J. A recombinant extracellular domain of the human interleukin 4 receptor inhibits the biological effects of interleukin 4 on T and B lymphocytes. Eur J Immunol 1991; 21:1365–1368.
264. Nasert S, Millner M, Enssle KH, Wahn U, Renz H. Differential modulation of T cell functions by soluble IL-4R (sIL-4R) in two cases of severe atopic dermatitis. Pediatr Allergy Immunol 1996; 7(2):91–94.
265. Cooper KD, Kang K, Chan SC, Hanifin JM. Phosphodiesterase inhibition by Ro 20-1724 reduces hyper-IgE synthesis by atopic dermatitis cell in vitro. J Invest Dermatol 1985; 84:477–482.
266. Butler JM, Chan SC, Stevens S, Hanifin JM. Increased leukocyte histamine release with elevated cyclic AMP-phosphodiesterase activity in atopic dermatitis. J Allergy Clin Immunol 1983; 71:490–497.
267. Van Leent EJ, Graber M, Thurston M, Wagenaar A, Spuls PI, Bos JD. Effectiveness of the ascomycin macrolactam SDZ ASM 981 in the topical treatment of atopic dermatitis. Arch Dermatol 1998; 134(7):805–809.

# 8

## Urticaria and Angioedema

**Malcolm W. Greaves**
*United Medical and Dental School of Guy's and St. Thomas' Hospitals, King's College, London, England*

## I. INTRODUCTION

Although it is likely that the eruption we nowadays call urticaria masqueraded under a variety of different Greek, Latin, and Arabic titles in Greco-Roman and medieval times, the word urticaria first seems to have been used by Frank in his treatise "De Curandis Hominum Morbis Epitome" in the eighteenth century. In the English language the condition was previously termed by Heberden "nettle rash." Robert Willan, a nineteenth century enthusiast for morphological classification of rashes, used the term urticaria and recognized febrile, transitory, persistent, confluent, subcutaneous, and tuberous varieties. Angioedema was described in detail by John Laws Milton [1], the founder of St. John's Institute of Dermatology, although Quincke [2] usually has his name attached to the disease. The unfortunate but widely used term angioneurotic oedema appeared in the literature in the 1880s, and in 1888 Osler [3] separated hereditary angioedema as a distinct entity.

Willan thought some forms of urticaria were dietary in origin—a view that is still prevalent. However, the pathomechanisms of urticaria began to be studied scientifically following the report of Dale [4] of the actions of histamine and its involvement in anaphylactic hypersensitivity reactions and the observation by Lewis [5] of the similarities between the responses of human skin to histamine and the urticarial reaction (Lewis's "triple response"). That the histamine content of healthy skin mainly resides in the resident skin mast cells was established by Riley and West [6]. Although it has been assumed on the basis of indirect evidence that the wheals and itch of urticaria were caused by release of histamine from mast cells, the involvement of histamine, at least in chronic urticaria, was not convincingly demonstrated until Kaplan et al. [7] made direct measurements of tissue histamine in involved and uninvolved skin of chronic urticaria patients. This chapter covers all forms of urticaria and angioedema except for physical urticarias and angioedema due to C'1 esterase deficiency, which are dealt with in other sections. Urticaria vasculitis is also included for convenience.

## II. ACUTE URTICARIA

Acute urticaria is a model of IgE (type I, Gell and Coombs)–mediated hypersensitivity and can be conveniently defined as the occurrence of daily or almost daily short-lived

*171*

wheals usually with itching for less than 6 weeks. Patients may occasionally present with intermittent acute attacks of urticaria, separated by weeks or months (acute intermittent urticaria). Many of these patients never reach the attention of the specialist allergist or dermatologist because the precipitating cause (food, drug, infection) is self-evident to patient and physician alike.

## A.  Etiology

Published studies of aetiological factors in acute urticaria are biased by the type of population studied. A Japanese report suggested acute virus infections as a major cause in 50 patients with urticaria for less than 1 week. Thirty-one had a recent history of respiratory or gastrointestinal infection. Agents incriminated included cytomegalovirus, Coxsackie Ag, and hepatitis B viruses. More recently Zuberbier et al. [8] found that 40% of over 100 patients with acute urticaria also had an upper respiratory infection. In infancy allergic reactions to food items, especially dairy products, are important. In adults Zuberbier et al. found no instances of food allergy, but my own experience, in a presumably different pattern of referrals, is not the same. At least 50% of adult acute urticaria patients referred to me proved to have allergies to food items, including peanuts, shellfish, fruits, and sesame seed, confirmed by skin or serological testing. Association with intercurrent infections and reactions to drugs, especially aspirin and penicillin, amount for some of the remainder but in many the cause remains obscure. There does not appear to be an increased prevalence of atopy in acute urticaria [8] at least in adults, and few of these patients ever proceed to develop chronic urticaria.

## B.  Clinical Features

The individual wheals and swellings of acute urticaria and angioedema usually last less than 24 hours and are indistinguishable clinically from those of chronic urticaria and angioedema. However, there may be associated systemic symptoms including headache, gastrointestinal upset, and wheezing. Pruritus is usually prominent, and the angioedema may affect the oropharyngeal mucous membranes. Urticaria wheals are hot red and elevated with a well-defined margin. The center of the wheal is pale due to the blanching effect of dermal edema. The shape of the wheals is variable, including papules and annular lesions, which may merge together into large plaques with a geographic outline. That they last individually less than 24 hours and fade without leaving a mark distinguishes them from the otherwise similar wheals of urticaria vasculitis. Their consistency is firm but not indurated; the latter suggests heavy fibrin deposition characteristic of urticarial vasculitis. There may be a zone of pallor surrounding the wheal due to a ''steal'' effect of the increased blood flow through the lesion. Itching may be of a burning or pricking quality, but occasionally patients describe formication. Patients tend to rub rather than scratch skin affected by urticaria. I have never seen vesicles or bullae in true urticaria. Swellings of angioedema are subcutaneous, submucosal, and painless unless they occur on the hands or feet. They last less than 24 hours or slightly longer depending upon size. They may be skin colored or red, but they subside without visible damage to the skin. When affecting the lips or eyelids they can be especially disfiguring. In the mouth or throat they can cause dysphagia and stridor, causing acute fear and distress to the patient. Skin that has previously been affected by whealing is usually refractory to further whealing for a few days.

## C. Diagnosis

A history of raised inflammatory lesions, each individually lasting less than 24 hours, is diagnostic of urticaria. A careful history of food or drug intake may reveal a convincing relationship between a triggering event as outlined above and bouts of acute urticaria. Infection-provoked urticaria usually occurs on or around the day of onset of the infection [9]. Food- or drug-evoked urticaria normally occurs within hours of ingestion.

For acute urticaria (i.e., a history of no more than 6 weeks) prick tests may be worth doing to confirm a suggestion from the history of food allergy. Oral challenge tests are not recommended because of the risk of oropharyngeal angioedema. If available, radio allergosorbent tests (RAST) to food items may also be useful.

The differential white blood cell count, erythrocyte sedimentation rate (ESR), and total serum IgE are not helpful in the investigation of patients with acute urticaria.

## D. Treatment

Symptomatic treatment including a cool bedroom, light bedclothes, tepid shower, calamine lotion to reduce itching, and avoidance of heavy clothing, especially woollen garments, is usually helpful. Menthol cream 1% has valuable antipruritic qualities [10]. Identified culprit etiological factors (food items, aspirin, penicillin) should be withdrawn. Antihistamines given parenterally in acutely distressed patients or, more commonly, orally are valuable. The first-generation $H_1$ antihistamines (chlorpheniramine 4 mg; hydroxyzine 25 mg; promethazine 25 mg) combine effective $H_1$ receptor antagonism with a variable degree of sedation—often very useful in a patient who is highly agitated as a result of acute urticaria and angioedema. Administration of a sedative antihistamine at night is especially appropriate since the itch of acute urticaria frequently keeps the patient awake. For the acutely distressed and depressed patient, doxepin 25 mg at night is also useful; however, during the daytime a low-sedation antihistamine (cetirizine 10 mg; loratidine 10 mg) is often preferred. Patients receiving sedative antihistamines need to be warned to avoid alcohol and activities involving fine judgment, balance, and sharp reflexes. For angioedema of the oropharynx, adrenaline can be injected subcutaneously in dosage 0.5 mg in 0.5 ml. I have found nebulized 2% ephedrine in water applied locally very effective. A short tapering course of oral steroids can also be used (50 mg daily reducing by 5 mg every third day to zero) in situations where rapid relief is urgently needed. Prolonged systemic steroid treatment (longer than 3 weeks maximum) is not recommended [11]. Apart from cooling creams and lotions and menthol, topical antipruritics, antihistamines, or corticosteroids are not effective. Theoretically therapy directed at stabilizing cutaneous mast cells should be effective, but in vitro studies indicate that cutaneous mast cells are unresponsive to this class of compound, and there are no convincing reports that sodium cromoglycate or other agents with a similar action are superior to placebo in patients with urticaria.

## III. PHYSICAL URTICARIAS

Physical urticarias are defined as urticaria reactions to physical stimuli. The most important physical urticarias are listed in Table 1. Most but not all physical urticarias occur within

**Table 1**  Physical Urticarias

| Type of urticaria | Nature of stimulus |
| --- | --- |
| Symptomatic dermographism (factitious urticaria) | Shearing force |
| Delayed-pressure urticaria | Perpendicular force |
| Cold urticaria | Lowering of skin temperature |
| Heat urticaria | Raising of skin temperature |
| Solar urticaria | Exposure to sunlight |
| Vibratory urticaria | High frequency oscillation of skin |
| Cholinergic urticaria[a] | Rise in core temperature of body; emotion |
| Aquagenic urticaria | Wetting of skin |
| Aquagenic pruritus[b] | Wetting of skin |

[a] Not a true physical urticaria but included.
[b] No visible signs in involved skin.

minutes of provocation and last no more than 1 hour, the affected skin remaining insensitive to whealing for several hours subsequently.

The diagnosis of physical urticarias is normally confirmed by physical urticaria challenge testing. This is important because once the diagnosis has been confirmed and provided the physical urticaria is the main cause of the patient's symptoms, no further investigations are required. Allergy tests, exclusion diets, and immunological workups are not indicated in most physical urticarias. Symptomatic treatment with antihistamines should be instituted and the patient advised that in most cases spontaneous remission eventually occurs.

More than one physical urticaria can coexist in the same patient. Commonly encountered pairs include dermographism and cholinergic urticaria; delayed-pressure urticaria and dermographism; solar urticaria and heat urticaria; and cold urticaria and cholinergic urticaria. Delayed-pressure urticaria occurs in 37% of patients with chronic "idiopathic" urticaria [12]. A consensus view on criteria for diagnosis of physical urticaria has been published [13].

## A.  Symptomatic Dermographism (Factitious Urticaria)

Symptomatic dermographism affects at least 2% of the population and is the most common physical urticaria. It usually affects young adults who complain of a widespread burning itch made worse by rubbing or scratching. It does not affect the mucous membranes. It normally runs a course of 1–2 years before clearing spontaneously. There is a short-lived form of dermographism, which occurs as a transitory sequel of treated scabies and severe insect bite reactions. The diagnosis can be confirmed by firm stroking of the skin, which elicits within minutes a linear wheal with redness and intense itching in previously clinically normal looking skin. The differential diagnosis includes delayed-pressure urticaria (the wheal takes 2–6 hours to develop and lasts over 24 hours) and urticaria pigmentosa (cutaneous mastocytosis) (the wheal develops in clinically abnormal skin). Systemic symptoms hardly ever occur in this physical urticaria.

The sensitivity of the skin can be quantified using a calibrated spring-loaded dermographometer [14,15]. Photochemotherapy with 8-methoxy psoralen and UV-A (PUVA) may relieve the itching in some patients. Other measures tried include calcium channel blocking agents (ineffective) [16] and potent topical corticosteroid application (effective but impractical in most patients) [17].

## B. Delayed Pressure Urticaria

Delayed-pressure urticaria is common, affecting adults at any age and causing severe disability due to pain and tenderness, especially when it affects the palms or soles. Characteristically a painful swelling (often preceded by a tingling sensation) develops 2–6 hours after contact of the skin with a firm edge such as leaning against a table, carrying a heavy bag by a strap on the shoulder, and wearing a tight belt or tight shoes. The swelling persists for 24–48 hours and during this period systemic disturbance is common including fatigue arthralgia and "flu-like symptoms" [18]. Delayed-pressure urticaria is a cause of serious disability in manual workers (e.g., auto mechanics, construction workers) and can also cause troublesome marital problems [19]. Individual lesions are red, tender, hot, and indurated, but despite their long duration they rarely leave a mark on the skin. Pain is common, but itching may also occur and may predominate. When swellings develop near joints, stiffness may occur and may be mistaken for an acute arthritis. Delayed dermographism is probably an additional manifestation of delayed-pressure urticaria. Thirty-seven percent of patients with chronic "idiopathic" urticaria also have delayed pressure [12] and it is my impression that the latter rarely, if ever, occurs alone.

There is no elevated sedimentation rate, leucocytosis, or peripheral blood eosinophilia [20]. The longer time course of individual wheals compared with other physical urticarias is reflected in their specific histological features. The presence of large numbers of eosinophils in affected skin but not peripheral blood accompanied by increased numbers of dermal T lymphocytes (predominantly of the CD4 phenotype) is striking. Mast cells are present in normal numbers [21]. But in accordance with the prominent mononuclear infiltrate there was an upregulation of expression of vascular E-selectin. Delayed-pressure urticaria tends to be a persistent problem, the mean duration of the disease being 9 years [18].

The diagnosis is confirmed by pressure challenge testing in which pressure is applied perpendicularly to the skin by means of a weighted rod or spring-loaded dermographometer [22]. The test can be made fully quantitative if the cross-sectional area of the rod, the weight applied to it and duration of application are known. The site develops a wheal 2–6 hours after challenge lasting 24–48 hours. The differential diagnosis includes symptomatic dermographism (the wheal occurs within minutes of applying pressure to the skin and lasts less than 1 hour) and urticaria vasculitis (vide infra) in which wheals occur at sites of pressure and can only be clearly distinguished from delayed-pressure urticaria by the presence of histological evidence of vasculitis.

### 1. Etiology and Pathogenesis

The cause of delayed-pressure urticaria is unknown. The resemblance between the histological appearances of delayed pressure urticaria and late-phase reactions has been noted [23]. Mast cell degranulation is probably an early event, followed by release of pro-inflammatory mediators including interleukin-1 (IL-1), IL-6, and possibly TNF-α [24]. These mediators induce up regulation of adhesion molecule expression including E-selectin and VCAM-1 on vascular endothelium. The resultant dense inflammatory infiltrate consists of neutrophils, eosinophils, and mononuclear cells. Eosinophil major basic protein probably augments the reaction [25]. Transformation of arachidonic acid to its lipoxygenase and cyclooxygenase pro-inflammatory products does not appear to be involved [26].

### 2. Treatment

Delayed-pressure urticaria is poorly responsive to treatment and can be a major therapeutic problem, given its chronicity [18]. Indeed, of all the treatments tried, only large doses of systemic steroids are consistently effective and their long-term use is essentially precluded by toxicity. Treatments which I have found ineffective include indomethacin colchicine [18], dapsone [22], and pentoxifylline (M. W. Greaves, unpublished findings). Antihistamines are generally of little or no value. Cetirizine has been claimed to exert a specific therapeutic action in delayed pressure urticaria [27] but I have not been able to confirm this (M. W. Greaves, unpublished findings). Application of a potent topical steroid (clobestesol propionate 0.05% ointment) for 6 weeks in a randomized double-blind study reduced both skin reactivity and mast cell population density [28].

## C. Cold Urticaria

Cold urticaria is a rare physical urticaria, which can be classified as familial and acquired primary and secondary forms and which differs from other physical urticarias in a number of ways. Fatalities have been recorded following exposure to cold, especially after sea-bathing [29], due to the systemic effects of massive mediator release, including histamine, following whole body immersion. Unlike other physical urticarias, cold urticaria may rarely be a skin manifestation of systemic disease including primary and secondary acquired cryoglobulinemia (see below). However, in over 95% of patients presenting with cold urticaria no evidence of cryoglobulins can be found. Cold urticaria is defined clinically as the immediate onset of local whealing and itching at the site of cooling of the skin by contact with either cold surfaces or fluids.

Atypical cases of cold urticaria are occasionally seen in which widespread urticaria affects warm, covered, as well as exposed skin in response to cold environmental conditions. Termed cold reflex urticaria by Illig, local ice cube challenge testing is usually negative, but the rash can be triggered by placing the patient in a cold environmental chamber [30], which evokes widespread urticaria. Recently, a positive association between HIV infection and cold urticaria has been noted [31]. These patients have high serum IgG levels, presumably due to disordered immunoregulation.

### 1. Familial Cold Urticaria

This is a rare autosomal dominant condition first described in 1940 [32], with an onset in early life. Only 10 pedigrees have been reported, one having been recently described in detail [33]. Apart from its heritability, clinical and pathological features differ from those of ordinary acquired cold urticaria. These include the longer duration of individual lesions (several hours) and accompanying fever, arthralgia, and leukocytosis with elevated acute phase reactants. The ice cube challenge test is usually negative. Histologically biopsies of lesional skin show a prolific perivascular leukocytic infiltrate which falls short of vasculitis. It responds poorly to $H_1$ or $H_2$ antihistamines [33].

### 2. Acquired Secondary Cold Urticaria

This presents as a cold urticaria associated with cold precipitating serum proteins (usually IgG or IgM cryoglobulins), which enable passive transfer of the cold reactivity [34]. Underlying diseases include chronic lymphocytic leukemia, myelomatosis, and other types of benign or malignant lymphoreticular proliferative disorders. Both classical and alternate complement pathway components may be lowered. Histological evidence of leucocytoclastic vasculitis is normally seen in lesional skin biopsy material. The clinical picture is correspondingly different. Cold-induced wheals last longer than 24 hours and are frequently purpuric, leaving staining of the skin after the wheals fade. The diagnosis of underlying cryoglobulinemia can be confirmed by putting the patient's plasma (collected and separated warm) in the refrigerator at 4°C for at least 48 hours. A precipitate forms in cryoglobulin-positive patients. Cold urticaria associated with cryoglobulinemia responds poorly to antihistamine treatment, but the treatment of the underlying lymphoproliferative disorder must be a priority.

### 3. Acquired Primary (Essential) Cold Urticaria

Patients, usually children or young adults, complain of redness, itching, and swelling within minutes of cold exposure of the skin, lasting for one half to one hour. Change in temperature from warm to cold is usually more of a problem than the absolute temperature. Systemic symptoms range from none in most cases through headache, wheezing, and visual disturbance to loss of consciousness and anaphylactic shock with angioedema in rare severe cases following widespread cold exposure as in swimming in the sea or an unheated pool. The condition may develop after an acute virus infection (especially *Mycoplasma pneumoniae* or infectious mononucleosis), severe insect venom reactions or immunizations. The diagnosis is confirmed by ice cube challenge testing in which an ice cube, preferably wrapped in waterproof plastic film, is applied to the skin for 15–20 minutes. Upon removal the skin should be allowed to warm up before reading the result. A positive reaction occurs as itching, persistent redness, and palpable whealing at the challenge site. These symptoms and signs fade within an hour leaving no visible trace in the skin. False-positive ice cube challenge tests can occur in patients with dermographism or delayed-pressure urticaria. In these cases immersion of a hand in water at 4°C will produce no urticarial response. Histological examination of a biopsy from lesional skin does not show evidence of vasculitis [35] although repeated cold challenge at the same skin site may induce vasculitis in essential primary acquired cold urticaria [36]. However, examination of the serum reveals no evidence of circulating immunoreactants. As with most other physical urticarias, the natural history of the acquired essential cold urticaria is for spontaneous resolution in 1–2 years. Patients with a preceding history of virus infection or other identifiable precipitating aetiological factor usually experience more rapid improvement of symptoms.

    a.   Aetiology and Pathogenesis.

    Primary acquired cold urticaria is passively transferable by serum to nonhuman primates [37]. The transferable factor concerned may be an IgE immunoglobulin [38]. IgE auto antibodies directed against a cold-sensitive skin factor have also been proposed [39]. Histamine derived from cutaneous mast cells is clearly a major cause of cold-induced whealing and itching, but other mediators involved include prostaglandin $D_2$ [40,41] and eosinophilotactic factors [42].

    b.   Treatment.

    Patients should be warned to avoid abrupt transitions from warm to cold. Bathing in sea water or unheated pool water should be prohibited, and I usually advise patients that if they bathe in a heated pool they should be accompanied by someone who is aware of their disorder and its complications. Patients with cold urticaria requiring surgery should be protected from low temperature in the operating theatre and all IV fluids should be prewarmed. Most patients with primary (essential) acquired cold urticaria respond well to H1-antihistamine treatment. A single dose of a low-sedation $H_1$ antihistamine (cetirizine 10 mg; fexofenadine 180 mg; loratidine 10 mg) taken first thing in the morning is usually sufficient to suppress cold provoked symptoms in the early part of the day, although an additional dose may be required in the afternoon or later. Other drugs that have been proven effective in cold urticaria include oral doxantrazole [43] and a combination of oral salbatamol and aminophylline [44], both of which suppress histamine release from cutaneous mast cells. Oral prednisolone also causes suppression of cold-evoked histamine release in cold urticaria but was not found to lead to significant clinical improvement [45].

Cold tolerance has been used with success in patients with cold urticaria. This treatment is based upon the assumption that cold-evoked histamine release occurs from mast cell stores in the cold-challenged skin. Repeated evoked release of histamine from skin mast cells results in histamine depletion and reduced clinical responsiveness of tolerant skin to cold. Since mast cells rapidly resynthesize histamine, stores are soon replenished. Therefore patients using tolerance treatment have to expose their skin to cold challenge at least once daily. Compliance is, not surprisingly, poor [46,47]. However, strongly motivated patients find this treatment useful for limited periods of time, e.g., during vacations. Apart from $H_1$ antihistamines, no really satisfactory treatments are available for this annoying and occasionally serious disorder.

## D. Cholinergic Urticaria

Cholinergic urticaria was first described by Duke in 1924 [48]. Subsequently there have been a number of useful reviews [49–51]. It is a common form of urticaria, occurring, at least in a milder form (often referred to popularly as ''heat bumps''), in up to 12% of the population. In severe cases it can cause serious personal and occupational disability. Presenting more commonly in young adults, it frequently occurs against an atopic background [52]. Its average duration is 2–3 years, it is rarely seen in the elderly, and it is not characteristically familial, although I have occasionally seen familial cases.

In its classical presentation in a young adult, cholinergic urticaria consists of a widespread pruritic erythematous symmetrical eruption occurring abruptly. A rise in body temperature of about 1°C is sufficient to provoke an outbreak, and I have seen attacks occur in susceptible individuals due to mild febrile illnesses. That the eruption is associated with stimulation of eccrine sweating is underlined by the characteristic outbreak following emotional stress. Other common provoking stimuli include hot baths or showers, moving from a cold to a hot atmosphere, sexual activity, excitement (outbreaks were provoked in 1998 by watching World Cup football) [53], laughter, gustatory stimuli, alcohol, and any form of physical exertion. Individual lesions characteristically consist of punctate wheals surrounded by a bright red flare. The rash is transitory, lasting up to 30 minutes, and several outbreaks may occur in any one day. Occasionally the wheals may be much larger due to confluence of pinpoint wheals and may even resemble angioedema. However, mucous membranes are normally spared. The regions most frequently affected include the head and neck, trunk, lower legs, forearms and wrists. The hands and feet are rarely involved, but virtually any area can be affected. Systemic symptoms are frequent and include wheezing due to bronchospasm, abdominal symptoms, and headache. A reduced respiratory peak flow reading during attacks is common even in patients without respiratory symptoms.

The diagnosis can be confirmed by provocation testing (immersion in a bath at 42°C; exercise provocation; mental arithmetic) [49]. Intradermal injection of acetylcholine or other cholinergics, recommended by earlier authors as a local provocation test, is unhelpful.

Rare but important clinical variants of cholinergic urticaria include exercise-induced angioedema [54], persistent cholinergic erythema [55], and food and exercise-induced cholinergic urticaria [56]. Exercise-induced anaphylaxis may be another variant of cholinergic urticaria. Occasionally patients may present with heat, exercise, or emotion-evoked pruritus without visible evidence of a rash [57,58].

The differential diagnosis includes aquagenic pruritus (see below) in which there is no visible eruption, no provocation by emotional stress, and positive provocation by cold as well as hot water. Aquagenic urticaria (see below) manifests with an itchy rash, which closely resembles that of cholinergic urticaria but which, like aquagenic pruritus, is provoked by wetting the skin independently of temperature.

## 1. Etiology and Pathogenesis

Any stimulus that activates eccrine sweating can evoke the rash in susceptible individuals. As the name of this urticaria suggests, acetylcholine, the transmitter substance for sympathetic autonomically innervated sweat glands, plays a key role. Atropinization of a small area of skin by topical application of 6% aqueous hyoscine inhibits local sweating and also blocks the rash of cholinergic urticaria [59], implying either excessive production of acetylcholine or abnormal sensitivity to it. Histamine release is also involved as evidenced by the suppressive action of $H_1$ antihistamines and prior local mast cell degranulation [59]. A report that patients with cholinergic urticaria are "allergic" to their own sweat [60] has not been independently confirmed and could not be reproduced by this author.

A circulating serum factor may also play a part. Murphy et al. [61] successfully demonstrated passive transfer of cholinergic urticaria by serum from human to monkey in confirmation of early similar reports. How these different observations can be put together into an integrated molecular and cellular mechanism remains unclear.

## 2. Management

Patients with confirmed cholinergic urticaria should be advised that allergy tests, other laboratory tests, and special diets have no place in its management. The natural history is for gradual improvement, but chronicity is common. Occupational changes may be necessary in some patients, and reduction in day to day stress, alcohol consumption and exertion should be helpful. Some patients benefit from the anxiolytic actions of hydroxyzine 25 mg or doxepin 10–25 mg. Although tolerance does occur after an attack of cholinergic urticaria, it is too short-lived to make tolerance treatment a viable option (M. W. Greaves, unpublished observations).

Patients with cholinergic urticaria exhibit lowered plasma levels of protease inhibitors (PI) [62]. Elevation of PI by means of oral administration of the anabolic steroid danazol has been shown to be effective treatment in severely affected patients in a double-blind, placebo-controlled trial. This treatment is very useful [63] in male patients but less so in females due to troublesome menorrhagia, weight gain, deepening of voice, etc. In most patients, modification of lifestyle together with regular use of low-sedation antihistamines (cetirizine 10 mg; loratidine 10 mg, fexofenadine 180 mg) continues to be the mainstay of treatment.

## E.  Heat Urticaria

Better described as heat contact urticaria, to distinguish it from cholinergic urticaria, heat urticaria occurs as urticaria wheals localized to the precise site at which skin is warmed. It is very rare. I have reported two cases in some detail [64,65]. Any warm surface or radiant heat provokes local whealing, which lasts up to 1 hour after removal of the heat source. The threshold temperature to evoke whealing was 43°C in both patients (optimum 49°C) when applied for 3 minutes. Passive transfer to nonhuman primates by serum was unsuccessful. Dermal perfusion studies and analysis of venous effluent from heat-challenge skin elicited evidence of local release of histamine and prostaglandin D2. Local heat tolerance persisted for a week, and the condition was moderately responsive to H1 antihistamine therapy and can be treated by a heat-tolerance regime [66] but in most patients reported it tends to be very persistent. The etiology and pathogenesis are unclear. Clearly the end result is cutaneous mast cell degranulation, but the events linking warming of the skin with mast cell activation remain speculative.

## F.  Aquagenic Urticaria

Aquagenic urticaria is another rare, physical urticaria, occurring principally in young adults. One case has recently been reported in an HIV-positive individual [67]. The individual cutaneous wheals are indistinguishable from those of cholinergic urticaria, with a similar distribution and equally intense itch. Sytemic symptoms are much less common, and the rash only occurs when the skin is wetted, irrespective of the temperature of the water. Other physical stimuli are ineffective. In detailed studies of 2 patients we [68] demonstrated that protection of the water-challenged skin by Vaseline prevented elicitation of the rash and prior treatment of the water-challenged skin by organic solvents enhanced water-induced whealing. Acetylcholine is also involved as a transmitter substance since atropinisation of the skin blocked its responsiveness to water. Histamine is clearly the final mediator, based upon the response to $H_1$ antihistamines and the demonstration of elevated plasma levels of histamine following elicitation of the rash. Presumably wetting the skin liberates a water-soluble substance in the stratum corneum which, absorbed percutaneously, causes whealing.

The diagnosis is confirmed by wetting of the skin and observing local itching and punctate whealing. The differential diagnosis includes cholinergic urticaria (the rash is identical and cholinergic urticaria can be caused by hot baths or the exertion of swimming), cold urticaria (patients may complain of contact with water causing the rash, but it is the low temperature of the water that evokes the whealing; warm water is ineffective), and dermographism (the force of water jets from a shower head may cause whealing in dermographism as a mechanical effect). All these alternative diagnoses can be excluded by showing that the skin responses to gentle application of tepid water to the skin.

The natural history is usually characterized by improvement in less than 5 years. $H_1$ antihistamines are effective. Other treatments possibly successful include UV-B or PUVA (8 methoxy-psoralen-UV-A photochemotherapy) and stanazolol [67,69].

## G. Aquagenic Pruritus

Originally mentioned by Shelley [70] who also drew attention to its association with polycythemia vera, aquagenic pruritis was first described comprehensively by Greaves et al. [71]. It is actually quite common but is poorly recognized as an entity. Almost exclusively occurring in adults, most commonly in middle age, the condition is both chronic and unremitting. Intense itching without visible signs in the skin occur at the sites of contact of the skin with water at any temperature. Characteristically the irritation occurs after emerging from the bath or shower, while drying. It lasts about 40 minutes, is pricking in character, and causes intense distress. There are otherwise no associated systemic symptoms. A family history of the same symptoms occur in about one third of cases. An identical syndrome occurs in patients with polycythemia vera ("bath itch"), and it is important to carry out regular hematological checks. Because of the lack of visible evidence despite symptom severity, patients tend to be labeled as "psychoneurotic." However, objective evidence of mast cell degranulation and elevated plasma histamine levels have been observed during attacks [71]. The condition has been fully reviewed by Steinmann and Greaves [72], Kligman et al. [73] (where a clear distinction was drawn with water-induced itching of the elderly which is due to wetting a desiccated skin), Archer and Greaves [74], and Menage and Greaves [75]. Besides polycythemia vera, which may occasionally be preceded by aquagenic pruritus [76], other associated systemic diseases include juvenile xanthogranuloma [77] and myelodysplasia [78].

The diagnosis is based upon clinical evidence confirmed by challenge testing by contact with tepid water. It is readily distinguishable from water-induced itching of the elderly [73] because in the latter the skin is visibly dry and the itch is prevented by emollients. Aquagenic urticaria shows no visible whealing. The etiology is unknown. Changes reported in the water-challenged skin include mast cell degranulation and increased skin tissue fibrinolytic activity [71,79,80].

The condition responds poorly to $H_1$ antihistamines. Ultraviolet B (UV-B) phototherapy may be of value in some patients [81] but PUVA (psoralen photochemotherapy) is the treatment of choice, being effective in most patients although relapse occurs and re-treatment is often necessary [82].

## H. Solar Urticaria

Solar urticaria is rare. It was initially characterized clinically by Ive et al. [83]. Most patients have a long history, going back several years, of acute cutaneous reactivity to sunlight, without any evident underlying cause. Redness, a burning itch, and whealing develop in exposed skin no more than 2–3 minutes after exposure to sunlight. Widespread exposure may cause headache, faintness, and palpitations. The urticaria eruption usually fades within 1 hour, and repeated exposure may cause some degree of tolerance. According to the monochromator studies reported by Ive et al. [83], the action spectrum of solar urticaria ranges from medium-wavelength ultraviolet (UV-B) into the visible part of the spectrum.

The diagnosis is confirmed by exposure to either strong natural sunlight or a slide projector lamp which causes immediate whealing and itching. Use of window glass as a filter to remove UV-B is often useful as a guide to sunscreen treatment. Solar urticaria may be mimicked by the acute photosensitivity of erythropoietic protoporphyria. However, most confusion is caused by misdiagnosis of polymorphic light eruption. The latter condition comes on hours (not seconds) after sunlight exposure and persists for days even after sun avoidance. The rash of systemic lupus is also similarly persistent, with a prolonged latent period. Heat urticaria may be closely related to solar urticaria; bearing in mind the proximity of visible light and heat in the electromagnetic spectrum.

The pathogenesis of solar urticaria has been extensively investigated. Elevated histamine levels in venous blood effluent from irradiated skin accompanied by evidence of mast cell degranulation in the whealing skin substantiates the role of skin mast cell-derived histamine [84], the symptomatic response to $H_1$ antihistamines providing further support. It is proposed that irradiation of skin in susceptible patients causes a photoallergen to be produced. Leenutaphong et al. [85] demonstrated that intradermal injection of irradiated serum from solar urticaria patients induced whealing in unexposed but not tolerant skin of the same patients. They also proposed that the photoallergen occupies binding sites on the IgE adherent to mast cells in the skin during tolerance.

Avoidance of sunlight and use of sunscreens with an appropriate absorption spectrum may be helpful. Low sedation $H_1$ antihistamines may reduce the itching. However, tolerance induction is the preferred treatment. Ramsay [86] successfully treated nine patients by repeated exposures to artificial or natural sources of solar radiation. More recently 8-methoxypsoralen–UV-A photochemotherapy (PUVA) and plasmapheresis have been proposed to be effective [87,88], or even a combination of both [89].

## I. Vibratory Angioedema

One of the rarest but also one of the most striking forms of physical urticaria, vibratory angioedema, presents as itching redness and swelling in response to a local vibratory stimulus. The patient I studied [17] got angioedema after using a power lawnmower, or garden shears, jogging, and even repeated clapping of the hands. Symptoms appeared within 10 minutes of the vibratory stimulus and lasted for about half an hour. The reaction was associated with systemic symptoms including facial flushing, dyspnea, and chest tightness. There was no evidence of tolerance following repeated vibratory challenge. The diagnosis was confirmed by applying a whirlmix (13 cycles/second, 1 mm amplitude 10 min) to the forearm. Routine histological and electron microscopic examination of a biopsy from affected skin revealed no abnormality, mast cells appearing normal. Nevertheless, local histamine release has been demonstrated previously in this physical urticaria [90]. The condition has been reported to be hereditary [90,91], but there was no family history in my patient. She responded quite well to oral terfenadine.

## IV. CHRONIC URTICARIA AND ANGIOEDEMA

Chronic "idiopathic" urticaria, with or without angioedema, is commonly but arbitrarily defined as the occurrence of daily or almost daily urticaria for a minimum of 6 weeks. In fact, most patients referred with this diagnosis to our clinic have had urticaria for months if not years. Its incidence is unclear. The often quoted figure of 15% of the population suffering at least one bout of urticaria refers to urticaria of all types, including the much more frequent and trivial attacks of acute urticaria. Probably close to 5% of the U.K. population get chronic urticaria at some time in their lives [92]. It is an extremely disabling condition, causing personal, social, and occupational handicap at a level comparable with patients with triple coronary heart disease awaiting bypass intervention [93].

Apart from the length of history, the clinical appearances of the affected patient do not differ significantly from those already described for acute urticaria. Angioedema coexists with chronic urticaria in about 50% of patients [92], and has the same etiological basis. Delayed pressure urticaria occurs in 37% of patients with chronic idiopathic urticaria [12]. There is no significant increase in the incidence of atopy [92]. The natural history is for slow spontaneous improvement, 50% of patients having experienced sustained remission within about 5 years from onset [92].

## A. Etiology and Pathogenesis

The principal mediator is histamine derived from skin mast cells [7], although other mediators derived from mast and other infiltrating inflammatory cells play a part. Although mast cell numbers are not increased in chronic urticaria, there is evidence of degranulation, and a perivascular T-cell infiltrate is characteristic with a preponderance of CD4+ over CD8+ cells. There is no evidence of T-cell activation [21]. There is moderate upregulation of E-selectin and VCAM-1 adhesion molecule expression concurrently with the development of the leukocyte infiltrate [94]. Earlier reports of "ten times the number of mast cells in chronic urticaria biopsy sites" [95] could not be confirmed. However, some clinically indistinguishable patients with chronic urticaria show a perivascular predominantly neutrophilic infiltrate [96]. The uninvolved skin of patients with chronic urticaria does seem to show an augmented wheal and flare response to intradermal injection of histamine and other mediators [97], but this is probably nonspecific.

The causes of the cutaneous mast cell activation characteristic of chronic urticaria have until recently been essentially unknown (Fig. 1). Early reports that as many as 75%

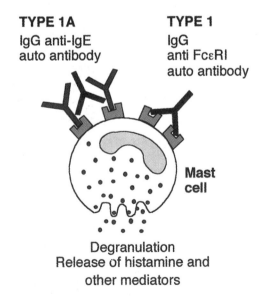

**TYPE 1A**
IgG anti-IgE
auto antibody

**TYPE 1**
IgG
anti FcεRI
auto antibody

Mast
cell

Degranulation
Release of histamine and
other mediators

**Figure 1**  Autoimmune chronic urticaria. (From Refs. 24, 25, 35.)

of patients with chronic urticaria could be demonstrated by oral challenge testing to be reacting to food preservatives and dyes [98] have not been confirmed, although aspirin undoubtedly nonspecifically exacerbates urticaria and may cause severe idiosyncratic reactions [99]. As pointed out by May [100] and more recently by Pastorello [101], the only procedure able to establish a correct diagnosis of specific food reaction is the double-blind, placebo-controlled food challenge. Using these rigorous criteria proven cases of food additive–evoked chronic urticaria represent less than 5% of the total chronic urticaria patients referred to my clinic.

## B. Role of Autoimmunity

There is now persuasive evidence from several different centers that autoimmunity plays a major role in the etiology of up to 50% of patients with chronic "idiopathic" urticaria. The possibility that circulating histamine-releasing factors might be involved in the pathogenesis was first hinted at by Rorsman [102] who reported basophil leukopenia in chronic urticaria. In 1974 Greaves et al. [103] reported reduced anti-IgE-evoked histamine release from basophil leukocytes in patients with chronic urticaria, compared to comparable healthy controls, suggesting the presence of circulating basophil-degranulating activity in at least some of these patients. No further progress was made until 1993, when a subset of patients with chronic urticaria was demonstrated to have functional IgG autoantibodies directed against the high-affinity IgE receptor (FcεRI) expressed by basophil leukocytes and mast cells [104] (Fig. 2). They represent about 25–30% of all chronic "idiopathic" urticaria patients in my series [105]. These functional histamine-releasing autoantibodies, which are only found to date in patients with chronic "idiopathic" urticaria, have now

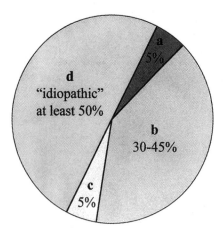

**Figure 2** Chronic "idiopathic" urticaria: frequency of identifiable causes. a = autoimmune (Type Ia) (anti-IgE); b = autoimmune (Type I) (anti-FcεRIα); c = confirmed reactivity to food additive by placebo-controlled challenge with reproduceability; d = no cause found (idiopathic).

been independently confirmed to be present in 33% [106] and over 50% [107] of patients. That anti-FcεRI autoantibodies are the cause of the disease in this subset of chronic urticaria patients is indicated by their ability to release histamine from normal human mast cells and basophils in vitro, their ability to cause a wheal-and-flare reaction when injected intradermally into uninvolved human skin, and the remission of chronic urticaria consequent upon their removal by plasmapheresis [108]. An additional smaller subset of chronic "idiopathic" urticaria patients (5% of my series) [105] have anti-IgE antibodies, which are probably functional and contribute to the pathogenesis of the disease in these patients. The autoimmune basis of patients with chronic urticaria is in keeping with the recognized positive relationship between chronic urticaria and autoimmune thyroid disease [109]. Patients with autoimmune chronic urticaria are clinically and histologically (as determined by skin biopsy) indistinguishable from those with no evidence of an autoimmune basis.

Diagnosis of autoimmune chronic urticaria is based upon obtaining a positive autologous serum skin test (intradermal injection of 50 μl of the patient's serum into the same patient's uninvolved skin causes a wheal and flare reaction) combined with the ability of the same serum to release histamine from normal donor basophil leukocytes [105]. Study of a large group of patients has revealed a close correlation between antibody levels determined by bioassay and by immunoblotting. The above evidence has recently been reviewed [110].

The cause of chronic urticaria in the remaining 50–60% of patients remains elusive. Proposed causes for which these is no confirmatory evidence include candidosis, *Helicobacter pylori* infection, parasite infestation, and HIV infection [111]. Less than 5% of these patients can be confirmed by placebo-controlled oral challenge testing to be reactive to certain food additives.

Preliminary evidence suggests that circulating nonimmunoglobulin histamine-releasing factors may be important. These include cytokines [112,113], and a mast cell-specific histamine releasing factor [114] which is currently undergoing full characterization. A paradigm for the investigation of a patient presenting with chronic urticaria is shown in Figure 2.

## C. Treatment

Treatment of chronic urticaria is supportive and symptomatic. Itching can be reduced by maintaining a cool environment and avoiding woollen clothes. A tepid shower is useful to avoid nocturnal itching. Alcohol, stress, overtiredness, and physical exertion should be avoided where possible. Aspirin and angiotensin convertasing enzyme inhibitors should also be avoided. The few cases in which a culprit food additive can be confirmed should be treated by a diet. Topical antipruritic creams (1% menthol cream, calamine cream) can be useful. A 2% ephedrine spray can be very valuable to suppress oropharyngeal angioedema.

However, the mainstay of treatment remains the use of oral $H_1$ antihistamines. Their use is fully reviewed by Simons and Simons [115]. A combination of low-sedation antihistamines (Loratidine 10 mg; cetirizine 10 mg) in the daytime and a sedative antihistamine at night (hydroxyzine 25 mg; doxepin 20 mg) is useful for severely affected patients. Terfenadine is also effective, but the rare complication of cardiac arrhythmia has limited its use, and it is now effectively replaced by its active derivative fexofenadine. $H_2$ antihistamines probably have little or no role in the management of chronic urticaria [116]. A short tapering course of oral steroids (prednisolone, starting dose 50 mg daily) is occasionally justified in special circumstances where for specific reasons rapid control is essential over a limited period. Prolonged systemic corticosteroid treatment invariably results in steroid toxicity coupled with poor control.

Although not a licensed indication, at least in the United Kingdom, cyclosporine (3.5–4.0 mg/kg/day) is effective in the majority of patients with chronic urticaria (but not physical urticarias) irrespective of the underlying cause [117]. It has proved to be more effective in autoantibody positive than non–autoantibody positive patients. Patients who are considered for cyclosporine normally have severe recalcitrant urticaria resistant to conventional antihistamine treatment. They have often received one or more courses of oral steroids and may have lost considerable time off work due to their urticaria. I usually prescribe a 3-month course of cyclosporine having first ensured that renal function and blood pressure readings are satisfactory and that there is no contraindication including a history of cancer or precancer. Remission is usually rapid, within days. Cyclosporine is not curative, and the urticaria may relapse following withdrawal although there is usually no rebound. Since after cyclosporine withdrawal urticaria is often more responsive to $H_1$ antihistamines than before cyclosporine, it may be unnecessary to give a further course. Cyclosporine is a mast cell–stabilizing agent, being inhibitory on evoked mediator release from human mast cells [118] in therapeutic concentrations. Patients proved to possess anti-FcεRIα autoantibodies may benefit from intravenous immunoglobulin or plasmapheresis [108,119].

## V.  URTICARIA VASCULITIS

Although only relatively recently characterized [120], urticaria vasculitis is becoming increasingly recognized as an important cause of an otherwise unremarkable clinical picture of chronic urticaria. Although originally believed to present classically as indolent-looking wheals, which slowly subside leaving staining of the skin, and associated with polyarthritis, hypocomplementaemia and histological appearances of vasculitis in the skin, it is now recognized to occur more commonly with a clinical picture indistinguishable from ordinary chronic idiopathic urticaria. The clinical spectrum of urticaria vasculitis has been comprehensively reviewed by O'Donnell and Black [121]. Urticaria vasculitis may occur as an isolated clinical entity or as an early warning presentation of systemic lupus. Depending upon the histological criteria for diagnosis, the incidence of urticaria vasculitis in chronic urticaria ranges from 2–20%.

Patients with urticaria vasculitis present with widespread wheals, which may be annular, papular, or plaque-like. They may itch but are often more tender and painful than in ordinary chronic urticaria. Characteristically individual wheals last longer than 24 hours, and when they eventually fade they may leave residual staining of the skin. Palpation often reveals an indurated consistency due to fibrin deposition. Angioedema is a common association with urticaria vasculitis. Wheals of urticaria vasculitis often occur at pressure points, e.g., the waistband, and given their long duration may closely resemble delayed-pressure urticaria clinically. Arthralgia is common, and other clinical features include livedo reticularis and episcleritis. The disease may be complicated by glomerulonephritis and chronic obstructive airways disease, although in my experience these systemic complications are rare.

Besides systemic lupus [122], other disease associations with urticarial vasculitis include Sjogren's syndrome [123], polycythaemia vera [124], Lyme disease [125], and serum sickness [126]. Urticarial vasculitis may also be associated with an IgM monoclonal gammopathy (Schnitzler's syndrome) [127], progesterone hypersensitivity, and hepatitis C infection with cryoglobulinaemia [128], and may also be an adverse reaction to oral methotrexate.

Diagnosis of urticarial vasculitis is based upon clinical and histological grounds. Any patient with chronic urticaria poorly responsive to antihistamines and with other atypical features (duration of individual wheals greater than 24 hours, lesional tenderness or pain, residual skin staining, associated joint symptoms) should have a skin biopsy to exclude urticarial vasculitis. Much has been written about the minimum histological criteria to confirm a diagnosis of urticarial vasculitis. Evidence of postcapillary venular endothelial damage is a sine qua non. However, this may be no more than endothelial cell swelling. Leukocytoclasis and red blood cell leakage are important confirmatory features but are frequently not present. Fibrin deposition is common but may occur in "ordinary" chronic urticaria.

Laboratory investigations may be helpful and include the ESR, plasma levels of complement CH50, C3, C4, and $C_1q$, circulating immune complexes, antinuclear factor, anti-Ro (SSA), hepatitis B and C serology, plasma protein electrophoretic analysis for paraproteinemia, and lung function tests.

Urticarial vasculitis responds poorly to treatment. $H_1$ antihistamines are usually ineffective. Oral steroids are usually unhelpful unless high doses are given, and then steroid toxicity is a problem. I have also found colchicine, dapsone, antimalarials, azathioprine, and nonsteroidal antiinflammatories to be effective in the occasional patient. Pentoxiphylline has also been disappointing, but I have one patient who responded dramatically to intramuscular gold injections [129]. I have no personal experience with the use of plasmapheresis or intravenous immunoglobin infusion, but they might be worth trying in this unstable and persistent disorder.

## REFERENCES

1. Milton JL. On giant urticaria. Edinburgh Medical Journal, 1876; 22:513.
2. Quincke H. Uber akutes Umschriebenes Hauntoderm. Monatshefte für praktische Dermatologie 1882; 1:129.
3. Osler W. Hereditary angioneurotic oedema. Am J Med Sci 1888; 95, 362.
4. Dale HH, Laidlaw PP. The physiological action of β-imino-azolyl ethylamine. J Physiol 1910; 41:318.
5. Lewis T. The blood vessels of the human skin and their responses. Shaw and Sons London, 1927, p 47.
6. Riley JF, West GB. Skin histamine. Its location in the tissue mast cells. Arch Dermatol 1956; 74:471–478.
7. Kaplan AP, Horakova Z, Katz SI. Assessment of tissue fluid histamine levels in patients with urticaria. J Allergy Clin Immunol 1978; 61:350–354.
8. Zuberbier T, Ifflander J, Simmler C, Czarnetzki BM. Acute urticaria-clinical aspects and therapeutic responsiveness. Acta Derm Venereol (Stockh) 1996; 76:295–297.
9. Aoki T, Kojima M, Horiko T. Acute urticaria: history and natural course of 50 cases. J Dermatol 1994; 21:73–77.

10. Bromm B, Scharein E, Darsow U, Ring J. Effects of menthol and cold on histamine induced itch and skin reactions in man. Neuroscience Letters 1995; 187:157–160.

11. Monroe EW. Urticaria: an updated review. Arch Dermatol 1977; 113:80–90.

12. Barlow RJ, Warburton F, Watson K, Black AK, Greaves MW. Diagnosis and incidence of delayed pressure urticaria in patients with chronic urticaria. J Am Acad Dermatol 1993; 29: 954–958.

13. Black AK, Lawlor F, Greaves MW. Consensus meeting on the definition of physical urticarias and urticarial vasculitis. Clin Exp Dermatol 1996; 21:424–426.

14. Breathnach SM, Allen R, Milford-Ward A, Greaves MW. Symptomatic dermographism: natural history clinical features, laboratory investigations and response to therapy. Clin Exp Dermatol 1983; 8:463–476.

15. Kaur S, Greaves MW, Eftekhari N. Factitious urticaria (dermographism) treatment by cimetidine and chlorpheniramine in a randomized double-blind study. Br J Dermatol 1981; 104: 185–190.

16. Lawlor F, Ormerod AD, Greaves MW. Calcium antagonists in the treatment of symptomatic dermographism. Dermatologica 1988; 197:287–291.

17. Lawlor F, Black AK, Murdoch RD, Greaves MW. Symptomatic dermographism: whealing mast cells and histamine are decreased in the skin following long term application of a potent topical corticosteroid. Br J Dermatol 1989; 121:629–634.

18. Dover JS, Black AK, Milford Ward A, Greaves MW. Delayed-pressure urticaria: clinical features, laboratory investigations, and response to therapy of 44 patients. J Am Acad Dermatol 1988; 18:1289–1298.

19. McFadden JP, Newton JA, Greaves MW. Dyspareunia as a complication of delayed pressure urticaria. Br J Sexual Med 1988; 15:61.

20. Winkelmann RK, Black AK, Dover J, Greaves MW. Pressure urticaria-histopathological study. Clin Exp Dermatol 1986; 11:139–147.

21. Barlow RJ, Ross EL, MacDonald DM, Black AK, Greaves MW. Mast cells and T-lymphocytes in chronic urticaria. Clin Exp Allergy 1995; 25:317–322.

22. Lawlor F, Black AK, Milford Ward A, Morris R, Greaves MW. Delayed-pressure urticaria, objective evaluation of a variable disease using a dermographometer and assessment of treatment using colchicine. Br J Dermatol 1989; 120:403–408.

23. Mekori YA, Dobozin BS, Schocket AL, Kohler PF, Clark RAF. Delayed pressure urticaria histologically resembles cutaneous late phase reactions. Arch Dermatol 1984; 124:230–235.

24. Lawlor F, Bird C, Camp RDR, Barlow R, Barr RM, Black AK, Judge MR, Greaves MW. Increased interleukin-6, but reduced interleukin 1 in delayed-pressure urticaria. Br J Dermatol 1993; 128:500–503.

25. Peters MS, Winkelmann RK, Greaves MW, Kephart GM, Gleich GJ. Extra cellular deposition of eosinophil granule major basic protein in pressure urticaria. J Am Acad Dermatol 1987; 16(3):513–517.

26. Lawlor F, Barr RM, Black AK, Cromwell O, Isaacs J, Greaves MW. Arachidonic acid transformation is not stimulated in delayed-pressure urticaria. Br J Dermatol 1989; 121:317–321.

27. Kontou-Fili K, Maniatakou G, Demaka P, Gonianakis M, Palaiologos G, Aromi K. Therapeutic effect of cetirizine in delayed-pressure urticaria: clinicopathologic findings. J Am Acad Dermatol 1991; 24:1090–1093.

28. Barlow RJ, MacDonald DM, Black AK, Greaves MW. The effect of topical steroid on delayed pressure urticaria. Arch Dermatol Res 1995; 287:285–288.

29. Horton BT, Brown GE, Roth GM. Hypersensitiveness to cold with local and systemic manifestations of a histamine-like character. Its amenability to treatment. JAMA 1936; 107:1263–1269.

30. Illig L, Paul E, Bruck K, Schwennicke HP. Experimental investigations on the trigger mechanisms of the generalized type of heat and cold urticaria by means of a climate chamber. Acta Dermato Venereol (Stockh) 1980; 60:373–380.

31. Lin RY, Schwartz RA. Cold urticaria and HIV infection. Brit J Dermatol 1993; 129:465–467.

32. Kile RL, Rusk HA. A case of cold urticaria with an unusual family history. J Am Med Assoc 1940; 114:1067–1068.

33. Zip CM, Ross JB, Greaves MW, Scriver CR, Mitchell JJ, Zoar S. Familial cold urticaria. Clin Exp Dermatol 1993; 18:338–341.

34. Constanzi JJ, Coltman JR, Donaldson VH. Activation of complement by a monoclonal cryoglobulin associated with cold urticaria. J Lab Clin Med 1969; 74:902–910.

35. Lawlor F, Black AK, Breathnach AS, McKee P. Sarathchandra A, Bhogal B, Isaacs JL, Greaves MW, Winkelmann RK. A timed study of the histopathology direct immunoflourescence and ultrastructural findings in idiopathic cold contact urticaria over a 24-h period. Clin Exp Dermatol 1989; 14:416–420.

36. Eady RAJ, Greaves MW. Induction of cutaneous vasculitis by repeated cold challenge in cold urticaria. Lancet 1978; I:336–337.

37. Misch K, Black AK, Greaves MW, Almosawi T, Stanworth DR. Passive transfer of idiopathic cold urticaria to monkeys. Acta Dermato Venereol (Stockh) 1983; 63:163–164.

38. Mathews KP. Exploiting the cold urticaria models. New Eng J Med 1981; 305:1090–1091.

39. Gruber BL, Baeza ML, Marchese MJ, Kaplan AP, Autoantibodies in urticaria syndromes. J Invest Dermatol 1988; 90:213–217.

40. Heavey DJ, Black AK, Barrow SE, Chappell CG, Greaves MW, Dollery CT. Protaglandin D2 and histamine release in cold urticaria. J Allergy Clin Immunol 1986; 78:458–461.

41. Ormerod AD, Black AK, Dawes J, Murdoch RD, Koro O, Barr RM, Greaves MW. Prostaglandin D2 and histamine release in cold urticaria unaccompanied by evidence of platelet activation. J Allergy Clin Immunol 1988; 82:586–589.

42. Wasserman SI, Austen KF, Soter NA. The functional and physicochemical characterisation of three eosinophilotactic activities released into the circulation by cold challenge in patients with cold urticaria. Clin Exp Immunol 1982; 47:570–578.

43. Bentley-Phillips CB, Eady RAJ, Greaves MW. Cold urticaria: inhibition of cold-induced histamine release by doxantrazole. J Invest Dermatol 1978; 71:266–268.

44. Keahey TM, Greaves MW. Cold urticaria: disassociation of cold evoked histamine release and urticaria following cold challenge. Arch Dermatol 1980; 116:174–177.

45. Black AK, Keahey TM, Eady RAJ, Greaves MW. Dissociation of histamine release and clinical improvement following treatment of acquired cold urticaria by prednisone. Br J Clin Pharmacol 1981; 12:327–331.

46. Bentley Phillips CB, Black AK, Greaves MW. Induced tolerance in cold evoked histamine release. Lancet 1976; ii:63–66.

47. Black AK, Sibbald RG, Greaves MW. Cold urticaria treated by induction of tolerance. Lancet 1979; ii:964.

48. Duke W. Urticaria caused specifically by the actions of physical agents. J Am Med Assoc 1924: 83:3–9.

49. Commens CA, Greaves MW. Test to establish the diagnosis cholinergic urticaria. Br J Dermatol 1978; 98:47–51.

50. Hirschmann JV, Lawlor F, English SJC, Louback JB, Winkelmann RK, Greaves MW. Cholinergic urticaria. Arch Dermatol 1987; 123:462–467.

51. Jorizzo JL. Cholinergic urticaria. Arch Dermatol 1987; 123:455–457.

52. Zuberbier T, Althaus C. Chantraine-Hess, Czarnetski BM. Prevalence of cholinergic urticaria in young adults. J Am Acad Dermatol 1994; 31:478–481.

53. Merry P. World cup urticaria. J R Soc Med 1987; 80:779.

54. Lawrence CM, Jorizzo JL, Black AK, Coutts A, Greaves MW. Cholinergic urticaria with associated angioedema. Br J Dermatol 1981; 105:543–550.

55. Murphy GM, Black AK, Greaves MW. Persisting cholinergic erythema: a variant of cholinergic urticaria. Br J Dermatol 1983; 109:343–348.

56.  Kivity S, Snech E, Greif J, Topilsky M, Mekori YA. The effect of food and exercise on the skin response to compound 48/80 in patients with food associated exercise induced urticaria angioedema. J Allergy Clin Immunol 1988; 81:1155–1158.

57.  Nomland R. Cholinergic urticaria and cholinergic itching. Arch Derm Syph 1944; 50:247–250.

58.  Berth-Jones J, Graham-Brown RAC. Cholinergic pruritus erythema and urticaria. A disease spectrum responding to danazol. Br J Dermatol 1989; 121:235–237.

59.  Herxheimer A. The nervous pathway mediating cholinergic urticaria. Clin Sci 1956; 15:194–205.

60.  Adachi J, Aoki T, Yamatodani A. Demonstration of sweat allergy in cholinergic urticaria. J Dermatol Sci 1994; 7:142–149.

61.  Murphy GM, Greaves MW, Zollman P, Stanworth D. Cholinergic urticaria. Passive transfer experiments from human to monkey. Dermatologica 1988; 177:338–340.

62.  Eftekhari N, Milford Ward A, Allen R, Greaves MW. Protease inhibitor profiles in urticaria and angioedema. Br J Dermatol 1980; 103:33–39.

63.  Wong E, Eftekhari N, Greaves MW, Milford Ward A. Beneficial effects of danazol on symptoms and laboratory charges of cholinergic urticaria. Br J Dermatol 1987; 116:553–556.

64.  Greaves MW, Sneddon IB, Smith AK, Stanworth DR. Heat urticaria. Br J Dermatol 1974; 90:289–292.

65.  Koro O, Dover JS, Francis DM, Black AK, Kelly RW, Barr RM, Greaves MW. Release of prostaglandin D2 and histamine in a case of localized heat urticaria and effects of treatments. Br J Dermatol 1986; 115:722–728.

66.  Leigh I, Ramsay CA. Localized heat urticaria treated by inducing tolerance to heat.

67.  Fearfield LA, Gazzard B, Bunker CB. Aquagenic urticaria and human immunodeficiency virus infection: treatment with stanazolol. Br J Dermatol 1997; 137:620–622.

68.  Sibbald RG, Black AK, Eady RAJ, James M, Greaves MW. Aquagenic urticaria: evidence of a cholinergic and histaminergic basis. Br J Dermatol 1981; 105:297–302.

69.  Martinez-Escribano JA, Quecedo E, de la Cuadra J, Frias J, Sanchez-Pedreno P, Aliaga A. Treatment of aquagenic urticaria with PUVA and asteminzole. J Am Acad Dermatol 1997; 36:118–119.

70.  Shelley WB. Questions and Answers. J Am Med Assoc 1970; 212:1385.

71.  Greaves MW, Black AK, Eady RAJ, Coutts A. Aquagenic pruritus. Br Med J 1981; 282:2007–2010.

72.  Steinman HK, Greaves MW. Aquagenic pruritus. J Am Acad Dermatol 1985; 13:91–96.

73.  Kligman AM, Greaves MW. Steinman H. Water induced itching without cutaneous signs. Arch Dermatol 1986; 122:183–186.

74.  Archer CB, Greaves MW. Aquagenic pruritus. Semin Dermatol 1988; 7:301–303.

75.  Menage H du P, Greaves MW. Aquagenic pruritus. Semin Dermatol 1995; 14:313–316.

76.  Archer CB, Camp RDR, Greaves MW. Polycythaemia vera can present with aquagenic pruritus. Lancet 1988; i:1451.

77.  Handfield-Jones SE, Hills RJ, Ive FA, Greaves MW. Aquagenic pruritus associated with juvenile xanthogranuloma. Clin Exp Dermatol 1993; 18:253–255.

78.  McGrath JA, Greaves MW. Aquagenic pruritus and myelodysplastic syndrome. Br J Dermatol 1990; 123:414–415.

79.  Lotti T, Steinman HK, Greaves MW, Fabril P, Brunetti L, Panconesi E. Increased cutaneous fibrinocytic activity in aquagenic pruritus. Int J Dermatol 1986; 25:508–510.

80.  Steinman HK, Black AK, Lotti TM, Brunetti L, Panconesi E, Greaves MW. Polycythaemia rubra vera and water induced pruritus. Blood histamine levels and cutaneous fibrinolytic activity before and after water challenge. Br J Dermatol 1987; 116:329–333.

81.  Greaves MW, Handfield-Jones, SE. Aquagenic pruritus-pharmacological findings and treatment. Eur J Dermatol 1992; 2:482–484.

82. Menage H du P, Norris PG, Hawk JLM, Greaves MW. The efficacy of psoralen photochemotherapy in the treatments of aquagenic pruritus. Br J Dermatol 1993; 129:163–165.
83. Ive H, Lloyd J, Magnus IA. Action spectra in idiopathic solar urticaria. Br J Dermatol 1965; 77:229–243.
84. Hawk JLM, Eady RAJ, Challoner AVJ, Black AK, Keahey TM, Greaves MW. Elevated blood histamine levels and mast cell degranulation in solar urticaria. Br J Clin Pharmac 1980; 9:183–186.
85. Leenutaphong V, Holzle E, Plewig G. Solar urticaria: studies on mechanisms of tolerance. Br J Dermatol 1990; 122:601–606.
86. Ramsay CA. Solar urticaria treatment by inducing tolerance to artificial radiation and natural light. Arch Dermatol 1977; 113:1222–1225.
87. Parrish JA, Jaenicke KF, Morison WL, Momtaz K, Shea C. Solar urticaria: treatment with PUVA and mediator inhibitors. Br J Dermatol 1982; 106:575–580.
88. Duschet P, Leyen P, Schwartz T, Hocker P, Greiter J, Gschnait F. Solar urticaria: effective treatment by plasmapheresis. Clin Exp Dermatol 1987; 12:185–188.
89. Hudson-Peacock MJ, Farr PM, Diffey BL, Goodship THJ. Combined treatment of solar urticaria with plasmapheresis and PUVA. Br J Dermatol 1993; 128:440–442.
90. Metzger WJ, Kaplan AP, Beaven MA. Hereditary vibratory angioedema: confirmation of histamine release in a type of physical hypersensitivity. J Allergy Clin Immunol 1976; 57:605–608.
91. Patterson R, Mellies CJ, Blankership ML, Pruzansky JJ. Vibratory angioedema: a hereditary type of physical hypersensitivity. J Allergy Clin Immunol 1972; 50:184–188.
92. Champion RH, Roberts SOB, Carpenter RG, Roger JH. Urticaria and angioedema—a review of 554 patients. Br J Dermatol 1969; 81:588–597.
93. O'Donnell BF, Lawlor F, Simpson J, Morgan M, Greaves MW. The impact of chronic urticaria on the quality of life. Br J Dermatol 1997; 136:197–201.
94. Barlow RJ, Ross EL, MacDonald D, Black AK, Greaves MW. Adhesion molecule expression and the inflammatory cell infiltrate in delayed pressure urticaria. Br J Dermatol 1994; 131:341–347.
95. Natbony SF, Phillips ME, Elias JM, Godfrey HP, Kaplan AP. Histological studies of chronic idiopathic urticaria. J Allergy Clin Immunol 1983; 71:177–183.
96. Peters MS, Winkelmann RK. Neutrophilic urticaria. Br J Dermatol 1985; 113:25–30.
97. Krause LB, Shuster S. Enhanced wheal and flare response to histamine in chronic urticaria. Br J Clin Pharmacol 1985; 20:486–488.
98. Michaelsson G, Juhlin L. Urticaria induced by preservatives and dye additives in food and drugs. Br J Dermatol 1973; 88:525–532.
99. Doeglas HMG. Reactions to aspirin and food additives in patients with chronic urticaria including the physical urticarias. Br J Dermatol 1975; 93:135–144.
100. May CD. Are confusion and controversy about food hypersensitivity really necessary? J Allergy Clin Immunol 1985; 75:329–333.
101. Pastorello EA. Evaluating new tests for the diagnosis of food allergy. Allergy 1995; 50:289–291.
102. Rorsman H. Basopenia in urticaria. Acta Allergologica 1962; 17:168–184.
103. Greaves MW, Plummer VM, McLaughlan P, Stanworth DR. Serum and cell bound IgE in chronic urticaria. Clin Allergy 1974; 4:265–271.
104. Hide M, Francis DM, Grattan CEH, Hakimi J, Kochan JR, Greaves MW. Autoantibodies against the high affinity IgE receptor, as a cause of histamine release in chronic urticaria. New Engl J Med 1993; 328:1599–1604.
105. Niimi N, Francis DM, Kermani F, O'Donnell BF, Hide M, Black AK, Winkelmann RK, Greaves MW, Barr RM. Dermal mast cell activation by autoantibodies against the high affinity IgE receptor in chronic urticaria. J Invest Dermatol 1996; 106:1001–1006.
106. Fiebiger E, Maurer D, Holub H, Reininger B, Hartmann G, Woisetschlager M, Kinet J-P,

Stingl G. Serum IgG autoantibodies directed against the alpha chain of FcεRI: a selective marker and pathogenetic factor for a distinct subset of chronic urticaria patients. J Clin Invest 1995; 96:2606–2612.

107. Tong LJ, Balakrishnan G, Kochan JP, Kinet J-P, Kaplan AP. Assessment of autoimmunity in patients with chronic urticaria. J Allergy Clin Immunol 1997; 99:461–465.

108. Grattan CEH, Francis DM, Slater NGP, Barlow RJ, Greaves MW. Plasmapheresis for severe unremitting chronic urticaria. Lancet 1992; 339:1078–1080.

109. Leznoff A, Sussman GL. Syndrome of idiopathic chronic urticaria and angioedema with thyroid autoimmunity: A study of 90 patients. J Allergy Clin Immunol 1989; 84:66–71.

110. Hide M, Francis DM, Grattan CEH, Barr RM, Winkelmann RK, Greaves MW. The pathogenesis of chronic idiopathic urticaria. New evidence suggests an autoimmune basis and implications for treatment. Clin Exp Allergy 1994; 24:626–627.

111. Friedman D, Picard-Dahan C, Grossin M, Belaich D. Chronic urticaria revealing HIV infection. Eur J Dermatol 1993; 5:40–41.

112. Claveau J, Lavoie A, Brunet C, Bedard P-M, Hibert J. Chronic idiopathic urticaria possible contribution of histamine releasing factor to the pathogenesis. J Allergy Clin Immunol 1993; 92:132–137.

113. MacDonald SM, Rafnar T, Langdon J, Lichtenstein LM. Molecular identification of an IgE-dependent histamine releasing factor. Science 1995; 269:688–690.

114. Kermani F, Niimi N, Francis DM, Greaves MW, Barr RM. Characterisation of a novel mast cell specific histamine releasing activity in chronic idiopathic urticaria. J Invest Dermatol 1995; 105:452 (ABS).

115. Simons FER, Simons KJ. The pharmacology and use of H1-receptor antagonist drugs. N Engl J Med 1994; 330:1663–1670.

116. Bleehen SS, Thomas SE, Greaves MW, Newton J, Kennedy CT, Hindley F, et al. Cimetidine and chlorpheniramine in the treatment of chronic idiopathic urticaria: a multicenter randomized double-blind study. Br J Dermatol 1987; 117:81–88.

117. Barlow RJ, Black AK, Greaves MW. Treatment of severe chronic urticaria with cyclosporine A. Eur J Dermatol 1993; 3:273–275.

118. Speer WF, Agis H, Czerwenka K, Valent P. Effect of cyclosporin A and FK 506 on stem cell factor-induced histamine secretion and growth of human mast cells. J Allergy Clin Immunol 1996; 98:389–399.

119. O'Donnell BF, Barr RM, Black AK, Francis DM, Kermani F, Niimi N, Barlow RJ, Winkelmann RK, Greaves MW. Intravenous immunoglobulin (IVIG) in autoimmune chronic urticaria. Br J Dermatol 1998; 138:101–106.

120. Soter RA, Austen AK, Gigli I. Urticarias and arthralgias as manifestations of necrotising angiitis (vasculitis), J Invest Dermatol 1974; 63:485–490.

121. O'Donnell BF, Black AK. Urticaria vasculitis. Int Angiol 1995; 14:1661–1674.

122. Provost T, Zone JJ, Synkowski D, Maddison PJ, Reichlin M. Unusual cutaneous manifestations of systemic lupus 1. Urticaria-like lesions correlation with clinical and serological abnormalities. J Invest Dermatol 1980; 75:495–499.

123. Alexander EL, Provost T. Cutaneous manifestations of primary Sjogrens Syndrome: a reflection of vasculitis and association with anti-Ro (SSA) antibodies. J Invest Dermatol 1983; 80:386–391.

124. Farell AM, Sabroe RA, Bunker CB. Urticarial vasculitis associated with polycythaemia ruba vera. Clin Exp Dermatol 1996; 21:302–304.

125. Olson JC, Esterly NB. Urticarial vasculitis and Lyme disease. J Am Acad Dermatol 1989; 22:1114–1116.

126. Lawley TJ, Bielory L, Gascon P, Yancey KB, Young NS, Frank MM. A study of human serum sickness. J Invest Dermatol 1985; 85:129s–132s.

127. Borradori L, Rybojad M, Puissant A, Dallot A, Verola O, Morel P. Urticarial vasculitis associated with a monoclonal IgM gammopathy Schnitzer's syndrome. Br J Dermatol 1990; 123: 113–118.
128. Kuniyuki S, Katoh H. Urticarial vasculitis with papular lesions in a patient with type C hepatitis and cryoglobulinaemia. J Dermatol 1996; 23:279–283.
129. Handfield-Jones SE, Greaves MW. Urticarial vasculitis: response to gold therapy. J R Soc Med 1991; 84:169.

# 9

## The Physical Urticarias

**E. Frances Lawlor**
*St. John's Institute of Dermatology, St. Thomas' Hospital, and Newham Healthcare,*
*St. Andrews Hospital, London, England*

The physical urticarias are those in which wealing occurs in response to a specific physical stimulus. The reaction can be considered as a physical "hypersensitivity" to the stimulus without implying that an immunological response occurs. These disorders are pathergic rather than allergic.

There are two main groups of physical urticaria: the contact type and the reflex type. In the contact type the reaction is confined to the area affected by the physical stimulus as in idiopathic cold contact urticaria, solar urticaria, delayed-pressure urticaria, and dermographism. In the reflex type both the site of contact and distant structures are affected as in cholinergic urticaria or vibratory angioedema. If the physical stimuli are sufficiently strong, the patient may suffer systemic upset. The physical urticarias are common and make up approximately 20% of all patients attending dermatology clinics [1].

If the mucous membranes are involved, angioedema occurs. The physical urticarias can be transmitted genetically or acquired. The provoking physical stimuli are divided into mechanical trauma, change in temperature, and exposure to water and to light. The diagnosis of a physical urticaria is made from the patient's history, clinical examination, and ideally by provoking the lesions if possible. Treatment can be divided into nondrug treatment, in which an explanation about the disease and avoidance of provoking factors, if possible, is stressed, and drug treatment. Drug treatment is helpful in some conditions and less so in others.

## I. CUTANEOUS RESPONSES TO MECHANICAL STIMULI

The cutaneous reactions that occur in response to mechanical stimuli are dermographism, immediate-pressure urticaria, delayed-pressure urticaria, and vibratory angioedema.

### A. Dermographism

The two most common forms of dermographism are simple dermographism, which may be regarded as physiological [2,3], and symptomatic dermographism, which is pathological. Rarer forms of dermographism include delayed dermographism, localized dermographism, red dermographism, transient dermographism, and drug-induced dermographism. Dermographism also occurs in normal skin in association with generalized cutaneous mastocytosis.

## 1.  Simple Dermographism

In simple dermographism, a weal and flare reaction without itching occurs in response to moderate stroking of the skin. People with this condition are aware of it. The condition has been noted in about 5% of normal young men without skin disease [2]. Lewis believed that a more severe frictional pressure, for example, a whiplash, would cause wealing in practically all young people. No treatment is necessary for this condition.

## 2.  Symptomatic Dermographism

In symptomatic dermographism (SD), there is itching associated with an itching and wealing response to a minor stroking pressure applied to the skin. The reaction maximal is within 5–10 minutes and disappears within 30–60 minutes [3,4]. The pattern of wealing matches the pattern of the stimulus and is often linear. Weals appear under belts, where clothes are tight, and at the site of scratching. In severely affected people, minimum friction like the movement of collars of cuffs on the skin or using a towel cause itching and wealing. Showering can cause symptoms as the jets of water impinge on the skin. Waves of itching also occur without visible wealing, and the itch, which is worse in the evening [5], often seems disproportionate to the wealing seen. The condition can occur at any age [5], has a mean duration of 5 years, and may last longer than 10 years in some [5]. There are no underlying medical problems, and SD is not increased in patients with chronic urticaria. The diagnosis is made by taking the history, from the pattern of visible wealing, and by stroking the skin lightly using a blunt instrument. The stroked site should be inspected 5 minutes later. Although the morphology and the numbers of mast cells present in the skin are normal [6], histamine is the major mediator in the reaction [6–8]. Treatment with H1 antihistamines is generally effective.

## 3.  Rarer Forms of Dermographism

Delayed dermographism, in which a wealing response occurs several hours after the stimulus, either with or without an immediate wealing response [9–12], may be a separate disorder or may be a manifestation of delayed-pressure urticaria. Localized dermographism that persists for a short time period may occur at sites of insect bites, tatoo marks, or where intradermal skin testing has been performed [13,14]. Cholinergic dermographism with erythema studded with tiny weals that happens within minutes of a stimulus occurs occasionally in cholinergic urticaria [3,13,15]. Transient dermographism, present for a short period of time, may occur after scabies, infestation, or penicillin treatment [13,16]. It also occurs in association with linear eczematous plaques after treatment with bleomycin [17]. Real dermographism is distinct in that the wealing response is broader, erythematous, and provoked by rubbing rather than by simple stroking pressure [18].

## B.  Immediate Pressure Urticaria

In this condition there is an immediate response to a perpendicular pressure stimulus applied to the skin. Itching occurs within seconds of the stimulus and is followed by a burning erythema and wealing developing within minutes. Lesions occur in the absence of dermographism and are provoked by leaning against furniture, resting the face on the arm, crossing the legs, or handling the steering wheel of a car. Pressure from fingers on the skin also causes the reaction. Lesions may be present for several hours. This condition may occur as an isolated physical urticaria, in conjunction with other urticarias [19], and in patients with the hypereosinophilic syndrome [20]. Histology of the skin shows dermal edema with a mild unremarkable perivascular infiltration of lymphocytes and histiocytes [19]. Antihistamines are an effective drug treatment.

## C. Delayed-Pressure Urticaria

A sustained pressure stimulus to the skin provokes delayed-pressure urticaria. Cutaneous erythema and edema in association with marked subcutaneous edema occurs between 30 minutes and 9 hours after the stimulus and may be present up to 48 hours [9]. Delayed-pressure urticaria usually occurs in patients who have chronic idiopathic urticaria (CIU), although both conditions may not always be present together at the same time [9,21–24].

This condition should be considered in all patients whose CIU is not responding to antihistamines. Direct questioning is necessary to obtain the relevant history. Certain activities provoke lesions. Sitting produces lesions on buttocks and thighs. Crossing the legs produces lesions on the knees, as does gardening. leaning against furniture, lying on hard beds, and wearing seat belts and tight clothing cause lesions. Walking, running, jogging, and climbing produce swelling of the feet indistinguishable from idiopathic angioedema. Using screwdrivers, carrying bags, and driving cause similar swelling of the hands. The lesions are itchy, painful, and burning, and arthralgia may occur in joints close to larger lesions. Some patients experience a flu-like illness with malaise, tiredness, and rigors [9,25].

Laboratory tests may show an increased erythrocyte sedimentation rate [23,26], and a neutrophil leucocytosis is frequent. Total antitrypsin and $\alpha_1$-antitrypsin are elevated [27]. Lesions can be reproduced by hanging a 15 Ib weight over the shoulders or thighs for 15 minutes [25], by using a calibrated dermographometer to reproduce lesions [23], or by using a specially constructed pressure instrument in which known weights rest on the back [4,24,29]. The pathogenesis of the disease is unclear.

The concomitant CIU is usually controlled using antihistamines, to which the pressure lesions are unresponsive, although there is one report suggesting that cetirizine is effective. There is no satisfactory drug treatment for the pressure-induced wealing [21,25]. Antihistamines, nonsteroidal anti-inflammatory drugs [9], and colchicine [23] are generally ineffective. Systemic steroids are not effective, but in occasional patients doses of >30 mg/day may improve the condition although wealing continues to occur [25]. This dosage might be used on a short-term basis for a specific occasion, but adverse effects would prohibit longer-term use. Anecdotal suggestions that dapsone may have an effect and that cyclosporine is effective await controlled trials. It is important to explain that the disease is one that ranges in severity over weeks to months [22,23] and that remits in time although it may be present for years [9]. Avoidance of pressure stimuli as far as possible is the best approach.

## D. Vibratory Angioedema

This is a reflex urticaria in which a vibratory stimulus applied to the skin causes acute, short-lived itchy swellings at the site of application and at distant sites. If the stimulus is sufficient, flushing, chest tightness, headache, and a generalized feeling of heat may occur [30,31]. The condition is transmitted genetically or acquired.

### 1.  Genetically Transmitted Vibratory Angioedema

Two families are reported in which this condition is recorded as an autosomal dominant trait with high penetrance [30,32]. This is a benign disorder recognized by those affected and by their relatives. Affected babies usually show signs when rubbed with a towel. In others the reaction is reproduced by massage, walking, running, scratching, and stroking. The response occurs within 5 minutes, disappears within 1 hour, and consists of erythema and cutaneous and subcutaneous edema. Mucosal and laryngeal involvement are not reported. The severity tends to decrease with time. There is no association with any other physical urticaria or underlying disease. Life is not shortened. Those affected usually limit their activities, and drug therapy is not usually necessary.

### 2.  Acquired Vibratory Angioedema

Sporadic cases of acquired vibratory angioedema have been reported in adults [31,33,34] The symptoms and signs are similar to the inherited variant. Lesions are produced by daily activities or work that causes vibration to the skin. The stimuli include riding motorbikes, mowing the lawn, using garden shears, metal grinding, clapping the hands, walking, or jogging. The areas of the body affected are those that are vibrated during a particular activity.

Lesions can be reproduced by performing these activities in the clinic setting, although for research purposes different vibrators have been used [30,33,34].

There is no known immunological basis for this reaction. No laboratory abnormalities have been reported. Skin mast cell numbers are normal. Plasma histamine levels rise during the reaction [33,34]. A positive therapeutic response to H1 antihistamines has been recorded [31].

A synopsis of the diagnosis of the mechanical urticarias is shown in Table 1.

## II.  CUTANEOUS RESPONSES TO CHANGES IN TEMPERATURE

### A.  Responses to Heat

### 1.  Cholinergic Urticaria

The eruption of cholinergic urticaria (CU) consists of intensely itchy weals that may occur anywhere in the body. CU is provoked by exercise, emotion, and warming the body [35]. These stimuli cause an increase in core body temperature to which the eruption is secondary [36]. The rash is provoked by any exercise such as jogging, running, cycling, or dancing. Passive warming of the body (e.g., going in to a warm room or taking a hot bath or shower) may also cause the rash. Brief and usually unpleasant emotion causes symptoms and signs. Lesions develop up to 10 minutes after the provoking factor has ceased [13]. The attack begins with itching, tingling, burning, warmth, or irritation. This is followed by the eruption, which may begin at any site and can involve all areas. The progression may be from punctate erythematous macules or blotchy macular erythema to confluent erythema and tiny weals. The weals may become as large as 2.5 cm. All patients itch. Attacks last between 5 minutes and 8 hours [37,38]. Some complain of dizziness, nausea, and irritability, while others experience faintness, abdominal cramps, or headache [13]. Occasionally, patients may develop angioedema and symptoms of anaphylaxis [39]. Wheezing may occur [3]. Significant decreases in forced expiratory volumes (FEVI) have been recorded [40]. A refractory period occurs after provoking the eruption during, which time the rash is less easily provoked [35]. CU is not associated with any systemic diseases.

**Table 1**  Clinical Diagnosis of the Mechanical Urticarias

| Urticaria | Clinical | Lesion induction |
|---|---|---|
| Symptomatic dermographism | Friction induced, frequently linear, itchy weals | Stroke skin lightly using a blunt instrument or dermographometer; inspect for itchy weal and flare reaction 5 minutes later |
| Immediate-pressure urticaria | Itchy burning lesions within minutes of pressure | Finger pressure on the skin, or blunt instrument or dermographometer pressure |
| Delayed-pressure urticaria | Urticaria and angioedema 30 minutes after application of sustained pressure to the skin | 1. A 15 lb weight suspended over shoulder or thigh for 15 minutes<br>2. A calibrated dermographometer applied to skin for a known time period<br>3. A special pressure instrument applied to the back or thighs; all sites inspected 6 hours later |
| Genetically transmitted vibratory angioedema | Lesions noted soon after birth, which occur within 5 minutes of stimulus; a positive family history | Rubbing with a towel; massaging the skin |
| Acquired vibratory angioedema | Itching, swelling, and wealing within minutes of jogging, walking, mowing the lawn, etc. | Jogging on the spot |

Acetylcholine or related cholinergic substances are considered important in the pathogenesis of the reaction [35,41,42], which can be blocked by the topical application of atropine sulfate and hyoscine hydrobromide [41,42]. Whether or not sweating is important is not clear [42–44]. Histamine is also important with increased reaction with increased plasma histamine levels found in vessels draining involved skin [45,46] and mast cell degranulation [6]. The diagnosis is made from the history and confirmed by reproducing the lesions. This is done by asking the patients to exercise or by passively raising the body temperature [38,40]. Patients may exercise until semi-exhausted by jogging on the spot, cycling on a stationary bicycle, running on a treadmill, or they may have a hot bath or shower.

Immersion in a bath kept at 40–41°C for 10–15 minutes is usually sufficient [13]. The "mecholyl test" is not reliable and is not necessary in clinical practice [47]. Antihistamines have an effect in CU. They increase the threshold at which the rash appears but do not control the disease completely. In the more severely affected patient, danazol [48] or stanozolol may be effective.

## 2.  Variants of Cholinergic Urticaria

These variants include cholinergic pruritus, familial CU, persisting cholinergic erythema, exercise-induced anaphylaxis, food-induced angioedema, and food-dependant exercise-induced urticaria, angioedema, and anaphylaxis.

### 3. Cholinergic Pruritus

In this condition, exercise, heat, and exertion provoke itching without rash [49,50]. The condition may progress in time to cholinergic urticaria. Antihistamines are the treatment of choice together with avoidance of the provoking stimuli.

### 4. Persisting Cholinergic Erythema

This variant of CU presents with pruritus and a macular erythema that is constant. The erythema is distributed maximally over the upper trunk and limbs. While each individual macule is of short duration, new macules appear both spontaneously and in response to exercise and hot baths [51,52].

### 5. Familial Cholinergic Urticaria

Four families are described in whom more than one member suffers from CU. An autosomal dominant inheritance is proposed. In these families any affected parents had suffered for several decades [53].

### 6. Exercise-Induced Anaphylaxis

Here some patients may have an urticarial eruption with or without symptoms of anaphylaxis. This syndrome may be distinguished from CU by the fact that it is provoked by exercise only. After exercise the core body temperature rises and plasma histamine levels increase as they do in CU. The distinguishing factor clinically is that patients with this syndrome do not develop symptoms after passive warming of the body [54]. A familial form has been described [55].

The emergency treatment is identical to that for anaphylaxis from other causes. Antihistamines may be helpful as maintenance therapy taken before exercise as they may decrease the severity of the attack. A self-administered injection of adrenaline should be carried out by the patient, who should not exercise alone and should stop exercising at the onset of the earliest premonitory symptoms [56]. It is wiser not to exercise until 4–6 hours after a meal and also to avoid aspirin and nonsteroidal anti-inflammatory drugs.

### 7. Angioedema Provoked by Food in Combination with a Rise in Body Temperature

One report exists documenting angioedema provoked by exercise or hot bath if taken within 2 hours of food ingestion. The patient was not allergic to any particular food, and the condition is secondary to the rise in core body temperature that occurs after the ingestion of food taken in conjunction with the further temperature rise that occurs after exercise or a hot bath. The symptoms in this case were blocked by ingestion of an anticholinergic drug, and a refractory period was induced by either exercising or taking a hot bath every morning [57].

### 8. Food and Drug-Dependent Exercise-Induced Anaphylaxis

Urticaria, angioedema, and full-blown anaphylaxis have been described not only after ingestion of any specific food but also after taking specific foods to which the patients demonstrate skin sensitivity [58]. In these cases it is suggested either that exercise lowers the threshold for mediator release to a specific IgE allergen or that antigens lower the threshold to exercise [59]. Similar reactions have occurred with gliadens in cereal where both skin prick tests and RASTs are positive to gliaden [60]. Ingestion of drugs followed by exercise also provokes exercise-induced anaphylaxis in some. Acetylsalicylic acid [61] and nufylpropion acid [62] have both been implicated.

### 9. Adrenergic Urticaria

This variant of urticaria is distinguished from cholinergic urticaria by the presence of a halo of blanched vasoconstricted skin that surrounds the urticarial weal. The reaction is induced by emotional stress and is reproduced by intradermal skin testing with noradrenaline (3–10 mg). Plasma noradrenaline and adrenaline levels are increased. In the cases described propanolol reduced the frequency and severity of attacks [63].

### 10. Localized Heat Urticaria

This condition is rare and is described in many single case reports. The patients experience pruritus and wealing, including angioedema, in areas directly in contact with heat. Sources of heat include sunlight, hot water, cooking utensils, and hot food and drink. The latter sometimes induce swelling of the lips and mouth. Patients have frequently presented following a hot bath or shower. Systemic symptoms of dizziness, faintness, headaches, nausea, and abdominal pain appear common, and collapse has occurred [64–67]. In the experimental situation, local heat at temperatures of between 39°C [66] and 56°C [65] have induced lesions, most being induced between 40 and 45°C. There are two types of reaction, an immediate reaction in which lesions occur within 15 minutes of the stimulus and in which they disappear within one hour, and a familial delayed-type reaction in which lesions occur after approximately 2 hours [74]. The pathogenesis of the disorder is unclear. Some workers have found a rise in plasma histamine levels during the reaction [66,68–70,72], other have found evidence of complement activation [67,71].

There is a partial response to H1 antihistamines and a reported response to combined H1 and H2 antihistamines [70]. Treatment using the induction of tolerance has been successful [73].

A summary of the diagnosis of the major physical urticarias induced by a rise in temperature is shown in Table 2.

## B. Cutaneous Wealing Reactions to Cold

The majority of patients with cold urticaria suffer from acquired idiopathic immediate cold contact urticaria. There are many rare types of cold urticaria. These include secondary cold urticaria, systemic types of cold urticaria, localized types of cold urticaria, and familial cold urticarias. The diagnosis of cold and other physical urticarias is shown in Table 3.

### 1. Acquired Idiopathic Immediate Cold Contact Urticaria

This is the most common form of cold urticaria, present in 96% of patients with this disease [75]. Clinically, exposure to cold produces itching and wealing on exposed sites. A combination of rain and wind is a potent provoking factor. Touching cold surfaces, washing up, using cold water, and removing food from a freezer may all provoke lesions. Swimming in a cold sea or outdoor pool almost invariably causes lesions and must be forbidden as histamine release causing systemic symptoms has been recorded as causing syncope and death by drowning [76]. The duration of cold exposure necessary to cause symptoms varies from less than one minute to 30 minutes. Lesions are normally present for up to 60 minutes and leave a normal-appearing skin [77]. Drinking cold liquids can cause edema of the oral mucosa and tongue in up to 25% of patients [78]. In sensitive patients, widespread exposure may be associated with systemic symptoms. Flushing, pal-

**Table 2**  Clinical Diagnosis of the Major Urticarias Induced by a Rise in Temperature

| Urticaria | Clinical | Lesion induction |
|---|---|---|
| Cholinergic urticaria | Itchy weals provoked by a hot room, exercise, hot bath, or short-lived emotion | 1. Jogging on the spot 2. Cycling on a stationery bicycle 3. Running on a treadmill 4. A hot bath at 40–41°C for 10–15 minutes (inspect up to 10 minutes later) |
| Exercise-induced anaphylaxis | Angioedema with associated systemic symptoms and signs | Exercise only Exercise challenge as for cholinergic urticaria |
| Angioedema provoked by food in combination with a rise in body temperature | Angioedema following a meal with a hot bath or exercise | Any food eaten followed by exercise challenge |
| Food, and drug-dependent exercise-induced anaphylaxis | Urticaria and angioedema which occurs if a specific food or drug is ingested and followed by exercise | The specific food or drug followed by exercise challenge; sometimes there is positive RAST testing to specific foods; skin testing may be positive |
| Localized heat urticaria | Itching wealing and swelling in areas in direct contact with heat | Lesion induction using a heat source, i.e., a beaker containing hot water kept at between 40° and 45°C |

pitations, headache, shortness of breath, wheezing, syncope, nausea, and abdominal pain may occur at some time in 50% of patients [75,78]. While cold urticaria may present at any age, presentation is most common during the second and third decades. This is a chronic disorder with a mean duration of 7.6 years [75]. There is a tendency to improvement over time.

While the disease is in an active phase, cold challenge can reproduce wealing in 90% of patients. The diagnosis may be confirmed by fixing an ice cube (at 1°C) to the flexor aspect of the forearm. If the ice cube is applied for 2 or 5 minutes, the positivity of the test if 30% and 51% respectively. If the ice cube is applied for 20 minutes, the positivity rate is 90% [70].

The diagnostic itching erythema and wealing occur generally while the skin is rewarming. This may occur up to 7 minutes after ice removal. If the history is atypical, the site should be inspected at 8 and 24 hours after ice removal to exclude a delayed form of cold contact urticaria [79]. Sometimes patients with other physical urticarias may develop wealing at the ice cube site from friction or pressure. Some may give a positive history with negative ice cube test. In both these groups of patients, testing may be performed by immersing the patient's hand and fingers in cold water kept at 10°C for 10 minutes. The reaction should be observed for 20 minutes after the hand is removed [75]. If a skin biopsy is performed, the changes detected on skin histopathology are slight. Direct immunofluorescence is negative. Electron microscopy shows mast cell degranulation, and exudate is seen between the keratinocytes, melanocytes, and collagen bundles [80].

The pathogenesis of the disease is unknown. However, in one series 50% of patients gave a positive family history [75]. The onset of cold urticaria following viral infections

**Table 3** Clinical Diagnosis of the Major Physical Urticarias Induced by Cold, Water, and Ultraviolet Light

| Urticaria | Clinical | Lesion induction |
|---|---|---|
| Acquired idipathic cold contact urticaria | Itching, redness, and wealing induced by cold air, rain, wind, and touching cold surfaces | 1. Ice cube at 1°C on the flexor forearm for 20 minutes (inspect 10 minutes after removal)<br>2. Immersion of hand, wrist, and part of forearm in cold water at 10°C for 10 minutes |
| Familial reflex delayed cold urticaria | Cold sensitivity noted in the neonatal period persisting throughout life | Induce systemic cooling by keeping in a cold room for 30 minutes or more; a neurtrophil leukocytosis during an attack is universal |
| Aquagenic urticaria | Itching and wealing on exposed areas after showering, bathing, or water-skiing | 1. A 10-minute shower<br>2. Place a wet gauze swab on the upper chest for 20 minutes |
| Solar urticarias | Itchy, burning, weals on exposed areas within minutes of ultraviolet radiation | Light testing using:<br>a) a slide projector<br>b) a UVB source<br>c) an AVA source<br>d) a visible light source<br>e) an argon pulsed dye laser |

streptococcal sore throats [75], infectious mononucleosis, and the possible higher incidence in HIV-positive patients suggests that a change in immune status may be responsible for the development of the disorder [81]. In the past, the disease has been transferred in humans [82], monkeys [83], and guinea pigs [84] using serum from affected individuals. The mast cell population density is similar to that found in normal skin [85]. Histamine is released during the reaction [45,86]. The precise significance of the reduction of the acute phase protein $\alpha_1$-antitrypsin is unknown [87].

Avoidance of cold stimuli as far as possible is the baseline treatment. Swimming in the cold sea or cold outdoor pools should be forbidden. There is usually an improvement if regular antihistamines are taken. The antihistamines of choice would be the newer minimally sedating antihistamines. In a severely affected, well-motivated patient, the induction of tolerance is a possibility [88].

## 2. Secondary Cold Urticaria

This is rare. Cryoglobulin was found in the serum of only 2 of 220 patients with cold urticaria [75] and 4 of 39 patients [89]. No cold hemolysins have been found in recent series.

## C. Rarer Cold Urticarias

### 1. Reflex Cold Urticaria (Systemic Cold Urticaria)

In this condition, generalized cooling of the body induces widespread wealing. If cooling is followed by sufficient exercise to raise the body temperature, wealing is reduced [90–92].

Patients usually recognize that their cold urticaria symptoms can be reproduced by exposure to cold air. The ice cube test is negative.

### 2. Cold-Induced Cholinergic Urticaria

In these patients, cooling of the body followed by exercise causes widespread wealing. The ice cube test is negative [93].

### 3. Delayed Cold Urticaria

Localized delayed responses to cold have been recorded. In affected patients erythema and induration may appear up to 24 hours after ice cube application and may persist for up to 48 hours [94].

### 4. Cold-Dependent Dermographism

Here, if the skin is cool a frictional stimulus will induce wealing as the skin temperature returns to normal [91].

## D. Localized Cold Urticarias

### 1. Localized Site-Specific Cold Urticaria

A wealing reaction to the application of cold to the skin has occurred, which is confined to areas where hyposensitization injections have been given [95].

### 2. Localized Cold Reflex Urticaria

Here weals do not develop at the precise site of cold stimulation, but in the surrounding area [96].

## E. Familial Cold Urticarias

### 1. Reflex Form (Systemic Form Familial Delayed Form)

Systemic cooling may induce generalized wealing in certain families. This disorder is dominantly inherited. Cold sensitivity is noted in the neonatal period and persists throughout life. The reaction begins at 30 minutes after exposure and may persist for up to 48 hours. Fever, headache, and arthralgia may occur. Leukocytosis constantly accompanies the symptoms and signs [97–99].

### 2. Localized Cold Urticaria (Familial)

A localized form of dominantly inherited disorder also occurs. Here cold challenge does not provoke any immediate symptoms or signs. Lesions develop hours after local cold challenge [100].

## III. CUTANEOUS WEALING REACTIONS TO WATER

Direct contact with water provokes urticaria in some people. Tap water, sea water, or water in rain, sweat, or tears may be the provoking stimulus. Aquagenic urticaria is rare. Presentation normally occurs after the occurrence of repeated attacks of wealing in exposed areas following activities such as water skiing, showering, or bathing. The original report suggested that the upper trunk and arms are the sites of predilection and that the lesions are follicular [101]. However, a longer exposure to water may induce weals on any area of the body, and weals of all sizes may occur [102]. Pruritus is usually intense.

Lesions occur within minutes of the stimulus and may be present for up to one hour. systemic symptoms do not occur, but drinking and tooth brushing are reported to cause shortness of breath or dysphagia on occasion.

The diagnosis is confirmed by giving the patient a 10-minute shower or by placing wet gauze swabs on the chest for 20 minutes. The condition may present at any age and may persist for up to two decades [104]. It has occurred in families, with father-son and aunt-niece being affected [105]. No associated underlying medical disorders have been described.

The pathogenesis and mechanism of the reaction are unknown, but histamine is considered important in the reaction. The generally satisfactory response to antihistamines supports this assertion. However, the therapeutic response to antihistamines may be one in which the wealing threshold is raised rather than one in which complete abolition of symptoms is achieved. It is common to suggest antihistamine treatment 1–2 hours before a bath or shower. If antihistamine treatment is ineffective, stanazolol has been found to be useful [102].

## IV.  SOLAR URTICARIA

Solar urticaria is an extremely rare physical urticaria provoked by light. The symptoms and signs develop within minutes of exposure to sun. All lesions occur within 30 minutes, and while most disappear within hours, all resolve within 24 hours. All patients experience itch, and some complain of a burning sensation. Occasionally pain occurs. Lesions appear in areas exposed to sunlight, the V of the neck and the arms being the most common sites. Other light-exposed areas as well as areas covered with clothing that permits light to penetrate to the skin may be affected. Lesions consist of an itchy erythema, urticarial weals, or a mixture of both morphological types [106,107]. Generally there is no spontaneous improvement or development of natural tolerance over a summer. If there is sufficient exposure to light, systemic symptoms including syncope may occur. The diagnosis can usually be confirmed by light testing. Testing is carried out to measure reactions to UVB, UVA, and visible light. Light testing is also frequently performed using a slide projector [107]. For those whose tests are negative and whose reaction is caused by long wavelengths, an argon-pulsed dye laser can be used at wavelengths of 610, 650, and 690 nm [108].

The differential diagnosis includes polymorphic light eruption, lupus erythematosis, and, in those who have suffered from a very young age, erythropoietic protoporphyria. The pathogenesis of the disorder is unknown. Treatment with sunscreens is not usuallly very helpful, even in those sensitive to UVB or shorter UVA wavelenghts. Antimalarial drugs, oral beta-carotene, and oral steroids have been used but are not particularly effective.

The newer minimally sedating antihistamines are the treatment of first choice and may reduce itching and wealing. In those whose response to antihistamines is unsatisfactory, phototherapy with narrow-band UVB, broad-band UVB, UVA, or a combination of UVB and UVA or visible light may be effective. The tolerance obtained with these treatments lasts only a few days; a longer-lasting tolerance for many weeks may be obtained using photochemotherapy. This treatment produces an increase in the minimal urticarial dose [107]. In specialized centers and with severely affected patients, plasmapheresis has been used [109,110].

## V.  CLUSTERING OF PHYSICAL URTICARIAS

Considering that many of the physical urticarias are uncommon, it is of interest that two or more are often present in a single individual. This phenomenon is termed "clustering." Exercise-induced anaphylaxis, delayed-pressure urticaria, cholinergic urticaria, and dermographism have all been documented in the same patient [111]. Other examples of mixed physical urticarias in the same individual include cold urticaria and delayed-pressure urticaria (in association with chronic urticaria) [112] and delayed-pressure urticaria occurring in a patient with vibratory angioedema [31]. Cold urticaria frequently occurs in association with other physical urticarias. The combination of both cold urticaria and cholinergic urticaria is well known. The first report of a patient with both cold and cholinergic urticaria, one who developed wealing after exposure to "cold, exercise and warming the body," was published in 1936 [35]. In the large series of 220 patients with cold urticaria described by Neittaanmaki, 17 had cholinergic urticaria [75]. In 1988 Ormerod et al. reported a series of 13 patients, all of whom suffered from both cold and cholinergic urticaria. Two of these patients also had symptomatic dermographism [113]. Localized heat urticaria and cold urticaria can coexist [114].

The presence of delayed pressure urticaria is frequently linked with that of delayed dermographism. This combination was first reported in 1950 [10] In the largest series of delayed pressure urticaria patients reported to date, 55% have delayed dermographism [9]. It is not yet clear whether delayed dermographism exists as an independent condition in association with delayed-pressure urticaria or whether it is a manifestation of it.

Many of these combinations may occur by chance, but this clustering encourages consideration of the hypothesis that certain people are predisposed to developing physical urticarias.

## VI.  CONCLUSION

The physical urticarias are a heterogeneous group of disorders. Delayed-pressure urticaria is different from the others in terms of clinical expression, histopathology, and response to treatment.

While histamine is released, it is of major importance only in those in which there is a therapeutic response to antihistamines. The pathogenesis and mechanism of the reaction in many of these disorders is unclear, and other mediators and mechanisms may be involved.

The diagnosis of the physical urticarias is clinical. Therefore careful clinical characterization of each different type of physical urticaria is necessary. It is important that "clustering" or the coexistence of more than one type of physical urticaria in the same patient is recognized.

In the past treatment of these disorders has been empirical. Therapeutic progress now depends on the accurate diagnosis and quantitative production of lesions using reproducible challenge techniques.

## REFERENCES

1. Champion RH. Urticaria: then and now. Br J Dermatol 1988; 119:427–436.
2. Lewis T. Vascular reactions to the skin to injury. I. Reaction to stroking: urticaria factition. Heart 1924; 11:119.
3. Warin RP, Champion RH, Rook A. Urticaria. Philadephia: WB Saunders Co, 1974.
4. Illig L, Kunick J. Klinik und Diagnostik der physikalischen Urticaria. Der Hautarzt 1969; 20(4):167.
5. Breathnach SM, Allen R, Milford Ward, Greaves MW. Symptomatic dermographism., clinical features laboratory investigations and responses to therapy. Clin Exp Dermatol 1953; 8: 463.
6. James MP, Eady RAJ, Kobza Black A, Hawk JLM, Greaves MW. Physical urticaria, a microscopical and pharmacological study of mast cell involvement. J Invest Dermatol 1980; 74: 451.
7. Greaves MW, Sondergaard J. Urticaria pigmentosa and factitious urticaria—direct evidence for release of histamine and other smooth muscle-contracting agents in dermographic skin. Arch Dermatol 1990; 101:418–425.
8. Lawlor F, Kobza Black A, Murdoch RD, Greaves MW. Symptomatic dermographism, wealing, mast cells and histamine are decreased in the skin following long term application of a potent topical corticosteroid. Br J Dermatol 1989; 121:629–634.
9. Dover JS, Kobza Black A, Milford Ward A, Greaves MW. Delayed pressure urticaria. J Am Acad Dermatol 1988; 18(6):1289
10. Kalz F, Bower CM, Prichard H. Delayed and persistent dermographia. Arch Derm Syph 1950; 61:772.
11. Baughman RD, Jillson OF. Seven specific types of urticaria. Ann Allergy 1963; 21:248.
12. Engelhardt AW. Zur Kenntnis der mechanischen Späturticaria. Derm Wechr 1961; 144:1084.
13. Czarnetzski BM. Urticaria. Berlin: Springer Verlag, 1986.
14. James MP, Warin RP. Factitious wealing at the site of previous cutaneous response. Br J Dermatol 1969; 81:882.
15. Mayou SC, Kobza Black A, Eady RAJ, Greaves MW. Cholinergic dermographism. Br J Dermatol 1986; 115:371.
16. Smith JA, Mansfield LE, Fokakis A, Nelson HS. Dermographia caused by IgE mediated penicillin allergy. Ann Allergy 1983; 51:30.
17. Lindae ML, Chung Hong H, Nickoloff B. Arch Derm 1987; 123.
18. Warin RP. Factitious urticaria. Red dermographism. Br J Dermatol 1981; 104:285–288.
19. Lawlor F, Kobza Black A, Greaves MW. Immediate pressure urticaria—a distinct disorder. Clin Exp Dermatol 1991; 16:155–157.
20. Parilo JE, Lawley TJ, Frank MM, Kaplan AP, Fauci AS. Immunologic reactivity in the hypereosinophilic syndrome. J Clin Immunol 1979; 64:3–12.
21. Sussman GL, Harvey RP, Schocker AL. Delayed pressure urticaria. J All Clin Immunol 1982; 70:5,337.
22. Warin RP. Clinical observations on delayed pressure urticaria. Br J Dermatol 1989; 121: 225.
23. Lawlor F, Kobza Black A, Milford Ward A, Morris A, Greaves MW. Delayed pressure urticaria, objective evaluation of a variable disease, using a dermographometer and assessment of treatment using colchicine. Br J Dermatol 1989; 120:403–408.

24. Barlow RJ, Warburton F, Watson K, Kobza Black A, Greaves MW. The diagnosis and incidence of delayed pressure urticaria in patients with chronic urticaria. J Am Acad Dermatol 1993; 29(6):954–958.

25. Ryan RJ, Shim-Young N, Turk JL. Delayed pressure urticaria. Br J Dermatol 1968; 80:485.

26. Czarnetzski BM, Meentken J. Rosenbach R, Poktopp A. Clinical, pharmacological and immunological aspects of delayed pressure urticaria. Br J Dermatol 1984; 111:315.

27. Doeglas HMG, Bleumink E. Plasma protease inhibitors in chronic urticaria. In Champion RH, Greaves MW, Kobza Black A, Pye RJ, eds. The Urticarias. London: Churchill Livingstone, 1985, pp. 59–69.

28. Estes SA, Yung CW. Delayed pressure urticaria, an investigation of some parameters of lesion indication. J Am Acad Dermatol 1981; 5:25.

29. Lawlor F. Arachidonic acid transformation is not stimulated in delayed pressure urticaria. Br J Dermatol 1989; 121(3):317–321.

30. Patterson R, Mellies CJ, BlanKenship ML, Pruzanski JJ. Vibratory angioedema, a hereditary type of physical hypersensitivity. J Allergy Clin Immunol 1972; 50:184.

31. Lawlor F, Kobza Black A, Melford West A, Morris A, Greaves MW. Vibratory angioedema: lesion induction, clinical features, laboratory and ultra structural findings. Br J Dermatol 1989; 120:403–408.

32. Epstein P, Kidd KK. Dermodistortive urticaria. An autosomal dominant dermatologic disorder. Am J Med Genet 1981; 9:307.

33. Ting S, Reiman BEF, Rer Nat, Rauls DU, Mansfield LE. Nonfamilial vibration induced angioedema. J Allergy Clin, Immunol 1983; 71(6):546.

34. Wener WH, Metzger WJ, Simon RA. Occupationally acquired vibratory angioedema, with secondary carpel tunnel syndrome. Ann Int Med 1983; 94:44.

35. Grant RT, Pearson RSB, Comeau WJ. Observations in urticaria provoked by emotion by exercise and by warming the body. Clin Sci 1936; 2:254–271.

36. Illig L, Heinike A. Zur pathogenesis der cholinergischen urticaria. Arch Klin Exp Dermatol 229:285.

37. Lawrence CM, Jorizzo JL, Kobza Black A, Coutts A, Greaves MW. Cholinergic urticaria with associated angio-oedema. Br J Dermatol 1981; 105:543–549.

38. Hirschmann JV, Lawlor F, English JSC, Loubeck JB, Winkelmann RK, Greaves MW. Cholinergic urticaria. A clinical and histologic study. Arch Derm 1989; 123:462–467.

39. Kaplan AP, Natbony SF, Tawil AP. Fructer L, Foster M. Exercise induced anaphylaxis as a manifestation of cholinergic urticaria. J Allergy Clin Immunol 1981; 68(4):319–324.

40. Soter NA, Wassermann SI, Austen KF, Regis McFadden E. Release of mast cell mediators and alterations in lung function in patients with cholinergic urticaria. N Engl J Med 1980; 302(1):604–608.

41. Herxheimer A. The nervous pathway mediating cholinergic urticaria. Clin Sci. 1956; 15:195–205.

42. Morgan JK. Observations on cholinergic urticaria. J Invest Dermatol 1953; 21:173–182.

43. Kay DM, Maibach HI. Pruritus and acquired anhydrosis: two unusual cases. Arch Dermatol 1969; 100:291.

44. Adachi J, Aoki T, Yamatodani A. Demonstration of sweat allergy in cholinergic urticaria. J Dermatol Surg 1994; 7:142–149.

45. Kaplan AP, Beavan MA. In vivo studies of the pathogenesis of cold urticaria, cholinergic urticaria on vibration induced swelling. J Invest Dermatol 1976; 67:327.

46. Soter NA, Wassermann SI. Physical urticaria/angioedema. An experimental model of mast cell activation in humans. J Allergy Clin Immunol 1980; 66:358.

47. Commens CA, Greaves MW. Tests to establish the diagnosis in cholinergic urticaria. Br J Dermatol 1978; 98:47–51.

48. Wong E, Eftekhari N, Greaves MW, Milford Ward A. Beneficial effects of danazol on symptoms and laboratory changes in cholinergic urticaria. Br J Dermatol 1987; 116:553.

49. Nomland R. Cholinergic urticaria and cholinergic itching. Arch Derm Syph 1944; 50:247–256.

50. Berth Jones J, Graham-Brown RAC. Cholinergic pruritus, erythema and urticaria: a disease spectrum responding to danazol. Br J Dermatol 1989; 121:235–235.

51. Murphy GM, Kobza Black A, Graves MW. Persisting cholinergic erythema: a variant of cholinergic urticaria. Br J Dermatol 1983; 109:343–348.

52. Kleinhaus D, Brandle I. Sog persistier Endes cholinergisches Erythem. Akt Dermatol 1986; 12:5–7.

53. Onn A, Levo Y, Kivity S. Familial cholinergic urticaria. J Allergy Clin Immunol 1996; 98:847–849.

54. Casale TB, Keahey TM, Kaliner M. Exercise induced anaphylactic syndromes JAMA 1986; 225(15):2049–2053.

55. Longley S, Panush RS. Familial exercise-induced anaphylaxis. J All Clin Immunol 1987; 58:257–259.

56. Volcheck GW, Li James TC. Exercise-induced urticaria and anaphylaxis. Mayo Clin Proc 1997; 72:140–147.

57. Zuberbier T, Bohm M, Czarnetzki BM. Food intake in combination with a rise in body temperature: a newly identified cause of angioedema. J All Clin Immunol 1993; 91:1226–1227.

58. Kidd JN, Cohen SH, sosman AJ, fink JN. Food dependent exercise-induced anaphylaxis. J Allergy Clin Immunol 1983; 71(4):407–411.

59. Kivity S, Sneh E, Creif J, Topilsky M, Mekori YA. Compound 48/80 in patients with food-associated exercise-induced urticaria-angioedema. J All Clin Immunol 1988; 81(6):1155–1158.

60. Varjonen E, Vainio E, Kalimo K. Life-threatening recurrent anaphylaxis caused by allergy to gliaden and exercise. Clin Exp Allergy 1997; 27:162–166.

61. Shaeffer Al, Austen KF. Exercise induced anaphylaxis. J Allergy Clin Immunol 1980; 66(2):106–111.

62. Gerth van Wijk R, de Groot H, Bougaard JM. Drug dependent exercise induced anaphylaxis. Allergy 1995; 50:992–994.

63. Shelley WB, Shelley ED. Lancet 1985; 1031–1032.

64. Greaves MW, Sneddon IB, Smith AK, Stanworth DR. Heat urticaria. Br J Dermatol 1974; 90:259.

65. Weiss NS, Dodell P, Brown HF. Thermal urticaria: an unusual case. Ann Allergy 1976; 37(1):55–57.

66. Atkins PC, Zweimen B. Mediator release in local heat urticaria. J Allergy Clin Immunol 1981; 68(4):286–289.

67. Daman L, Lieberman P, Gauier M, Hashimoto K. Localised heat urticaria. J Allergy Clin Immunol 1978; 61(4):273–278.

68. Higgins EM, Fiedmann PS. Clinical report and investigation of a patient with localised heat urticaria. Acta DV 1991; 71:434–436.

69. Babu T, Nomura K, Hanada K, Hashimoto I. Immediate-type heat urticaria, repeat of a case and study of plasma histamine release, Br J Dermatol 1998; 138:326–328.

70. Irwin RB, Liebermann P, Friedman MM, Kaliner M, Kaplan R, Bale G, Treadwell G, Yoo TJ. Mediator release in local heat urticaria. Protection with combined H1 and H2 antagonists. J Allergy Clin Immunol 1985; 76.

71. Johansson E, Reunala T, Kostimies S, Lagerstedt A, Kauppinenk K, Timonen K. Localised heat urticaria associated with a decrease in serum complement factor $B(C_3$ proactivator). Br J Dermatol 1984; 110:227–231.

72. Andrew Grant J, Findlay SR, Thueson DO, Fine DP, Kruger GG. Local heat urticaria/angioedema: evidence for histamine release without complement activations. J Allergy Clin Immunol 1981; 67(1):75–77.

73. Leigh IM, Ramsey CA. Localised heat urticaria treated by inducing tolerance to heat. Br J Dermatol 1975; 92:191–194.

74. Michaelsson G, Ros AM. Familial localised heat urticaria of delayed type. Acta Dermatovener 1971; 51:279–283.

75. Neittaanmaki HJ. Cold urticaria. Clinical findings in 220 patients. Am Acad Dermatol 1985; 13:636.

76. Horton BT, Brown GE, Roth GM. Hypersensitiveness to cold with local and systemic manifestations of a histamine-like character, its amenability to treatment: J Am Med Assoc 1936; 107:2663.

77. Kobza Black A. Cold urticaria. Semin Dermatol 1987; 6(4):292.

78. Kobza Black A. A clinical and investigational review of patients with acquired cold urticaria. Br J Dermatol 1980; 114:311.

79. Kobza Black A. Cold urticaria. In Champion RH, Greaves MW, Kobza Black A, Pye RJ, eds. The Urticarias. Edinburgh: Churchill Livingstone, 1985:168.

80. Lawlor F, Kobza Black A, Breathnach AS, McKee P, Sarachandra P, Bhogal B, Isaacs J, Winkelmann RK, Greaves MW. A timed study of the histology, direct immunofluorescence and ultrastructural findings in idiopathic cold contact urticaria, over a 24 hour period. Clin Exp Dermatol 1989; 14:416.

81. Lin RY, Schwartz RA. Cold urticaria and HIV infection. Br J Dermatol 1993; 129:465–467.

82. Houser DD, Arbesman CE, Kohi I, Wicher K. Cold urticaria (immunologic studies). Am J Med 1970; 49:20.

83. Misch K, Kobza Black A, Greaves MW, Almosdoi T, Stanworth DR. Passive transfer of idiopathic cold urticaria to monkeys. Acta Dermatovener 1983; 63:163.

84. Kalayama I, Doi T, Nishioka K. Possibility of passive transfer of cold urticaria to guinea pigs. J Dermatol 1984; 11:259.

85. Pastricha JS, Roy S, Khandhari KC. Study of cutaneous mast cells in patients of physical urticarias. Indian J Med Res 1974; 62(11):1967.

86. Soter NA, Wasserman SI, Austen KE. Cold urticaria. Release into the circulation of histamine and eosinophil chemotactic factor of anaphylaxis during cold challenge. N Engl J Med 1971; 294(13):687.

87. Doeglas HMG, Bleumink E. Protease inhibitors in patients with chronic urticaria. Arch Dermatol 1975; 111:979.

88. Bentley-Phillips CB, Kobza Black A, Greaves MW. Induced tolerance in cold urticaria caused by cold evoked histamine release. Lancet 1976; 2:63–66.

89. Doeglas HMG, Rijnten WJ, Schroder F, Schirm J. Cold urticaria and virus infections. A clinical and serological study in 39 patients. Br J Dermatol 1986; 114:311.

90. Illig L, Paul E, Bruek K, Schwennicke HP. Experimental investigations on the trigger mechanism of the generalised type of heat and cold urticaria by means of a climatic chamber. Acta Dermatovener 1986; 60:373.

91. Kaplan AP. Unusual cold induced disorders: cold dependent dermographism and cold urticaria. J Allergy Clin Immunol 1984; 73:453–456.

92. Kivity S, Schwartz Y, Wolf R, Topilsky M. Systemic cold induced urticaria. Clinical and laboratory characterisation. J All Clin Immunol 1998; 85:53–54.

93. Kaplan AP, Garofolo J. Identification of a new physically induced urticaria-cold induced cholinergic urticaria. J Allergy Clin Immunol 1981; 68:438.

94. Sarkany I, Turk JL. Delayed hypersensitivity to cold. Proc Roy Soc Med 1965; 58:622.

95. Solomon LM, Strauss H, Leznoff A. Localised secondary cold urticaria. Arch Dermatol 1966; 94:156.

96. Czarnetzki BM, Frosch PJ, Strekler R. Localised cold reflex urticaria. Br J Dermatol 1981; 104:83.

97. Doeglas HM, Bleumink E. Familial cold urticaria. Arch Dermatol 1974; 110:382–358.

98. Tindell JP, Becker SK, Rosse WF. Familial cold urticaria. Arch Int Med 1969; 124:129.

99. Vlagopoulos T, Townley R, Villacombe G. Familial cold urticaria. Ann Allergy 1975; 34: 366.

100. Soter NA, Joshi NP, Twaroq FJ, Zeiger RS, Rothman PM, Colten HR. Delayed cold-induced urticaria. A dominantly inherited disorder: J Allergy Clin Immunol 1977; 59:294.

101. Shelley WB, Rawnsley HM. Aquagenic urticaria. Contact sensitivity reaction to water. J Am Med Assoc 1964; 89(12):895.

102. Fearfield LA, Gazzard B, Bunker CB. Aquagenic urticaria and human immunodeficiency virus infection: treatment with stanozolol. Br J Dermatol 1997; 137:620.

103. Gimoner-Arnau A, Sera-Baldrich E, Camarasa JG. Chronic aquagenic urticaria. Acta Dermatovener 1992; 72:389.

104. Czarnetzki BM. In Urticaria. Berlin: Springer-Verlag, 1986.

105. Bonnet-Blanc JM, Andrieu-Pfaul F, Merand JP, Roux J. Familial aquagenic urticaria. Dermatologica 1979; 158:468.

106. Torinuki W. Two patients with solar urticaria manifesting pruritic urticaria. J Dermatol 1992; 9:635–637.

107. Rychaert S, Roelandts R. Solar urticaria: A report of 25 cases and difficulties in phototesting. Arch Dermatol 1988; 134:71–74.

108. Alora MBT, Taylor CR. Solar urticaria: case report and phototesting with lasers. J Am Acad Dermatol 1998; 38(2):341–343.

109. Duschet P, Leyen P, Schwarz T, Höcker P, Greiter J, Gschnait F. Solar urticaria—effective treatment by plasmapheresis. Clin Exp Dermatol 1987; 12:185–188.

110. Hudson-Peacock MJ, Farr PM, Diffey BL, Goodship THJ. Combined treatment of solar urticaria with plasmapheresis and PUVA. Br J Dermatol 1993; 128:440–442.

111. Sonin L, Grammer LC, Patterson R. The occurrence of multiple physical allergies in the same patient: report of three cases. J Allergy Clin Immunol 1988; 75:705.

112. Lawlor F, Kobza Black A, Greaves MW. Delayed pressure urticaria, cold urticaria, chronic urticaria. Br J Dermatol 1988; 33:91.

113. Ormerod AD, Kobza Black A, Milford Ward A, Greaves MW. Combined cold urticaria and cholinergic urticaria—clinical characterisation and laboratory findings. Br J Dermatol 1988; 118:621.

114. Neittaanmaki H, Fraki JL. Combination of localised heat urticaria and cold urticaria. Release of histamine in suction blisters and successful treatment of heat urticaria with doxepin Clin Exp Dermatol 1988; 13:87.

# 10
# Immunology of Allergic Contact Dermatitis

**John McFadden**
*St. Thomas' Hospital, London, England*

## I. IMMUNOLOGICAL MECHANISMS

The process of allergic contact dermatitis depends upon four major processes: (1) penetration of contact allergen into skin, (2) haptenization or binding of a small protein in order to become allergenic, (3) the process of sensitization, whereby an immune response to the contact allergen builds to such an extent that an elicitation reaction can occur, and (4) elicitation reaction to a contact allergen.

### A. Clinical Features

In the acute stage one sees vesicles or small blisters, intense edema, and inflammation; in the chronic stages one sees fissuring, scaling, and lichenification or thickening of the epidermis; this is presumably secondary to the scratching, Any area of the skin that comes into contact with the offending allergen may become invoved; compared to the nonimmunological irritant dermatatitis, there may be spread from the primary sites; transfer by hand can occur. Secondary infection may produce crusting and oozing, as with other forms of eczema. Clinical features can give clues to the nature of the offending allergen (see below).

### B. Histological Features

Histological features of allergic contact dermatitis vary according to severity and acuteness of eruption. Perivascular lymphocytes and monocytes are seen within 6 hours of exposure to the allergen. The infiltration may be accompanies by considerable edema of the epidermis; subsequently edema develops in the epidermis with subsequent spongiosis. During these later stages (48–72 hours after onset) basophils may constitute 5–15% of the cells; eosinophils may also be present but to a lesser extent.

### C. Haptens

Haptens are classically of low molecular weight and lipid soluble so that they are able to penetrate through the skin barrier. They bind to proteins to form allergenic conjugates.

In the case of nickel they tend to bind to the peptide occupying the antigenic groove, making them allergenic [1], whereas some other allergens may bind onto larger proteins. Potential allergenicity of contact allergens may depend to some extent on their ability to bind to amino acid peptides, and computer models have been devised to predict potential allergenicity (OSAR) [2]. Consideration of the chemical processes of a wide variety of known sensitizers concludes that in most cases the binding of the sensitizer to protein acting as a nucleophile and the sensitizer acting as an electrophile [3]. Catechol derivatives such as poison ivy are readily oxidized to orthoquinones, which are highly electrophilic; hydroquinones can sensitize via an analogous mechanism being oxidized to orthoquinones; oxidation of a primary or secondary alcohol group can produce an ultimate sensitizer if the resulting aldehyde or ketone group is electrophilic enough to form a Schiff's base–like conjugate with proteins; in the case of nickel salts they are known to form square planar complexes with histidine.

In the classical case of antigen recognition, the hapten is presented on an antigenic peptide and is involved in T-cell selection; in some cases the cross-reactivity seen conforms with structural similarities such as with steroids [4]. Cells cloned to nickel will not react with cobalt—this proves ground for the presumption that double sensitization as seen with cobalt and nickel involves concomitant sensitizers rather than cross-reactors; as with the triadcortyl components neomycin, ethylenediamine, nystatin, and adcortyl; however, molecular mimicry can occur, as has been reported with nickel and palladium.

## D. Langerhans Cells

Langerhans cells are bone marrow derived but reside in the epidermis. Langerhans cells are the antigen-presenting cells of the epidermis; they carry contact allergens to the local lymph node, where sensitization occurs; migration appears to be under cytokine control, including TNF-$\alpha$ and IL-1 [5]. When the adhesion molecule cadherin-1 is lost, then the Langerhans cell may migrate to the local lymph node; whether this is an active or passive migration is a subject of speculation. Birbeck granules may be involved in this process [6] Langerhans cells possess class II molecule. After hapten application to the skin there is enhanced expression of class II molecules as well as increased T-cell stimulatory capacity by Langerhans cells [7]. Interleukin-1$\beta$ from Langerhans cells and IL-10 from keratinocytes are released in response to hapten application on the skin [8].

Macatonia et al. [9] demonstrated that an increased number of dendritic cells appeared in regional lymph nodes 24 hours after application, implying that Langerhans cells migrate from the skin to regional lymph nodes. In guinea pigs removal of the draining lymph node up to 5 days after application of the allergen will prevent sensitization [10].

## E. Sensitization

Potential allergens have to stay in the skin for several hours in order to drive sensitization. It has been shown in guinea pigs that if the skin is excised within 8 hour of application sensitization does not occur (Fig. 1).

In the paracortical areas of the lymph node, conditions are ideal for the Langerhans cell to present antigen to T cells; in the nonsensitized subject very few T cells will recognize the antigen, but the dendritic morphology of the Langerhans cell allows it to interact with many T cells. T cells proliferate, secreting the autocrine interleukin-2 and forming

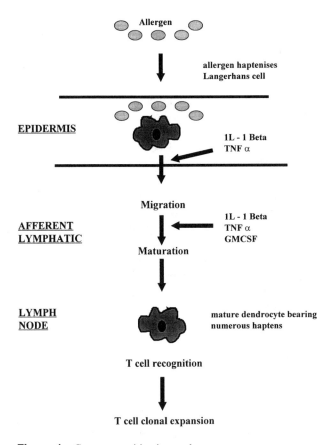

**Figure 1**   Contact sensitization pathway.

many blast cells. The expanded T-cell clone now disseminate, throughout the body and is in the general circulation.

When sensitization has occurred experimentally in animals there is often a flare at the site of application on the skin. Sensitization from a single dose can take 7–20 days to occur, but after that elicitation can occur after 24–96 hours. Important variables in the onset of sensitization include (1) increasing the concentration of the allergen, (2) increasing the number of exposures, and (3) concomitant allergen exposure resulting in allergic contact dermatitis.

## F.   Allergic Contact Dermatitis

For elicitation to occur the size of the T-cell clone should be able to initiate an inflammatory reaction at the primary site of allergen application; in nonsensitized individuals, not enough T cells locally react with the antigen in order to produce inflammation. T cells travel throughout the body continuously, whereby the lymphocytes move through the curculation; when T cells move into the skin, the CLA ligand on the T cell binds to E selectin on the postcapillary venule; only a minority of circulating T cells are CLA+, and therefore there is a pool of T-cell skin-homing lymphocytes [11]. In nickel-sensitive subjects the circulating memory–responsive T cells were almost exclusively CLA or skin-homing, suggesting a mechanism of sorting particular T cells specific into homing receptor-defined subsets [12].

The nature of the T cells that mediate contact sensitivity has gradually become more evident. It was shown that T cells can transfer allergic contact dematitis [13] and that these cells were primarily T-helper cells [14]. Although cytotoxic T cells can mediate distinct skin damage in ACD, the helper subset is held to be primarily responsible for mediating delayed hypersensitivity in ACD. The major subset of effector T cells are (CD45RO) [15].

After hapten painting distinct helper T cells are generated. Helper T cells have been shown to passively transfer allergic contact dermatitis, and most recently it was shown that a distinct subset, Th1, produces IL-2 and IFN-$\gamma$ [16]. Specific supressor cells are generated after sensitization with haptens [17]. Tolerance is at least in part due to T-specific supressor cells [18]. Several studies show an admixture of helper and supressor-cytotoxic cells, with helper cells predominating [19]. Only a small percentage of the T cells infiltrating a cutaneous DTH response have specificity for the antigen; the majority of cells are nonspecifically recruited [20]. Keratinocytes may participate in the inflammation by producing TNF and IL-1 by induction of ICAM I Langerhans cell migration and lymphocyte chemotaxis. Class II expression in keratinocytes may induce a degree of supression of allergic contact dermatitis [21] or at least a means of controlling the contact dermatitis reaction.

Presentation of allergen by class II molecules does not provide sufficient binding strength. Additional sets of adhesion molecules are necessary for full binding and activation of T cells. The CD4 molecule has affinity for a constant region of the class II molecule; also, LFA-1 is abundantly present on T cells, and one of its counterstructures (ICAM-1) is present on Langerhans cells; the T-cell molecule CD2 also binds to the LFA3 anchored in the membrane of most nucleated cells. The CD28/B7 is also an important adhesion molecule for full T-cell–antigen presenting cell interaction.

## II. PATCH TESTING

Patch testing was first performed by Jadassohn in 1896 with mercuric chloride, but it was only used as a clinical tool several decades later. Patch testing is the only current means of identifying allergic contact dermatitis in clinical practice and is an underused procedure.

All subjects should be patch tested using (1) the European standard battery, (2) any relevant additional battery (e.g., dental, hairdressers), and (3) the subject's own samples. These may need to be diluted. Generally substances applied to the skin, such as moisturizing cream, can be applied undiluted. Substances that are washed off, such as shampoos, need to be diluted, (e.g., 2%).

Other substances that need to be diluted include coolant oils (5–10%).

Allergens are usually sequenced so that those frequently causing strong, cross-, or concomitant reactions are spaced apart. Allergens in petroleum should be applied across the diameter of the chamber. Liquid preparations are applied to a filter disc that fits into the aluminum chamber.

The usual patch tests used are Finn chambers (8 mm aluminium discs) and scanpore (a relatively nonallergic tape). Finn chambers are supplied in strips of 10 chambers on tape—two parallel rows of five chambers. Patches should be applied to the upper back. The outline of the patches are marked with a skin pen.

Patients should not be tested if on prednisolone ($\geq$20 mg/day) or if their eczema is very active, as this increases the risk of false-negative or false-positive reactions. Patches should be taken off and read at either 2 or 3 days. There should also be a second reading between 4 and 7 days. The authors usually read patches at 2 and 4 days. When taken off the back the patches should be left for at least 10 minutes to allow any tape reaction to settle and to let any reaction become clearly visible.

The following scoring system should be used (recommended by the International Contact Dermatitis Research Group):

| | |
|---|---|
| + | Doubtful reaction; faint erythema only |
| + | Weak positive reaction; erythema, infiltration, possibly papules |
| ++ | Strong positive reaction; erythema, infiltration, papules, vesicles |
| +++ | Extreme positive reaction; intense erythema and infiltration and coalescing vesicles |
| IR | Irritant reaction of different types |
| NT | Not tested |

An allergic reaction can often give a gradually increasing reaction when read at 2 and 4 days. False reactions can occur so the patches should be read with care. Causes of false-positive reactions include too high a concentration for that patient; impure or contaminated substance; the vehicle is an irritant (especially solvents); excess test preparation applied (unlikely); the test substance is unevenly applied; recent dermatitis at site; current dermatitis at distant skin sites; pressure effects; mechanical irritation of solid test material or adhesive tape reaction or an allergic reaction to the aluminum (extremely rare!). It may be an artefact; the nurses may have wrongly numbered the site! Or, alternatively, the doctors have misread the site number!

False-negative reactions can also occur, the causes of which are insufficient penetration of allergen, too low a test concentration for that particular patient, the test substance is not released from the vehicle or retained by the filter paper, there is insufficient amount of test preparation applied or insufficient occlusion; the duration of contact too brief (the test strip has fallen off!); the test was not applied to the upper back; the reading is made too early (e.g., corticosteroid allergic reaction); the test site has been treated with steroids or UV irradiation; systemic treatment with steroids ($\geq$20 mg/day). Cyclosporine does not seem to have an effect. Antihistamines are thought to not have an effect, although one study did show a reduction in patch test reactivity.

Complications of patch testing can occur but are rare. They include:

1. Patch test sensitization
2. Irritant reactions from nonstandard allergens or substances bought up by the patient
3. Flare of previous dermatitis
4. Depigmentation
5. Pigmentation, sometimes after sunlight exposure of test sites; postinflammatory pigment change, especially in dark-skinned patients

6.  Scars, keloids
7.  Anaphylactic reactions or shock
8.  Infection

Other tests are sometimes used in addition to patch testing. Some of there are:

1.  Open Test (Use Test): usually means that a product, as is, is dropped onto the skin and allowed to spread freely. No occlusion is applied. Usual site is volar forearm. Used when substance is poorly defined.
2.  Use Test (Provocation Test): intended to evaluate the clinical significance of ingredient(s) of a formulated product previously found reactive by ordinary patch testing.
3.  Repeated Open Application Test (ROAT): uses arm or scapular area of back. The area used is either 5 × 5 cm (1 ml substance) or 10 × 10 cm (1 ml substance). Substance is applied twice daily for 7 days. A positive response appears within 2–4 days.

It is recommended to obtain protocols of chemical analysis and data on purity of samples. (Word of warning—totoally unknown substances should not be applied to skin.) Most allergens are tested in the concentration range 0.01–10%. If in doubt one should start testing at lower concentrations and increase (by a factor of 10).

## III.  STANDARD ALLERGENS

Patients subjected to patch testing in the United Kingdom are usually subjected to the European standard series, a commercially available series of allergens designed to screen for the most common contact sensitizers. Patients may also be subjected to a specialized series (e.g., a hairdressers or medicament series) and may be tested using substances they themselves bring along. Their individual items may need to be diluted (e.g., shampoos) or can be applied "as is" (e.g., moisturiser, most perfumes). Obviously some substances they bring to the clinic (e.g., solvents) may be too inherently irritant for testing. If a complex, such as a cosmetic moisturizer, is patch-test positive but the European and other series of allergens are negative, it may then be necessary to obtain the individual items from the manufacturer to test to identify the causative contact allergen(s).

The European standard series contains eight different classes of allergens.

### A.  Metals

Nickel is found in metal jewelry. It may cause a rash on earlobes, wrists (watches and bracelets), and under rings. Nickel dermatitis was first described in relation to suspender dermatitis, and it may still be seen in relation to clothing; "jean button" dermatitis is very commonly seen. Dimethylglyoxime solution will turn pink on reacting with nickel; this is a useful test for the presence of nickel. Nickel is also present on some utensils and in electroplating. Cobalt is usually seen as a cosensitizer and is found along with nickel in metallic jewelry and clothing items. It is also found in ceramics and in blue paint and tattoo dye. Chromate is the chief allergen in cement but can now be seen commonly in relation to leather, ceramics, alloys, and in green paint and tattoo dye.

## B.   Preservatives

Formaldehyde is an ubiquitous chemical, which can cause dermatitis through consumer and occupational use. It is used in a wide variety of cosmetics including shampoos, deoderants, blushes, hair tonics, and nail hardeners. It is also contained in household products such as disinfectants and detergents. Formaldehyde can cause dermatitis through resin-treated or permanent-press clothing. Workers are exposed through its use as a preservative for pathology specimens, embalming fluid, cooling solutions, and cutting oils. Formaldehyde allergy may be difficult to predict before patch tests. As an additional complicating factor, several preservative products contain and can release formaldehyde, so that anyone allergic to formaldehyde must avoid these as well; the main such preservatives are quaternium-15, imidazolidinyl urea, diazolidinyl urea, 2-bromo-2-nitropropane-1,3-diol, and DMDM hydantoin.

Quaternium 15 (Dowicil 200) is incorported into a large number of cosmetic products, particularly rinse-off formulations where there is a high water content. Occupational cases of imidazolidinyl urea (germall 115) are rare but may be reported as it is incorporated into some soaps and lotions. The vast majority of cases are due to its use in cosmetics and medicines. 2-Bromo-2-nitropropane-1,3-diol (bronopol) is still used as a preservative in cosmetics, particularly shampoos. Paraben esters are patch tested as a mixture of different varieties. They are generally considered safe and of low allergenicity, but their subsequent high usage has resulted in a significant number of cases of sensitization. They are also used in medicaments, especially in sunscreen agents, where it is difficult to avoid paraben exposure. Methyl(chloro)isothiazilinone (MI/MCI, Kathon CG) is a highly effective preservative but has caused a large number of cases of cosmetic allergy. It does not release formaldehyde. As is common with other contact allergens, it has a significant irritant potential.

## C.   Fragrances

The commonly used screen is known as the Larsen fragrance mix. Those contained the perfume chemicals amyl cinnamicaldhyde, cinnamic alcohol, cinnamic aldehyde, eugenol, isoeugenol, geraniol, hydroxycitronellal and oak moss, tested in the emulsifier sorbitan sesquioleate. This screen picks up 75% of subjects who are fragrance allergic. Perfume allergy can present as an obvious dermatitis reaction to a perfume, aftershave, or deodarant, but alternatively can present as a more subtle rash when the perfume is contained in a toiletry such as a moisturizing cream or a shampoo.

Balsam of Peru is a fragrance substance derived from a tree native to El Salvador. Allergic subjects may need to avoid fragranced chemicals, but they also need to avoid certain flavored foods, such as citrus peels, cola, and artifical flavors, and also spices.

## D.   Medicaments

Neomycin and clioquinol are topically applied antibiotics used in treating skin infections or combined with topical steroids in treating inflammatory skin disorders; sensitization is frequent. Benzocaine is a topically applied local anesthetic that can also sensitize; subjects allergic to benzocaine usually can take lignocaine as these do not cross-react. Ethylenediamine is sold in the United Kingdom as triadcortyl cream. Allergic subjects should also avoid aminophylline, as this contains ethylenediamine, as do the antihistamines hydroxyzine hydrochloride, cyclizine, and piperazine. Ethylenediamine is also used in floor polish removers, epoxy hardeners, and coolant oil.

## E. Adhesives

*p*-Tert-butylphenol-formaldehyde resin (PTBP) is made by reacting the substituted phenol, *p*-tert-butylphenol, with formaldehyde. It is a useful adhesive which sticks rapidly; it is used in shoe construction and in leather goods. It is used in other contact adhesives such as those used in laminating surfaces and is often formulated with neoprene. It is used in car assembly plants, and can sensitize in leather watch straps and plastic fingernail adhesives.

Epoxy resin consists of 95% of a glycydyl ether group formed by the reaction of bisphenol A with epichlorhydrin. Recently there has been a divergence in the chemical compositions of epoxy resins used as a wider variety of different preparations are required. Epoxy resins can be used in paints and in the impregnation of carbon fiber cloth.

Colophony is a widespread, naturally occurring material, which is the residue left after distilling off the volatile oil from the oleoresin obtained from the trees of the Pinacea. Colophony is composed of about 90% resin acids and 10% neutral substances. The principal allergens have not yet been determined, but abeitic acid and dehydroabietic acid have been identified as allergens. Colophony is present in glues, adhesives, as well as paper printing inks, soldering flux, and polishes.

## F. Rubber Allergens

The thiuram mix used in standard series contain four different thiurams; thiurams are accelerators used in the manufacture of rubber that are retained in small quantities. It is the most common cause of glove allergy. Thiurams have also been used as fungicides, in agricultural purposes, as well as in wallpaper adhesives and paints. Mercaptobenzathiazole is present in many rubbers and is used as an accelerator in the manufacture of rubber. Three other mercaptos are tested in the *mercapto-mix*. Mercapto- allergy is the most common cause of rubber dermatitis to shoes. *N*-Isopropyl-*N*-phenylediamine (IPPD) is used in black rubber as an antiozonant to reduce the effects of weathering or perishing.

## G. Plants

Primin (2-mothoxy-6-pentylbenzoquinone) is the major allergen in primula dermatitis; it is an important allergen in northern European countries; primula leaves are covered with visible fine hairs, and primin is present as a powerful sensitiser within the hairs. Other plants and woods containing quinones may show cross-reactivity with primin.

Sesquiterpene lactone mix contains three different lactones. The sesquiterpene lactones are contact allergens present in Compositae plants, which constitute one of the largest flowering plant families in the world. Plants include chrysanthemum, marguerite, marigold, goldenrod, African marigold, sunflower, and many common weeds such as milfoil, tansy, mugwort, and wild chamomile.

## H. Other Allergens

Lanolin (wool alcohol) is a natural product from sheep hair and is a complex mixture of esters and polyesters of high molecular weight and fatty acids. Lanolin and wool alohols are weak allergens, and experimental sensitisation is difficult to achieve. However, their widespread use leads to a sensitization rate of more than 1% in patch test populations.

*p*-Phenylediamine (PPD) is a compound that acts as a primary intermediate in hair dyes. It is oxidized by hydrogen peroxide and then polymerized within the hair by a coupler. Patients with PPD allergy can cross-react with bezocaine, IPPD, sulfonamide, and PABA derivatives. Cross-reactions do occur to other related hair dyes, and finding a suitable alternative dye may be a problem.

## REFERENCES

1.  Emtestam L, Olerup O. On T cell recognition of nickel as a hapten. Acta Derm Venereol 1996; 76:344–347.
2.  Roberts DW, Williams DL. The derivation of quantitative correlations between skin sensitisation and physicochemical parameters from alkylating agents, and their application to experimental data for sulfones. J Theor Biol 1982; 99:807–825.
3.  Roberts DW, Lepoittevin J-P. Hapten-protein interactions. In: Lepoittevin J-P, Basketter DA, Goossens A, Karlberg A-T, eds. Allergic Contact Dermatitis. Heidelberg: Springer-Verlag, 1998:81–111.
4.  Lepoittevin J-P, Drieghe J, Dooms-Goosens A. Studies in patients with corticosteroid contact allergy: understanding cross-reactivity among different steroids. Arch Dermatol 1995; 131:31–37.
5.  Cumberbatch M, Dearman RJ, Kimber I. Langerhans cells migration requires signals from both TNF alpha and interleukin 1 beta for migration. Immunology 1997; 92:388–395.
6.  Schuler G, ed. Epidermal Langerhans Cells. Boca Raton, FL: CRC Press, 1991.
7.  Aiba S, Katz SI. Phenotypic and functional characteristics of in vivo activated Langerhans cells. J Immunol 1990; 145: 2791.
8.  Enk A, Katz SI. Early molecular events in the induction of contact sensitivity Proc Natl Acad Sci USA 1992; 89:1398.
9.  Macatonia SE, et al. Localization of antigen on lymph node dendritic cells after exposure to the contact sensitiser fluorescein isothiocyanate. Functional and morphological studies. J Exp Med 1987; 166:1654.
10. Frey JR, Wenk P. Experimental studies on the pathogenesis of contact sensitization in the guinea pig. Int Arch Allergy 1957; 11:81–100.
11. Picker Lj Kishomoto TK, Smith CW, et al. ELAM-1 is an adhesion molecule for skin-homing T cells. Nature 1991; 349:796–799.
12. Babi LFS, Picker LJ, Soler MTP, et al. Circulating allergen-reactive T cells from patients with atopic dermatitis and allergic contact dermatitis express the skin-homing receptor "the cutaneous lymphocyte antigen." J Exp Med 1995; 181:1935–1940.
13. Polak L. Immunological aspects of contact sensitivity. An experimental study. Monogr Allergy 1980; 15:4–60.
14. Bergstrasser PR. Sensitisation and elicitation of inflammation in contact dermatitis. In: Norris DA, ed. Immune Mechanisms in Cutaneous Disease. New York: Marcel Dekker, 1989:219–246.
15. Sanders S, Akgoba MW, Shaw S. Human naïve and memory T cells; reinterpretation of helper-inducer and supressor—inducer subsets. Immunol Today 1988; 9:195–198.

16. Hauser C, Katz SI. Activation and expansion of hapten- and protein-specific T helper cells from non-sensitized mice. Proc Natl Acad Sci USA 1988; 85:5625.

17. Knop J, Reichmann R, Macher E. Modulation of supressor mechanisms in allergic contacder-matitis. J Invest Dermatol 1981; 76:193.

18. Elmets CA, et al. Analysis of the mechanisms of unresponsiveness produced by haptens painted on skin exposed to low dose ultraviolet radiation. J Exp Med 1983; 158:781.

19. Kanerva L, Ranki A, Lauharanta J. Lymphocytes and Langerhans cells in patch tests. Contact Dermatitis 1984; 11:150.

20. McCluskey RT, Benacerraf B, McCluskey JW. Studies on the specificity of the cellular infil-trate in delayed hypersensitivity reactions. J Immunol 1963; 90:466.

21. Gaspari AA, Jenkins MK, Katz SI. Class II bearing keratinocytes induce antigen-specific unre-sponsiveness for hapten-specific TH1 cells. J Immunol 1991; 141:2216–2220.

# 11

## Chronic Actinic Dermatitis

**Hélène du Peloux Menagé**
*Lewisham University Hospital and St. Thomas' Hospital, London, England*

**John L. M. Hawk**
*St. Thomas' Hospital, London, England*

## I. DEFINITION

Chronic actinic dermatitis (CAD) is a rare photodermatosis, often associated with allergic contact dermatitis, sometimes to multiple allergens. It is characterized predominantly by eczema, mainly on light-exposed sites, induced by ultraviolet B (UVB), sometimes also ultraviolet A (UVA), and occasionally also visible light. The pathogenesis of the condition is not fully understood, but recent studies support the view that it may be a delayed-type hypersensitivity response, possibly to an ultraviolet-related antigen.

The term chronic actinic dermatitis was coined by Hawk and Magnus [1] and is used synonymously with the term photosensitivity dermatitis (PD) actinic reticuloid (AR) syndrome (PD/AR), coined by Frain-Bell and colleagues [2]. The label CAD/PD/AR encompasses four diagnoses: persistent light reactivity [3], actinic reticuloid [4], photosensitive eczema [5], and photosensitivity dermatitis [2]. These were originally described as distinct disorders but are now accepted as variants of the one disorder. The terms persistent light reactivity, actinic reticuloid, photosensitive eczema, and photosensitivity dermatitis are no longer generally in clinical use, but are explained below for clarity.

Persistent light reactivity (PLR) was coined by Wilkinson in 1962 [3] and referred to eczema on light-exposed sites following an episode of topical photoallergic contact dermatitis, which in the original description of the disorder was tetrachlorsalicylanilide in a germicidal soap. This developed despite avoidance of the original photocontact allergen and irrespective of whether or not the affected sites had previously been exposed to allergen. The wavelengths responsible for induction of lesions lay not only in the UVA (315–400 nm), generally responsible for photoallergic responses, but extended into the UVB (280–315 nm) as well. PLR has been reported following sensitization to other halogenated phenols (tribromosalicylanilide) [3], to the agents fentichlor and bithionol used in soaps, antiseptics and toiletries in the 1960s and early 1970s [6], and to the fragrance musk ambrette, a synthetic musk used widely in aftershave. These products have now been withdrawn. Isolated cases have also been reported following sensitization to quinoxaline-*N*-dioxide in animal foodstuffs [7], to zinc pyrithione [8], and to bleaching agents [9]. Generally speaking, however, cases of PLR are nowadays very rarely observed, none having been observed in our unit in recent years, although there is an isolated report following photosensitivity to sunscreen ingredients and another following use of olaquindox in animal feed in pig breeders [10].

The term actinic reticuloid was coined by Ive et al. in 1969 [4]. The clinical hallmark of the condition was infiltrated erythematous plaques (hence reticuloid) arising on eczematous or normal skin in elderly males. The histopathological features were suggestive of cutaneous T-cell lymphoma, and photosensitivity extended from the UVB into the visible wavelengths. Clinical similarity was noted to severe cases of photoallergic contact dermatitis, suggesting that persistent exposure to allergen might account for the exaggerated clinical features. Photopatch tests were negative. Such cases are still observed within the CAD spectrum but less frequently, conceivably because, with heightened awareness of the condition, it is diagnosed and treated at an earlier stage, before intense photosensitivity develops.

Photosensitive eczema, described by Ramsay and Kobza-Black in 1973 [5], referred to an eczematous eruption with no preceding photoallergy. Features of actinic reticuloid were observed in some patients, but the action spectrum differed and was in the UVB region alone.

Photosensitivity dermatitis, reported by Frain-Bell and colleagues, described a similar eczematous eruption, but with photosensitivity often also extending to include the UVA wavelengths [2]. In 1979, however, Hawk and Magnus showed that there was significant overlap between photosensitive eczema and actinic reticuloid patients, describing patients with the histological features of eczema and the photobiological abnormalities associated with actinic reticuloid. They also confirmed that transition could be observed between these disease states [2,11] and therefore coined the unifying term CAD. More recently, it has observed that transition may occur from persistent light reactivity to actinic reticuloid [12] and that there was overlap between persistent light reactivity and the CAD spectrum. In 1990 it was therefore proposed that persistent light reactivity should be encompassed within the term CAD [13,14]. The terms persistent light reactivity, actinic reticuloid, photosensitive eczema, and photosensitivity dermatitis are now predominantly of historical interest. Introduction of unifying diagnostic criteria has also reduced confusion and facilitated diagnosis and progress in understanding of the condition [13,15,16].

## II.  CLINICAL ASPECTS

### A.  Clinical Features

The precise incidence of CAD is not known but has been estimated at 1:6000 in northern Scotland [17]. It is therefore an uncommon condition, although probably underdiagnosed. Originally diagnosed as a disease of males, females are now known to make up 10–22% of patients [17,18]; the average age at diagnosis is 65 years [18], although exceptionally atopic eczema may predispose to early-onset disease under the age of 50 years [19]. Although CAD is triggered by exposure to sunlight, the relationship to ultraviolet exposure is not always evident to the patient or physician, particularly early on in the evolution of the disorder. The eruption may thus be delayed for hours to days following exposure and, although generally worse in the spring and summer months, may persist into the winter months and may become generalized and be complicated by the features of associated contact dermatitis. Classical cases show chronic or subacute eczema, predominantly of the light-exposed sites. In patients with severe light sensitivity, the eruption frequently spreads to affect covered areas as well, and episodes of erythroderma may develop. Lichenification is often observed while in again more severely affected patients infiltrated papules and plaques mimicking cutaneous lymphoma may develop [4]. Palmar and occasionally plantar eczema may also be a feature. Areas of hyperpigmentation or hypopigmentation may sometimes develop during the course of the disease, the latter sometimes closely resembling widespread vitiligo and attributed to the cytotoxic destruction of melanocytes [20]. Loss of eyebrow and scalp hair may also occur, or hair may become grey prematurely.

Originally described in white Caucasians, CAD is not limited to this racial group. Thus in London it is frequently observed in Asians [18] and has also been reported in the Japanese [12] and in Afro-Caribbeans [18,21]. Outdoor workers, particularly gardeners, appear more likely to be affected, perhaps because they have greater cumulative exposure to sunlight and to exacerbating allergens. A report of onset after accidental UVC exposure suggests that any form of excessive ultraviolet exposure may be contributory [22]. However, a careful study of cumulative ultraviolet exposure in affected individuals has yet to be performed.

## B. Predisposing Factors

CAD is occasionally observed in patients previously on potentially photosensitizing systemic drugs, including thiazide diuretics [23]. Intake of potentially photosensitizing medication is, however, common in the age group of patients who develop CAD, and it remains unclear whether these systemic agents may occasionally predispose to the development of the disorder. CAD has also been reported in association with human immunodeficiency virus (HIV) infection and predated the onset of AIDS-defining disorders; the immunological mechanisms underlying this observation are not understood [24]. Some patients with CAD give a history of preceding endogenous eczema including palmar and plantar eczema [18]. The majority (about 75%) have associated contact dermatitis [18,25,26]; only 12% of patients have neither associated contact or photocontact allergies nor associated eczema [18]. Contact allergy has been documented to precede the development of photosensitivity [27], but in most cases the diagnosis of contact allergy is made from concurrent patch testing at the time when formal phototesting confirms a diagnosis of CAD. The main allergens implicated are Compositae plant extracts, fragrance compounds, colophony, metals and rubber, and occasionally epoxy resins, phosphorus sesquisulfide, medicaments, preservatives, and vehicle bases [18,26,28–31]. These reactions have been shown to be persistent and reproducible and do not simply represent increased cutaneous reactivity [32]. Contact dermatitis may also complicate the management of CAD, and sensitivity to sunscreens has been reported during the course of the disease [33]. Photoallergic contact dermatitis as well is historically associated with CAD, the condition having been reported to evolve from it (so-called PLR—see above), but this is only rarely observed.

## C. Diagnosis and Differential Diagnosis

The diagnosis of CAD is suggested by the clinical findings, supported by the histological features of eczema, sometimes pseudo-lymphomatous in severe cases. Phototesting of unaffected skin to broad-band or monochromatic irradiation is always necessary to confirm the diagnosis and is almost invariably abnormal: there is a reduction in the minimum dose required to induce a response at 24 hours, and the response is often of abnormal morphology, with papular or eczematous lesions characteristic of the disease itself [2]. However, very rarely, such phototest abnormalities may not become manifest for some months after onset of the disease, and retesting may therefore be advisable in clinically suggestive cases with negative phototests. Patients generally react abnormally to the UVB wavelengths, and in the majority there is extension to the UVA wavelengths; a minority respond to the visible wavelengths as well [2,18]. Occasionally, however, abnormalities are detected in the UVA alone; these cases do not fulfill the original diagnostic criteria [1,14] and are rare, although increasingly recognized [34–36].

Phototesting to monochromatic or broad-band sources is generally only available in specialist centers. Nonetheless it is essential for a confident diagnosis of CAD, as it enables exclusion of a number of other eczematous conditions. Thus, contact dermatitis, particularly to airborne allergens, and photocontact dermatitis may closely mimic CAD but are distinguished by normal monochromatic irradiation tests, and both may also occur in association with CAD. In addition, light-exacerbated atopic or seborrheic eczema can generally be distinguished clinically, but in more difficult cases cutaneous irradiation tests should be performed and generally give normal responses. Erythrodermic CAD may be distinguished from other erythrodermas by normal irradiation tests, but clearance of the eruption must be achieved prior to testing to avoid false-positive responses, and nursing of the patient in a light protected room is helpful to achieve this and preferred to immunosuppressive therapy, which may also modify the phototest response. Systemic drug-induced photosensitivity is associated with normal cutaneous irradiation tests or abnormalities in the UVA range only, and withdrawal of the drug generally results in progressive resolution of the clinical and phototest abnormalities over a period of about 6 months [37].

Cutaneous T-cell lymphoma may occasionally be clinically and histologically indistinguishable from severe CAD, in some instances patients with erythrodermic CAD having circulating Sézary cells in the peripheral blood [38]. However, morphometry using electron microscopy and image analysis generally distinguishes the Sézary syndrome from CAD [39]. Cutaneous irradiation tests are usually, albeit not invariably, negative in cutaneous T-cell lymphoma (CTCL); abnormalities, if detected, are generally minor [40] and out of keeping with the severity of clinical disease. In difficult cases the ratio of CD4+ to CD8+ circulating lymphocytes may be helpful in distinguishing the two conditions with CD8+ predominance in CAD, particularly severe variants [41] and CD4+ cells in cutaneous T-cell lymphoma [42]. T-cell receptor gene studies may also be helpful, as abnormalities have not been reported in CAD [41,43]. Quantitative phenotypic analysis of the cutaneous T-cell infiltrate may also be of value: epidermal CD8 predominance has been reported in CAD and CD4 predominance reported in CTCL, and discordance between CD3 and BF-1 expression may be observed in CTCL but not in CAD [44]. There remain nonetheless isolated reports of cutaneous lymphoma developing in patients with CAD [45–49], and it remains unclear whether these are coincidental, confusions in diagnosis, or genuine associations. It has also been suggested that persistent abnormal cellular response to antigen, such as is postulated to occur in CAD, may predispose to T-cell lymphoma [50], but neither clinical [17] nor experimental evidence supports this as a regular phenomenon. Thus, comparison with sex-matched national morbidity data has not confirmed an increased risk of lymphoma [51], while a flow cytometric study showed no evidence of DNA aneuploidy in the cutaneous infiltrate of patients with actinic reticuloid [52], and T-cell receptor and immunoglobulin gene rearrangement studies have demonstrated no evidence of a clonal lymphoid population in CAD [41,43]. If present at all, the risk of lymphomatous transformation is therefore likely to be small.

## III. PATHOGENESIS OF THE CAD RESPONSE TO LIGHT

## A. Autoimmunity

In order to explain the various features of CAD, it has been proposed that ultraviolet light irradiation may alter a normal skin constituent such that it is no longer regarded as self, thus provoking a delayed hypersensitivity–like response (see Fig. 1). Evidence in support of this theory, at least in relation to progression of photoallergic contact dermatitis to CAD, comes from a 1977 study by Kochevar and Harber [53], who showed that, in vitro, tetrachlorsalicylanilide binds strongly to human albumin and promotes the oxidation of the histidine moiety of albumin, rendering it weakly antigenic; subsequent absorption of UV radiation by albumin alone in the absence of the initiating exogenous photosensitizer then produced oxidized protein. The same phenomenon could occur in vivo, and, because albumin is widely distributed throughout the skin, this could explain the potential for a delayed-type hypersensitivity response at all skin sites in the absence of the initial photosensitizer.

Three types of evidence can be marshaled to establish that a human disease is autoimmune in origin. They include direct evidence from transfer of pathogenic T cells (or antibodies), indirect evidence based on reproduction of autoimmune disease in experimental animals, and circumstantial evidence from clinical clues [54]. Direct proof of autoimmunity in CAD does not exist, and because cell transfer requires major histocompatibility complex (MHC) compatibility, is not feasible from human to human or human to animal.

There is, however, significant indirect evidence through reproduction of the disease in experimental animal models by Katsumura and colleagues [55] and Ichikawa and colleagues [56]. Ichikawa et al. treated guinea pigs with intradermal injections of adjuvant (desiccated mycobacteria or muramyl dipeptide) followed by the topical application of hapten (5% benzocaine solution) and UVA irradiation. Skin reactions could subsequently be elicited by UVA irradiation in the absence of hapten application. This enhanced UVA sensitivity persisted for more than 2 years and was associated with increased sensitivity to UVB. Of note, both groups also induced UV sensitivity in the absence of hapten application using only injections of adjuvant and UVA in the immunization procedure [54,55], thus providing a model for the development of CAD in the absence of photoallergic contact dermatitis (when contact or endogenous dermatitis may be heightening immune reactivity and acting as "adjuvant"). They found that the induction of photosensitivity was strain dependent, indicating that it was influenced by genetic background [56]. They went on to show adoptive transfer of photosensitivity through the transfer of peritoneal exudate cells (but not with spleen cells, suggesting that the T cells responsible are more prevalent in the peritoneal exudate). A proliferative response was observed when peritoneal exudate cells were cultured with lymph node cells in the presence of sera that had been irradiated with UVA in vitro, and, furthermore, positive skin reactions with erythema were elicited in the photosensitive guinea pigs by intradermal injections of UVA-exposed sera from *both* photosensitive *and* normal guinea pigs, suggesting that the antigen triggering the response was generated from normal serum components following UV exposure [56].

Circumstantial evidence that a disease is autoimmune can be obtained from (1) favorable response to immunosuppression, (2) lymphocytic infiltration of the target organ, (3) association with other autoimmune diseases in the same individual or the same family, and (4) statistical association with a particular MHC haplotype or aberrant expression of MHC class II antigens in the affected organ [54]. Some circumstantial evidence has already established that CAD may be an autoimmune disease. Thus T-cell immunomodulatory therapy with azathioprine [57] or cyclosporin A [58] is of established value in the management of resistant cases, and there are two isolated reports of the efficacy of α-interferon, which downregulates suppressor T cells [59]. It has also been established that a T-cell lymphocytic infiltrate is found in lesional skin and that the time course and detailed nature of the infiltrate is comparable with other previously established cellular responses to antigen (see below). However, there have been no reports of family association of CAD, and there are no formal studies on genetic susceptibility. Furthur, human leukocyte antigen (HLA) studies have failed to establish an HLA association; a possible association with patch test–positive CAD and HLA-DQ1 is likely to be related to an immunogenetic relationship to Compositae sensitivity than to CAD itself (H. du P. Menagé, R. W. Vaughan, J. L. M. Hawk, unpublished observations).

## B.   Evidence for a Delayed Hypersensitivity Reaction

### 1.   Histology

Clinically, histologically, and experimentally, lesions of CAD are compatible with a process of cell-mediated hypersensitivity. Clinically, the lesions resemble those of allergic contact dermatitis. Histologically, the changes are very similar to those in allergic contact dermatitis, with epidermal spongiosis and a variable degree of acanthosis, and a lympho-histiocytic infiltrate with occasional plasma cells and eosinophils, predominantly in the upper dermis in a perivascular distribution and extending into the epidermis. In the pseudolymphoma or actinic reticuloid stage, the infiltrate is much heavier, with atypical lymphocytes with convoluted nuclei (Sézary-like cells) and Pautrier-like microabscesses in the epidermis. Similar changes have been reported in certain forms of chronic contact dermatitis, so-called lymphomatoid contact dermatitis [60], suggesting that the pseudolymphomatous lesions represent a severe stage in the spectrum of CAD, presumably occurring after persistent antigenic stimulation.

### 2.   Immunophenotype

A number of immunohistochemical studies have been performed to characterize the dermal infiltrate in lesions of chronic actinic dermatitis. This consists predominantly of T cells, both in fully evolved [61–65] and in induced lesions [66,67], together with Langerhans cells, interdigitating reticulum cells, and monocyte-macrophages including CD36 (OKM5+), factor XIIIa+, CD11b+, CD11c+, and CD14+ cells [66,67]. Leukocyte epidermotropism is observed, and keratinocytes express MHC class II antigens in induced lesions [66,67]. The relative proportion of CD4+ (T-helper/inducer) and CD8+ (T-suppressor/cytotoxic) cells in the dermal infiltrate has varied in different studies; in some a predominance of CD4+ cells has been reported [62,67], while in others equal ratios [62,63] or a predominance of CD8+ cells was found [64,66], particularly in lesions with more florid histological changes [65]. Most studies agree that CD4+ T cells predominate over CD8+ T cells in the early stages of allergic contact dermatitis and the tuberculin response [68,69], with an increase in CD8+ cells occurring in the late stage [66]. The kinetics of the inflammatory cell infiltrate in induced lesions of CAD is consistent with a delayed-type hypersensitivity response [69] with a peak in the intensity of infiltrate, including dermal and epidermal activated T cells, epidermal Langerhans cells, and monocyte-macrophages, at 24–48 hours [67], and the pattern of the infiltrate distinct from that following UVB irradiation alone when T-cell and Langerhans cell epidermotropism is not observed [70].

Analysis of circulating lymphocyte subsets in CAD has given variable results. In some patients they have been normal [65,71], while in others a reduction in the CD4+: CD8+ ratio has been observed [63,65,66], generally due to a predominance of CD8+ circulating lymphocytes, most marked in patients with the actinic reticuloid variant of CAD [41]. The latter finding correlates with the reported increase in CD8+ cells in the cutaneous infiltrate of more florid cases of CAD [65].

## 3. Adhesion Molecule Expression

Specific changes in the kinetics and pattern of cell surface adhesion molecule expression have been reported in the delayed-type hypersensitivity response and similar changes documented in CAD. Following purified protein derivative (PPD) injection, prolonged expression of endothelial leukocyte adhesion molecule 1 (ELAM-1), expression of vascular cell adhesion molecule 1 (VCAM-1) by perivascular and dermal interstitial cells, and early intercellular adhesion molecule 1 (ICAM-1) expression by keratinocytes have been reported [72]. Similar changes have been found in allergic contact dermatitis: keratinocyte ICAM-1 expression occurs early in the induction of lesions, and upregulation of ICAM-1, VCAM-1, and ELAM-1 is observed on dermal perivascular cells [73]. Time-course biopsies following 8 to 10 minimal response doses of solar simulated irradiation (less than 1 minimal erythema dose in normals) in five patients with CAD revealed upregulation of perivascular ICAM-1, VCAM-1, and ELAM-1, and of dermal interstitial VCAM-1 and ICAM-1, from 1 to 5 hours on, persisting at 5–7 days. There was also increased expression of ICAM-1 by basal keratinocytes and focally throughout the epidermis at 1 hour, persisting at 5–7 days [74]. These changes are not simply a function of ultraviolet radiation; following UVB irradiation, the expression of ELAM-1 is less prolonged, and induction of VCAM-1 and induction of keratinocyte ICAM-1 is not observed, and following combined UVB and UVA irradiation expression of ICAM-1 on keratinocytes in vitro is delayed by 48 hours [72,75]. Thus, the pattern of adhesion molecule expression observed in CAD is likely to be of significance in the development of lesions and suggests delayed-type hypersensitivity.

## 4. Cytokine Expression

Studies on the role of cytokines in the pathogenesis of the lesions of CAD are limited. However, an immunohistochemical time-course study of the expression and distribution of IL-1$\alpha$, its type 1 receptor (IL-1R), and the inhibitor of IL-1 (IL-1RA) during the evolution of induced lesions of CAD, compared to those changes seen after solar simulated irradiation in normals, support a proposed pro-inflammatory role for IL-1$\alpha$ in CAD mediated via its receptor, distinct from that following UV irradiation alone, and comparable to that observed in a delayed-type hypersensitivity response [76].

## 5. Functional Studies

Preliminary studies of dermal and epidermal extracts of lesional skin from patients with CAD have shown no evidence of proliferation in the autologous mixed epidermal cell

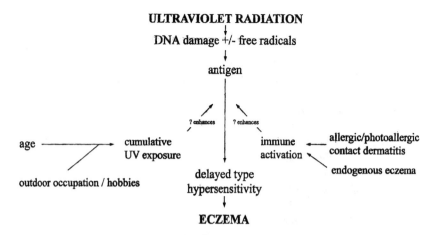

**Figure 1**   Possible mechanism for chronic actinic dermatitis.

leukocyte culture response [77]. Confirmatory evidence of an antigen driven process is therefore still required.

## IV. CANDIDATE ALLERGENS FOR THE CAD RESPONSE

Willis and Kligman in 1968 induced local photosensitivity to halogenated salicyl-anilides and related compounds and by studying the UV absorption spectra of skin extracts from these patients showed persistence of the original photosensitizer in the skin for months and occasionally a year or more [78]. It was therefore proposed that small persistent amounts of exogenous photoallergen were triggering the photosensitivity in CAD. However, this theory does not explain the development of generalized reactivity, nor does it explain spread beyond the original UVA elicitation spectrum of photoallergic contact dermatitis to include UVB sensitivity in CAD, nor the pathogenesis of CAD arising in all but the occasional patient in the absence of documented exogenous photoallergy.

Kynurenic acid is an endogenous protein that is a metabolic by-product of tryptophan metabolism and has been shown to cause phototoxic oxidation of histidine in vitro [79]. Levels of kynurenic acid were found to be increased in the skin of one patient with CAD [79], while another study revealed abnormal tryptophan metabolism with accumulation of kynurenic acid [80], suggesting that it may be acting as an endogenous photosensitizer in CAD patients. However, these findings have not proved reproducible [81].

The autoimmune theory of the pathogenesis of CAD is generally held, therefore, to be the most attractive [82]. Study of the biological response curve to UV irradiation in CAD (so-called action spectrum for induction of lesions) has shown that the shape of the action spectrum for induction of lesions resembles that for induction of UV erythema in normals although considerably displaced in magnitude [83]. This implies that the chromophores (or chemical absorbers) responsible for the changes of CAD are the same as that/

those responsible for the sunburn response in normal UV-irradiated skin, for which the chromophore is suspected to be DNA. Therefore the antigen responsible for CAD may indeed be an altered self protein, conceivably altered DNA. Why self-reactivity to such a protein should develop is not understood, but it may be a function both of cumulative UV exposure and of persistent T-cell stimulation from coexistent contact, photocontact, or endogenous eczema (see Fig. 1). Alternatively, as ultraviolet irradiation is well known to diminish cutaneous immune reactivity and, in particular, the induction phase of delayed hypersensitivity [84], both CAD and the frequently associated contact dermatitis may represent a fundamental dysregulation of normal UV suppressor mechanisms. Finally, in vitro studies have suggested a possible hypersensitivity of CAD fibroblasts to both UVA and UVB irradiation [85–88]. Evidence is conflicting [86,89] and a role for cellular hypersensitivity to UVR in the pathogenesis of CAD remains to be established but would not necessarily be incompatible with the autoimmune hypothesis of CAD causation, such susceptibility hypothetically increasing antigen load which in turn triggers the hypersensitivity response (see Fig. 1).

## V. TREATMENT

CAD is a disabling condition and prior to the introduction of immunotherapy was said to be associated with significant psychological morbidity. Ultraviolet avoidance is the cornerstone of management, although the longer wavelengths are particularly difficult to protect against. Thus, outdoor exposure should be minimized, particularly in the middle of the day when irradiance is high, and protective clothing should be worn in conjunction with high sun protection factor sunscreens with good UVA protection. Nonirritant reflectant sunscreen preparations are generally preferable in view of the risk of contact allergy to chemical preparations. Ultraviolet screening blinds in the home and in the car may be helpful to limit exposure to long-wavelength ultraviolet radiation. Careful avoidance of associated contact allergens is, however, also essential, and apparent worsening of the condition may be due to the development of new or additional contact or photocontact allergies, sunscreens being particularly notorious [33]. Acute flares of the disease may require nursing in light-protected cubicles, generally only available in specialist units, while emollients and topical or short term oral corticosteroids are helpful adjunctive therapy.

For persistent or frequently relapsing cases, immunosuppressive therapy or psoralen and ultraviolet A (PUVA) may also be required. PUVA therapy is often poorly tolerated in the early phase of treatment even under systemic steroid cover. Maintenance therapy, possibly restricted to light-exposed sites, is generally also required [90,91]. The mode of action is unknown but is likely to involve modification of the immune response, in addition possibly to the induction of protective skin thickening and melanogenesis. Azathioprine is generally effective if tolerated [57], as is cyclosporin A [58], which prevents the clonal expansion of activated T cells through inhibition of interleukins 1 and 2. Danazol has also been reported to be effective in an isolated patient with associated $\alpha_1$-antitrypsin deficiency, but this has yet to be confirmed [92]. There are also two isolated reports of the efficacy of $\alpha$-interferon, which downregulates suppressor T cells [59]. Although immunotherapy appears to control the inflammatory response, it is not clear if such treatments modify the underlying photosensitivity.

CAD is often a persistent disorder. However, clinical improvement does occur, although the phototest abnormalities may nonetheless persist [16]. The chances of resolution of both clinical photosensitivity and phototest abnormalities increase with time and have been estimated to be as high as 50% after 16 years [93]. Long-term life expectancy is probably unaffected (A. Ive, unpublished observations), although it has been reported to be reduced in those with erythroderma [94]. Careful management can thus generally allow the patient to maintain a satisfactory lifestyle.

## VI. SUMMARY

CAD is characterized by extreme sensitivity to ultraviolet radiation, which initiates an inflammatory eczematous process resembling delayed-type hypersensitivity. It is possible that an endogenous photoallergen is responsible for the process, although there is as yet only circumstantial and no direct support for this. A state of heightened reactivity of the skin immune system, due to coexistent eczema, may favor the development of the disease, but the mechanisms remain undefined. The disorder may respond to a combination of ultraviolet and contact allergen avoidance but often also requires oral immunomodulatory therapy or PUVA.

## REFERENCES

1. Hawk JLM, Magnus IA. Chronic actinic dermatitis—an idiopathic photosensitivity syndrome including actinic reticuloid and photosensitive eczema. Br J Dermatol 1979; 101(suppl 17): 24.
2. Frain-Bell W, Lakshmipathi T, Rogers J, Willock J. The syndrome of chronic photosensitivity dermatitis and actinic reticuloid. Br J Dermatol 1974; 91:617–634.
3. Wilkinson DS. Patch test reactions to certain halogenated salicylanalides. Br J Dermatol 1962; 74:302–306.
4. Ive FA, Magnus IA, Warin RP, Wilson Jones E. 'Actinic reticuloid'; a chronic dermatosis associated with severe photosensitivity and the histological resemblance to lymphoma. Br J Dermatol 1969; 81:469–485.
5. Ramsay CA, Kobza-Black A. Photosensitive eczema. Translations of the St John's Hospital Dermatological Society 1973; 59:152–158.
6. Jillson OF, Baughman RD. Contact photodermatitis from bithionol. Arch Dermatol 1963; 88: 409–418.
7. Zaynoun S, Johnson BE, Frain-Bell W. The investigation of quindoxin photosensitivity. Contact Dermatitis 1976; 2(6):343–352.
8. Yates VM, Finn OA. Contact allergic sensitivity to zinc pirithione followed by the photosensitivity dermatitis and actinic reticuloid syndrome. Contact Dermatitis 1980; 6:349–350.
9. Burckhardt W. Photoallergic eczema due to blankophores (optic brightening agents). Hautartz 1957; 8:486–488.
10. Schauder S, Schroder W, Geier J. Olaquindox-induced airborne photoallergic contact dermatitis followed by transient or persistent light reactions in 15 pig breeders. Contact Dermatitis 1996; 35:344–354.
11. Hawk JLM, Magnus IA. Resolution of actinic reticuloid with transition to photosensitive eczema. J Roy Soc Med 1978; 71:608–610.
12. Horio T. Actinic reticuloid via persistent light reactivity from photoallergic contact dermatitis. Arch Dermatol 1982; 118:339–342.
13. Lim HW, Buchness MR, Ashinoff R, Soter N. Chronic actinic dermatitis: study of the spectrum of chronic photosensitivity in 12 patients. Arch Dermatol 1990; 126:317–323.

14. Norris PG, Hawk JL. Chronic actinic dermatitis: a unifying concept. Arch Dermatol 1990; 126:376–378.

15. Milde P, Holzle E, Neumann N, Lehmann P, Trautvetter U, Plewig G. Chronic actinic dermatitis. Concept and case examples. Hautartz 1991; 42:617–622.

16. Roelandts R. Chronic actinic dermatitis. J Am Acad Dermatol 1993; 28:240–249.

17. Ferguson J. Photosensitivity dermatitis and actinic reticuloid syndrome (chronic actinic dermatitis). Semin Dermatol 1990; 9:47–54.

18. du P. Menagé H, Ross J, Hawk JLM, White I. Contact and photocontact sensitisation in chronic actinic dermatitis: sesquiterpene lactone mix is an important allergen. Br J Dermatol 1995; 132:543–547.

19. Russell SC, Dawe RS, Collins P, Man I, Ferguson J. The photosensitivity dermatitis and actinic reticuloid syndrome (chronic actinic dermatitis) occurring in seven young atopic dermatitis patients. Br J Dermatol 1998; 138:496–501.

20. Von Den Driesch P, Fartasch M, Hornstein OP. Chronic actinic dermatitis with vitiligo-like depigmentation. Clin Exp Dermatol 1992; 17:38–43.

21. Kingston TP, Lowe NJ, Sofen HL, Weingarten DP. Actinic reticuloid in a black man: successful treatment with azathioprine. J Am Acad Dermatol 1987; 16:1079–1083.

22. Roelandts R, Huys I. Broad-band and persistent photosensitivity following accidental ultraviolet C overexposure. Photodermatol Photoimmunol Photomed 1993; 9:144–146.

23. Robinson HN, Morison WL, Hood AF. Thiazide diuretic therapy and chronic photosensitivity. Arch Dermatol 1985; 121:522–524.

24. Pappert A, Grossman M, Deleo V. Photosensitivity as the presenting illness in four patients with human immunodeficiency viral infection. Arch Dermatol Res 1994; 130:618–623.

25. Frain-Bell W. Photosensitivity and Compositae dermatitis. Clin Dermatol 1986; 4:122–126.

26. Hannuksela M, Suhonen R, Forstrom L. Delayed contact allergies in patients with photosensitivity dermatitis. Arch Dermatovenereol (Stockholm) 1981; 61:303–306.

27. Murphy GM, White IR, Hawk JLM. Allergic airbourne dermatitis to Compositae with photosensitivity—CAD in evolution. Photodermatol Photoimmunol Photomed 1990; 7:38–39.

28. Frain-Bell W, Hetherington A, Johnson BE. Contact allergic sensitivity to chrysanthemum and the photosensitivity dermatitis and actinic reticuloid syndrome. Br J Dermatol 1979; 101:491–501.

29. Addo HA, Sharma SC, Ferguson J, Johnson BE, Frain-Bell W. A study of Compositae plant extract reactions in photosensitivity dermatitis. Photodermatology 1985; 2:68–79.

30. Addo HA, Ferguson J, Johnson BE, Frain-Bell W. The relationship between exposure to fragrance materials and persistent light reaction in the photosensitivity dermatitis with actinic reticuloid syndrome. Br J Dermatol 1982; 107:261–274.

31. Thune P. Contact allergy due to lichens in patients with a history of photosensitivity. Contact Dermatitis 1977; 3:267–272.

32. Addo HA, Frain-Bell W. Persistence of allergic contact sensitivities in subjects with the photosensitive dermatitis and actinic reticuloid syndrome. Br J Dermatol 1987; 117:555–559.

33. Green C, Catterall M, Hawk JLM. Chronic actinic dermatitis and sunscreen allergy. Clin Exp Dermatol 1991; 16:70–71.

34. Healy E, Rogers S. Photosensitivity dermatitis/actinic reticuloid syndrome in an Irish population: a review and some unusual features. Acta Dermato-Venereologica 1995; 75:72–74.

35. Lim HW, Morison WL, Kamide R, Buchness MR, Harris R, Soter NA. Chronic actinic dermatitis: an analysis of 51 patients evaluated in the United States and Japan. Arch Dermatol Res 1994; 130:1284–1289.

36. Patel DC, McGregor JM, Ross JS, Hawk JLM. UVA associated eczematous photosensitivity and multiple contact allergies: a further form of chronic actinic dermatitis (abstr). Br J Dermatol 1998; 139(S):27.

37. Bisland D, Ferguson J. Management of chronic photosensitive eczema. Arch Dermatol 1991; 127:1065(letter).

38. Neild VS, Hawk JLM, Eady RAJ, Cream JJ. Actinic reticuloid with Sézary cells. Clin Exp Dermatol 1982; 7:143–148.

39. Preesman AH, Schrooyen SJ, Toonstra J, van der Putte SCJ, Rademakers LHMP, Willemze R, van Vloten WA. The diagnostic value of morphometry in blood lymphocytes in erythrodermic actinic reticuloid. Arch Dermatol 1995; 131:1298–1303.

40. Volden G, Thune PO. Light sensitivity in mycosis fungoides. Br J Dermatol 1977; 97:279–284.

41. du P. Menagé H, Whittaker SJ, Ng YL, Hamblin A, Smith NP, Hawk JLM. Analysis of T-cell receptor genes in chronic actinic dermatitis: no evidence of clonality (abstr). J Invest Dermatol 1992; 98:546.

42. Chu AC, Robinson D, Hawk JLM, Meacham R, Spittle MF, Smith NP. Immunologic differentiation for the Sézary syndrome due to cutaneous T-cell lymphoma and chronic actinic dermatitis. J Invest Dermatol 1986; 98:134–137.

43. Bakeks V, van Oostveen JW, Preesman AH, Meijer CJ, Willemze R. Differentiation between actinic reticuloid and cutaneous T cell lymphoma by T cell receptor gamma gene rearrangement analysis and immunophenotyping. J Clin Pathol 1998; 51:154–158.

44. Heller P, Wieczorek R, Waldo E, Meola T, Buchness MR, Soter NA, Lim HW. Chronic actinic dermatitis: an immunohistochemical study of its T-cell antigenic profile, with comparison to T-cell lymphoma. Am J Dermatopathol 1994; 165:510–516.

45. Jensen NE, Sneddon IB. Actinic reticuloid with lymphoma. Br J Dermatol 1970; 82:287–291.

46. Thestrup-Pedersen K, Zachariae C, Kaltoft K, Pallesen G, Sogaard H. Development of cutaneous pseudolymphoma following ciclosporin therapy of actinic reticuloid. Dermatologica 1988; 177:376–381.

47. Thomsen K. The development of Hodgkins disease in a patient with actinic reticuloid. Clin Exp Dermatol 1977; 2:109–113.

48. Ashinoff R, Buchness MR, Lim HW. Lymphoma in a black patient with actinic reticuloid treated with PUVA: Possible aetiologic considerations. J Am Acad Dermatol 1989; 21:1134–1137.

49. Meynadier J, Peyron JL, Barneon G, Guillot B, Habib A, Guilhou J-J. Hodgkin's disease complicating actinic reticulosis. Ann Dermatol Venereol 1984; 111:999–1003.

50. Tan RSH, Butterworth CM, McLaughlin H. Mycosis fungoides—a disease of antigen persistence. Br J Dermatol 1974; 91:607–611.

51. Bilsland D, Crombie IK, Ferguson J. Is the photosensitivity dermatitis/actinic reticuloid syndrome associated with cutaneous lymphoma (abstr)? Br J Dermatol 1993; 129(S);42.

52. Norris PG, Newton JA, Camplejohn RS. A flow cytometric study of actinic reticuloid. Clin Exp Dermatol 1989; 14:128–131.

53. Kochevar IE, Harber LC. Photoreactions of 3′, 3′, 4′, 5-tetrachlorosalicylanilide with proteins. J Invest Dermatol 1977; 68:151–156.

54. Rose N, Bona C. Defining criteria for autoimmune diseases (Witebsky's postulates revisited). Immunol Today 1993; 14:426–430.

55. Katsumura Y, Tanaka J, Icikawa H, Kato S, Kobayashi T, Horio T. Persistent light reaction: induction in the guinea pig. J Invest Dermatol 1986; 87:330–333.

56. Ichikawa H, Osaka T, Sato Y, Fukushima S. Adjuvant-induced persistent photosensitivity models in guinea pigs. I & II. Characterisation of immunological mechanisms. J Dermatol Sci 1995; 9:1–11.

57. Murphy GM, Maurice PM, Norris PG, Morris RW, Hawk JLM. Azathioprine in the treatment of chronic actinic dermatitis: a double-blind controlled trial with monitoring of exposure to ultraviolet radiation. Br J Dermatol 1989; 121:639–646.

58. Norris PG, Camp RDR, Hawk JLM. Actinic reticuloid: response to cyclosporin. J Am Acad Dermatol 1989; 307:21–22.

59. Parodi A, Gallo R, Guarrera M, Rebora A. Natural alpha interferon in chronic actinic dermatitis. Acta Dermato-Venereologica 1995; 75:80.

60. Orbeneja JG, Diez LI, Lozano JLS, Salazar LC. Lymphomatoid contact dermatitis: a syndrome produced by epicutaneous hypersensitivity with clinical features and a histopathologic picture similar to that of mycosis fungoides. Contact Dermatitis 1976; 2:139–143.

61. Braathen LR, Førre Ø, Natvig JB. An anti-human T-lymphocyte antiserum: in situ identification of T cells in the skin of delayed type hypersensitivity reactions, chronic photosensitivity dermatitis, and mycosis fungoides. Clin Immunol Immunopathol 1979; 13:211–219.

62. Ralfkiaer E, Lange Wantzin G, Stein H, Mason DY. Photosensitive dermatitis with actinic reticuloid syndrome: an immunohistological study of the cutaneous infiltrate. Br J Dermatol 1986; 114:47–56.

63. Takigawa M, Tokura Y, Shirahama S, Sugimoto H, Yamada M. Actinic Reticuloid: an immunohistochemical study. Arch Dermatol 1987; 123:296–297 (letter).

64. Toonstra H, van der Putte SCJ, van Wichen DF, van Weeldon H, Henquet CJM, van Vloten WA. Actinic reticuloid: immunohistochemical analysis of the cutaneous infiltrate in 13 patients. Br J Dermatol 1989; 120:779–786.

65. Norris PG, Morris J, Smith NP, Chu AC, Hawk JLM. Chronic actinic dermatitis: An immunohistologic and photobiologic study. J Am Acad Dermatol 1989; 21:966–971.

66. Fujita M, Miyachi Y, Horio T, Imamura S. Immunohistochemical comparison of actinic reticuloid with contact dermatitis. J Dermatol Sci 1990; 1:289–296.

67. du P. Managé H, Sattar N, Hawk JLM, Breathnach SM. Immunophenotyping of the inflammatory cell infiltrate during the evolution of induced lesions of chronic actinic dermatitis (abstr). J Invest Dermatol 1993; 100:482.

68. Gawkrodger DJ, McVittie E, Carr MM, Ross JA, Hunter JAA. Phenotypic characterisation of the early cellular responses in allergic and irritant contact dermatitis. Clin Exp Immunol 1986; 66:590–598.

69. Poulter LW, Seymour GJ, Duke O, Janossy G, Panayi G. Immunohistological analysis of delayed type hypersensitivity in man. Cell Immunol 1982; 74:358–369.

70. Vandervleuten CJM, Kroot EJA, Dejong EMJ, Vanderkerkhof PCM. The immunohistochemical effects of a single challenge with an intermediate dose of ultraviolet B on normal human skin. Arch Dermatol Res 1996; 288:510–516.

71. Kofoed ML, Munch-Petersen B, Larsen JK, Lange Wantzin G. Non-replicative DNA synthesis detected in peripheral lymphocytes from a patient with actinic reticuloid. Photodermatology 1986; 3:158–163.

72. Norris DA, Bradley-Lyons M, Middleton MH, Yohn JJ, Kashihara-Sawani M. Ultraviolet radiation can either suppress or induce expression of intercellular adhesion molecule 1 on the surface of cultured human keratinocytes. J Invest Dermatol 1990; 95:132–138.

73. Griffiths CEM, Barker JNWN, Kunkel S, Nickoloff BJ. Modulation of leukocyte adhesion molecules, a T-cell chemotactin (IL-8), and a regulatory cytokine (TNF-$\alpha$) in allergic contact dermatitis (rhus dermatitis). Br J Dermatol 1991; 124:519–526.

74. du P. Menagé H, Sattar N, Haskard DO, Hawk JLM, Breathnach SM. A study of the kinetics and pattern of adhesion molecule expression in induced lesions of chronic actinic dermatitis. Br J Dermatol 1996; 134:262–268.

75. Norris PGN, Poston RN, Thomas DS. The expression of endothelial leukocyte adhesion molecule-1 (ELAM-1), intercellular adhesion molecule-1 (ICAM-1), and vascular cell adhesion molecule-1 (VCAM-1) in experimental cutaneous inflammation: a comparison of ultraviolet B erythema and delayed type hypersensitivity. J Invest Dermatol 1991; 96:763–770.

76. du P. Menagé H, Kristensen M, Chu CQ, Brennan FM, Hawk JLM, Breathnach SM. Upregulation of interleukin 1$\alpha$, its receptor and interleukin 1 receptor antagonist levels in induced lesions of chronic actinic dermatitis (abstr). Br J Dermatol 1992; 127(S):429.

77. Sepulveda-Merill C, du P. Menagé H, Hawk JLM, Breathnach SM. Functional studies of antigen presentation in induced lesions of chronic actinic dermatitis (abstr). J Invest Dermatol 1994; 102:603.

78. Willis I, Kligman AM. The mechanism of the persistent light reactor. J Invest Dermatol 1968; 51:385–394.

79. Swanbeck G, Wennersten G. Evidence for kynurenic acid as a potential photosensitiser in actinic reticuloid. Acta Dermato-Venerologica (Stockh) 1973; 53:109–113.

80. Binazzi M, Calandra P. Actinic reticuloid pathogenic aspects. Arch Dermatol Forsch 1971; 241:391–395.

81. Vonderheid EC, Sobel EL, Hoeldtke RD, Faeber GJ, Sardi VS. Kynurenic acid and xanthurenic acid excretion after tryptophan loading in actinic reticuloid. Int J Dermatol 1987; 26: 33–41.

82. Harber LC, Bickers DR. Persistent light reactivity. In: Photosensitivity Disease: Principles of Diagnosis and Treatment. 2d ed. Philadelphia: B.C. Decker Inc., 1989:181–183.

83. du P. Menagé H, Harrison GI, Potten CS, Young AR, Hawk JLM. The action spectrum for induction of chronic actinic dermatitis is similar to that for sunburn inflammation. Photochem Photobiol 1995; 62:976–979.

84. Baadsgaard O. In vivo ultraviolet irradiation causes profound perturbation of the immune system. Arch Dermatol 1991; 127:99–109.

85. Gianelli F, Botcherby PK, Marimo B, Magnus IA. Cellular hypersensitivity to UVA: a clue to the aetiology of actinic reticuloid? Lancet 1983; 1:88–91.

86. Johnson BE, Walker EM, Ferguson J, Frain-Bell W. Cellular sensitivity to UVA in photosensitivity dermatitis/actinic reticuloid (PD/AR) (abstr). Br J Dermatol 1988; 118:286.

87. Gibbs NK, Botcherby PK, Morris RW, Young AR, Gianelli F. UVA dose response of normal and actinic reticuloid cell fibroblasts: a statistical analysis (abstr). Br J Dermatol 1988; 118: 289.

88. Applegate LA, Frenk E, Gibbs N, Johnson B, Ferguson F, Tyrell RM. Cellular sensitivity to oxidative stress in the photosensitivity dermatitis/actinic reticuloid syndrome. J Invest Dermatol 1994; 102:762–767.

89. Kondo S, Nishioka K. Hypersensitivity of skin fibroblasts from patients with chronic actinic dermatitis to ultraviolet B (UVB), UVA and superoxide radical. Photodermatol Photoimmunol Photomed 1991; 8:212–217.

90. Hindson C, Spiro J, Downey A. PUVA therapy of chronic actinic dermatitis. Br J Dermatol 1984; 113:156–160.

91. Hindson C, Downey A, Sinclair S. PUVA therapy of chronic actinic dermatitis: a 5 year follow-up. Br J Dermatol 1990; 123:273 (letter).

92. Humbert P, Drobacheff C, Vigan M, Quencez E, Laurent R, Agache P. Chronic actinic dermatitis responding to danazol. Br J Dermatol 1991; 124:195–197.

93. Dawe R, Crombie I, Ferguson J. The natural history of the photosensitivity dermatitis and actinic reticuloid syndrome (abstr). Br J Dermatol 1998; 139(S):51.

94. Sigurdsson V, Toonstra J, Hezemans-Boer M, van Vloten WA. Erythroderma. A clinical and follow-up study of 102 patients, with a special emphasis on survival. J Am Acad Dermatol 1996; 35:53–57.

# 12

## Latex Allergy

**James S. Taylor and Penpun Wattanakrai**
*Cleveland Clinic, Cleveland, Ohio*

**B. Lauren Charous**
*Milwaukee Medical Clinic, Milwaukee, Wisconsin*

**Dennis Ownby**
*Medical College of Georgia, Augusta, Georgia*

## I. INTRODUCTION

Natural rubber latex (NRL) is a ubiquitous part of life today. Because of its strength, elasticity, flexibility, and barrier properties, NRL is the main constituent of numerous medical and consumer products, although this fact is not always obvious when the products are examined (Table 1). Two types of allergic reactions to rubber products are now known.

The first, delayed-type hypersensitivity (type IV Gell and Coombs classification) [1], is caused mainly by chemicals added during the manufacturing of natural or synthetic rubber [2]. Commonly known as allergic contact dermatitis, this reaction has been known for nearly 60 years, is cell-mediated, and is diagnosed by patch testing [3].

The second, immediate-type hypersensitivity (type I Gell and Coombs classification) [1], was first reported in Germany in 1927 [3] and not again until 1979 in England by Nutter [4] and in 1980 in Finland by Förström [5]. Köpman and Hannuksela were the first to suggest an IgE-mediated mechanism in 1983 based on a positive passive transfer test in two subjects [6], and later Turjanmaa et al. [7], using radioimmunoassay, was able to find specific IgE antibodies against latex in two female nurses experiencing anaphylactic symptoms while undergoing gynecological operations. Although there are approximately 240 separate proteins in NRL, less than 25% show reactivity with IgE antibodies. IgE antibodies in the serum can be quantitated by the radioallergosorbent test (RAST). IgE antibodies fixed to cells may be quantitated by the response of the cells when challenged with the specific latex protein allergens—either in vivo, as in the cutaneous skin test, or in vitro, as in the basophil histamine release test [8]. Thus the term ''latex allergy'' generally refers to this IgE-mediated immediate hypersensitivity reaction to NRL proteins with protean clinical manifestations ranging from contact urticaria to fatal anaphylaxis. With the increasing number of cases, NRL allergy has become a major medical, occupational health, medicolegal, and financial problem [2,9–17].

**Table 1**  Products That May Contain Natural Rubber Latex

General medical products
  Gloves
  Finger cots
  Elastic bandage
  Adhesive tape
  Dressings
  Blood pressure cuffs, tubing
  Stethoscope tubing
  Oral, nasal airways
  Syringes
  Electrode pads
  Electrocardiographic pads
  Tourniquets
  Hot water bottles
  Elastic support stockings
  Wound drains (rubber, Penrose)
  Gastrostomy tubes
  Feeding tubes
  Intestinal tubes
  Catheters
  Wheelchair tires
  Absorbent bed pads
  Rubber sheets, pillows
  Crutches (arm and hand pads)
  Enema kits
  Enema retention cuffs
  Ileostomy bags
  Urine bags and straps
  Eye dropper bulbs
  Reflex hammers
  Soft casts
  Vascular stockings
Anesthesia/respiratory supplies
  Endotracheal tubes
  Face masks
  Airways
  Rubber suction catheters
  Teeth protectors
  Ambu bags
  Ventilator bellows
  Ventilator tubing
  Breathing circuits
  Reservoir breathing circuits
  Manual resuscitators
  Pulse oximeters
Intravenous supplies
  Rubber tops of multidose vials
  PRN adaptor (heparin lock)
  Bags, intravenous tubing (latex
    injection ports)

  Medication pumps
  Infusion sets
  Y-sites
  Buretrol ports
Dental supplies
  Dental dams
  Coffer dams
  Bite blocks
  Teeth protectors
  Orthodontic elastic
  Prophy cups
  Root canal materials
Obstetric/gynecological products
  Condoms
  Cervical caps
  Diaphragms
  Cervical dilators
  Rubber vaginal vibrators
  Douche bulbs
Personal protective equipment
  Gloves
  Surgical masks
  Disposable hats, shoe covers
  Goggles
  Respirators
  Rubber aprons
Office supplies
  Rubber bands
  Pencil erasers
  Stamps
  Art and craft supplies (paints, glue,
    fabric paints)
Household and consumer products
  Household gloves
  Balloons
  Automobile tires
  Motorcycle, bicycle handgrips
  Carpet backing and pads
  Swimming goggles
  Swim caps
  Snorkeling/scuba equipment
  Sport racquet handles
  Shoe soles
  Expandable fabric
  Stretch textile
  Waistbands
  Underwear elastic
  Pacifiers
  Baby bottle nipples
  Infant toothbrushes—gum massagers

**Table 1**  Continued

| | |
|---|---|
| Rubber toys | Disposable diapers, incontinence pads |
| Rubber balls | Rubber pants |
| Raincoats | Rubber cement |
| Shower curtains | Halloween masks |
| Bath mats | Zippered plastic storage bags |
| Window insulation | |
| Air mattresses | |
| Whoopee cushions | |
| Squash balls | |
| Foam rubber | |

*Source*: Refs. 9, 13, 158, 251, 265.

Since early 1990, there has been a disproportional increase in type I allergies to NRL, which may be due to several factors including [9,12,13,18]:

1. Increased frequency and duration of exposure to NRL-containing barrier devices, mostly latex gloves, as a result of the Centers for Disease Control (CDC) recommendation of "universal precautions" on August 21, 1987 [19].
2. Changes in the manufacturing process for latex gloves. Due to increased demands, many new, inexperienced manufacturers of NRL gloves began production in the 1980s. In some cases this probably resulted in poorly compounded and inadequately leached products with higher allergen content.
3. Bias of ascertainment or increased recognition of NRL by clinicians and improved diagnostic techniques.
4. Increased awareness of NRL allergy by latex-exposed health-care workers or individuals routinely exposed to rubber products.
5. Possibly a true increase in latex allergy parallel to increased atopy and sensitivity to many allergens in western populations.

## II.  NOMENCLATURE

Terminology established by the Latex Task Force of the Health Industry Manufacturers Association (HIMA) identifies natural latex as a milky fluid of agricultural origin produced by the *Hevea brasiliensis* tree; natural rubber latex (NRL) refers to products made directly from water-based natural latex emulsions [9,13]. Gloves, balloons, tourniquets, and condoms are examples of products produced by dipping porcelain forms into liquid latex. Dry rubber latex refers to products made from processed, dried, or milled sheets of latex rubber. Syringe plungers, vial stoppers, and baby nipples are examples of extruded or compression-molded dry products. Most immediate-type reactions result from exposure to NRL products that are dipped. A study by Yunginger et al. [20] confirmed that dry-molded rubber products contain lower residual latex protein levels or have less easily extracted proteins than do dipped products produced from NRL.

The biology, source, composition, and processing of natural latex have been extensively reviewed by Hamann [13] and Warshaw [9].

## III.  EPIDEMIOLOGY AND RISK FACTORS

Prevalence measures the total number of people sensitized at a point in time, whereas incidence describes the frequency of new cases occurring during a time period within a defined population [13]. Most epidemiological studies published to date have been confined to single time-point prevalence assessments, with prevalence rates widely varying due to the study design, study population, sample size, and diagnostic testing methodology used. The incidence of NRL allergy is still unknown, with only one prospective study by Sussman et al. [21] estimating 1% incidence of sensitization in hospital personnel using latex gloves. Further longitudinal and case-control studies are needed to determine the incidence, prevalence, and risk factors of NRL allergy.

It is generally known that high prevalence rates have been found in health-care workers, spina bifida patients, and atopic populations. But anyone with repeated exposure to gloves or other NRL products are at risk. Other significant risk factors include atopy, multiple surgical procedures, preexisting hand eczema, food and fruit allergy, and female gender [2,4,9–15].

### A.  General Population

The prevalence of NRL in the general population has generally been quoted to be low— less than 1–2% [14,22–27]. Turjanmaa et al. [23] found only one (0.12%) of 804 unselected adult Finns prick-tested before surgery to have NRL allergy. In contrast to this, other studies of preoperative patients, annual check-up patients, and blood donors found a prevalence of 6–8% [28–32]. Of importance is that not all persons diagnosed as being sensitized to NRL, by either SPT or presence of IgE-mediated antibodies, will have clinical symptoms; the clinical relevance of these findings needs further evaluation.

### B.  Spina Bifida

Children with spina bifida (SB)/meningomyelocele (MM) are known to have the highest prevalence of latex allergy. After the first cases were reported in 1989 by Slater [17], who described two SB children with perioperative latex-induced anaphylactic shock, many others followed. In 1991, the CDC alerted medical personnel of this high-risk group [33]. The high prevalence rates in this group ranges from 30 to 65% [26,34–47].

In contrast to these high prevalence rates, a study of 93 SB patients in Venezuela showed a low rate of sensitization, with only 4 patients (4.3%) having NRL allergy by skin testing. The authors concluded that this was due to a low level of rubber exposure as a result of socioeconomic factors, best exemplified by the use of nonlatex catheters, by frequently washed and resterilized surgeons' gloves, and by low numbers of operations per patient [43].

The high prevalence of latex allergy in most SB patients is related to repeated exposure to NRL via multiple surgical, therapeutic, and diagnostic procedures. Many studies have shown that the main risk factors for latex sensitization in this unique patient group are multiple operations and atopic predisposition (either asthma, food allergy, or elevated total IgE) [37–39,42,44,46]. Likewise, patients with a history of multiple surgical interventions and/or multiple congenital anomalies are also at risk of sensitization to NRL [29,37].

Although these prevalence rates are high, not all of the sensitized SB patients will have clinical symptoms; however, these children may later progress to have severe reactions including life-threatening anaphylaxis. The risk of anaphylactic reactions in the operating room was greater than 500-fold in spina bifida patients when compared to controls, and the rate of anaphylaxis in patients with spina bifida was estimated approximately to be 13.5% [9,45].

## C. Occupational Exposure

Anyone in an occupation that requires them to routinely wear protective gloves or regularly exposes them to NRL may develop NRL allergy. Most prevalence studies have been done in health-care workers [48–68], where overall rates of sensitization range from as low as 1% to to as high as 16%. Sensitization rates are significantly higher, 30–70% [69–73], in symptomatic health-care workers.

Other, non–health-care occupations with regular exposure to NRL gloves have comparable rates of sensitization [74–78]. These include kitchen workers; cleaners; rubber band, surgical glove, and latex-doll manufacturing workers; paper mill workers; secretaries; caregivers; dairy farmers; artists; cashiers; and horse farmers [10–12,23].

## D. Atopic Population

Atopy is most often defined as evidence of a person having developed IgE antibodies to one or more common allergens. In most epidemiological studies, this means that a person has one or more positive skin or in vitro tests for IgE antibodies. Atopy is common among latex-sensitive individuals and has been considered as a risk factor for latex sensitivity. The prevalence of latex allergy in various studies in the atopic-allergy population is summarized in References 23, 25, 27, 56, and 79–83.

## E. Hand Eczema

Associated or preexisting hand eczema is common in patients with NRL allergy and is often mentioned as a significant risk factor for NRL allergy [12,13,15,84–86]. Chronic hand eczema and atopy often coexist, [84] and individuals with hand eczema and atopic dermatitis often wear NRL gloves, which increases their exposure to NRL protein allergens. In Turjanmaa's series of 124 adults [11], 75% of the health-care workers and 81% of those in other occupations had a personal history of atopy and, with the same frequency, hand eczema, but not always in the same person at the same time. Eighty-three of the 124 with NRL allergy were patch tested, with 11 (13%) having positive reactions to rubber chemical or mixes [11]. In Taylor and Praditsuwan's series of 44 patients with NRL allergy, also in a dermatology department, 36 had hand eczema with 26 having relevant positive patch test results, especially to glutaraldehyde, rubber chemicals, latex gloves, and preservatives [10]. Thus, it is important to emphasize that concomitant type IV and type I allergy to rubber products may co-exist in the same patient [10,13,87–90].

Preexisting hand eczema—either atopic, irritant, or allergic contact dermatitis in nature—may mask signs of contact urticaria, and NRL allergy should be suspected when symptoms of pruritus, burning, and stinging occur on donning NRL gloves or after exposure to other NRL devices [10,13]. Additionally, some glove-wearing NRL-allergic patients may present with only persistent hand eczema [14].

## F. Female Gender

Women predominate in most reports of NRL glove allergy, and female gender may increase the incidence of NRL sensitivity. This has been postulated to occur because women wear gloves more frequently than men and predominate in the nursing professions [9,15]. However, recent studies found that male gender increases the risk of latex sensitization in ambulatory surgical patients and in volunteer blood donors [28,30,31].

## IV. NRL ALLERGENS

Allergic reactions to natural rubber products are due to IgE-binding antibodies directed against a wide range of NRL constituent polypeptides [91–107]; details are summarized in several comprehensive reviews [108–111]. An international convention has been developed for naming individual pure allergens [126]. The allergen is named using the first three letters of the genus name, followed by the first letter of the species name, followed by an Arabic numeral. This first allergen should be a dominant allergen, meaning that it is recognized by a majority of persons allergic to the crude allergen. Thus, for latex coming from *Hevea brasilensis*, the first purified allergen, from the crude mixture of latex allergens, would be named Hev b1, the second allergen Hev b2, etc. Table 2 lists the currently recognized latex allergens. Within this list of allergens is the cluster of Hev b6. This cluster is the result of the same allergic portion of a molecule remaining intact as a protein is altered within the plant. The initial protein is preprohevein, which is cleaved to prohevein and then cleaved to hevein. The N-terminal fragment of prohevein is cleaved off as hevein and has significant allergenicity. The C-terminal fragment also has some allergenicity. Considerable efforts have been expended over the last several years at isolating, purifying, and molecular sequencing of these allergenic peptides in NRL. These proteins are found both in ammoniated raw latex and in extracts from manufactured products. In addition to proteins formally recognized by the IUIS, hevamine, Class I and III chitinases, manganese superoxide dismutase, enolase, a lysozyme [112], as well as an isomerase and proteasome subunit have been identified [109]. Many of these antigens are plant stress

**Table 2** Allergenic Proteins of Natural Rubber Latex[a]

| Allergen | Common name | Molecular weight | % Reactivity |
|---|---|---|---|
| Hev b1 | Rubber elongation factor (REF) | 14.6, 58 | 22 |
| Hev b2 | β-1-3-Gluconase | 34–36 | ? |
| Hev b3 | Prenyltransferase | 24–27 | ? |
| Hev b4 | Microhalix | 100,110,115 | ? |
| Hev b5 | Acidic protein | 16–24 | 62 |
| Hev b6 | | | |
| 6.01 | Prohevein | 20 | 60 |
| 6.02 | Hevein | 14 | 60 |
| 6.03 | Pro-hevein C domain | 5 | 60 |
| Hev b7 | Patatin homolog | 43–46 | 23 |
| Hev b8 | Proflin | 15–16 | ? |

[a] Allergen designation by the International Union of Immunological Societies (IUIS).
*Source*: Adapted from Refs. 119, 231.

proteins, which are widely conserved in the botanical world, a fact that helps explain the extensive number of cross-reacting foods and plants that have been identified.

The pattern of reactivity to latex antigens appears to vary predictably among distinct allergic populations. Children with spina bifida appear to preferentially develop IgE antibodies to 24 kDa and 27 kDa proteins [103,113], while health-care workers are most commonly sensitized to a 46 kDa protein [101]. Whether these differences are due to antigenic variability in the latex products to which individuals are exposed or to differences in the mode of exposure remains under active investigation. In this regard, one preliminary study showed that a prior history of contact dermatitis in health-care workers did not alter the pattern of sensitivity [114].

The unanticipated and epidemic nature of latex allergy has suggested that some cofactor, hapten, or adjuvant may contribute to the sensitizing process. One possibility is that neo-antigens are formed during vulcanization and processing; however, no antigens or epitopes that are unique to finished NRL products have thus far been identified. Evidence for the participation of chemicals and other substances found in rubber products either as alternate antigens or as adjuvants has been aggressively sought, but no definitive proof confirming that other substances play such a role has emerged. Despite some initial reports suggesting that corn starch proteins might serve as a second primary allergen [115,116], convincing confirmatory studies are lacking. Alternatively, the capacity of several chemicals used in rubber manufacture, such as thiuram and mercaptobenzothiazole, to generate immunologically specific cell-mediated reactions has raised similar but equally unanswered questions regarding their potential contribution as haptens to atopic sensitization to latex proteins.

It has recently been proposed that endotoxin, which is a frequent and measurable contaminant in latex gloves, may serve as a potent adjuvant [117]. Endotoxin possesses several properties that appear relevant for a potential role as a cofactor in the pathogenesis of latex allergy and occupational asthma. Endotoxin has proinflammatory properties and can act as both an adjuvant and B-cell mitogen for IgE responses to the latex allergen Hev b5 in BALB/c mice [118]. Taken together, these effects serve as a plausible explanation for the observed generation of IgE antibodies directed at a wide range of latex constituent proteins found in many individuals with latex allergy. However, the preliminary nature of these findings suggests that a substantial amount of additional work is needed to confirm this hypothesis. Additional data concerning the amounts of endotoxin present in hospitals and operating rooms must be collected and shown to reach significant levels. Furthermore, while the adjuvant and pro-inflammatory effects of endotoxin seen in vitro murine systems are of interest, they cannot be uncritically assumed to have direct relevance for human in vivo responses. In humans, endotoxin is not a B-cell mitogen, its ability to act as an immune adjuvant is unknown, and its ability to augment atopic responses remains to be demonstrated. The nature, extent, and length of exposure required to generate these putative effects must be carefully evaluated [119].

## V. FOOD AND FRUIT ALLERGY

Allergists have recognized cross-reactivity between certain allergens for a number of years. As commonly used, the term cross-reactivity means that IgE antibodies produced to one allergen will also recognize a second allergen to a variable degree. Cross-reactivity may or may not be clinically significant. In some cases, cross-reactivity appears to cause allergic disease when a person is exposed to either the primary allergen or the cross-reactive allergen. In other cases, disease is only associated with the primary allergen. Cross-reactivity may occur in several ways. Since most crude allergens are mixtures of many different proteins, it is possible that the same or a very similar protein exists in both allergens. It is also possible for two different proteins to have sections that are substantially the same, either in primary amino acid sequence or in three-dimensional conformation [120–128].

Allergic reactions to multiple foods appear to occur with an unusual frequency and severity in latex-allergic individuals. Initial reports described reactions to tropical fruits such as banana, kiwi, and avocado as well as to European chestnuts [129–131]. The list of foods cross-reacting with NRL has expanded to become the most extensive of any known allergen and now includes melons, peaches, plums, and other stone fruits, celery, carrot, apple, pear, papaya, mango, citrus fruits, fig, wheat germ, hazelnut, potato, and tomato [132,133]. In addition, several reports document an association between latex allergy and sensitization to latex from the weeping figs (*Ficus benjamina*) [134,135].

Immunological cross-reactivity between proteins in NRL and other proteins widely conserved in the botanical world, such as the plant stress proteins patatin and chitinase, at least partially explains the unexpected prevalence of food allergy in latex allergy patients [136,137].

Allergic reactions to cross-reactive foods should be anticipated in latex-allergic individuals. Inasmuch as the initial manifestation of food allergy can be anaphylaxis, patients should be educated about the risk of food allergy and be instructed to always carry a personal epinephrine syringe. The degree of sensitivity to latex allergen is a poor predictor both of the risk of developing food allergy and of the severity of a reaction. In the event of a food reaction more severe than oral itching or swelling, which necessitates the use of epinephrine, patients should proceed immediately to an emergency room for observation, since late, even fatal, reactions can occur up to 4–6 hours postingestion of food allergen. In the event of a reaction, patients should avoid closely related foods (e.g., peaches, plums, cherries, nectarines, apricots) [120–128].

Patients with oral allergy syndrome (oral itching and swelling) provoked by cross-reacting foods appear to be at increased risk of latex sensitization [138,139]. Descriptions of heightened reactions or a widening range of provoking foods should be viewed as potential warning signs of latex allergy. In this event appropriate diagnostic evaluation and safeguards should be initiated.

## VI. CLINICAL MANIFESTATIONS

Clinical symptoms of NRL allergy are dependent on individual susceptibility to the allergen, the mode and route of exposure, and the amount of bioavailable protein allergen. Symptoms usually result from direct contact with a NRL product but may also result from inhalation of aerosolized powder containing NRL protein. The spectrum of symptoms and signs ranges from nonspecific pruritus, burning, and localized urticaria to generalized urticaria, allergic rhinitis, allergic conjunctivitis, angioedema asthma, and anaphylaxis. Localized symptoms of NRL allergy may be superimposed on preexisting, chronic irritant or allergic eczematous hand dermatitis. The skin is most frequently involved, followed by nasal, ocular, and pulmonary symptoms. Less common but also reported are gastrointestinal and cardiovascular symptoms [2,4,9–17,23,56,73,78,140–168].

## A.  Contact Urticaria

The skin is frequently involved in NRL allergic reactions, presumably because of frequent and prolonged cutaneous exposure to latex allergens. Contact urticaria presents as a spectrum of cutaneous manifestations—pruritus, burning, erythema, and edema (urticaria)—usually starting within 15 minutes of exposure and disappearing without treatment within 1–2 hours. Initially, symptoms may be limited to itching and mild erythema [59]. As sensitivity or exposure increases, urticaria and edema may develop [149]. In sensitive health-care workers, symptoms may appear more rapidly if the hands or gloves are wet or if the gloves produce significant pressure [149]. Urticaria may initially be limited to areas of direct latex contact, but it may spread to contiguous skin and become generalized. Health-care workers often give a history of first noticing itching of the hands following gloving. With continued use of gloves over weeks or months, the symptoms often develop sooner after donning gloves, and urticaria may develop. After additional weeks, generalized urticaria may develop along with other accelerated type I allergic symptoms. In some individuals, symptoms do not extend beyond the hands, but the pruritus and edema become more intense to the point of being described as immediate burning [162].

In addition to symptoms of contact urticaria, some NRL-allergic patients may present with a chronic hand eczema [10,12,14,66,69,169]. Sixty-seven percent of Turjanmaa's NRL-allergic hospital employees were found to have hand eczema. After the withdrawal of latex gloves, the eczema resolved in several patients despite the fact that they did not have type IV contact allergy to rubber chemicals [169]. Dyshidrosis and eczematous changes similar to protein contact dermatitis has also been described in cases with latex allergy [10,15].

Patients presenting with hand eczema as the only manifestation of NRL allergy may be easily misdiagnosed, as they may be clinically identical to irritant and allergic contact dermatitis [11,12].

Protein contact dermatitis was a term introduced by Hjorth and Roed-Petersen to describe patients with recurrent eczema who demonstrated immediate reactions when affected skin is exposed to certain protein-containing foods, as observed in bakers, butchers, kitchen workers, and veterinarians [170]. Within 30 minutes to 6 hours of exposure, the patient experiences clinical features ranging from pruritus, erythema, burning to urticaria, and in some cases dyshidrotic vesicles [170]. Secondary eczematous changes, suggested to represent an IgE-mediated late-phase reaction, may develop at the area of contact 6–48 hours later [171]. Latex-induced protein contact dermatitis was first described by Kleinhans [172] in a 23-year-old nurse with hand eczema and urticaria thought to be caused by latex gloves. Similar reports from Turjanmaa and Reunala seem to confirm this clinical entity [173]. Some of Taylor and Praditsuwan's 44 patients with NRL allergy presented with localized skin reactions consistent with protein contact dermatitis [10].

## B.  Respiratory and Anaphylactic Reactions

The clinical variability in presentation of NRL allergy is noteworthy. Perhaps the most striking feature is the exquisite degree of sensitivity reflected in the occurrence of severe reactions experienced by a substantial number of sensitized individuals. Reports of contact urticaria and angioedema resulting from casual contact with donning powder residue on furniture surfaces or clothing, respiratory difficulties elicited by the snapping of powdered gloves in the proximity of sensitized individuals, and anaphylaxis induced by exposure to trace amounts of latex carried home on clothing or on food handled with powdered latex gloves all underline the usual propensity of this allergen to evoke potentially catastrophic reactions in allergic individuals [169,170].

Mucosal swelling is a typical symptom after oral, vaginal, or rectal exposure to NRL products such as balloons, gloves, and condoms or after dental, rectal, or gynecological exams [15,141–147].

Although cutaneous exposure to NRL usually results in contact urticaria, some cases of anaphylaxis have been reported [147,174]. In contrast, mucosal, visceral, and parenteral exposures are associated with the greatest risk for developing severe systemic reactions [144,145,166–168]. In the United States, exposure to latex balloons used during retention barium enemas caused several anaphylactic deaths [151,175,176]; these have now been replaced with synthetic devices [150,153].

In addition, anaphylactic reactions have been documented in patients, particularly in patients undergoing surgical [147,177–179], dental [17,180,181], gynecological or obstetrical [144,167,168], or urological examination or procedures [179,182]. Latex condoms may induce acute reactions via vaginal mucosal exposure [94,147,183,184]. Other reported medical devices causing anaphylaxis include Foley catheters, latex balloon trip catheters, dental cofferdams, endotrachial tubes, and electrocardiographic pads [177]. However, reports of anaphylaxis outside the health-care system do occur (i.e., from toy balloons, baby bottle nipples/pacifiers, squash balls, food handled with latex gloves, rubber vaginal vibrators, expelled air from a whoopee cushion, and condoms) [177,180].

Latex causes at least 10% of intraoperative reactions [148,149]. The diagnosis of latex-induced intraoperative anaphylaxis may be easily missed because its manifestations may be limited to mild to moderate hypotension and increased airway resistance due to bronchospasm; other, more suggestive signs of an acute allergic reaction, such as urticaria and angioedema, may not occur in a hypotensive anesthetized patient. In this setting, intraoperative difficulties may be incorrectly attributed to other causes, such as a reaction to an anesthetic agent, ethylene oxide, or a drug given earlier, such as an antibiotic. Thus, the differential diagnosis of any case of intraoperative or unexplained anaphylaxis must include an allergic reaction due to latex exposure in a patient with unsuspected latex allergy.

Latex anaphylaxis has also been reported among patients with no recognizable risk factors, thus mandating a cautious attitude on the part of health-care givers who provide procedures that expose patients' mucosal and/or serosal surfaces to high concentrations of latex antigens [26,30,31,139,154].

Allergic rhinoconjunctivitis and asthma have been described in workers exposed to latex aeroallergens. Such diagnoses are suggested by the onset of nasal congestion, rhinorrhea, sneezing or lacrimation, ocular injection or mucosal pruritus occurring on exposure at work. Asthmatic symptoms, including chest tightness, persistent cough, shortness of breath, or wheezing, occur with long-term exposure and may persist beyond immediate exposures and thus may not be as readily perceived as related to latex exposure. Although respiratory symptoms can be the initial manifestation of latex allergy, more commonly these symptoms occur in workers with contact urticaria and represent a progression and generalization of sensitization due to ongoing exposure to latex aeroallergen [69]. Latex-containing aerosols may be generated in some industrial settings (manufacturing facilities for latex gloves and dolls) sufficient to induce asthma [78,185,186]. However, the preponderance of respiratory illness appears to be linked to the use of powdered latex gloves. Donning glove powders bind latex allergen [187,188] resulting in the production of measurable aeroallergen levels [189–191] that have been shown to be directly dependent on active use of powdered gloves [190].

According to several recent reports [78,186,192,193], occupational asthma, induced by ongoing respiration of these allergens, already affects 2.5% or more of exposed health-care and manufacturing workers. Vandenplas reported that nearly half of latex skin-test–positive workers demonstrated bronchospasm on specific inhalation challenge with latex gloves even in the absence of any workplace asthmatic complaints [194]. These observations suggest that persistent exposure to latex aeroallergen may place latex allergic workers at risk of development of occupational asthma, which, in turn, may result in persistent asthmatic symptomatology even after cessation of occupational exposure [195–198].

Symptoms of occupational asthma usually worsen at work. However, a lack of correlation between presumed exposure and perceived symptoms may be due to the uneven and intermittent nature of latex aeroallergen exposure and the persistence of asthmatic symptoms after exposure. Further confusion results from failure to recognize that sufficient latex aeroallergen may be generated when coworkers wear powdered latex gloves, causing asthma in allergic employees who follow recommended measures of personal NRL avoidance [15].

## VII. DIAGNOSTIC TESTING FOR LATEX ALLERGY

While latex allergy is most frequently suggested by characteristic symptoms, confirmation of the diagnosis rests on the demonstration of latex-specific anti-IgE antibodies. Diagnostic tests can rely on either in vitro measurements using RAST, enzyme-linked immunosorbent assay (ELISA), Western blot assays, or in vivo prick skin tests. Studies suggest that significant differences in specificity and sensitivity may exist between various commercial U.S. Food and Drug Administration (FDA)–approved in vitro assays. A recent preliminary report showed discordant positive results in 9–25% of assays between three FDA-licensed reagents, a finding that recommends caution in overreliance on these test results [199]. Attempts to increase reliability by the addition of IgE Western blots as a further in vitro diagnostic test have not proved rewarding [200].

As compared to in vitro methods, skin prick testing appears substantially more sensitive [26,34,201,202]. Two earlier studies reported skin testing with either a standard ammoniated latex preparation (Bencard, Mississauga, Ontario, Canada) or with glove extract to be approximately 25–35% more sensitive than commercial in vitro assays, without apparent loss of specificity [203,204]. Current research into the development of a standardized validated NRL extract is proceeding [205–207]. In a recent multicenter trial involving 134 subjects, one such extract developed by Hamilton and colleagues at Johns Hopkins University and Greer Laboratories showed a 95% sensitivity and 96% specificity at 100 µg/ml concentration at an acceptable rate of complications limited to at most only mild systemic reactions. Initial comparison of this standardized reagent with in vitro tests verified superior sensitivity of skin testing as compared to two commonly used in vitro assays, the Pharmacia-UpJohn CAP and the Diagnostic Products Corporation's AlaSTAT assays. Despite the diagnostic difficulties engendered by the limited sensitivity of in vitro testing, skin testing with uncharacterized extracts made from NRL products is discouraged due to significant variations in allergenic concentration [208], which may provoke severe reactions [208]. Instead, in cases where suspicions of latex allergy are not confirmed by in vitro testing and an adequate skin test reagent is not available, use of a validated glove provocation procedure [209] should be considered but should probably be limited to specialized centers capable of managing severe reactions.

In latex-allergic workers who have symptoms of airway obstruction and supporting findings of bronchial hyperresponsiveness, the diagnosis of occupational asthma should be entertained. In some cases, the repetitive and witnessed conjunction of acute urticaria, rhinoconjunctivitis, and asthma or anaphylaxis occurring on passive exposure to powdered latex gloves is sufficient for diagnosis. In the majority of cases, confirmation that asthmatic symptoms are due to latex exposure on the job is most frequently accomplished by use of serial monitoring of pulmonary functions. Preshift, mid-shift, and postshift peak expiratory flows or spirometric studies should be compared to baseline values obtained during weekends or, in more severe cases, after cessation of exposure for one or more weeks. Characteristic decreases in expiratory flows or changes in the PC20 values on methacholine challenge following exposure substantiate the existence of a causal relationship between exposure to latex aeroallergen and asthmatic responses. Specific inhalation challenge with powdered gloves offers a definitive diagnostic method [210] but should only be offered in specialized centers capable of dealing with acute severe reactions.

## VIII.  CONDOM ALLERGIES

Most condoms, like rubber gloves, contain both NRL and rubber chemical allergens [211–215]. Accordingly, condom allergies may also manifest in two distinct varieties: delayed eczematous (type IV) allergies and immediate urticarial (type I) allergies, which may be accompanied by syncope, anaphylaxis [213]. There has also been an increase in the use of condoms, which most likely should be accompanied by an increased incidence of condom reactions similar to latex glove allergy [213].

Condom allergies may occur in either partner and have been reported in both men and women. The reactions may be localized to the genital area or may be widespread, including thighs, lower abdomen, perianal area, anal area, cheilitis, and stomatitis. In men, there is usually a clear relationship with intercourse, and the condition is commonly seen as itching and penile edema. Type I condom allergy was seen in 7 (24%) of 29 Finnish women with NRL glove allergy. Because of mucosal exposure, symptoms were more severe than with cutaneous contact alone. Condom reactions may also cause eczematous dermatitis, which may spread to the scrotum, inguinal area, inner thighs, as well as to more distal locations. Symptoms in women may range from mild pruritus and burning vaginal sensation to more severe reactions, with redness and edema of the vulva or eczematous dermatitis of adjacent skin [214].

Other chemicals that are added to condoms should also be considered in the differential diagnosis of condom reactions. These include spermicide (nonoxynol 9), corn starch (may cause contact urticaria), local anesthetics, ''dry'' lubricant (silicone-based), ''wet'' lubricant (surgical jelly containing preservatives such as paraben or Bronopol®), propylene glycol used as a lubricant, perfumes, and flavoring agents, as well as other chemical contraceptive agents and hygienic sprays [212].

Some patients may be reluctant to mention or inquire about problems related to condom allergy. Physicians should always consider this possibility, especially in patients reporting reactions to other NRL products. Questions about condom-related reactions and dermatitis should be included in the evaluation of a putative latex-sensitive person. Alternative contraceptive devices and HIV protection should be discussed with sexually active latex-allergic patients.

Most condoms are made from latex rubber. Nonlatex alternative condoms for NRL allergic patients include [214,215]:

1.  Nonrubber ''skin'' condoms, made of processed sheep intestine such as Kling Tite®, Fourex®, or Lambskin®, cost several times more than latex condoms. However, due to the natural membrane's porosity, lamb skin condoms should not be used for preventing transmission of sexually transmitted diseases, especially viral pathogens.
2.  Polyurethane condoms [215]: the polyurethane male condom, the Avanti® (Schmidt Laboratories), has been approved by FDA since May 1994. Polyurethanes are resins formed by a combination of isocyanates reacting with a group of polyalcohols. The final resins are very rare contact sensitizers. Polyurethane condoms may be used to prevent the sexual transmission of viral diseases, such as HIV and herpes simplex. The polyurethane vaginal pouch (female condom) (Reality Pouch®, Wisconsin Pharmacal; Jackson, Wisconsin) has been approved by the FDA since May 1993 and has also proved effective in preventing sexually transmitted diseases [169].
3.  Tactylon® condoms: Tactylon® medical-grade gloves have been sold since 1990. Four versions of Tactylon® condoms have been cleared by FDA for sale in the United States. The manufacturers anticipate sale in the fourth quarter of 1999 (Hans Sleeuwenhoek, Safeskin Sensicon Corporation, Vista, California, personal communication). Tactylon® is a nonthermoplastic elastomer, and Tactylon® condoms have been approved for prevention of transmission of sexually transmitted diseases including HIV. They contain no antioxidants or antiozonants that may act as type IV allergens [216,217] and are unaffected by contact with petrolatum and ozone, conditions that may cause deterioration of NRL condoms [211].

In 1991, Fisher proposed that NRL-sensitive men wear a lambskin condom under a NRL condom and that the condom order be reversed if the partner is sensitive to NRL [166]. Hamann and Kick postulated that a pore large enough to permit passage of a viral particle could possibly permit passage of the much smaller latex protein allergen [211]. Because of potential systemic symptoms from mucosal exposure to NRL, we believe the risk of error with this two-condom approach mitigates against its use.

## IX. METHODS OF NRL ALLERGEN MEASUREMENT

The best way to prevent NRL allergy is to eliminate the allergens from NRL devices or more practically to decrease further sensitization by the use of low-allergen–containing NRL devices. In order to accomplish this goal, standardized methods to measure NRL allergen levels in latex products are required. Data from two studies indicate that there are many differences between the allergen levels of gloves made by different manufacturers, between different glove brands, and even between different glove batches from the same manufacturer [20,218]. Powdered gloves contain higher allergen levels than nonpowdered gloves, and nonsterile exam gloves contain higher allergen levels than sterile surgical or chemotherapy gloves. Yunginger et al., using extractable allergen and protein levels, found that allergen levels varied 3000-fold among gloves from different manufacturers and also confirmed the fact that gloves labeled as "hypoallergenic" contained measurable NRL allergens [20].

Specific methods for measuring NRL allergen levels in manufactured rubber products include [219] skin prick testing, total protein measurement, IgE-inhibition assays and the LEAP assay.

Skin prick testing (SPT), the "gold standard" for diagnosing type I latex allergy [14,219], may also be used to measure total allergen content of extracts of manufactured NRL products in vivo in NRL-allergic subjects. Although not practical for routine measurement of allergen levels, information from SPT is essential in validating the specificity and sensitivity of other in vitro assays for allergen measurement [219].

Significant correlation between total protein content and allergen levels of NRL product extracts, based on both in vivo and in vitro assays, has been shown in a number of studies [20,219–221]. However, total protein content and IgE-binding capacity of certain allergen preparations may show no correlation and, therefore, may not predict the allergenicity of a certain product [218]. Additionally, there is no safe level of NRL proteins that will not sensitize exposed persons or cause reactions in NRL-allergic patients. Even though correlation coefficients between NRL proteins and NRL allergens are statistically significant [220,221], they are still not accurate enough to use the levels of extractable proteins as representative of quantitative allergen levels in the extracts. Not all proteins are common allergens, and the presence of other glove proteins, such as casein, may lead to incorrectly high levels [22,218]. On the other hand, total protein quantification is technically easy and possible to standardize, thus making it is feasible to use while other specific methods for measuring NRL allergens are being developed. FDA and the CEN (The European Committee for Standardization) have acknowledged that the measurement of total protein is a simple option for glove manufacturers to monitor their products; however, due to technical limitations values less than 50 µg/g cannot be reported [15,219]. The measurement of total protein levels during the various phases of product manufacturing is also proposed to be helpful in the development of less allergenic products.

In the in vitro IgE-inhibition assay (i.e., RAST inhibition assay [222,223]), soluble allergens in latex extracts compete for binding to latex-specific IgE in pooled sera from latex allergic patients [159] and ELISA inhibition [219]. Both methods have pitfalls in that they depend on the properties of the IgE antisera used and on the composition of the reference NRL preparation. Palosuo et al.'s study [219] found that both the ELISA and RAST inhibition assays correlated well with each other and highly significantly with SPT. They noted that the ELISA method was sensitive, reproducible, technically easy, inexpensive, free from the hazards of radioisotopes, and suitable for the analysis of a large number of NRL products. The Finnish Medical Devices Centre of the National Agency for Medicines has used the IgE-ELISA inhibition assay to monitor levels of allergen content in latex gloves in a market surveillance study of medical gloves sold and used in Finland in 1994, 1995, and 1997 [224]. Each survey covered more than 90% of the locally available medical gloves with results communicated to the medical community, users of latex gloves, and manufacturers. Gloves were defined as low-allergen gloves (allergen content of less than 10 AU/ml), moderate-allergen gloves (10–100 AU/ml), and high-allergen gloves (more than 100 AU/ml). During 1994–1997, they found that the proportion of high-allergen gloves decreased, that of moderate-allergen gloves increased, while low-allergen gloves retained more than half of the market. The mean allergen content in gloves also decreased. Such nationwide market analysis by national health authorities may offer an effective means of directing glove purchase and use toward low-allergen gloves, which in turn is expected to cause future decrease in NRL sensitivity.

The latex ELISA for antigenic protein (LEAP) is an indirect ELISA technique using rabbit antiserum to measure the immunogenic latex protein content in commercial products [159]. Wrangsjö and Lundberg did not find good correlation between the LEAP assay and latex-specific IgE antibody inhibition assay [225]. Palusuo et al. commented that this assay also detects nonallergenic proteins, which may have little relevance to induction of symptoms in latex-allergenic patients [219].

## X. LATEX AEROALLERGENS

Baur and Jäger [226] suggested that NRL allergens are transferred to glove powder, which becomes airborne during glove use, producing symptoms via inhalation. Other studies have confirmed the importance of NRL aeroallergens, especially in medical centers [2,23,226,227]. Thus, symptoms of mucosal allergy in patients with NRL allergy may be provoked not only by touch contact of the mucous membrane during dental or gynecological exams or during surgery, but also by inhalation of airborne latex proteins [13,226]. Initial sensitization to latex is also possible by direct mucosal exposure to NRL allergens [18]. Studies in animals have shown that NRL sensitivity may be induced by administrating the allergen via subcutaneous, intranasal, intratracheal, or intraperitoneal routes [228,229]. A study on quantification of latex allergens at the Mayo Clinic by Swanson et al. [189] found that latex aeroallergen levels were highest (range 13–208 ng/m$^3$) in work areas where powdered NRL gloves were in frequent use and lowest (range 0.3–1.8 ng/m$^3$) in work areas where powder-free or synthetic gloves were in use. The allergens were airborne only when there was activity in the work area, with levels becoming undetectable at the end of weekdays and on weekends, when the rooms were not in use. In this study, latex aeroallergen levels were similar in an operating room with high laminar flow air-exchange rate compared with one with conventional air-exchange rates. Use of a laminar flow glove changing station in one work area did not reduce latex aeroallergen levels. This contrasts with Baur et al.'s study [192], which found that the aeroallergen level in a room did not always reflect total glove use and that rooms with well-functioning ventilation systems and a fresh air supply were found to have no or much lower concentration of latex aeroallergens, even though using more gloves per day. This study, involving 145 subjects working in 32 hospitals or operating rooms, concluded that symptoms and presence of latex-specific IgE antibodies in subjects were significantly associated with measurable levels of latex aeroallergens. They proposed a critical latex aeroallergen threshold limit level of 0.6 ng/m$^3$ of room air, which, if exceeded, was more likely to be associated with the development of latex-specific IgE antibodies and occupational respiratory reactions (e.g., conjunctivitis, rhinitis, and asthma) [192]. There is no standardized method to quantify NRL aeroallergens; different results may be obtained from the same air sample, depending on the methods and reference standard extracts used for antigen detection. Other reports support the importance of latex aeroallergen levels in initiating symptoms of latex allergy and that individuals working in environments with a high level of latex aeroallergens have more symptoms than those in environments with undetectable latex aeroallergens [94,189,192,230,231]. A latex-sensitive technician, keeping a symptom diary, reported an asthma episode on a day when the latex allergen concentration was 12 ng/m$^3$, while showing no symptoms in the laboratory where no allergen was detectable in air samples [189].

Another report by Tarlo et al. [230] demonstrated that NRL allergen levels in the range of 39–311 ng/m$^3$ were associated with latex-related anaphylaxis and asthma. Comparing the impact of substituting low-allergen for high-allergen gloves on NRL aeroallergen levels in a single operating room, a prospective study by Heilman et al. [190] demonstrated significantly lower levels during low-allergen glove use. Latex aeroallergen levels correlated with the total number of gloves used on high-allergen glove use days. Substituting low-allergen–for high-allergen–containing gloves can reduce levels of NRL aeroallergen by more than 10-fold, similar to that found for the substitution of synthetic gloves for NRL gloves [77].

Donning and doffing powdered NRL gloves regularly results in detectable levels of latex aeroallergens in room air. Latex aeroallergen levels are determined by the amount of latex glove allergen and the presence of glove powder [190,226,227]. Additionally, a reservoir of settled allergenic dust found on laboratory surfaces, surgical gowns, anesthesia scrub suits, and laboratory coats may also be responsible for NRL symptoms even causing secondary exposure at home or to other family members [189,190]. The use of powder-free [20,230] or low-allergen–containing NRL products are effective in the control and prevention of exposure to airborne NRL particles, which serves as a major route of exposure [189,192,227].

Airborne latex particles, aside from being an important cause of allergen exposure and occupational asthma in the medical setting, has also been detected as an aeroallergen causing symptoms of latex allergy in the general environment [232]. Latex antigens were extractable from rubber tire fragments, which are found in particulate air pollutants from urban air samples and should be considered as a possible cause of respiratory tract diseases associated with air pollution [233].

## XI. HYPOALLERGENIC GLOVES

The term "hypoallergenic" was previously used by manufacturers to describe gloves that had a reduced risk of producing DTH reactions and was based on results of a skin sensitization study (Shelanski or modified Draize evaluation). The preferred modified Draize test included the application of skin patches of glove material to the forearm of 200 human volunteers for a specified period of time; to "pass" there must have been no adverse skin reactions, meaning the product did not induce delayed-type hypersensitivity [159]. The term "hypoallergenic" did not measure the ability of a product to prevent a potentially fatal IgE antibody response to NRL [13,20]. Hypoallergenic gloves still contained NRL [20,218], and the term was thought to confuse or put NRL-sensitive users with immediate allergy at risk for serious adverse reactions. Wolf reported a latex-sensitive nurse who developed anaphylaxis to sterile surgical gloves labeled "specially formulated for hands allergic to latex," which the manufacturer claimed to refer to the removal of the chemical that caused DTH [234,235]. FDA also received reports of allergic reactions to medical gloves labeled as "hypoallergenic" [236]. Regulatory authorities in both Europe and the United States generally agree with the importance of improved labeling and warning state-

**Table 3** Glove Usage in U.S. Hospitals

| Year | Billions of gloves |
|------|--------------------|
| 1978 | 0.8 |
| 1990 | 2.0 |
| 1992 | 3.0 |
| 1998 | 6.5 |

*Source*: Milt Hench, London International, Norcross, Georgia; March 11, 1999.

ments about NRL products. FDA ordered removal of the term ''hypoallergenic'' on labels of medical devices containing natural rubber and, in the same ruling, also mandated other user labeling requirements. Specifically, labels of NRL medical devices must state ''Caution: This product contains natural rubber latex, which may cause allergic reactions'' and dry natural rubber medical devices must be labeled ''This product contains dry natural rubber'' [9,236,237]. Labeling will also be required for packaging of NRL-containing medical devices and of dry natural rubber that contacts humans. These rulings were effective September 30, 1998 [236].

In a ''Guidance'' document for industry and FDA reviewers and staff issued on January 13, 1999, FDA approved two new labeling options and testing requirements to replace the ''hypoallergenic'' label. These are ''low dermatitis potential'' and ''low thiuram, and/or carbamate, and/or thiazole.'' Both labels also require a warning that the product should not be used in patients with a known allergy to natural rubber protein. The first claim is based on a negative modified Draize 95 test on at least 200 nonsensitized human subjects. The second claim is based on data to support the first claim plus a negative patch test on 25 individuals who are allergic to the major chemical sensitizers in natural rubber products.

FDA and the CEN are also developing standards for powder-free latex devices. FDA additionally believes it is prudent to warn glove users of the presence of donning powder on examination gloves. The CEN is drafting requirements to indicate the type of donning powder present and, for surgical gloves, the need for its removal [238].

Table 3 shows the dramatic increase in hospital glove usage over 20 years. Table 4 illustrates the projected decrease in the use of latex-powdered gloves accompanied by an increase in latex powder–free and synthetic gloves. Table 5 lists alternative glove materials for NRL-allergic patients.

**Table 4** Exam Gloves: U.S. Market Percentage, Actual and Projected

|  | 1994 | 1998 | 2004 |
|------|------|------|------|
| Latex-powdered | 65 | 30 | 6 |
| Latex powder–free | 26 | 47 | 63 |
| Free synthetic | 7 | 22 | 36 |

*Source*: Milt Hench, London International, Norcross, Georgia; March 11, 1999.

**Table 5**  Non-NRL Glove Alternatives

Vinyl
Nitrile
Neoprene
Block polymers
   Styrene-butadiene-styrene
   Styrene-ethylene-butylene-styrene
Polyethylene

## XII.  MANAGEMENT

The cardinal principle for managing NRL allergy is *avoidance*, but it is difficult to implement because NRL is ubiquitous in medical and nonmedical environments. According to Sussman and Ownby, latex-avoidance precautions are indicated in high-risk children from birth, in patients diagnosed with NRL allergy, and in patients with known risk factors and suggestive histories [239].

Current recommendations are that all SB children, including nonallergic patients, should avoid contact with NRL to prevent sensitization and a NRL-safe environment should be used for all of their medical and surgical procedures. The efficacy of latex prophylaxis in spina bifida patients was studied by Cremer et al. in a longitudinal follow-up study measuring IgE antibodies against latex [47]. Sixty-seven SB patients were instructed about NRL avoidance and were provided with a NRL-free environment for surgery and reevaluated 0.6–4.1 years later. Results showed that 37% did develop latex antibodies during the follow-up period; 27% showed decreased antibody levels (12% to nondetectable levels), 19% had an increase in latex antibody levels (6% newly sensitized), and 9% had no change in latex antibody levels. In SB patients, prophylactic measures may reduce mild sensitization to nondetectable antibody levels.

Patients with type I NRL allergy should avoid direct contact not only with NRL products but also with airborne latex allergen. They should be educated regarding the identification and sources of NRL in the home and in the workplace (Table 1). Lists and reviews of substitute synthetic non-NRL surgical and examination gloves, low-allergen latex gloves, and DTH allergens in gloves are available [9,13,73,159,240], as are lists of latex-safe alternatives for hospital and home consumer products [241].

We provide our latex-allergic patients with general information available from various latex support groups [9,140]: (1) ELASTIC (Education for Latex Allergy Support Team and Information Coalition), who publishes Latex Allergy News at 800-482-6869, (2) ALERT (Allergy to Latex Education and Resource Team) at 414-677-9707, and (3) Spina Bifida Association of America at 800-621-3141 or 202-944-3285.

Latex allergy information is also available on the internet [9,40]. Lists of latex allergy organizations, publications, news sources, and internet web sites have been summarized by Warshaw [9].

We recommend that our latex-allergic patients obtain Medic-Alert bracelets and inform health-care providers of their diagnosis. We provide them with lists of substitute non-NRL gloves, other non-NRL devices, potentially allergenic cross-reacting fruits, and occult sources of NRL exposure, such as dog and child toys and dental dams and prophylaxis cups, and provide them with the Cleveland Clinic Foundation's protocol for latex-safe anesthesia procedures.

Since continued exposure may result in increasing sensitivity over time, treatment with antiallergic medications such as antihistamines should not be prescribed as an alternative to allergen avoidance. Their use may also mask early expression of allergic reactions from inadvertent exposure. Patients with systemic symptoms should carry their own epinephrine syringe, and the use of B-blocking drugs is contraindicated in NRL-allergic patients [239].

Treatment of concomitant hand eczema is also important. Irritant contact dermatitis from moisture, sweat, heat, and friction under gloves can be minimized by wearing a soft breathable glove liner (e.g., cotton liners) under NRL gloves [158]. Other useful measures include reducing exposure to other irritants, appropriate hand-washing techniques, the use of nonirritating skin cleansers, frequent use of nonsensitizing moisturizers/lubricants, and treatment with topical corticosteroids.

In type IV contact allergy to NRL gloves, avoidance of the causative allergens is important. Patch testing should be done to identify specific allergenic rubber accelerators or antioxidants. Alternative gloves that do not contain the patch test–positive allergen may be substituted [158]. Lists of specific accelerators used in the manufacture of different brands of latex gloves have been published [73,159,242]. Vinyl gloves or other synthetic gloves may also be utilized.

Natural rubber latex gloves with an inside coating of hydrogel or polyurethane have been tolerated by some NRL-allergic patients [73,243]. However, these "hypoallergenic gloves" should *not* be worn by NRL-allergic patients [244] because of potential serious adverse reactions, even to low levels of latex proteins [244].

The use of skin-protection creams has been shown in a study by Baur et al. [245] to increase the frequency of allergic reaction to latex gloves, probably by serving as a vehicle for allergen transmission from gloves or glove powder.

Recommendations for workers with occupational asthma have emphasized personal avoidance of latex products, particularly glove use [246]. Several reports have determined that use of lower allergen or nonpowdered gloves has a protective effect on occupational asthma [231,247,248] in studies of aeroallergen levels in a single laboratory or location. However, a more recent study by Charous and coworkers [249] strongly suggests that such personal measures of avoidance may give inadequate protection to latex allergic workers. In their study of aeroallergen levels in a dental practice setting, latex aeroallergen dispersion from areas using powdered gloves to "safe" areas containing only nonpowdered latex occurred in quantities sufficient to worsen occupational asthma [249].

Based on the above considerations, employers and institutions should consider adopting exclusive use of nonlatex or nonpowdered latex gloves in lieu of powdered latex gloves as recommended by the American College of Allergy, Asthma and Immunology and the Latex Committee of the American Academy of Allergy, Asthma and Immunology [250]. The introduction of such policies would reduce both costs of workers compensation claims as well as replacement costs associated with the loss of highly skilled workers. Moreover, it would reduce the risks to latex-allergic patients of inhalant exposure during medical procedures or during emergency room visits for acute illness. Adoption of exclusive use of nonpowdered gloves appears to result in virtual elimination of latex aerosol from noncarpeted rooms within one month. Cleaning of surfaces likely to serve as allergen repositories, such as carpeting, rugs, and upholstery, concomitant with introduction of nonpowdered latex gloves seems appropriate [249].

## XIII.  PREVENTION/PROPHYLAXIS

Many organizations such as the National Institute of Occupational Safety and Health (NI-OSH) [251]; the American Academy of Dermatology [158]; the American College of Allergy, Asthma, and Immunology (ACAAI); and the American Academy of Allergy, Asthma and Immunology (AAAAI) [154,250] have developed position statements concerning latex allergy. Selected recommendations are reviewed here.

Nonsensitized individuals in high-risk groups should use non-NRL or low-allergen NRL gloves and avoid other rubber contact as much as possible [12]. The importance of aeroallergen exposure to NRL in glove powder is emphasized, and powder-free, low-NRL allergen substitute gloves are suggested for coworkers of health-care workers with NRL allergy. This is especially important to accommodate those NRL patients with mucosal and respiratory symptoms [2,10,16,252,253]. Children with spina bifida or multiple congenital anomalies who are undergoing multiple surgeries and multiple catheterizations should minimize the risk of sensitization with NRL avoidance such as through latex-safe operating rooms and utilizing nonlatex hospital supplies, i.e., urinary catheters [13]. The unnecessary use of NRL gloves should be discouraged. Because vinyl and other synthetic gloves may not always possess the same barrier protection as NRL gloves [254,255], NRL gloves should be used only when appropriate barrier protection is necessary as in handling infectious material. The routine use of NRL gloves by food handlers, housekeeping, and transport and medical personnel in low-risk situations (e.g., food handling, bed transport, routine physical examination) should be discouraged [250]. NRL gloves should not be used as ''hand protection'' in persons with chronic hand eczema. Nonlatex gloves should always be used when there is little potential for contact with infectious material. If latex gloves are required, the use of reduced-protein, low-allergen latex gloves will not only reduce the occurrence of reactions among sensitized workers but also should reduce the rate of sensitization [20,94,189,192,230,231,250,256,257].

Turjanmaa stated that powdered, low-allergen gloves were satisfactory because minimal allergen levels probably would not contaminate the glove powder [11]. However, position statements by several groups recommend the use of powder-free gloves to reduce latex aeroallergens levels and exposure [231,250,258,259].

Other recommendations include suggested clinical strategies in medical institutions:

1. Allergic or high-risk individuals should be identified.
2. Health-care facilities should offer latex-safe environments for patients with NRL allergy. The American Academy of Dermatology's position paper on latex allergy defines a latex-safe environment as [258]:
   a)  No one in the area wears latex gloves with powder.
   b)  Only nonlatex gloves are used to examine the patient.
   c)  All NRL objects that routinely directly or indirectly contact mucosa, nonintact skin, and internal body spaces (e.g., catheters, medicine stoppers, endotracheal tubes) should be removed or made latex safe (e.g., by covering).
   d)  Products made of dry-molded NRL (e.g., wheelchair tires, tool handles) do *not* need to be removed from the area. If direct contact with these objects is routine, then the object should be covered or the patient should wear non-latex gloves, such as when wheeling self in a wheelchair.
   e)  Hospital dietary services should offer latex-safe meals that lack cross-reacting foods. Hospitals should also have latex-safe equipment carts and one operating room that is latex safe.

3. NRL-allergic patients should be educated regarding identification and avoidance of NRL.

4. Health-care facilities are encouraged to use powder-free low-allergen latex gloves.

5. Medical facilities should consider using latex-safe operating rooms for trauma surgery.

6. Medical facilities should use vinyl or other non-NRL gloves for physical examinations (especially mucosal exams).

7. Since most serious reactions result from mucosal exposure to latex, all food-preparation facilities (e.g., cafeterias, food-processing plants, restaurants) should be encouraged to use only nonlatex gloves to prepare foods.

8. Health-care facilities are encouraged to form multidisciplinary committees to deal with NRL-allergic patients and employees.

In addition to allergists and dermatologists, all health-care providers, but especially surgeons, gynecologists, anesthesiologists, and dentists, should be familiar with latex allergy. All high-risk groups should be increasingly informed and have access to educational programs about latex allergy.

Manufacturers should make an effort to manufacture products with decreased allergen content.

## XIV. OCCUPATIONAL DISABILITY ASSOCIATED WITH LATEX ALLERGY

Several studies have shown that NRL-allergic patients, especially occupationally sensitized health-care workers, may have decreased work ability and continuing symptoms at work due to their latex allergy. In an average 7-year follow-up on 25 (93%) of 27 latex allergic health-care workers, Wrangsjö reported that 10 (40%) had quit working or changed jobs because of the latex allergy, while 15 (79%) of 19 workers remaining on the same job reported work-related symptoms [260]. Taylor and Praditsuwan's series [10] showed that one (2%) of 41 latex allergic patients quit working and 8 others (20%) had changed jobs or tasks to reduce NRL exposure. Twelve (31%) had lost work time because of significant and sometimes incapacitating symptoms. Kujala et al. [261] studied 32 female health-care workers with occupational latex allergy compared with nonsensitized control subjects to find that work ability index (WAI) scores were on average lower among the sensitized subjects as compared with their nonsensitized controls. Ten health-care workers (31%) had changed occupation, and one early retirement occurred after NRL sensitization.

Taylor [262] estimated the costs of device-related occupational illness. Direct costs include the purchase of powder-free or latex-free gloves, the substitution of other hospital equipment containing latex, and the cost of installing an air filtration/laminar flow changing station. Indirect costs that are worker-related include job relocation to other sites in the hospital, job change without retraining, or retraining and reeducation for a new ''nonclinical'' placement.

Some hospitals have estimated that the cost of adopting latex-free policies would be ''arduous'' and ''burdensome.'' The cost of implementing a dust- and latex-free working environment at California Pacific Medical Center has been estimated at between $75,000 and $200,000/year. At the Mayo Clinic, a one-time savings of more than $200,000 was achieved by consolidation of glove purchases among fewer vendors and by negotiating prices to replace high-allergen latex gloves with low-allergen gloves. The Mayo Medical Center found no correlation between the latex allergen level in the glove and the cost of the glove [263].

Latex allergy is an important occupational health concern, especially considering the issues of employee safety and disability. This may lead to further medicolegal and financial costs, not only for employees but also for employers, in order to achieve adequate employee accommodation or pay for workers' compensation.


## XV.  THE FUTURE OF LATEX ALLERGY

Many unresolved issues remain: while the risk groups and major symptoms have been identified, asymptomatic NRL-allergic patients are a diagnostic challenge. In addition, the mechanisms of NRL sensitization are still poorly understood.

Several major allergens have been purified from natural rubber latex. Partial or complete amino acid sequences have been determined and the DNA encoding for some of these proteins has been isolated. Despite this progress, questions persist about the relative importance of the identified allergens and about additional allergens that have not been as yet identified. A well-accepted standardized test for the specific measurement of NRL allergens should lead to the manufacturing of low-allergen–containing products. FDA and the CEN have acknowledged the measurement of total protein as a simple indicator for glove manufacturers to monitor their products.

Ideally, all NRL-containing medical products as well as consumer goods should be adequately labeled demonstrating latex content and other potentially sensitizing rubber chemicals.

Hopefully, a commercially available standardized NRL skin test allergen will be approved and marketed soon in the United States. Other commercial latex reagents have proved safe and useful in other areas such as in France (Stallergènes Lab.), Canada (Bencard), and Scandinavian countries (ALK) [9].

New approaches to prevention are needed. These include changing to synthetic devices as well as minimizing levels of bioavailable NRL allergens in medical and consumer products. Immunotherapy with peptide eptiope–based allergens or naked DNA vaccines is under investigation [264].

In conclusion, NRL latex allergy is caused by potent allergens from an unexpected source. Although only recognized for the past 20 years, NRL allergy occurs in new risk groups and is accompanied by unique cross-reactions [264].


## REFERENCES

1.  Coombs RRA, Gell PGH. The classification of allergic reactions underlying disease. In: PGH Gell, RRA Coombs, eds. Clinical Aspects of Immunology. Philadelphia: FA Davis, 1969: 317.
2.  Slater JE. Allergic reactions to natural rubber. Ann Allergy 1992; 68:203–211.
3.  Downing JG. Dermatitis from rubber gloves. N Engl J Med 1933; 208:196–198.
4.  Nutter AF. Contact urticaria to rubber. Br J Dermatol 1979; 101:597–598.
5.  Förström L. Contact urticaria from latex surgical gloves. Contact Dermatitis 1980; 6:33–34.

6. Köpman A, Hannuksela M. Contact urticaria to rubber. Duodecim 1983; 99:221–224.

7. Turjanmaa K, Reunala T, Tuimala R, Kärkkäinen T. Severe IgE-mediated allergy to surgical gloves. Proceedings from the SV Nordic Congress of Allergology, Turku (abstr). Allergy 1984; 2(suppl):35.

8. Leynadier F. Pathophysiological and clinical aspects of immediate hypersensitivity to latex. Clin Rev Allergy 1993; 11:371–380.

9. Warshaw EM. Latex allergy. J Am Acad Dermatol 1998; 39:1–24.

10. Taylor JS, Praditsuwan P. Latex allergy review of 44 cases including outcome and frequent association with allergic hand eczema. Arch Dermatol 1996; 132:265–271.

11. Turjanmaa K. Contact urticaria from latex gloves. In: GA Mellstrom, JR Wahlberg, HI Maibach, eds. Protective Gloves for Occupational Use. Boca Raton, FL: CRC Press, Inc., 1994: 241–254.

12. Turjanmaa K. Update on occupational natural rubber latex allergy. Dermatol Clin 1994; 12(3):561–567.

13. Hamann CP. Natural rubber latex protein sensitivity in review. Am J Contact Dermatitis 1993; 4:4–21.

14. Turjanmaa K, Alenius H, Mäkinen-Kiljunen S, Reunala T, Palosuo T. Natural rubber latex allergy. Allergy 1996; 51:593–602.

15. Sussman GL, Beezhold DH. Allergy to latex rubber. Ann Intern Med 1995; 122:43–46.

16. Fink JN, ed. Latex allergy. Immunol Allergy Clin North Am 1995; 15:1–179.

17. Slater JE. Rubber anaphylaxis. N Engl J Med 1989; 17:1126–1130.

18. Brehler R, Kolling R, Webb M, Wastell C. Glove powder a risk factor for the development of latex allergy? Eur J Surg 1997; 579(suppl):23–25.

19. Centers for Disease Control. Recommendations for the prevention of HIV transmission in health-care settings. MMWR 1987; 36(suppl 2):15–185.

20. Yunginger JW, Jones AT, Fransway AF, Kelso JM, Warner MA, Hunt LW. Extractable latex allergens and proteins in disposable medical gloves and other rubber products. J Allergy Clin Immunol 1994; 93:836–842.

21. Sussman GL, Liss GM, Deal K, Brown S, Cividino M, Siu S, Beezhold DH, Smith G, Swanson MC, Yunginger J, Douglas A, Holness DL, Lebert P, Keith P, Waserman S, Turjanmaa K. Incidence of latex sensitization among latex glove users. J Allergy Clin Immunol 1998; 101:171–178.

22. Turjanmaa K. Allergy to natural rubber latex—a growing problem. Ann Med 1994; 26:297–300.

23. Turjanmaa K, Mäkinen-Kiljunen S, Reunala T, Alenium H, Palosuo T. Natural rubber latex allergy—the European experience. Immunol Allergy Clin North Am 1995; 15:71–88.

24. Bernardini R, Novembre E, Ingargiola A, Veltroni M, Mugnaini L, Cianferoni A, Lombardi E, Vierucci A. Prevalence and risk factors of latex sensitization in an unselected pediatric population. J Allergy Clin Immunol 1998; 101(5):621–625.

25. Liebke C, Niggemann B, Wahn U. Sensitivity and allergy to latex in atopic and non-atopic children. Pediatr Allergy Immunol 1996; 7(2):103–107.

26. Moneret-Vautrin DA, Beaudouin E, Widmer S, Mouton C, Kanny G, Prestat F. Prospective study of risk factors in natural rubber latex hypersensitivity. J Allergy Clin Immunol 1993; 92:668–677.

27. Cremer R, Hoppe A, Korsch E, Kleine-Diepenbruck U, Blaker F. Natural rubber latex allergy: prevalence and risk factors in patients with spina bifida compared with atopic children and controls. Eur J of Pediatr 1998; 157(1):13–16.

28. Lebenbom-Mansour MH, Oesterle JR, Ownby DR, Jennett MK, Post SK, Zaglaniczy K. The incidence of latex sensitivity in ambulatory surgical patients: a correction of historical factors with positive serum IgE levels. Anesth Analg 1997; 85:44–49.

29. Theissen U, Theissen JL, Mertes N, Brenler R. EgE-mediated hypersensitivity to latex in childhood. Allergy: Eur J Allergy Clin Immunol 1997; 52(6):665–669.

30. Ownby DR, Ownby HE, McCullough J, Shafer AW. The Prevalence of anti-latex IgE antibodies in 1000 volunteer blood donors. J Allergy Clin Immunol 1996; 97:1188–1192.

31. Merrett TG, Merrett J, Bhambri S, Kekwick R. Prevalence of latex specific IgE antibodies in the UK (abstr). J Allergy Clin Immunol 1995; 95:154.

32. Porri F, Lemiere C, Birnbaum J, Guilloux L, Lanteaume A, Didelot R, Vervloet D, Charpin D. Prevalence of latex sensitization in subjects attending health screening—implications for a periooperative screening. Clin Exp Allergy 1997; 27(4):413–417.

33. Centers for Disease Control. Latex allergy. Letter to health professionals, Atlanta, July 1991.

34. Kelly K, Kurup V, Zacharisen M, Resnick A, Fink J. Skin and serologic testing in the diagnosis of latex allergy. J Allergy Clin Immunol 1993; 91:1140–1145.

35. Mathew SN, Melton A, Wagner W. Latex hypersensitivity: prevalence among children with spina bifida and immunoblotting identification of latex proteins (abstr). J Allergy Clin Immunol 1992; 89:225.

36. Yassin MS, Sanyurah S, Lien MB. Evaluation of latex allergy in patients with meningomyelocele. Ann Allergy 1992; 69:207–211.

37. Michael T, Niggemann B, Muers A, Seidel U, Wahn U, Scheffner D. Risk factors for latex allergy in patients with spina bifida. Clin Exp Allergy 1996; 26(87):934–939.

38. Nieto A, Estornell F, Mazó A, Reig Ni C, Garcia-Ibarra F. Allergy to latex in spina bifida: a multivariate study of associated factors in 100 consecutive patients. J Allergy Clin Immunol 1996; 98:501–507.

39. Shah S, Cawley M, Gleeson R, O'Connor J, McGeady S. Latex allergy and latex sensitization in children and adolescents with meningomyelocele. J Allergy Clin Immunol 1998; 101: 741–746.

40. Sandberg ET, Slater JE, Roth DR. Rubber specific IgE in children enrolled in a spina bifida clinic (abstr). J Allergy Clin Immunol 1992; 89:223.

41. Alter JE, Mostello LA, Shaer C. Rubber-specific IgE in children with spina bifida. J Urol 1991; 146:578–579.

42. Porri F, Pradal M, Lemiere C, Birnbaum J, Mege JL, Lanteaume A, Charpin D, Vervloet D, Comboulives J. Association between latex sensitization and repeated latex exposure in children. Anesthesiology 1997; 86(3):599–602.

43. Capriles-Hulett A, Sanchez-Borges M, Von-Scanzoni C, Medina JR. Very low frequency of latex and fruit allergy in patients with spina bifida from Venezuela: influence of socioeconomic factors. Ann Allergy Asthma Immunol 1995; 75:62–64.

44. Mazon A, Nieto A, Estornell F, Reig C, Garcia-Ibarra F. Factors that influence the presence of symptoms caused by latex allergy in children with spina bifida. J Allergy Clin Immunol 1997; 99:600–604.

45. Kelly KJ, Pearson ML, Kurup VP, Havens PL, Byrd RS, Setlock ME. A cluster of anaphylactic reactions in children with SB during general anesthesia: epidemiologic features, risk factors, and latex hypersensitivity. J Allergy Clin Immunol 1994; 94:53–61.

46. Mazón A, Nieto A, Estornell F, Nieto A, Reig C, Garcia-Ibarra F. Factors that influence the presence of symptoms caused by latex allergy in children with spina bifida. J Allergy Clin Immunol 1997; 99:600–604.

47. Cremer R, Hoppe A, Kleine-Diepenbruck U, Bläker F. Longitudinal study on latex sensitization in children with spina bifida. Pediatr Allergy Immunol 1998; 9:40–43.

48. Harfi H, Tipirneni P, Mohammed GH, Lonnevig VG. Latex hypersensitivity: prevalence among health care personnel measured by SPT, CAP, and challenge (abstr). J Allergy Clin Immunol 1997; 99(suppl):S160.

49. Kibby T, Akl M. Prevalence of latex sensitization in a hospital employee population. Ann Allergy Asthma Immunol 1997; 78(1):41–44.

50. Yassin MS, Lierl MB, Fischer TJ, O'Brien K, Cross J, Steinmetz C. Latex allergy in hospital employees. Ann Allergy 1994; 72:245–249.

51. Liss GM, Sussman GL, Deal K, Brown S, Cividino M, Siu S, Beezhold DH, Smith G, Swan-

son MC, Yunginger J, Douglas A, Holness DL, Lebert P, Keith P, Wasserman S, Turjanmaa K. Latex allergy: epidemiological study of 1351 hospital workers. Occup Environ Med 1997; 54(5):335–342.

52. Eriksen P, Nissen D, DuBuske LM, Sheffer A, Skov PS, Cielewicz G. Comparison latex-specific IgE binding of various latex extracts in hospital personnel (abstr). J Allergy Clin Immunol 1997; 99(suppl):S156.

53. Kaczmarek RG, Silverman BG, Gross TP, Hamilton RG, Kessler E, Arrowsmith-Lowe JT, Moore RM. Prevalance of latex-specific IgE antibodies in hospital personnel. Ann Allergy Asthma Immunol 1996; 76(1):51–56.

54. Akasawa A, Matsumoto K, Saito H, Sakaguchi N, Tanaka K, Obata T. Incidence of latex allergy in atopic children and hospital workers in Japan. Int Arch Allergy Immunol 1993; 101:177–181.

55. Wrangsjö K, Osterman K, van Hage-Hamsten M. Glove related skin symptoms among operating theatre and dental care unit personnel (II). Clinical examination, tests and laboratory findings indicating latex allergy. Contact Dermatitis 1994; 30:139–140.

56. Turjanmaa K. Incidence of immediate allergy to latex gloves in hospital personnel. Contact Dermatitis 1987; 17:270–275.

57. Cormio L, Turjanmaa K, Talja M. Toxicity and immediate allergenicity of latex gloves. Clin Exp Allergy 1993; 23:618–623.

58. Mace SR, Sussman GL, Liss G, Stark DF, Beezhold D, Thompson R, Kelly K. Latex allergy in operating room nurses. Ann Allergy Asthma Immunol 1998; 80(3):252–256.

59. Lagier F, Vervloer D, Lhermet I, Poyen D, Chapin D. Prevalence of latex allergy in operating room nurses. J Allergy Clin Immunol 1992; 90:319–322.

60. Grzybowski M, Ownby DR, Peysen PA, Johnson CC, Schork MA. The prevalence of antilatex IgE antibodies among registered nurses. J Allergy Clin Immunol 1996; 98:535–544.

61. Douglas R, Morton J, Czarny D, O'Hehir RE. Prevalence of IgE-mediated allergy to latex in hospital nursing staff. Aust NZ J Med 1997; 27(2):165–169.

62. De Groot H, de Jong NW, Duijster E, Geth Van Wijk R, Vermeulen A, Van Toorenenbergen AW, Geursen L, van Joost T. Prevalence of natural rubber latex allergy (type I and type IV) in laboratory workers in The Netherlands. Contact Dermatitis 1998; 38(3):159–163.

63. Salkie ML, Chir B. The prevalence of atopy and hypersensitivity to latex. In medical laboratory technologists. Arch Pathol Lab Med 1993; 117:897–899.

64. Hamann CP, Turjanmaa K, Rietschel R, Siew C, Owenby D, Gruninger SE, Sullivan KM. Natural rubber latex hypersensitivity: Incidence and prevalence of type I allergy in dental professionals. J Am Dent Assoc 1998; 129:43–54.

65. Tarlo SM, Sussman GL, Holness DL. Latex sensitivity in dental students and staff. A cross-sectional study. J Allergy Clin Immunol 1997; 99:396–401.

66. Arellano R, Bradley J, Sussman G. Prevalence of latex sensitization among hospital physicians occupationally exposed to latex gloves. Anesthesiology 1992; 77:905–908.

67. Konrad C, Fieber T, Gerber H, Schuepfer G, Muellner G. The prevalence of latex sensitivity among anesthesiology staff. Anesthesia Analg 1997; 84(3):629–633.

68. Safadi GS, Corey EC, Taylor JS, Wagner WO, Pien LC, Melton AL Jr. Latex hypersensitivity in emergency medical service providers. Ann Allergy Asthma Immunol 1996; 77:39–42.

69. Charous BL, Hamilton R, Yunginger J. Occupational latex exposure: characteristics of contact and systemic reactions in 47 workers. J Allergy Clin Immunol 1994; 94:12–18.

70. Jones RT, Bubak ME, Grosselin VA, Yunginger JW. Relative latex allergen contents of several commercial latex gloves (abstr). J Allergy Clin Immunol 1992; 89:225.

71. Bubak ME, Reed CE, Fransway AF, Yunginger JW, Jones RT, Carlson CA. Allergic reactions to latex among health-care workers. Mayo Clin Proc 1992; 67:1075–1079.

72. Hunt LW, Fransway AF, Reed CE, Miller LK, Jones RT, Swanson MC, Yunginger JW. An epidemic of occupational allergy to latex involving health care workers. J Occup Environ Med 1995; 37(10):1204–1209.

73. Heese A, von Hintzenstern J, Peters KP, Koch HU, Hornstein OP. Allergic and irritant reactions to rubber gloves in medical health services: spectrum, diagnostic approach and therapy. J Am Acad Dermatol 1997; 25:831–839.

74. Sussman GL, Lem D, Liss G, Beezhold D. Latex allergy in housekeeping personnel. Ann Allergy 1995; 74:415–418.

75. Van Der Walle HB, Brunsveld VM. Latex allergy among hairdressers. Contact Dermatitis 1995; 32:177.

76. Carrillo T, Blanco C, Quiralte J, Castillo R, Cuevas M, Rodriguez de Castro F. Prevalence of latex allergy among greenhouse workers. J Allergy Clin Immunol 1995; 96:699–701.

77. Pisati G, Baruffini A, Bernabeo F, Falagiani P. Environmental and clinical study of latex allergy in a textile factory. J Allergy Clin Immunol 1998; 101:327–329.

78. Tarlo SM, Wong L, Roos J. Occupational asthma caused by latex in a surgical glove manufacturing plant. J Allergy Clin Immunol 1990; 85:626–631.

79. Hadjiliadis D, Khan K, Tarlo S. Skin test responses to latex in an allergy and asthma clinic. J Allergy Clin Immunol 1995; 96:431–432.

80. Reinheimer G, Ownby DR. Prevalence of latex-specific IgE antibodies in patients being evaluated for allergy. Ann Allergy 1995; 74:184–187.

81. Rheff F, Thomas P, Reissig G, Przybilla B. Natural rubber-latex allergy in patients not intensely exposed. Allergy Eur J Allergy Clin Immunol 1998; 53:(4):445–449.

82. Ylitalo L, Turjanmaa K, Palosuo T, Reunala T. Natural rubber latex allergy in children who had not undergone surgery and who had undergone multiple operations. J Allergy Clin Immunol 1997; 100:606–612.

83. Shield S, Blaiss MS, Gross S. Prevalence of latex sensitivity in children evaluated for inhalant allergy (abstr.). J Allergy Clin Immunol 1992; 89:223.

84. Rystedt I. Hand eczema in patients with history of atopic manifestations in childhood. Acta Derm Venereol 1985; 65:305–312.

85. Field EA, King CM. Skin problems associated with routine wearing of protective gloves in dental practice. Br Dent J 1990; 168:281–285.

86. Boxer M. Hand dermatitis: A risk factor for latex hypersensitivity. J Allergy Clin Immunol 1996; 98:855–856.

87. van Ketal WG. Contact urticaria from rubber gloves after dermatitis from thiurams. Contact Dermatitis 1984; 11:323–324.

88. Kanerva L, Estlander T, Jolanki R. Mechanism of concomitant type I and type IV allergic skin reactions. In: T Menne, HI Maibach, eds. Exogenous Dermatoses: Environmental Dermatitis. Boca Raton, FL: CRC, Press, 1991:120.

89. Von Krogh G, Maibach HI. The contact urticaria syndrome: updated review. J Am Acad Dermatol 1981; 8:328–342.

90. Placucci F, Vincenzi C, Ghedini G, Piana G, Tosti A. Coexistence of type I and type IV allergy to rubber latex. Contact Dermatitis 1996; 34:76.

91. Alenius H, Reunala M, Lukka T, Turjanmas K, Yip E, Makinen-Kiljunen S, Palosuo T. Prohevein from the rubber tree (*Hevea brasiliensis*) is a major latex allergen. Clin Exp Allergy 1995; 25:659–665.

92. Alenius H, Reunala T, Turjanmaa K, Palosuo T. The main IgE-binding epitope of a major latex allergen, prohevein, is present in its N-terminal 43-amino acid fragment, hevein. J Immunol 1996; 92:690–697.

93. Chambeyron C, Leynadier F, Pecquet C, Thao TX. Study of the allergenic fractions of latex. Allergy 1992; 47:92–97.

94. Jaeger D, Kleinhans D, Czuppon A, et al. Latex-specific proteins causing immediate-type cutaneous, nasal, bronchial and systemic reactions. J Allergy Clin Immunol 1992; 89(3):759–768.

95. Makinen-Kiljunen S, Palosuo T, Reunala T. Characterization of latex antigens and allergens

in surgical gloves and natural rubber by immunoelectrophoretic methods. J Allergy Clin Immunol 1992; 90:230–235.

96. Beezhold DH, Kostyal DA, Sussman GL. IgE epitope analysis of the hevein preprotein; a major latex allergen. Clin Exp Immunol 1997; 108:114–121.

97. Slater JE, Arthur-Smith A, Trybul DE, Kekwick RGO. Identification, cloning and sequence of a major allergen (Hev b 5) from natural rubber latex (*Hevea brasiliensis*). J Biol Chem 1996; 271:25394–25399.

98. Sunderasan EHS, Hamid S, Ward MA, Yeang HY, Cardoasa MJ. Latex B-serum β-1,3-glucanase (Hev b 11) and a component of the microhelix (Hev b IV) are major latex allergens. J Nat Rubb Res 1995; 10:82–89.

99. Kurup VP, Alenium H, Kelly KJ, et al. A two-dimensional electrophoretic analysis of latex peptides reacting with IgE and IgG antibodies from patients with latex allergy. Int Arch Allergy Immunol 1996; 109:58–67.

100. Czuppon A, Chen Z, Rennert S, et al. The rubber elongation factor of rubber trees (*Hevea brasiliensis*) is the major allergen in latex. J Allergy Clin Immunol 1993; 92(5):690–697.

101. Beezhold D, Sussman G, Kostyal D, et al. Identification of a 46-kD latex protein allergen in health care workers. Clin Exp Immunol 1994; 98:408–413.

102. Akasawa A, Martin BM, Liu T, Lin Y. A novel acidic allergen, Hev b 5, in latex. Purification cloning and characterization. J Biol Chem 1996; 271:25389–25393.

103. Alenius H, Palosuo T, Kelly K, et al. IgE reactivity to 14-kd and 27-kd natural rubber proteins in latex-allergy children with spina bifida and other congenital anomalies. Int Arch Allergy Immunol 1993; 102:61–66.

104. Yeang H, Ward M, Zamri A, et al. Amino acid sequence similarity of Hev b 3 to two previously reported 27 and 23-kDa latex proteins allergenic to spina bifida patients. Allergy 1998; 53:513–519.

105. Chen Z, Raulf-Heimsoth M, Baur X. Allergenic and antigenic determinants of latex allergen Hev b 1: peptide mapping of epitopes recognized by human, murine and rabbit antibodies. Clin Exp Allergy 1996; 26:406–415.

106. Vallier P, Balland S, Harf R, et al. Identification of profilin as an IgE-binding component in latex from *Hevea brasiliensis*: clinical implications. Clin Exp Allergy 1995; 25:332–339.

107. Kostyal D, Hickey V, Noti J, et al. Cloning and characterization of a latex allergen (Hev b 7); homology to patatin, a plant PLA2. Clin Exp Immunol 1998; 112:355–362.

108. Slater J, Chhabra S. Latex antigens. J Allergy Clin Immunol 1992; 89:673–678.

109. Breiteneder H, Scheiner O. Molecular and immunological characteristics of latex allergens. Int Arch Allergy Immunol 1998; 116:83–92.

110. Posch A, Chen Z, Raulf-Heimsoth M, et al. Latex allergens. Clin Exp Allergy 1998; 28:134–140.

111. Nel A, Gujuluva G. Latex antigens: identification and use in clinical and experimental studies, including cross reactivity with food and pollen allergens. Ann Allergy Asthma Immunol 1998; 81:388–398.

112. Yagami T, Nakamura A, Shono M. One of the rubber latex allergens is a lysozyme. J Allergy Clin Immunol 1995; 96:677–686.

113. Alenius H, Lukka M, Turjanmas K, Reunala T, Makinen-Kiljunen S, Palosuo T. Purification and partial amino acid sequencing of a 27-kD natural rubber allergen recognized by latex-allergic children with spina bifida. Int Arch Allergy Immunol 1995; 106:258–262.

114. Charous B, Steven G, Breezhold D. Anti-latex IgE specificity does not correlate with clinical history (abstr). J Allergy Clin Immunol 1995; 95(1):156.

115. Van der Meeren H, van Erp P. Life-threatening contact urticaria from glove powder. Contact Dermatitis 1986; 14:190–191.

116. Seggev J, Mawhinney T, Yunginger J, et al. Anaphylaxis due to cornstarch surgical glove powder. Ann Allergy 1990; 65:152–155.

117. Williams P, Halsey J. Entotoxin as a factor in adverse reactions to latex gloves. Ann Allergy Asthma Immunol 1997; 79:303–310.

118. Slater J, Paupore E, Elwell M, et al. Lipopolysaccharide augments IgG and IgE responses of mice to the latex allergen Hev b 5. J Allergy Clin Immunol 1998; 102:977–983.

119. Charous B, Beezhold D, Adler W, et al. Endotoxin: a role in latex allergy? Ann Allergy Asthma Immunol 1997; 79:277–280.

120. Blanco C, Diaz-Perales A, Collada C, Sanchez-Monge R, Aragoncillo C, Castillo R, Ortega N, Alvarez M, Carrillo T, Salcedo G. Class I chitinases as potential panallergens involved in the latex-fruit syndrome J Allergy Clin Immunol 1999; 103:507–513.

121. Brehler R, Abrams E, Sedimayer S. Cross-reactivity between *Ficus benjamina* (weeping fig) and natural rubber latex. Allergy 1998; 53:402–406.

122. Chen Z, Posch A, Cremer R, Raulf-Heimsoth M, Baur X. Identification of hevein (Hev b 6.02) in *Hevea latex* as a major cross-reacting allergen with avocado fruit in patients with latex allergy. J Allergy Clin Immunol 1998; 102:476–481.

123. Diaz-Perales A, Collada C, Blanco C, Sanchez-Monge R, Carillo T, Aragoncillo C, Salcedo G. Class I chitinases with hevin-like domain, but not class II enzymes, are relevant chestnut and avocado allergens. J Allergy Clin Immunol 1998; 102:127–133.

124. Diez-Gomez ML, Quirce S, Aragoneses E, Cuevas M. Asthma caused by *Ficus benjamina* latex: evidence of cross-reactivity with fig fruit and papain: Ann Allergy Asthma Immunol 1997; 80:24–30.

125. Fuchs T, Spitzauer S, Vente C, Hevler J, Kapiotis S, Rumpold H, Kraft D, Valenta R. Natural latex, grass pollen, and weed pollen share IgE epitopes. J Allergy Clin Immunol 1997; 100: 356–364.

126. King TP, Hoffman D, Lowenstein H, Marsh DG, Platts-Mills TAE, Thomas W. Allergen nomenclature. J Allergy Clin Immunol 1995; 96:5–14.

127. Ross BD, McCullough J, Ownby DR. Partial cross-reactivity between latex and banana allergens: J Allergy Clin Immunol 1992; 90:409–410.

128. Yiltalo L, Alenium H, Turjanmaa K, Palosuo T, Reunala T. IgE antibodies to prohevein, hevein and rubber alongation factor in children with latex allergy. J Allergy Clin Immunol 1998; 102:659–664.

129. Raihi LM, Charpin D, Pons A, et al. Cross-reactivity between latex and banana. J Allergy Clin Immunol 1991; 87:129.

130. Rodriguez M, Vega F, Farcia M, et al. Hypersensitivity to latex, chestnut and banana. Ann Allergy 1993; 70:31–34.

131. Fernandez de Corres L, Munoz D, Bernaola G, Fernandez E, Audicana M, Urrutia I. Sensitization from chestnut and bananas in patients with urticaria and anaphylaxis from contact with latex. Ann Allergy 1993; 70:35–39.

132. Blanco C, Carrillo T, Castillo R, et al. Latex allergy: clinical features and cross-reactivity with fruits. Ann Allergy 1994; 73(4):309–314.

133. Beezhold DH, Sussman G, Liss G, et al. Latex allergy can induce clinical reactions to specific foods. Clin Exp Allergy 1996; 26:416–422.

134. Axelsson JS, Larsson PH, Zetterström O. Characterization of allergenic components in sap extract from the weeping fig (*Ficus benjamina*). Int Arch Allergy Appl Immunol 1990; 91: 130–135.

135. Delbourg MF, Guilloux L, Ville G. Hypersensitivity to latex and *Ficus benjamina* allergens. Ann Allergy Asthma Immunol 1995; 75:496–500.

136. Mikkola J, Alenius H, Kalkkinen N, et al. Hevein-like protein domains as a possible cause for allergen cross-reactivity between latex and banana. J Allergy Clin Immunol 1998; 102: 1005–1012.

137. Nel A, Gujuluva G. Latex antigens: identification and use in clinical and experimental studies, including crossreactivity with food and pollen allergens. Ann Allergy Asthma Immunol 1998; 81:388–398.

138. Sorfva R, Suvilehto K, Juntunen-Backman K, Haahtela T. Latex allergy in children with no known risk factors for latex sensitization. Pediatr Allergy Immunol 1995; 6:36–38.

139. Charous B. Latex sensitivity in low-risk individuals (abstr). Ann Allergy Asthma Immunol 1994; 74:50.

140. Taylor JS. Latex allergy update: four vignettes. Am J Contact Dermatitis 1998; 9:1–4.

141. Taylor JS, Cassettari J, Wagner W, Helm T. Contact urticaria and anaphylaxis to latex. J Am Acad Dermatol 1989; 21:874–877.

142. Taylor JS, Evey P, Helm T, Wagner W. Contact urticaria and anaphylaxis from latex. Contact Dermatitis 1990; 23:277–278.

143. Assalve D, Cicioni C, Perno P. Contact urticaria and anaphylactoid reaction from cornstarch surgical glove powder. Contact Dermatitis 1988; 19:61.

144. Axelsson JGK, Johansson SGO, Wrangsjö. IgE-mediated anaphylactoid reactions to rubber. Allergy 1987; 42:46–50.

145. Gerber AC, Jorg W, Zbinden S, Seger A, Dangel PH. Severe intraoperative anaphylaxis to surgical gloves: lattex allergy, an unfamiliar condition. Anesthesiology 1989; 71:800–802.

146. Morales C, Basomba A, Carreira J. Anaphylaxis produced by rubber glove contact. Case reports and immunological identification of the antigens involved. Clin Exp Allergy 1989; 19:425–430.

147. Zenarola P. Rubber latex allergy: unusual complication during surgery. Contact Dermatitis 1989; 21:197–198.

148. Nguyen DH, Burns MW, Shapiro GG, Mayo ME, Murrey M, Mitchell ME. Intraoperative cardiovascular collapse—secondary to latex allergy. J Urol 1991; 146:571–574.

149. Pecquet C, Leynadier F, Dry J. Contact urticaria and anaphylaxis to natural latex. J Am Acad Dermatol 1990; 22:631–633.

150. Food and Drug Administration. Allergic reactions to latex-containing medical devices. Rockville, MD: FDA Medical Bulletin, July 1991.

151. Ownby DR, Tomlanovich M, Sammons N. Anaphylaxis associated with latex allergy during barium enema examinations. J Allergy Clin Immunol 1991; 156:903–908.

152. Gelfand DW. Barium enemas, latex balloons and anaphylactic reactions. Am J Radiol 1991; 156:1–2.

153. Barton EC. Latex allergy: recognition and management of a modern problem. Nurse Pract 1993; 18:54–58.

154. Latex allergy—an emerging healthcare problem. American College of Allergy, Asthma & Immunology position statement. Ann Allergy Asthma Immunol 1995; 75:19–21.

155. Taylor JS. Other reactions from gloves. In: Mellstrom GA, Wahlberg JE, Maibach HI, eds. Protective Gloves for Occupational Use. Boca Raton, FL: CRC Press, Inc., 1994:255–265.

156. Wrangsjö K, Mellström G, Axelsson G. Discomfort from rubber gloves indicating contact urticaria. Contact Dermatitis 1986; 15:79–84.

157. Taylor JS. Rubber. In: AA Fisher, ed. Contact Dermatitis. 3d ed. Philadelphia; Lea & Febiger, 1986:603–643.

158. Cohen D, Scheman A, Stewart L, Taylor J, Pratt M, Trotter K, Prawer S, Warshaw E, Rietschel R, Watsky K, Schwarzberger K, Zug K, Sharma S, Godwin L, Kosann MK, Wilson BA. American Academy of Dermatology's position paper on latex allergy. J Am Acad Dermatol 1998; 39:98–106.

159. Field EA. Hypoallergenic gloves. Int Dent J 1995; 45:339–346.

160. Wilkinson SM. An appraisal of contact allergens in glove users (abstr). Jadassohn Centenary Congress. European Society of Contact Dermatitis/American Contact Dermatitis Society, London, October 1996, pp. 9–12.

161. Heese A, Peters KP, Koch HU. Type I allergies to latex and the aeroallergen problem. Eur J Surg 1997; (suppl 579):19–22.

162. Ownby DR. Manifestations of latex allergy. Immunol Allergy Clin North Am 1995; 15:31–45.

163. Groves CJ, Edwards C, Marks R. The occlusive effects or protective gloves on the barrier properties of the stratum corneum. In: P Elsner, HI Maibach, eds. Irritant Dermatitis. New Clinical and Experimental Aspects. Karger: Basel, 1995:87–94.

164. Thelin A, Tegler Ö, Rylander R. Lung reactions during poultry handling related to dust and bacterial endotoxin levels. Eur J Respir Dis 1984; 65:266–271.

165. Shmunes E, Darby T. Contact dermatitis due to endotoxin in irradiated latex gloves. Contact Dermatitis 1984; 10:240–244.

166. Tomazic VJ, Withrow TJ, Fisher BR, Dillard SF. Latex associated allergies and anaphylactic reactions. Clin Immunol Immunopathol 1992; 64:89–97.

167. Mansell PI, Reckless JPD, Lovell CR. Severe anaphylactic reaction to latex rubber surgical gloves. BMJ 1994; 308:246–247.

168. Turjanmaa K, Reunala T, Tuimala P, Kärkkäinen T. Allergy to latex gloves: unusual complication during delivery. BMJ 1988; 297:1029.

169. Turjanmaa K. Latex glove urticaria. Thesis, University of Tampere, Finland 1988. Acta Universitatis Temperensis series A, vol. 254, 1–86.

170. Hjorth N, Roed-Petersen J. Occupational protein contact dermatitis in food handlers. Contact Dermatitis 1976; 2:24–42.

171. Gleich GJ. The late phase of the immunoglobulin E-mediated reaction: a link between anaphylaxis and common allergic disease? J Allergy Clin Immunol 1982; 70:160–169.

172. Kleinhans D. Soforttyp-Allergie gegen Latex: Kontakt Urtikaria and Ekzem. AKT Dermatol 1984; 10:227–228.

173. Turjanmaa K, Reunala T. Latex-contact urticaria associated with delayed allergy to rubber chemicals. In: Frosch PJ, Dooms-Goossens A, Lachapelle JM, eds. Current Topics in Contact Dermatitis. Berlin: Springer, 1989:460–464.

174. Beuers U, Baur X, Schraudolph M, et al. Anaphylactic shock after game of squash in atopic woman with latex allergy. Lancet 1990; 335:1095.

175. Sussman G, Tarlo S, Dolovich J. The spectrum of IgE-mediated responses to latex. J Am Med Assoc 1991; 265–284.

176. Sussman G, Beezhold D. Allergy to latex rubber. Ann Int Med 1995; 122(1):43–46.

177. Gerber A, Jorg W, Zbinden S. Severe intraoperative anaphylaxis to surgical gloves: Latex allergy, an unfamiliar condition. Anesthesiology 1989; 71:800–802.

178. Kelly K, Setlock M, Davis J. Anaphylactic reactions during general anesthesia among pediatric patients—United States, January 1990–January 1991. MMWR 1991; 40:437–443.

179. Leynadier FPC, Dry J. Anaphylaxis to latex during surgery. Anaesthesia 1989; 44:547–550.

180. Blinkhorn A, Leggate E. An allergic reaction to rubber dam. Br Dent J 1984; 156:401–403.

181. Grattan C, Kennedy C. Angioedema during dental treatment. Contact Dermatitis 1985; 13: 333–349.

182. Laurent JMR, Smiejan JM, Madelenat P, Herman D. Latex hypersensitivity after natural delivery. J Allergy Clin Immunol 1992; 89:779–780.

183. Turjanmaa K, Reunala T. Condoms as a source of latex allergen and cause of contact urticaria. Contact Dermatitis 1989; 17:270.

184. Belsito D. Contact urticaria caused by rubber. Dermatol Clin 1990; 8:61–66.

185. Orfan NARR, Dykewicz MS, Ganz M, Kolski GB. Occupational asthma in a latex doll manufacturing plant. J Allergy Clin Immunol 1994; 94:826–830.

186. Zuskin E, Mustajbegovic J, Kanceljak B, et al. Respiratory function and immunological status in workers employed in a latex glove manufacturing plant. Am J Ind Med 1998; 33:175–181.

187. Beezhold D, Beck W. Surgical glove powders bind latex antigens. Arch Surg 1992; 127: 1354–1357.

188. Tomazic V, Shampanie E, Lamanna A, et al. Cornstarch powder on latex products is an allergen carrier. J Allergy Clin Immunol 1994; 93(4):751–758.

189. Swanson MC, Mark E, Bubak ME, Hunt LW, Yuninger JW, Warner MA, Reed CE. Quanti-

fication of occupational latex aeroallergens in a medical center. J Allergy Clin Immunol 1994; 94:445–551.

190. Heilman DK, Jones RT, Swanson MC, et al. A propspective controlled study showing that rubber gloves are the major contributor to latex aeroallergen levels in the operating room. J Allergy Clin Immunol 1996; 98:325–330.

191. Swanson MC, Yunginger JW, Reed CE. Immunochemical quantification of airborne natural rubber allergens in medical and dental office buildings. In: Maroni M, ed. Ventilation and Indoor Air Quality in Hospitals. Kluwer Academic Publishers, Boston, 1996:257–262.

192. Baur X, Chen Z, Allmers H. Can a threshold limit value for natural rubber latex airborne allergens be defined? J Allergy Clin Immunol 1998; 101:24–27.

193. Vandenplas O, Delwiche J-P, Evrard G, et al. Prevalence of occupational asthma due to latex among hospital personnel. Am J Respir Crit Care Med 1995; 151:54–60.

194. Vandenplas O. Occupational asthma due to natural rubber latex. Eur Respir J 1995; 8:1957–1965.

195. Brugnami G, Marabini A, Siracusa A, et al. Work-related late asthmatic response induced by latex allergy. J Allergy Clin Immunol 1995; 96:457–464.

196. Gassert T, Hu H, Kelsey K, et al. Long-term health and employment outcomes of occupational asthma and their determinants. J Occup Environ Med 1998; 40:481–491.

197. Paggiaro P, Vagaggini B, Bacci E, et al. Prognosis of occupational asthma. Eur Respir J 1994; 7:761–767.

198. Vandenplas O, Charous B, Tarlo S. Latex allergy. In: Bernstein D, Berstein I, Chan-Yeung M, Malo J-L, eds. Asthma in the Workplace. 2d ed. 1999, Marcel Dekker, pp. 425–444.

199. Biagini RE, Krieg EF, Sharpnack DD, et al. Performance of FDA-cleared serologic assays for latex specific IgE antibody (abstr). J Allergy Clin Immunol 1999; 103:5124.

200. Grüber C, Wahn U, Niggerman B. Is there a role for western blots in the diagnosis of latex allergy? (abstr). J Allergy Clin Immunol 1999; 103:S124.

201. Turjanmaa K, Reunala T, Räsänen L. Comparison of diagnostic methods in latex surgical glove contact urticaria. Contact Dermatitis 1988; 19:251–257.

202. Hamilton RG, Adkinson NF Jr. Natural rubber latex skin testing reagents, safety and diagnostic accuracy of nonammoniated latex, ammoniated latex, and latex rubber glove extracts. J Allergy Clin Immunol 1996; 98:872–883.

203. Kadambi A, Field S, Charous B. Diagnostic testing in latex allergy (abstr). J Allerg Clin Immunol 1997; 99:S503.

204. Kim K, Safadi G, Sheikh K. Diagnostic evaluation of type latex allergy. Ann Allergy Asthma Immunol 1998; 80:66–70.

205. Hamilton R, Nadkinson, MLSTST Force. Diagnostic natural rubber latex allergy: multicenter latex skin testing efficacy study. J Allergy Clin Immunol 1998; 102:482–490.

206. Turjanmaa K, Palosuo T, Alenium H, et al. Latex allergy diagnosis: in vivo and in vitro standardization of a natural rubber latex extract. Allergy 1997; 52:41–50.

207. Wai Y, Tarlo S. A comparison of the skin test bioequivalence of ammoniated raw latex and a filtered glycerinated extract. Can J Allergy Clin Immunol 1997; 2:110–113.

208. Fink J, Kelly K, Elms N, et al. Comparative studies of latex extracts used in skin testing. Ann Allergy Asthma Immunol 1996; 52:41–50.

209. Hamilton R, Adkinson N. Validation of the latex glove provocation procedure in latex-allergic subjects. Ann Allergy Asthma Immunol 1997; 79:266–272.

210. Vandenplas O. Occupational asthma due to natural rubber latex. Eur Respir J 1995; 8:1957–1965.

211. Hamann CP, Kick SA. Update, immediate and delayed hypersensitivity to natural rubber latex. Cutis 1993; 52:307–311.

212. Fisher AA. Condom conundrums: Part I. Cutis 1991; 48:359–360.

213. Fisher AA. Condom conundrums: Part II. Cutis 1991; 48:433–434.

214. Fisher AA. Condom dermatitis in either partner. Cutis 1987; 39:281–285.

215. Fisher AA. The new female and male polyurethane condoms. Cutis 1995; 56:82.

216. Trussell J, Warner DL, Hatcher R. Condom performance during vaginal intercourse: comparison of Trojan-enz® and Tactylon® condoms. Contraception 1992; 45:11–19.

217. Hamann CP, Nelson JR. Permeability of latex and thermoplastic elastomer to the bacteriophage II × 174. Am J Infect Control 1993; 21:289–296.

218. Turjanmaa K, Laurila K, Mäkinen-Kiljunen S, Reunala T. Rubber contact urticaria allergenic properties of 19 brands of latex gloves. Contact Dermatitis 1988; 19:362–367.

219. Palosuo T, Mäkinen-Kiljunen S, Alenius H, Reunala T, Yip E, Turjanmaa K. Measurement of natural rubber latex allergen levels in medical gloves by allergen-specific IgE-ELISA inhibition, RAST inhibition and skin prick test. Allergy 1998; 53:59–67.

220. Beezhold D, Pugh B, Liss G, Sussman G. Correlation of protein levels with skin prick test reactions in patients allergic to latex. J Allergy Clin Immunol 1996; 98:1097–1102.

221. Yip E, Turjanmaa K, Ng PH, Mok KL. Allergic responses and levels of extractable proteins in NRL gloves and dry rubber products. N Nat Rubber Res 1994; 9:79–86.

222. Mäkinen-Kiljunen S, Turjanmaa K. Comparison of latex allergen activity from in vivo and in vitro testing. Proceedings Latex Allergy Symposium (abstr). Toronto: 1994:35.

223. Yip E, Turjanmaa K, Mäkinen-Kiljunen S. The non-allergenicity of NR dry rubber products with reference to type I protein allergy. Rubber Dev 1995; 48:48–52.

224. Palusüo T, Turjanmaa K, Reinikka-Railo H. Allergen content of latex gloves. A market surveillance study of medical gloves used in Finland in 1997. Pub Natl Agency Med 1997; 9: 1–12.

225. Wrangsjö K, Lundberg M. Prevention of latex allergy. Allergy 1996; 51:65–67.

226. Baur X, Jäger A. Airborne allergens from latex gloves. Lancet 1990; 335:912.

227. Beezhold D, Beck WC. Surgical glove powders bind latex antigens. Arch Surg 1992; 127: 1354–1357.

228. Reijula KE, Kelly KJ, Kurup VP, Choi H, Bongard RD, Dawson CA, Fink JN. Latex-induced dermal and pulmonary hypersensitivity in rabbits. J Allergy Clin Immunol 1994; 94:891–902.

229. Kurup UP, Kumar A, Choi H, Muraly PS, Resnik A, Kelly KT, Fink JN. Latex antigens induce IgE and eosinophils in mice. Int Arch Allergy Immunol 1994; 103:370–377.

230. Tarlo SM, Sussman G, Contela A, Swanson MC. Control of airborne latex by use of powder-free latex gloves. J Allergy Clin Immunol 1994; 93:985–989.

231. Vanderplas O, Delwiche JP, Depelchin S, Sibille Y, Vande Weyer R, Delaunois L. Latex gloves with a lower protein content reduce bronchial reactions in subjects with occupational asthma caused by latex. Am J Respir Crit Care Med 1995; 151:887–891.

232. Ruëff F, Thomas P, Przybilla B. Natural rubber latex as an aeroallergen in the general environment. Contact Dermatitis 1996; 35:46–47.

233. Williams PB, Buhr MP, Weber RW, Volz MA, Koepke JW, Selner JC. Latex allergen in respirable particulate air pollution. J Allergy Clin Immunol 1995; 95:88–95.

234. Wolf BL. Anaphylactic reaction to latex gloves (letter). N Engl J Med 1993; 329:279–280.

235. Truscott W. Anaphylactic reaction to latex gloves (letter reply to Wolf). N Engl J Med 1993; 329:280.

236. Natural rubber-containing medical devices: user labeling. Fed Reg 1997; 62:51021–51030.

237. Stigi J, Lowery A, Cardamae T. Department of Health and Human Services, Center for Devices and Radiological Health (US). Regulatory requirements for medical gloves. Rockville, MD: HHS Publication, May 1993.

238. Premarket Notification [510 (k)]. Submission for testing for skin sensitization to chemicals in natural rubber products. U.S. Food and Drug Administration Center for Devices and Radiological Health, Rockville, MD, January 13, 1999.

239. Sussman GL, Ownby DR. Latex Allergy: Clinical perspectives. Breakfast seminar syllabus. Am Acad Allergy Asthma and Immunology, Orlando, FL, March 2, 1999.

240. Maso MJ, Goldberg DJ. Contact dermatoses from disposable glove use: a review. J Am Acad Dermatol 1990; 23:733–737.

241. Product list. Latex Allergy News 1997; 5–9.

242. Mellström GA, Wahlberg JE, Maibach HI. Protective gloves for occupational use. Boca Raton, FL: CRC Press; 1994:150–151.

243. Tanglertsampan C, Patrakarn S, Vassansiri E. Double use test for latex allergy. Contact Dermatitis 1997; 36:311–312.

244. Kwangsukstith C, Maibach HI. Contact urticaria from polyurethane-membrane hypoallergenic gloves. Contact Dermatitis 1995; 33:200–201.

245. Baur X, Chen Z, Raulf-Heinsoth M. Results of wearing test with two different latex gloves and without the use of skin protection cream. Allergy 1998; 53:441–444.

246. Charous B, Banov C, Bardana EJ, et al. Latex allergy—an emerging healthcare problem. Ann Allergy Asthma Immunol 1995; 75:19–21.

247. Siu SR, Smith GJ, Sussman GL, et al. Reduction of airborne latex protein exposure by use of low protein powder-free gloves (abstr). J Allergy Clin Immunol 1996; 97:325.

248. Tarlo SM, Sussman G, Contala A, et al. Control of airborne latex by use of powder-free gloves. J Allergy Clin Immunol 1994; 93:985–989.

249. Charous B, Scheunemann P, Swanson M. Dispersion of latex aeroallergen (abstract). J Allergy Clin Immunol 1998; 101:S160.

250. AAAA1 and ACAA1 joint statement concerning the use of powdered and non-powdered natural latex gloves. Ann Allergy Asthma and Immunol 1997; 79:487.

251. Preventing allergic reactions to natural rubber latex in the workplace. National Institute for Occupational Safety and Health, Cincinnati, Ohio, Pub. No 97–135, 1997.

252. Kelso JM, Yunginger JW, Jones RT, Fransway AF, Warner MA, Hunt LW. Extractable latex allergens and proteins in disposable medical gloves and other rubber products. J Allergy Clin Immunol 1994; 93:836–842.

253. Taylor JS, Hamann CP, Yoon HA. Latex avoidance: a multidisciplinary approach. In: International Latex Conference: Sensitivity to Latex and Medical Devices. Baltimore, MD: U.S. Food and Drug Administration, 1992.

254. Kotilainen HR, Brinker JP, Avato JL. Latex and vinyl examination gloves. Arch Intern Med 1989; 149:2749–2753.

255. Korniewicz D, Laughan B, Cry W, Lytle D, Larson E. Leakage of virus through used vinyl and latex examination gloves. J Clin Microbiol 1990; 28:787–788.

256. Jones R, Scheppmann D, Heilman D. Prospective study of extractable latex allergen contents of disposable medical gloves. Ann Allergy 1994; 73:321–325.

257. Patterson P. Allergy issues complicate buying decisions for gloves. OR Manager 1995; 11(6).

258. Cohen D, Scheman A, Stewart L, Taylor J, Pratt M, et al. American Academy of Dermatology position paper on latex allergy. J Am Acad Dermatol 1998; 39:98–106.

259. Sine S, Smith G, Sussman G. Reduction of airborne latex protein exposure by use of low protein, powder-free gloves. J Allergy Clin Immunol 1996; 97:325.

260. Wrangsjö K. IgE-mediated latex allergy and contact allergy to rubber. In: Clinical Occupational Dermatology. Stockholm: National Institute of Occupational Health, 1993.

261. Kujala VM, Karvonen J, Läärä E, Kanerva L, Estlander T, Reijula KE. Postal questionnaire study of disability associated with latex allergy among health care workers in Finland. Am J Int Med 1997; 32:197–204.

262. Taylor M. Cost of latex device-related occupational illness, workmen's compensation and legal issues. Eur J Surg 1997; (suppl 579):49–57.

263. Hunt LW, Boone-Orke JL, Fransway AF, Fremstad CE, Jones RT, Swanson MC, McEvoy MT, Miller LK, Majerus ET, Luker PA, Scheppmann DL, Webb NJ, Yunginger JW. A medical-center-wide multidisciplinary approach to the problem of NRL allergy. J Occup Environ Med 1996; 38:765–770.

264. Slater JE. Is immunotherapy an option? Syllabus Latex allergy, thinking ahead workshop. Am Acad Allergy, Asthma and Immunology, Orlando, FL, March 1, 1999.

265. Melton AL. Managing latex allergy in patients and health care workers. Cleve Clin J Med 1997; 64(2):76–82.

# 13
## Reactions to Stinging and Biting Insects

**Pamela W. Ewan**
*MRC Centre & Addenbrooke's Hospital, University of Cambridge Clinical School, Cambridge, United Kingdom*

Arthropoda is the largest phylum in the animal kingdom. It contains insects (the class Insecta or Hexapoda) and arachnids (the class Arachnida). Arachnids—spiders, scorpions, mites, and ticks—are carnivorous invertebrates. Certain venomous spiders and scorpions are dangerous to humans, but most are harmless. Insects are distinguished from other arthropods by their body (divided into head, thorax, and abdomen), by having three pairs of legs (all other arthropods have four or more pairs), and by (usually) bearing wings (all other arthropods are wingless). There are many insect groups, including the orders Hymenoptera (bee, wasp/yellow jacket, and ant), Diptera (midges, gnats, mosquitoes and horseflies), Phthiraptera (lice), and Siphonaptera (flea). This chapter will concentrate on bee and wasp stings, as they are important causes of allergic disease, and will cover some of the insect and arachnid bites. When patients describe reactions to bites or stings, they usually refer to all of the above as insects.

## I. HYMENOPTERA

Hymenoptera (bee or wasp) stings can cause severe allergic reactions and are an important cause of anaphylaxis.

### A. Hymenoptera Classification

The Hymenoptera are subdivided into families, which include the Apidae (honeybee and bumblebee) and the Vespidae (wasp or yellow jacket, hornets, and paper wasps). The wasp is a more common cause of allergic reactions than the honey bee in the United Kingdom, the northeast United States, Scandinavia, and parts of Europe. Of the Apidae, the vast majority of allergic reactions are due to the honeybee. Allergic reactions to the bumblebee are rare but have been described as an occupational hazard in greenhouse workers in Holland since the introduction of bumblebees for pollination. Of the Vespidae, most reactions are due to the species *vespula*, known as yellow jacket (in the United States) or wasp (in the United Kingdom). Polistes cause fewer reactions, and these occur mainly in the southern part of Europe around the Mediterranean.

## B.  Hymenoptera Venoms

Bee and wasp venoms are distinct. They contain several well-defined major allergens as well as a number of less well-characterized proteins and many low molecular weight substances. The major allergens of bee venom are phospholipase $A_2$, hyaluronidase, and acid phosphatase, while mellitin and allergen C are weaker allergens [1–3]. Vespid venoms contain phospholipase (A and B), hyaluronidase, acid phosphatase, and antigen 5 [4–6]. There is cross-reactivity of venom from closely related insects, e.g., from the *Vespid* genus, polistes or paper wasp [7]. A minimal degree of immunogenic cross-reactivity has been demonstrated between *Apis mellifera* and vespid venoms [8], and this appears to be due to cross-reactivity between the hyaluronidases [9]; however, clinically it is unusual to find a patient allergic to bee and wasp.

Venom also contains biogenic amines and other low molecular weight substances, the most important of which is histamine. These account for 25% of the dry weight of bee venom, are not allergenic, but have biological effects. Vespid venom contains more histamine (4–5%) than honeybee venom. Venom also contains peptides; e.g., mellitin and mast cell degranulating peptide in bee venom and kinins in Vespidae venoms. The local swelling is primarily caused by biogenic amines and low molecular weight peptides, which increase tissue permeability and release histamine from mast cells.

## C.  Sensitization to Hymenoptera Venom

Most people are rarely stung by wasps, perhaps once every 15 years, unless there is some specific occupational hazard (bakery worker, fruit farm worker, etc.). Patients developing wasp venom allergy have usually been stung infrequently: one study found this to be an average of two to three stings [10]. In contrast, bee venom allergy occurs mainly in bee-keepers, their relatives, and sometimes their neighbors—people who are frequently stung. This suggests that the degree of exposure to venom before the onset of allergic reactions is different in bee and wasp allergy, bee venom–allergic patients usually requiring a larger number of stings before sensitization [10].

## D.  Mechanism

Hymenoptera venom allergy is an IgE-mediated type I hypersensitivity reaction. Venom IgE binds to the surface of mast cells via high-affinity receptors for the Fc piece of IgE (FceRI). After a sting, venom rapidly enters the circulation. When venom cross-links two adjacent venom-specific IgE antibody molecules bound to mast cells, the mast cell is activated and mediator release occurs. Stored mediators including histamine are released in minutes, but production of the newly synthesized mediators (including leukotrienes and prostaglandins) follows quickly. These cause mucosal or subcutaneous edema, increased capillary permeability, and smooth muscle contraction. The resulting clinical features depend on the site of the venom-IgE interaction and the degree of mast cell activation.

It has been suggested that in a minority of patients systemic reactions to stings may occur through a non-IgE mechanism [11,12] because a small number of patients studied within a year of a reaction did not have detectable serum venom-specific IgE. In support of this, some patients had apparently reacted to their first sting. The reaction may have been due to direct effects of vasoactive substances in venom. However, it is possible that the serum assay was not sensitive enough to detect very low levels of venom-specific IgE or that all of this was bound to mast cells. Patients with negative radioallergosorbent tests for serum venom-specific IgE but positive intradermal venom skin tests have been shown to have venom IgE in the serum by immunoblotting [13].

## E. Clinical Features

Hymenoptera stings can cause local or systemic (generalized) allergic reactions (Table 1).

### 1. Local Reactions

The normal reaction to a sting is immediate pain followed in 10–15 minutes by a small area of erythema and edema, a few centimeters in diameter, which resolves in a few hours. Local reactions consist of much larger edematous reactions around the site of the sting, lasting over 24 hours. Swelling develops over several hours, and the area becomes erythematous, edematous, tender, and often pruritic. Once established, local reactions take several days to resolve. The size varies, but severe local swellings can involve part or most of a limb. Local reactions are uncomfortable but not dangerous, unless they compromise the airway; e.g., local swelling from a sting in the mouth may cause marked respiratory difficulty. Swellings of the face, lips, or eyelids look more alarming and cause more distress than larger swellings of the limbs or trunk.

### 2. Systemic Reactions

A variety of symptoms may occur in a systemic reaction. These include erythema, flushing, intense generalized pruritus, urticaria, angioedema, dyspnea, and palpitations. The dyspnea is commonly due to laryngeal edema (patients describe a tightness or feeling of obstruction in the throat or neck) but may be due to asthma. Patients may become light-headed or weak, sometimes with visual disturbances, and may faint or lose consciousness, depending on the degree of hypotension. Rhinitis or conjunctivitis may occur. Vomiting is a less common feature, and central chest pain, similar to angina, fitting, or incontinence occurs rarely. In the more severe reactions, it is common for patients to suffer a sense of foreboding or impending doom: they feel they are going to die. The pattern of reaction varies greatly and depends on the site and degree of mast cell activation. Some or all of the above features may be present. Some patients begin with cutaneous features, then progress over 20 or so minutes to more serious symptoms, whereas others have few prodromal symptoms and then rapidly become hypotensive with loss of consciousness. The clinical features of 56 consecutive patients with systemic reactions to bee or wasp stings are shown in Table 2 [10].

It is useful clinically to classify systemic reactions as mild, moderate, or severe (Table 1), as this influences management.

**Table 1** Clinical Features of Allergic Reactions to Bee or Wasp Stings

| Type | Severity | Features |
|------|----------|----------|
| Local | Varies | Angioedema at/adjacent to site of sting |
| Systemic | Mild | Pruritus, urticaria, angioedema, rhinitis |
| (generalized) | Moderate | Mild asthma, more severe angioedema, abdominal pain, vomiting |
| | Severe | Respiratory difficulty (asthma/laryngeal edema), hypotension, collapse, loss of consciousness |

**Table 2**  Clinical Features in 56 Consecutive Patients with Systemic Reactions to Bee or Wasp Stings

| Feature | Number | % |
|---|---|---|
| Generalized pruritus | 30 | 56 |
| Urticaria | 30 | 56 |
| Angioedema | 31 | 57 |
| Laryngeal edema | 16 | 30 |
| Respiratory | 24 | 44 |
| Gastrointestinal | 21 | 39 |
| Hypotension without LOC | 21 | 39 |
| Loss of consciousness | 18 | 33 |

*Source*: Adapted from Ref. 10.

## F.  Natural History

Patients with a history of a severe systemic reaction to a bee or wasp sting may have no reaction to a subsequent sting, i.e., spontaneous resolution occurs. A number of studies confirm this clinical observation. In the first controlled trial of pure venom immunotherapy in patients with systemic reactions to stings, only 60% of the placebo group developed a systemic reaction to a challenge sting: thus the improvement rate was about 40% [15]. This might represent spontaneous improvement or a placebo effect, but the latter seems less likely.

In studies of natural history, where the endpoint was the response to a random field sting, spontaneous improvement was also demonstrated. Ewan [10] showed that 74% (20/27) of wasp-allergic and 80% (16/20) of bee-allergic patients had a further systemic reaction, and some of these repeat reactions were of reduced severity. Settipane and Chafee [16] found that about 44% of patients were "better" when restung: most of these had local reactions; some had systemic reactions of reduced severity.

A number of studies show the risk of a further systemic reaction to be quite variable, occurring in 20–80% of patients (Table 3) [10,15,17–23]. Those with mild systemic reactions appear to show the greatest improvement rate (e.g., 80%) [17,19–21], but even in those with severe reactions there is a definite spontaneous improvement rate [23]. The interval from the previous sting may also be a factor—the longer the interval, the less-severe the reaction. There seems to be a higher rate of repeat reactions following field stings [10] than challenge stings [18].

There are very few studies of natural history in children, but the risk of repeated reactions seems low. In a study of accidental stings in 242 children with a history of mild systemic reactions (mainly urticaria), only about 9% of those who had not received immunotherapy had further systemic reactions (SRs) [24]. [It should be noted that a patient who has shown spontaneous improvement after a sting might still react to a later sting.]

The reasons for change in response to sequential stings are not clear. Possible factors are differences in the dose of venom injected, and the site of the sting (which will influence absorption and distribution of venom), and changes in the immune response with time.

There are not many studies on the outcome in patients with large local reactions. Many continue to have local reactions only, but two studies showed that 40% of patients had systemic reactions to subsequent stings [25,26].

**Table 3** Spontaneous Improvement May Occur After a Systemic Allergic Reaction to a Bee or Wasp Sting

| Nature of the index reaction | Systemic reaction to subsequent sting (%) | Ref. |
| --- | --- | --- |
| Mild systemic | 20 | 17 |
| | 0 | 21 |
| | 20 | 19 |
| | 14 | 20 |
| Systemic | 58 | 15 |
| | 28 | |
| | | 18 |
| | 74–80 | 10 |
| | 50 (of patients) | 22 |
| | 35 (of stings) | |
| Severe systemic | 21 | 21 |
| | 61 (of patients) | 23 |
| | 39 (of stings) | |

## G. Investigation

A detailed history is essential. It is important to check the information that led the patient to conclude that the insect was a bee or wasp/yellow jacket, since patients may confuse these or the insect may not have been seen. In the United Kingdom, most bee-allergic patients are beekeepers or their relatives. Details of the site of sting, clinical features, and their time of onset, as well as the outcome and therapy required, should be obtained. It is important to ascertain whether this was a single sting or multiple stings, since a reaction to a large dose of venom does not necessarily mean that the patient would have the same reaction to a single sting. The number of previous stings by either bee or wasp and their effect should be noted. A general allergy history, including history of asthma, should be obtained. Specific enquiry should be made about cardiovascular disease, hypertension, or beta-blocker therapy, factors that may have a bearing on treatment of anaphylaxis and indications for venom immunotherapy.

Specific IgE to venom can be determined either by skin tests or measurement of specific IgE antibodies in serum. Skin prick tests are the standard test but, with venom, have the disadvantage of producing small wheals, which can be difficult to read [27], and a series of dilutions are needed. For this reason some investigators use intradermal skin tests, which give more clear-cut responses. The disadvantages are that some patients develop late local swelling, and they carry a greater risk of inducing a systemic reaction, although this is rare. It is important to test for both bee and wasp venom.

There are a variety of commercial assays for serum venom-specific IgE, e.g., the radioallergosorbent test (RAST) and its successor, the ImmunoCAP or UniCAP system (CAP-RAST).

Occasional patients are seen with a clear history of systemic reaction to a sting in whom the intradermal skin test is positive but venom-specific IgE in serum is negative. One author demonstrated that all such patients had specific IgE on immunoblotting [13].

It is probable that these patients would have been negative on skin prick test, so this and/or a negative RAST does not necessarily mean venom IgE is absent.

Since the introduction of the more sensitive CAP system, more double positives (for bee and wasp/yellow jacket) when the patient is allergic to only one insect have been seen: 30% were double positive on CAP testing compared to 6% on RAST testing [28]. It is therefore important not to measure IgE to a single venom only unless the insect has been identified with certainty, as the wrong diagnosis may be made.

## H.  Treatment

### 1.  Local (Swelling) Reactions

Oral antihistamines taken immediately after the sting before the local reaction is established are usually effective and are the mainstay of treatment. Early treatment is essential, because antihistamines taken after swelling is established have less effect. A variety of nonsedative antihistamines are available, and it is important to choose one with a quick onset of action. For more severe swellings, oral steroids, usually requiring only one or a few doses, may occasionally be prescribed. Urgent intervention may be required for a local reaction involving the airway. Parenteral chlorpheniramine and hydrocortisone (intramuscularly or by slow intravenous injection) are usually sufficient, but adrenaline (intramuscularly or subcutaneously) will rapidly reduce mucosal edema.

Immunotherapy is not indicated for local reactions.

### 2.  Systemic Reactions

There are two options: patients may carry drugs to treat reactions should they occur or be desensitized.

a.  Drug Treatment.  The drugs required will depend on the nature and severity of the reaction. An oral antihistamine should be taken as soon as any symptom appears. If the reaction is cutaneous only, this is usually all that is required. Sometimes further treatment with injected chlorpheniramine and hydrocortisone is required.

Severe reactions with definite respiratory difficulty or hypotension must be treated with parenteral adrenaline [29–31]. The adult dose is 0.5 mg [0.5 ml of 1 in 1000 strength (1 mg/ml)] intramuscularly or subcutaneously. Preloaded adrenaline syringes (Epi-pen and Epi-pen Junior) are available for self-administration (administering a fixed dose of 0.3 mg for adults and 0.15 mg for children).

Intermediate reactions of moderate severity such as mild laryngeal edema or lightheadedness may require parenteral chlorpheniramine and hydrocortisone and, if asthma occurs, inhaled $\beta_2$-agonists and oxygen. However, if in doubt, adrenaline (IM) should be given. Inhaled adrenaline is highly effective for laryngeal edema but is not a substitute for injected adrenaline if the reaction is severe.

Early treatment by the patient means that reactions are usually easier to control. Patients should still seek medical help in an emergency department in case further treatment is required. It is helpful if they have written treatment plans setting out when the various drugs should be administered, and they must be taught how to use the Epi-pen. This approach has the advantage that reactions are only treated if they occur. Patients may not be stung for many years and the allergy may have resolved.

b.  Venom Immunotherapy (Desensitization).  Before discussing indications for immunotherapy, it is important to consider efficacy, side effects, as well as the risk of a future reaction.

*Efficacy.*   Venom immunotherapy (VIT) is highly effective—more effective than immunotherapy with other allergens. The previously used whole body extracts of bee or wasp were shown to be no better than placebo [15]. The first double-blind placebo-controlled trial of pure venom immunotherapy in a small number of patients with a history of systemic reactions treated for 10 weeks showed that 95% of the actively treated group no longer reacted to a challenge sting [15]. In contrast, about 40% of the placebo group had no systemic reaction, and there was a similar outcome in the group treated with whole body extract. Many studies followed showing similar high efficacy rates for pure venom, e.g., 97% in a larger series of patients with wasp venom allergy [32]. Efficacy seems to be higher in wasp allergy than in bee sting allergy [22,33–35]. Müller [34] showed that after VIT, 28% of bee-allergic patients and 9% of yellow jacket–allergic patients developed systemic reactions to sting challenge.

*Side Effects.*   Immunotherapy with any allergen carries the risk of inducing allergic reactions including anaphylaxis, and fatal reactions have occurred [36,37]. In VIT the incidence of side effects will vary with the type of desensitizing vaccine (aqueous versus depot) and the dose schedule.

A multicenter retrospective study in the United States in 1400 patients, coordinated by the American Academy of Allergy, found the incidence of SRs was 12% [38]. The severity of the SR to immunotherapy did not correlate with the severity of reactions to previous field stings or to the diagnostic criteria for venom allergy.

Prospective studies are likely to give a more accurate indication of side effects than retrospective studies, and two have been reported from the United Kingdom [39,40]. In the first, a total of 727 injections were given to 11 bee- and 15 wasp-allergic patients, and the overall incidence of systemic reactions was 23% in the wasp group and 10% in the bee group [39]. The second study involved 109 patients, and systemic reactions occurred after 7.5% of injections during the initial phase and 2.1% of maintenance injections. Reactions were more frequent after bee than after wasp venom injections [40]. In both prospective studies, the patient's initial reaction to field sting had mainly been classified as severe, in line with indications for venom immunotherapy in the United Kingdom.

Although SRs occur more frequently in the initial course, about one third of SR occurred during maintenance therapy [39]. The more severe SRs usually occurred in the initial course. Of the 727 injections, 8 (1.1%) led to reactions severe enough to require systemic treatment, 4 of which (0.5%) required adrenaline. Twenty-one SR were classified as severe or potentially severe and included anaphylaxis (3), asymptomatic hypotension (3), light-headedness (1), mild laryngeal-edema (12), and profound lethargy (2). Most of these reactions occurred early, in the first 30 minutes after injection, but 5 began after 30 minutes. The anaphylactic reactions (severe reactions requiring adrenaline) began 3, 7, and 17 minutes after injection. These data suggest that a 1-hour observation period after each injection on a VIT schedule is necessary, as recommended in the U.K. guidelines on immunotherapy [41]. In one of these studies the higher incidence of SR in the wasp group was because a small number of patients developed repeated but severe late lethargy, beginning several hours after injection and lasting 1–2 days [39]. These reactions would only be picked up in a prospective study. Reisman [42] has described similar pronounced fatigue reactions following VIT. Most studies report more side effects in bee than wasp VIT, e.g., SRs in 41% of bee patients compared to 25% in yellow jacket patients [34].

*What Is the Risk of a Future Reaction?*   The studies of natural history discussed above show there is a considerable chance of no further SR, although this is variable. It is perceived but not proven that the risk of further SR is greater if the index reaction was severe. There is a very high incidence of no further SR when the index reaction was a mild systemic one. Twenty-nine patients with systemic reactions were followed over 10 years for the response to resting: those with a mild response had no reactions (100% spontaneous improvement), while 21% (3/14) of those with severe SRs had a further SR [21]. However, in other studies the outcome is similar whether the index sting caused a mild or a severe SR (Table 3). Between one third and one quarter of the patients in Savliwala and Reisman's study had lost their venom-specific IgE over the follow-up period, depending on whether this was assessed by skin test or RAST [21]. The risk of a further systemic reaction appears to fall with the interval from the last sting, and Settipane and Chafee [16] showed that an interval of at least 5 years was associated with a better outcome. The risk of being stung again is low unless there is a risk factor such as beekeeping, proximity to beehives, fruit farm worker, bakery worker, etc. In the studies of natural history, there will be many variables, such as interval from the last sting, dose of venom injected, and site of sting. The difficulty is that these variables are unpredictable in an individual patient so that the risk of a further systemic reaction can only be assessed in general terms.

*Venom IgG Levels.*    There has been a search for a test that would predict the reaction to a future sting. It was proposed that a high level of venom-specific IgG would be protective, because in early studies on venom immunotherapy, high levels of venom IgG were found after treatment [43]. However, subsequently a considerable body of evidence showed that venom IgG levels cannot be used to predict reactions to sting. Several studies show no correlation between levels of venom-specific IgG, IgG1, IgG4, or IgE, or the IgG:IgE ratios and the reaction to a sting [17,18,44].

In addition, beekeepers had systemic reactions to stings despite high bee venom IgG titers [44,45]. Thus, whereas in wasp allergy, wasp IgG levels are usually low before VIT and rise after treatment, most bee-allergic patients present with high titers, which change little or show a small further rise with VIT [44].

*Venom IgE Levels.*    Similarly, the severity of the allergic reaction is not directly related to the level of the venom-specific IgE. When patients with markedly elevated titers of venom-specific IgE were compared with patients with low titers, the nature of the allergic reaction (whether local, mild systemic, or severe systemic) was similar [46].

*Provocation Tests.*    A provocation test is the most useful test to predict a future reaction. It can be performed either by giving a subcutaneous injection of pure venom or by challenge sting, and it is argued that these are not identical, as a challenge sting may contain more vasoactive low molecular weight substances. The disadvantage is the risk of inducing a severe SR, but the former is safer since one can begin with a small dose. However, a provocation test simply delineates the response at the time of the test, which may not be the same as the outcome of a field sting at some future date, e.g., the provocation test might resensitize the patient.

Provocation tests can be useful in the assessment of patients in whom indications for immunotherapy are not clear-cut. A negative provocation may mean that in patients in whom indications for VIT were borderline (a history of a systemic reaction of moderate severity), immunotherapy can be avoided [47].

## I.    Indications for Venom Immunotherapy

Practice varies in different countries. Position papers on venom immunotherapy from the European Academy of Allergy and Clinical Immunology [48] and on allergen immunotherapy from the British Society for Allergy and Clinical Immunology [41] give similar recommendations. It is essential to demonstrate the presence of venom-specific IgE by skin testing or in serum.

In deciding whether VIT is indicated, factors to be considered are the severity of reaction, the risk of future stings, the general health of the patient, and other relevant disorders.

Patients with local reactions only should not be desensitized. It is helpful to categorize systemic reactions according to severity when considering VIT (Table 1). In the United Kingdom, a conservative approach is taken [41]. Severe systemic reactions with significant respiratory difficulty or collapse are usually an indication for VIT. Mild systemic reactions (cutaneous reactions with erythema, urticaria, or angioedema or rhinitis) do not require VIT. The main difficulty is in deciding how to manage patients who have had moderately severe systemic reactions. Desensitization is sometimes indicated, but often not. In some countries any systemic reaction is considered to be an indication for VIT. Factors relevant to the individual should also be considered, e.g., risk of further stings, accessibility of medical help, ability to self-administer adrenaline, etc. Children rarely need to be desensitized because the incidence of spontaneous improvement is so high.

## J. Administration of VIT

### 1. Which Venom?

Pure venom must be used, and it is important to determine the insect (e.g., honeybee or yellow jacket) causing the reaction and use the appropriate venom.

### 2. Treatment Regimes

A variety of regimes are available: conventional, rush, and semi-rush. These have evolved arbitrarily. The conventional regime involves an initial course, starting with very low dose and increasing weekly to reach the top dose, equivalent to about two stings, in about 3 months. Maintenance injections of the same dose are then given at longer intervals, usually monthly, for about 3 years. The optimal regime, maintenance interval, or duration of treatment is not known.

a. *Maintenance Interval.* Lichtenstein's group showed 6-weekly maintenance to be as good as monthly [49]. Two studies looked at the efficacy of 3-monthly maintenance injections, but because they took 19 months and 17 months, respectively, to reach or switch to the longer maintenance interval, they are difficult to interpret [50,51]. Both found no loss of efficacy on 3-monthly maintenance.

b. *Duration of Venom Immunotherapy.* In some countries, including the United States, a longer total course of 5 years or more is given. The standard duration of VIT is 3 years in the United Kingdom and Europe. A study from the United States tried to determine whether there is an optimal duration of treatment [52]. Fifty-one patients who had received from 2 to 10 years VIT stopped VIT if sting challenge was negative, then were followed up after 1 year with a further sting challenge. Only 2 of 51 (4%) patients developed SRs: both had a history of severe SR to the original sting and had been treated for less than 5 years. The authors suggest that VIT should be continued for 5 years in patients in whom the original field sting reaction was severe (grade IV). Since the overall outcome was so good, larger numbers of patients would be needed before this conclusion could be drawn.

In another study, 30 patients who had received VIT for at least 5 years stopped treatment. Venom IgG levels fell over the next 9 months. Sting challenge, performed in 29 patients after 12 months without therapy, caused no systemic reaction [53].

C.  Maintenance Dose.   The standard maintenance dose is 100 μg, equivalent to about two stings, and presumably this is to ensure that a patient would be well desensitized in the event of a single sting. Reisman and Livingston [54] suggest that a maintenance dose of 50 μg would be sufficient in most patients. In their study 108 patients received a maintenance dose of 50 μg over 10 years, and 258 restings occurred, 1 month to 8 years after starting VIT. Only three systemic reactions occurred, two of which were very mild (a reaction rate of 2.7% per patient or 1.2% per sting). The original reaction in 44 of the 108 patients was severe anaphylaxis.

d.  Aqueous Versus Depot Extracts.   Venom preparations are available as aqueous or depot extracts. Depot extracts release allergen more slowly and are likely to be safer. Most studies on venom immunotherapy are with aqueous extracts of pure venom. A study of aluminum hydroxide–adsorbed extracts in 30 patients found these to be safe (no severe reactions and a mild reaction rate of 1 in 139 injections) and effective (95%, with 1 mild SR in 19 restings) [55].

e.  Rush Immunotherapy.   In rush induction of immunotherapy, the initial course is condensed into one or a few days. There are various regimes, and injections may be given at $1/2$- to 2-hour intervals. The dose reached after the rush period is either the top dose or a little less, in which case further increments are given over the next few weeks. A dose of 50 μg or greater is usually reached in the first few days. Patients then continue on maintenance therapy, as in conventional regimes. Semi-rush or cluster regimes are slower versions of rush induction and take about 7 days.

Bernstein et al.'s [56] rush regime involves a cumulative dose of 58 μg on day 1, followed by an accelerated build-up over 3 weeks to a maintenance dose of 100 μg. Mild SRs occurred in 4 of 77 patients (5%) on day 1. The efficacy was 100%, calculated from responses to restings in 21 patients at a mean of 1 year after treatment.

Vervloet's group [57] compared three different rush protocols. Two hundred and eighty-four patients, allergic to either bee or yellow jacket, were treated with a 4-day protocol (cumulative dose 527 μg), a 6-hour protocol (cumulative dose 226 μg), or a 210-minute protocol (cumulative dose 101 μg). Side effects occurred in 28, 28, and 9% of these groups, respectively. They concluded that the safest regime was to give a low cumulative dose over a short period. Efficacy was not examined.

### 3.  Administration of Immunotherapy

Practice and regulations vary in different countries. IT should only be given by experienced medical and nursing staff. In the United Kingdom it can only be given in centers where there are facilities for resuscitation. A full general medical history must be obtained before the decision to start immunotherapy is made. Patients should be reviewed before each injection to determine whether the dose schedule can be followed or needs to be modified. Enquiry should be made about late reactions after the previous injection, infection, other intercurrent illness, or active allergy and whether they are taking any medication. If these factors are present, dose modification or even omission may be required. If patients are taking β-blockers, it is advisable to change to an alternative drug before starting IT, as β-blockers may modify the response to adrenaline.

Before the injection is given, blood pressure and ideally the peak expiratory flow rate must be measured in all patients. Adrenaline must always be immediately available (preferably drawn up in a syringe), and any other drugs likely to be needed to treat an allergic reaction should be on hand (including parenteral antihistamines, hydrocortisone, inhaled and nebulized $\beta_2$-agonists, oral antihistamines, IV fluids, and oxygen).

It is important to check the dose (concentration of venom in the vial, and volume) with another person: errors in dosage are a major cause of serious and fatal reactions to IT. The venom is given by slow subcutaneous injection.

### 4. Monitoring After Injection

Patients need to be watched carefully after injection to detect systemic allergic reactions as soon as they begin, as early intervention is important. In some centers blood pressure and peak flow in asthmatics are monitored after 30 minutes and 1 hour. Large local reactions often occur and may require oral antihistamines. It is important to treat systemic reactions early and aggressively. Anaphylaxis can usually be quickly reversed by prompt administration of intramuscular adrenaline. It is wise to follow this with IM hydrocortisone to minimize the risk of later relapse. Minor SR, e.g., rhinitis, slight urticaria, or angioedema, should be treated with oral antihistamines. Moderate SRs, e.g., more marked urticaria/angioedema or slight asthma/laryngeal edema, should be treated with injected chlorpheniramine and hydrocortisone or inhaled adrenaline or inhaled $\beta_2$-agonists, as appropriate.

Late-onset reactions (>2 hours) may occur. Late enlargement of local swelling is common, particularly early in the course of VIT, and if severe may persist for a few days. Late local reactions usually decrease as the course of immunotherapy progresses. Late systemic reactions are unusual and are usually mild, e.g., a few urticarial lesions.

The duration of monitoring required varies from country to country. In the United Kingdom this is 1 hour after the last injection [58], because of the risk of severe and life-threatening systemic reactions. However, serious reactions occur early, and most systemic reactions, irrespective of severity, occur by 30 minutes, although a few mild SRs begin up to 60 minutes from injection [39].

## K.  The Mechanism of Venom Immunotherapy

Although immunotherapy has been used for about 90 years, its mechanism is still not completely established. Initially studies focused on antibody, particularly IgG, but recent studies have looked at T-cell and cytokine changes.

### 1. Specific IgG Antibody

For many years it was thought that venom immunotherapy worked through the generation of specific IgG antibody, acting by blocking the access of allergen to specific IgE bound to mast cells. From the initial studies with pure venom immunotherapy a typical pattern of antibody response was reported, with a pronounced rise in venom IgG antibody titers, which then plateaued [59]. Further, the level of venom IgG was the only parameter associated with success of VIT [43]. However, subsequent studies correlating clinical outcome with venom IgG and IgE levels have shown that the relationship between antibody levels and clinical status is far from simple. Other studies, in untreated patients with systemic reactions, show no correlation between venom-specific IgG, IgG subclass or IgE levels, or the IgG:IgE ratio and the reaction to a sting [17–19,44,60]. Venom IgG4 and IgE levels, measured just before sting challenge in over 300 patients, failed to show any correlation with outcome [61]. Similarly, in patients on maintenance bee venom immunotherapy, phospholipase $A_2$–specific IgE, IgG, or IgG subclass levels failed to predict the outcome of a sting challenge [62].

A study from the United Kingdom found that the level of venom-specific IgG was high in untreated bee-allergic patients with systemic reactions to stings [44], against a protective role. There was no correlation between the severity of the GR in untreated patients, graded 1–8, and the venom IgG level [44]. The level of bee venom IgG appeared to be related more to the degree of immunization with venom, since most patients were beekeepers or their relatives, and frequently stung. In wasp-allergic patients who received only occasional stings, venom-IgG levels were low. After VIT, in the bee group the venom-specific IgG rose only a little, whereas in the wasp group there was a striking rise of similar pattern to that reported by Lichenstein (most of the patients reported by this group were allergic to yellow jacket). Kemeny et al. [45] have also described a different IgG pattern in bee compared with wasp VIT.

The Lichtenstein group produced further data supporting the concept of a protective role for IgG [63]. Patients on immunotherapy were divided into groups depending on the venom IgG levels—either below or greater than 3 µg/ml—then given a sting challenge. They found that more treatment failures occurred in the low-IgG group (10% SRs compared to 1.6%), but only in the first 4 years of immunotherapy with vespid or yellow jacket venom. IgG levels had no predictive value in patients who had received more than 4 years of immunotherapy or in bee venom allergy.

Other evidence that might support a role for IgG comes from studies where infusion of hyperimmune serum from beekeepers to patients with systemic reactions to stings rendered them unresponsive to a sting (but venom IgG levels was not measured or did not rise in all of these) [64]. Similarly, patients on immunotherapy stopped having adverse reactions following infusion of beekeeper gammaglobulin [65,66].

It is difficult to reconcile these variable findings on the protective role of venom IgG. Total venom-specific IgG levels in serum may be too crude a parameter, and levels near mast cells or even IgG responses to components of venom may be more relevant. However, in studies of IgG and IgE antibody responses to individual venom antigens by immunoblotting, although variations in the pattern of antibody responses were seen and occasional patients had missing bands, it was rare to find IgE bands without the corresponding IgG band [67,68].

### 2. Th1 and Th2 Cytokine Responses

T-helper cells can be subdivided into subsets—Th1 and Th2 cells—based on their cytokine-secreting profile [69,70]. Venom-allergic patients have a Th2 dominant response to venom, but a Th1 response to nonspecific antigens [71,72]. Peripheral blood mononuclear cells (PBMC), when stimulated with venom in vitro, secreted interleukin 4 (IL-4), a Th2 cytokine, but not interferon-gamma (IFN-γ), a Th1 cytokine, whereas stimulating with a nonspecific antigen such as streptokinase-streptodornase (SK-SD) led to secretion of IFN-γ but not IL-4. This Th2 response to allergen has been described in other allergic disorders (e.g., house dust mite rhinitis or asthma) using PBMC [73,74] or allergen-specific T-cell clones [75,76].

Conventional and rush venom immunotherapy led to marked changes in cytokine secretion patterns after VIT [72,77,78]. After conventional VIT, there is a significant loss of IL-4 and induction of IFN-γ secretion over 2–3 months. IL-4 secretion was undetectable by 6 months [72]. Using a different stimulation system, Jutel et al. [79] showed similar cytokine changes during bee VIT.

These cytokine changes, particularly the loss of IL-4 secretion, will in the long term lead to reduction of IgE production. However, this cannot explain the mechanism of VIT, since clinical desensitization is achieved long before significant falls in venom-specific IgE occur. It is possible that there are other cytokine or chemokine changes that alter the local milieu, so that naive T cells recruited into the late-phase responses and local lymph nodes are driven to a Th1 rather than a Th2 phenotype. In this respect Carballido et al. [80] have shown that the dose of antigen may be important. Bee venom phospholipase $A_2$ (PLA) can elicit different Th cytokine production from PLA-specific T-cell clones depending on the dose of antigen used, low-dose antigen causing Th2 (IL-4) and high-dose antigen causing Th1 (IFN-γ) cytokine production.

In patients who had stopped VIT after 5 years of treatment, sting challenge caused venom-specific IgG but not IgE titers to rise [53]. This suggests that VIT leads to isotype-specific suppression of the venom IgE response.

The mechanism of the rapid desensitization achieved in rush VIT is difficult to explain. The cytokine and chemokine changes may have other effects such as modulation of mast cell or basophil mediator release (e.g., IL-4, IL-3, and MCAF/MCP-1 enhance histamine release in vitro [81,82]), but this is not established.

## II. OTHER HYMENOPTERA: FIRE ANTS

Most ants are harmless, but some ants sting. Fire ants (*Solenopsis invicta* and *Solenopsis richteri*) have been imported to the southeastern United States and, because of resistance to chemicals, can overwhelm their environment. They usually cause simple stings, but there are rare reports of anaphylaxis after multiple stings [83], and fire ant venom–specific IgE has been demonstrated.

## III. DIPTERA

Flying insects, including midges, gnats, and mosquitoes, commonly bite humans and may all cause local swelling reactions. In some patients these can be severe. The mechanism is not always clear. Mild to moderate reactions should be treated with oral antihistamines, and these are more effective if taken early, at the onset of the reaction. Severe reactions with intense edema may be complicated by blistering, weeping or cellulitis. Treatment is with parenteral H1 blockers, steroids, and antibiotics if required, plus elevation.

### A. Midge

The green nimitti midge, a chironomid midge, is an important cause of immediate hypersensitivity reactions, particularly asthma and rhinitis, in the Sudan [84]. The allergen is inhaled. The disorder was first shown to be IgE mediated by positive skin prick tests with an extract of the green nimitti midge [85]; in subsequent studies the allergen was characterized and two major allergens appear to be hemoglobins [86].

### B. Horsefly

Horsefly bites cause local pain and a wheal. There are rare anecdotal reports of anaphylactic reactions, including fatal reactions (Bousquet and Ewan, personal communications) but the cause is not always confirmed because of the lack of assays, although specific IgE has sometimes been demonstrated.

## C. Mosquito

Local cutaneous reactions to mosquito bites are common. Both immediate and delayed reactions occur, either alone or together [87–89]. The appearance and time course of the immediate whealing reaction is consistent with an IgE-mediated (type I) reaction. It is thought that the delayed (swelling) hypersensitivity reactions may either be T-cell–mediated (type IV) or Arthus reactions (local IgG immune-complex reactions [89]). The allergens are present in saliva, and immunoblot analysis has shown 3–16 salivary allergens in each of 10 species studied, with both species-shared and species-specific allergens [90]. Although commercial extracts are available for diagnosis, some of these are of poor quality, containing few salivary antigens [91]. Seasonal exposure to mosquito bites leads to an increase in IgE, IgG4, and IgG1 responses, as is seen in pollen allergy [92]. Naturally acquired desensitization to mosquito bites occurs during long-term exposure [89].

Systemic reactions to mosquito bites are rare. A case of asthma has been described, thought to be IgE-mediated, which responded to desensitization with mosquito extract [93]. Two cases of anaphylaxis have been reported, and desensitization with whole body extract was effective [94].

## IV.  SIPHONAPTERA (FLEAS)

Fleas are small, wingless, blood-sucking insects. Fleas do not live on humans as a primary host but in crevices in the ground, bedding, walls, and furniture. Species that attack humans include the cat flea, the dog flea, the human flea (*Pulex irritans*), and the jigger flea. Infestation by fleas may cause severe inflammation of the skin and intense pruritus. The flea typically produces a cluster of wheals and papules due to its habit of sampling several adjacent spots when feeding on the skin. The female jigger flea burrows into the skin of its host, particularly on the feet, and lives within a cyst. Intense itching occurs as the cyst enlarges to the size of a pea. Fleas are important carriers of disease, including murine typhus, a rickettsial disease of humans, tapeworm of dogs and cats, and bubonic plague.

## V.  PHTHIRAPTERA (LICE)

The human louse, one of the biting lice, is a carrier of typhus and relapsing fever. Pediculosis is the skin disorder caused by various species of blood-sucking lice that infect the scalp, pubic area, and body. Lice are found in hairy areas, and infestations cause intense pruritus. The lice live on or close to the skin and attach their eggs to the hair. Early studies in 1943 suggested sensitized subjects had positive intradermal skin tests to extracts of lice head and lice feces, but the basis of this reaction is not clear [95]. Head lice (*Pediculus humanus capitis*) are transmitted by direct contact, and outbreaks are common in schools. The only symptom is itching of the scalp. The diagnosis is made by finding nits (egg cases) and/or eggs on the hair shaft. Eggs are difficult to see, but the egg cases, which remain after hatching, are pearly white and much more obvious. Body lice (*Pediculus humanus corporis*) cause red macules, particularly on the back and axilla, and severe pruritus. Pubic lice (*Pthirus pubis*) infest only areas with short hairs, especially the pubis but also the axillae and eyebrows. This louse is transmitted by sexual contact. Severe pruritus is the only symptom and may take up to 30 days after infestation to develop. Small blue-grey macules are characteristic on the thighs, suprapubic region, and buttocks, thought to be due to a reaction between louse saliva and blood [96]. Treatment of head, body, and pubic lice require killing of both adult lice and eggs with pediculicidal agents.

## VI. ARACHNIDS

### A. Spiders

Spiders have fangs and inject venom when they bite, but only a few of the many species bite humans. The venom may have toxic effects, but spider bites do not produce allergic reactions. In the United States, only tarantulas, widow spiders, and recluse spiders may be dangerous to humans. The widow spider venom contains a neurotoxin, but reactions are not usually fatal. They begin with mild local erythema, followed by muscle cramps, then severe rigidity, nausea, vomiting, salivation, weakness, and other systemic symptoms. The brown recluse bite causes severe pain followed by localized necrosis. This heals slowly with scarring.

### B. Scorpions

About 25 species of scorpion possess venom capable of killing humans, but these are not allergic reactions. Apart from snakes and bees or wasps, scorpions cause more deaths than any other nonparasitic group of animals—estimated at more than 5000 deaths each year. Some species are more dangerous, and these are found in certain parts of the world, including parts of Africa, India, the Middle East, and South America. These species all belong to the family Buthidae and produce a neurotoxin. Stings from these species cause convulsions, paralysis, and arrhythmia, then death. Antivenoms are available for most of the lethal species.

The majority of scorpion venoms do not cause life-threatening reactions. Interestingly the sting is less painful than a bee or wasp sting. These hemotoxins cause local effects with edema, pain, and purple discoloration, which resolve quickly.

### C. Scabies Mites

Scabies is an inflammatory skin disease caused by the mite *Sarcoptes scabiei*. The mite itself provokes little dermatitis. The rash and itch associated with scabies are probably manifestations of the immune response [97]. However, the immunology is not well defined. Falk and Bolle [98] first demonstrated IgE-mediated hypersensitivity by intracutaneous skin testing with an extract of scabies mites. Patients who had had scabies within one year had positive tests, whereas tests were negative in those with infection more than a year before. Scabies-specific IgE was further confirmed by Prausnitz-Kustner testing. A more recent study confirmed that at least half the patients with active scabies have *Scaroptes scabiei* IgE, whereas most patients cured of scabies lack this IgE response [99]. Antibodies to scabies also recognize Dermatophagoides house dust mites, a common cause of allergic asthma, rhinitis, and eczema [99]. Scabies infection seems to stimulate the production of IgE antibodies, but this is transient [99,100].

Scabies mites are spread by skin-to-skin contact, but mites can survive for a few days in clothing. The female mite burrows under the surface of the skin to lay its eggs in a tunnel that can be seen as a dark wavy line. After an incubation period of up to 2–4 weeks, intense pruritus occurs and the scratching leads to secondary skin lesions including papules, pustules, and crusting. Scabies is particularly seen in the interdigital webs and in skinfolds. Subsequent infestations result in an immediate rash in these areas. Rarely scabies presents with urticaria [101,102].

## REFERENCES

1.  Hoffman DR, Shipman WH. Allergens in bee venom: 1. Separation and identification of the major allergens. J Allergy Clin Immunol 1976; 58:551–562.
2.  King TP, Sobotka AK, Kochoumian L, Lichtenstein LM. Allergens of honey bee venom. Arch Biochem Biophys 1976; 172:661–671.
3.  Hoffman DR. Insect allergy, immunology and immunotherapy. In: Tu AT, ed. Insect Poisons, Allergens and Other Invertebrate Venoms. New York: Marcel Dekker, 1982:187–223.
4.  King TP, Sobotka AK, Alagon A, Kochoumian L, Lichtenstein LM. Protein allergens of white-faced hornet, yellow hornet and yellow jacket venoms. Biochemistry 1978; 17:5165–5174.
5.  Hoffman DR. Allergens in Hymenoptera venom XIV. IgE binding activities of venom proteins from three species of vespids. J Allergy Clin Immunol 1985; 75:606–609.
6.  Einarsson R, Karlsson R, Olsson R, Uhlin T, Oehman S. Crossed immunoelectrophoresis and crossed radio immunoelectrophoresis analysis of yellow jacket—common wasp (*Vespula* spp). Allergy 1985; 40:257–263.
7.  Hoffman DR, McDonald CA. Allergens in Hymenoptera venom IX species specificity to Polistes (paper wasp) venoms. Ann Allergy 1982; 47:223–237.
8.  Reisman RE, Mueller UR, Wypych JI, Lazell MI. Studies of co-existing honeybee and vespid venom sensitivity. J Allergy Clin Immunol 1984; 73:246–252.
9.  King TP. Insect allergens: venoms. In: Lockey RF, Kukantz SC, eds. Allergen Immunotherapy. New York: Marcel Dekker, 1991:103–118.
10. Ewan PW. Clinical features, natural history and immunological studies in insect sting allergy. QJ Med 1984; 52:542–543.
11. Clayton WF, Georgitis JW, Reisman RF. Insect sting anaphylaxis in patients without detectable serum venom specific IgE. Clin Allergy 1985; 15:329–333.
12. Reisman RE, Osur SR. Allergic reactions following first insect sting exposure. Ann Allergy 1987; 59:429–432.
13. Ewan PW, Deighton J, Lachmann PJ. Detection of IgE antibody to venom antigens by Western blotting in patients with negative RAST. Eur J Allergy Clin Immunol 1993; 48 (suppl 16):116.
14. Ewan PW. Allergy to insect stings: a review. J Roy Soc Med 1985; 78:234–239.
15. Hunt KJ, Valentine MD, Sobotka AK, Benton AW, Amodio FJ, Lichtenstein LM. A controlled trial of immunotherapy in insect hypersensitivity. N Engl J Med 1978; 299:157–161.
16. Settipane GA, Chafee FH. Natural history of allergy to hymenoptera. Clin Allergy 1979; 9:385–390.
17. Blaauw PJ, Smithuis LOMJ. The evaluation of the common diagnostic methods of hypersensitivity for bee and yellow jacket venom by means of an in-hospital insect sting. J Allergy Clin Immunol 1985; 5:556–562.
18. Kampelmacher MJ, van der Zwan JC. Provocation test with a living insect as a diagnostic tool in systemic reactions to bee and wasp venom: a prospective study with emphasis on the clinical aspects. Clin Allergy 1987; 17:317–327.

19. Engel T, Heinid JH, Weeke ER. Prognosis of patients reacting with urticaria to insect sting. Results of an in-hospital sting challenge. Allergy 1988; 43:289–293.

20. Van der Zwan JC. Anaphylactic reactions to bee or wasp stings: results of 308 sting provocations. Schweiz Med Wschr 1991; 121 (S40/I):62.

21. Savliwala MW, Reisman RF. Studies of the natural history of stinging insect allergy: long-term follow up of patients without immunotherapy. J Allergy Clin Immunol 1987; 80:741–745.

22. Reisman RE, Dvorin DJ, Randolph CC, Georgitis JW. Stinging insect allergy: natural history and modification with venom immunotherapy. J Allergy Clin Immunol 1985; 75:735–740.

23. Lantner R, Reisman MD. Clinical and immunologic features and subequent course of patients with severe insect-sting anaphylaxis. J Allergy Clin Immunol 1989; 84:900–906.

24. Valentine MD, Schuberth KC, Kagey-Sobotka A, Graft DF, Kwiterovich KA, Szklo M, Lichtenstein LM. The value of immunotherapy with venom in children with allergy to insect stings. N Engl J Med 1990; 323:1601–1603.

25. Graft DF, Schuberth KC, Kagey-Sobotka A, Kwiterovich KA, Niv Y, Lichtenstein LM, Valentine MD. A prospective study of the natural history of large local reactions after hymenoptera stings in children. J Pediatr 1984; 104:664–668.

26. Mauriello PM, Barde SH, Georgilis JW, Reisman RE. Natural history of large local reactions from stinging insects. J Allergy Clin Immunol 1984; 74:494–498.

27. Green-Graif Y, Ewan PW. Evaluation of skin prick tests in the diagnosis of insect sting allergy. Clin Allergy 1987; 7:431–438.

28. Egner W, Ward C, Brown DL, Ewan PW. The incidence and clinical significance of specific IgE to both wasp (Vespula) and bee (Apis) venom in the same patient. Clin Exp Allergy 1998; 28:26–34.

29. Ewan PW. Treatment of anaphylactic reactions. Prescriber's J 1997; 87:125–132.

30. Ewan PW. ABC of allergies. Anaphylaxis. BMJ 1998; 316:1442–1445.

31. Ewan PW. ABC of allergies. Venom allergy. BMJ 1998; 316:1365–1368.

32. Golden DPK, Meyers DA, Kagey-Sobotka A, Valentine MD, Lichtenstein LM. Dose dependence of Hymenoptera venom immunotherapy. J Allergy Clin Immunol 1981; 67:370–374.

33. Gillman SA, Cummins LH, Kozak PP, Hoffman DR. Venom immunotherapy: comparison of "rush" vs "conventional" schedules. Ann Allergy 1980; 45:351–354.

34. Müller U, Halbina A, Berchtold E. Immunotherapy with honey bee and yellow jacket venom is different regarding safety and efficacy. J Allergy Clin Immunol 1992; 89:529–535.

35. Mosbech HM, Malling HJ, Biering I, Bowadt H, Soborg M, Weeke B, Lowenstein H. Immunotherapy with yellow jacket venom. A comparative study including three different extracts: one adsorbed to aluminum extract and two unmodified. Allergy 1986; 41:95–103.

36. Committee on Safety of Medicines. CSM update: desensitizing vaccines. Br Med J 1986; 293–948.

37. Lockey RF, Benedict LM, Turkeltaub PC, Bukantz SC. Fatalities from immunotherapy and skin testing. J Allergy Clin Immunol 1987; 79:660–667.

38. Lockey RF, Turkeltaub PC, Olive ES, Hubbard JM, Baird-Warren JA, Bukantz SC. The hymenoptera venom study III: safety of venom immunotherapy. J Allergy Clin Immunol 1990; 86:775–780.

39. Ewan PW, Stewart AG. A prospective study of systemic reactions to venom immunotherapy (VIT). Clin Exp Allergy 1993; 23 (suppl 1):82.

40. Youlten LJF, Atkinson BA, Lee TH. The incidence and nature of adverse reactions to injection immunotherapy in bee and wasp venom allergy. Clin Exp Allergy 1995; 25:159–165.

41. Position paper on allergen immunotherapy: report of a British Society for Allergy and Clinical Immunology Working Party. Clin Exp Allergy 1993; 23 (suppl 3):19–22.

42. Reisman RE. Unusual reactions to insect venoms. Allergy Proc 1991; 12:395–399.

43. Golden DBK, Meyers DA, Kagey-Sobotka A, Valentine MD, Lichtenstein LM. Clinical relevance of the venom-specific IgG antibody level during immunotherapy. J Allergy Clin Immunol 1982; 69:489–493.

44. Ewan PW, Deighton J, Wilson AB, Lachmann PJ. Venom specific IgG antibodies in bee and allergy: lack of correlation with protection from stings. Clin Exp Allergy 1993; 23:647–660.

45. Kemeny DM, Lessof MH, Patel S, Youlten LJ, Williams A, Lambourn E. IgG and IgE antibodies after immunotherapy with bee and wasp venom. Int Arch Allergy Appl Immunol 1989; 88:247–249.

46. Reisman RE, DeMasi JM. Relationship of serum venom-specific IgE titers to clinical aspects of stinging insect allergy. Int Arch Allergy Appl Immunol 1989; 9:67–70.

47. Ewan PW, Stewart AG. Evaluation of provocation tests in assessing the need for venom immunotherapy. Abstracts XV ICACI and EAACI Meeting 1994. Clin Immunol News 1994; (suppl 2):124.

48. Subcommittee on Insect Venom Allergy of the European Academy of Allergology and Clinical Immunology. Immunotherapy with hymenoptera venoms: position paper. Allergy 1993; 48 (suppl 14):36–46.

49. Golden DBK, Meyers DA, Kagey-Sobotka A, Valentine MD, Lichtenstein LM. Prolonged maintenance interval in Hymenoptera venom immunotherapy. J Allergy Clin Immunol 1981; 67:482–484.

50. Kochuyt AM, Stevens EA. Safety and efficacy of a 12 week maintenance interval in patients treated with Hymenoptera venom immunotherapy. Clin Exp Allergy 1994; 24:35–41.

51. Goldherd A, Confino Cohen R, Mekori YA. Deliberate bee sting challenge of patients receiving maintenance venom immunotherapy at 3 month intervals. J Allergy Clin Immunol 1994; 93:997–1001.

52. Keating MV, Kagey-Sobotka A, Hamilton RG, Yunginger JW. Clinical and immunological follow up of patients who stop immunotherapy. J Allergy Clin Immunol 1991; 88:339–348.

53. Valentine MD, Lichtenstein LM. Prospective observations on stopping prolonged venom immunotherapy. J Allergy Clin Immunol 1989; 84:162–167.

54. Reisman RF, Livingston A. Venom immunotherapy: 10 years of experience with administration of single venoms and 50 µg maintenance doses. J Allergy Clin Immunol 1992; 89:1189–1195.

55. Wyss M, Scheitlin T, Stadler BM, Wuthrich B. Immunotherapy with aluminium hydroxide adsorbed insect venom extracts (Alutard SQ): immunological and clinical results of a prospective study over 3 years. Allergy 1993; 48:81–86.

56. Bernstein JA, Kaoen SL, Bernstein DI, Bernstein IL. Rapid venom immunotherapy is safe for routine use in the treatment of patients with Hymenoptera anaphylaxis. Ann Allergy 1994; 73:423–428.

57. Birnbaum J, Charpin D, Vervloet D. Rapid Hymenoptera venom immunotherapy: comparitive safety of three protocols. Clin Exp Allergy 1993; 23:226–230.

58. Committee on Safety of Medicines. Desensitising vaccines: new advice. Curr Problems Pharmacovigilance 1994; 20:5.

59. Lichtenstein LM, Valentine MD, Sobotka AK. Insect allergy: the state of the art. J Allergy Clin Immunol 1979; 64:5–12.

60. Wilson AB, Deighton J, Lachmann PJ, Ewan PW. A comparative study of IgG subclass antibodies in patients allergic to wasp or bee venom. Allergy 1994; 49:272–280.

61. Van der Linden PW, Hack CE, Struyvenberg A, van der Zwan JC. Insect sting challenge in 324 subjects with a previous anaphylactic reaction: current criteria for insect-venom hypersensitivity do not predict the occurrence and severity of anaphylaxis. J Allergy Clin Immunol 1994; 94:151–159.

62. Müller U, Helbling A, Bischof M. Predictive value of venom-specific IgE, IgG and IgG subclass antibodies in patients on immunotherapy with honey bee venom. Allergy 1989; 44: 412–418.

63. Golden DB, Lawrence ID, Hamilton RH, Kagey-Sabotka A, Valentine MD, Lichtenstein LM. Clinical correlation of the venom-specific IgG level during maintenance venom immunotherapy. J Allergy Clin Immunol 1992; 90:386–393.

64. Lessof MH, Sobotka AK, Lichtenstein LM. Effects of passive antibody in bee venom anaphylaxis. Johns Hopkins Med J 1978; 142:1–7.

65. Müller UR, Morris T, Bischof M, Friedli H, Skarvil F. Combined active and passive immunotherapy in honey-bee-sting allergy. J Allergy Clin Immunol 1986; 78:115–122.

66. Bousquet J, Fontez A, Aznar R, Robinet-Levy M, Michel FB. Combination of passive and active immunisation in honey venom immunotherapy. J Allergy Clin Immunol 1987; 79: 947–954.

67. Deighton J, Lachmann PJ, Ewan PW. Western blotting reveals the diversity of IgE and IgG response to bee venom antigens. BSACI Annual Meeting, Book of Abstracts 1993, p. 34.

68. Ewan PW, Deighton J, Lachmann PJ. An analysis of the IgE and IgG response to wasp venom antigens before and after venom immunotherapy. BSACI Annual Meeting, Book of Abstracts 1993, p. 34.

69. Mosmann TR, Cherwinski H, Bond MM, Giedari MA, Coffman RL. Two types of murine helper T cell clones: 1. Definition according to the profiles of lymphokine activities and secreted proteins. J Immunol 1986; 136:2348–2357.

70. Romagnani S. Human $T_H1$ and $T_H2$ cells: doubt no more. Immunol Today 1991; 12:256–257.

71. McHugh SM, Wilson AB, Lachmann PJ, Ewan PW. PBMC of bee venom allergic patients produce high levels of IL-4 to a venom extract in vitro. BSACI Annual Meeting Book of Abstracts 1993, p. 34.

72. McHugh SM, Deighton J, Stewart AG, Lachmann PJ, Ewan PW. Bee venom immunotherapy induces a shift in cytokine responses from a $T_H2$ to a $T_H1$ dominant pattern: comparison of rush and conventional immunotherapy. Clin Exp Allergy 1995; 25:828–838.

73. McHugh SM, Lachmann PJ, Ewan PW. Peripheral blood mononuclear cells from house dust mite allergic patients produce IL-2 in response to specific allergen challenge. Clin Exp Allergy 1993; 23:137–144.

74. McHugh SM, Wilson AB, Deighton J, Lachmann PJ, Ewan PW. IL-2, IL-6 and IFN-γ profiles from peripheral blood mononuclear cells of house dust mite allergic patients: a role for IL-6 in allergic disease. Eur J Allergy Clin Immunol 1994; 49(9):751–759.

75. Wierenga EA, Snoek M, de Groot C, Chretien I, Bos JD, Jansen HM, Kapsenberg ML. Evidence for compartmentalisation of functional subsets of CD4+ T lymphocytes in atopic patients. J Immunol 1990; 44:4651–4656.

76. Parronchi P, Macchia D, Piccini M-P. Allergen- and bacterial antigen-specific T cell clones established from atopic donors show a different profile of cytokine production. Proc Natl Acad Sci USA 1991; 88:4538–4542.

77. McHugh SM, Wilson AB, Deighton J, Stewart AG, Ewan PW. Bee venom immunotherapy induces $T_H2$ to $T_H1$ cytokine switch (abstract). Eur J Allergy Clin Immunol 1993; 48 (suppl 16):97.

78. McHugh SM, Wilson AB, Deighton J, Stewart AG, Ewan PW. $T_H2$ cytokine responses to hymenoptera venom in vitro are switched to a $T_H1$ type during specific venom immunotherapy. Abstracts XV ICACI and EAACI Meeting 1994. Allergy and Clinical Immunology News, Suppl 2, p. 44.

79. Jutel M, Pichler WJ, Skrbic D, Urwyler A, Dahinden C, Muller UR. Bee venom immunotherapy results in decrease of IL-4 and IL-5 and increase of IFN-γ secretion in specific allergen stimulated T cell cultures. J Immunol 1995; 154:4187–4194.

80. Carballido JM, Carballido-Perrig N, Terres G, Heusser CH, Blaser K. Bee venom phospholipase $A_2$ specific T cell clones from human allergic and non-allergic individuals: cytokine patterns change in response to the antigen concentration. Eur J Immunol 1992; 22:1357–1363.

81. Coleman JW, Holliday MR, Kimber I, Zesbo KM, Galli SJ. Regulation of mouse peritoneal mast cell secretory function by stem cell factor, IL-3 or IL-4. J Immunol 1993; 150:556–562.

82. Kuna P, Reddigari SR, Rucinski D, Oppenheim JJ, Kaplan AP. Monocyte chemotactic and activating factor is a potent histamine-releasing factor for human basophils. J Exp Med 1992; 175:489–493.

83. Prahlow JA, Barnard JJ. Fatal anaphylaxis to fire ant stings. Am J Forensic Med Pathol 1998; 19:137–142.

84. Kay AB, MacLean CM, Wilkinson AH, Gad-El-Rab MO. The prevalence of asthma and rhinitis in a Sudanese community seasonally exposed to a potent airborne allergen (the 'green nimitti' midge, Cladotanytarsus lewisi). J Allergy Clin Immunol 1983; 71:345–352.

85. Cranston PS, Gad-El-Rab MO, Tee RD, Kay AB. Immediate-type skin reactivity to extracts of the 'green nimitti' midge, (Cladotanytarsus lewisi), and other chironomids in asthmatic subjects in the Sudan and Egypt. Ann Trop Med Parasitol 1983; 77:527–533.

86. Tee RD, Cranston PS, Kay AB. Further characterization of allergens associated with hypersensitivity to the 'green nimitti' midge (Cladotanytarsus lewisi, Diptera: Chironomidae). Allergy 1987; 42:12–19.

87. Reunala T, Brummer-Korvenkontio H, Lappalainen P, Rasanen L, Palosuo T. Immunology and treatment of mosquito bites. Clin Exp Allergy 1990; 20 (suppl 4):19–24.

88. Oka K, Ohtaki N. Clinical observations of mosquito bite reactions in man; a survey of the relationship between age and bite reaction. J Dermatol 1989; 16:212–219.

89. Peng Z, Yang M, Simons FE Immunologic mechanisms in mosquito allergy: correlation of skin reactions with specific IgE and IgG antibodies and lymphocyte proliferation response to mosquito antigens. Ann Allergy Asthma Immunol 1996; 77:238–244.

90. Peng Z, Li H, Simons FE. Immunoblot analysis of salivary allergens in 10 mosquito species with worldwide distribution and the human IgE responses to these allergens. J Allergy Clin Immunol 1998; 101:498–505.

91. Peng Z, Simons FE. Comparison of proteins, IgE, and IgG binding antigens, and skin reactivity in commercial and laboratory-made mosquito extracts. Ann Allergy Asthma Immunol 1996; 77:371–376.

92. Palosuo K, Brummer-Korvenkontio H, Mikkola J, Sahi T, Reunala T. Seasonal increase in human IgE and IgG4 antisaliva antibodies to Aedes mosquito bites. Int Arch Allergy Immunol 1997; 114:367–372.

93. Gluck JC, Pacin MP. Asthma from mosquito bites. A case report. Ann Allergy 1986; 56: 492.

94. McCormack DR, Salata KF, Hershey JN, Carpenter GB, Engler RJ. Mosquito bite anaphylaxis: immunotherapy with whole body extracts. Ann Allergy Asthma Immunol 1995; 74: 39–44.

95. Peck SM, Wright WH, Gant JQ Jr. Cutaneous reactions due to the body louse (*Pediculus humanus*). JAMA 1943; 123:821.

96. Elgart ML. Pediculosis. Dermatol Clin 1990; 8:219.

97. Dahl MV. The immunology of scabies. Ann Allergy 1983; 51(6):560–566.

98. Falk ES, Bolle R. In vitro demonstration of specific immunological hypersensitivity to scabies mite. Br J Dermatol 1980; 103(4):367–373.

99. Morgan MS, Arlian LG, Estes SA. Skin test and radioallergosorbent test characteristics of scabietic patients. Am J Trop Med Hyg 1997; 57(2):190–196.

100. Falk ES. Serum IgE before and after treatment for scabies. Allergy 1981; 36(3):167–174.

101. Chapel TA, Krugel L, Chapel J, Segal A. Scabies presenting as urticaria. JAMA 1981; 246(13):1440–1441.

102. Witkowski JA, Parish LC. Scabies: a cause of generalized urticaria. Cutis 1984; 33(3):277–279.

# 14

## Cutaneous Vasculitis

**Nicholas A. Soter**
*New York University School of Medicine, Charles C. Harris Skin and Cancer Pavilion,
and Tisch Hospital—The University Hospital of New York University,
New York, New York*

## I. INTRODUCTION

Necrotizing angiitis or vasculitis comprises disorders of the blood vessels that combine segmental inflammation with necrosis. Clinical syndromes are defined by criteria [1] that include the gross appearance and the histopathological alterations of the vascular lesions, the caliber of the affected blood vessels, the frequency of involvement of specific organs, and the presence of laboratory abnormalities. Necrotizing vasculitis may be a primary disease, may develop as a feature of a systemic disorder, or may be idiopathic.

Although all sizes of blood vessels may be involved in the skin, necrotizing vasculitis involves predominantly venules and is known as cutaneous necrotizing venulitis and leukocytoclastic vasculitis. Cutaneous necrotizing venulitis may occur in association with an underlying chronic disease, may be precipitated by infections or drugs, or may develop for unknown reasons (Table 1) [2].

Systemic involvement of the small blood vessels in concert with cutaneous lesions has been classified as hypersensitivity angiitis or vasculitis, which includes cutaneous necrotizing venulitis and microscopic polyangiitis [3]. Systemic necrotizing vasculitis that involves blood vessels of various sites and is accompanied by skin lesions but that does not fit any diagnostic category is termed systemic polyangiitis [4]. Although IgA-mediated small-vessel necrotizing vasculitis has been proposed as a nosologic entity, at the present time an immunopathobiological classification of necrotizing vasculitis is not possible. This chapter will focus on cutaneous necrotizing venulitis.

## II. PATHOGENESIS

The most frequently postulated mechanisms in the production of cutaneous necrotizing venulitis are the local deposition of circulating immune complexes formed during antigen excess and the formation of immune complexes in situ in the skin. Certain types of immune complexes may activate the complement system and lead to the generation of C5a anaphylatoxin, which attracts neutrophils that release lysosomal enzymes and that produce reac-

**Table 1**   Cutaneous Necrotizing Venulitis

Associated chronic disorders
  Rheumatoid arthritis
  Sjögren's syndrome
  Systemic lupus erythematosus
  Hypergammaglobulineimic purpura
  Paraneoplastic vasculitis
  Cryoglobulinemia
  Inflammatory bowel diseases of the colon
  Cystic fibrosis
  Behçet's disease
  Antineutrophil cytoplasmic or antiphospholipid antibody
    syndromes
Precipitating events
  Bacterial, viral, and mycobacterial infections
  Therapeutic and diagnostic agents
Idiopathic disorders
  Henoch-Schönlein syndrome
  Acute hemorrhagic enema of childhood
  Urticarial vasculitis and variants
  Erythema elevatum diutinum
  Nodular vasculitis
  Livedoid vasculitis
  Sneddon's syndrome
  Genetic complement deficiencies
  Eosinophilic vasculitis

tive oxygen products. These enzymes and oxygen products cause tissue damage. The generation of the chemoattractant leukotriene $B_4$ ($LTB_4$) from infiltrating neutrophils would further enhance the influx of neutrophils. An infiltrate composed predominantly of neutrophils in lesional skin biopsy specimens of patients with cutaneous necrotizing venulitis is an observation that is consistent with tissue damage induced by immune complexes that activate the complement system.

In patients with cutaneous necrotizing venulitis, circulating immune complexes have been demonstrated as mixed-type cryoglobulins and by assays that detect C1q precipitins, materials that bind to complement receptors on human lymphocytoid (Raji) cells or to monoclonal rheumatoid factor, and substances that function in the antibody-dependent cellular cytotoxicity inhibition assay. Further evidence implicating immune complexes and complement activation are the presence of serum hypocomplementemia with activation of the classic activating pathway and the detection of increased plasma levels of C4a and C3a anaphylatoxins and of the IgG autoantibody C3 nephritic factor [5].

Immune complexes have been detected in lesional tissues by ultrastructural observation as electron-dense subendothelial deposits. The membrane-attack complex, C5b-9, of the complement system was expressed on the surface of endothelial cells and infiltrating neutrophils. Decay-accelerating factor, a regulatory complement protein that prevents the assembly of the membrane-attack complex, was not present on the surface of endothelial cells of the upper dermal microvasculature. Tissue immune complexes also have been detected by direct immunofluorescence techniques as deposited immunoglobulins and complement proteins. In time-course studies of the evolution of cutaneous vascular lesions, immune reactants have been detected in lesions less than 24 hours old but rarely in lesions that have persisted for more than 24 hours. The antigen has been identified in only a few instances as bacterial, viral [6], mycobacterial, or rickettsial proteins that have been detected by direct immunofluorescence techniques or the polymerase chain reaction (PCR).

A role for lymphocytes and mononuclear cells in the production of cutaneous necrotizing venulitis is suggested by a perivenular infiltrate in lesional skin biopsy specimens that is rich in lymphocytes and by a prominence of mononuclear cells in the vascular skin lesions of patients with cutaneous necrotizing venulitis and Sjögren's syndrome. Lymphocytes may be activated by immune complexes, by cellular immune mechanisms, or by primary activation in autoimmune disease to produce lymphokines. Endothelial cells also may present antigens to and activate T lymphocytes. Activated macrophages secrete chemokines and lysosomal enzymes. Gamma/delta T cells have been detected in cutaneous necrotizing venulitis with an infiltrate rich in neutrophils and with a documented infectious etiology [7,8]. In these specimens, a 72 kDa heat-shock protein was expressed by endothelial cells and antigen-presenting cells.

The participation of mast cells in cutaneous necrotizing venulitis is suggested by the presence of hypogranulated mast cells with shed extracellular granules in lesional biopsy specimens and by the development of vascular lesions after the intracutaneous injection of histamine in patients developing active lesions of cutaneous necrotizing venulitis. Interendothelial cell gaps have been noted in venules in patients with cutaneous necrotizing venulitis. Mast cell–derived factors chemotactic for eosinophils and neutrophils as well as neutral proteases and acid hydrolases of mast cells may play a role. The mast cell may also release tumor necrosis factor-$\alpha$ (TNF-$\alpha$) that could increase the expression of E-selectin on endothelial cells [9]. The participation of other cytokines produced by cutaneous mast cells remains unexamined.

Early in the evolution of necrotizing vasculitis, endothelial cells show increased expression of intercellular adhesion molecule-1 (ICAM-1) and E-selectin. Since E-selectin is an adhesion molecule for neutrophils and skin-homing, memory T lymphocytes [10], the increase in E-selectin is consistent with a neutrophilic infiltrate within the first 24 hours [11]. CD11b on neutrophils (Mac-1) may bind to ICAM-1 [11]. In skin biopsy specimens of patients with idiopathic cutaneous vasculitis, hypersensitivity vasculitis, urticarial vasculitis, and Henoch-Schönlein purpura, E-selectin was detected on endothelial cells of lesions less than 48 hours old and was associated with an infiltrate of neutrophils bearing CD11b. Further evidence of endothelial cell activation was demonstrated by increased plasma levels of tissue plasminogen activator antigen and von Willebrand factor antigen in some patients with livedoid vasculitis [12]. Diminished fibrinolysis has been demonstrated in patients with cutaneous necrotizing vasculitis, and the subsequent reduction in fibrinolytic activity may lead to fibrin deposition.

Cutaneous nerve fibers contain neuropeptides, such as substance P, neurokinin A, and calcitonin gene–related peptide (CGRP), which can cause vasodilation. Substance P can activate mast cells and macrophages and can increase fibrinolytic activity mediated by plasminogen activator. CGRP induces expression of endothelial E-selectin and is chemotactic for T lymphocytes.

Associations have been recognized between necrotizing vasculitis of the small blood vessels and autobodies termed antineutrophil cytoplasmic autoantibodies (ANCA), which have specificity for proteins of the cytoplasmic granules of neutrophils and the lysosomes of monocytes. Experimental animal models suggest that ANCA induce necrotizing vasculitis by activating circulating neutrophils and monocytes, which allows these cells to adhere to blood vessels and release reactive oxygen products that cause vascular injury [13]. Antiendothelial cell antibodies cause experimental vasculitis in BALB/C mice [14]. These antibodies have been detected in the sera of patients with systemic vasculitis, rheumatoid arthritis with vasculitis, microscopic polyangiitis [15], and Sneddon's syndrome [16].

An increased prevalence of the HLA haplotype HLA-A11, Bw35 was identified in patients with cutaneous necrotizing venulitis and associated connective-tissue disorders. This association suggests that genetic factors may be operative.

## III.  CLINICAL MANIFESTATIONS

Involvement of small arteries in the skin occurs in polyarteritis nodosa, which is recognized as nodular lesions along the course of an artery [17], and in giant-cell (temporal) arteritis, which may be present as erythema with or without necrosis overlying the affected vessel. Both allergic angiitis and granulomatosis (Churg-Strauss syndrome) [18] and Wegener's granulomatosis affect vessels of all sizes; the skin lesions in both disorders can be present as nodules with or without necrosis or as erythematous, edematous, purpuric, papular, vesicular, or pustular lesions.

In cutaneous necrotizing venulitis, erythematous papules that do not blanch when the skin is pressed and that are known as palpable purpura are the signature lesions (Fig. 1). Papules, urticaria and angioedema [19], pustules, vesicles, ulcers, necrosis, and livedo reticularis may occur.

The vascular eruption most often appears on the lower extremities or over dependent areas. Although the lesions may occur anywhere on the skin, they are uncommon on the face, palms, soles, and mucous membranes. The clinical lesions are episodic and may recur over weeks to years. Palpable purpura persists from 1 to 4 weeks and resolves at times with transient hyperpigmentation and/or atrophic scars. Lesional symptoms include pruritus, burning, and, less commonly, pain.

Pyrexia, malaise, arthralgias, or myalgias may occur with an episode of cutaneous vascular lesions. In patients with cutaneous necrotizing venulitis, systemic involvement of the small blood vessels most commonly occurs in the synovia, gastrointestinal tract, voluntary muscles, peripheral nerves, and kidneys.

## A.  Associated Chronic Disorders

Cutaneous necrotizing venulitis has been associated with rheumatoid arthritis, Sjögren's syndrome, systemic lupus erythematous (SLE), and hypergammaglobulinemic purpura. In patients with rheumatoid arthritis, the development of vascular lesions is related to the severity of the disease, which is usually but not always seropositive. Subcutaneous nodules and cutaneous ulcers often are present. Patients with rheumatoid arthritis may have involvement of larger vessels with associated peripheral neuropathy, nail fold infarcts, and digital gangrene.

In patients with SLE, the vasculitis occurs with exacerbations of the underlying disease. Vasculitis, however, is rare in patients with subacute cutaneous lupus erythematosus [20]. Approximately 5% of women with necrotizing vasculitis without connective tissue disease have anti-Ro antibodies, and their infants may be born with neonatal lupus erythematosus [20–23].

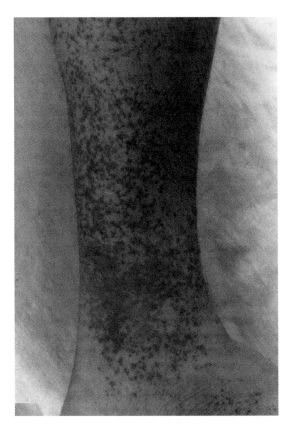

**Figure 1**   Palpable purpura over the lower legs of a patient with idiopathic cutaneous necrotizing venulitis.


In patients with Sjögren's syndrome, the vascular lesions are located predominantly on the lower extremities and appear after exercise. Both hyperpigmentation and cutaneous ulcers are common features. Hypergammaglobulinemic purpura occurs in older women and may be associated with Sjögren's syndrome, SLE, or a lymphoproliferative disorder. Dermatomyositis in children, but not in adults, may be associated with systemic vasculitis that involves the gastrointestinal tract.

Paraneoplastic vasculitis is a term that has been used to describe patients with cutaneous necrotizing vasculitis with associated malignant conditions, which include Hodgkin's disease, lymphosarcoma, adult T-cell leukemia, mycosis fungoides, myelofibrosis, acute and chronic myelogenous forms of leukemia, IgA myeloma, diffuse large-cell leukemia, hairy cell leukemia, squamous cell bronchiogenic carcinoma, prostatic carcinoma, renal carcinoma, and colon carcinoma.

Cryoglobulins [24], especially mixed types II and III, occur in patients with cutaneous necrotizing venulitis and associated connective tissue diseases, lymphoproliferative disorders, hepatitis A, B, and C virus infections [25–27], cystic fibrosis, inflammatory bowel diseases of the colon, Behçet's disease [28], and as an idiopathic condition.

Both ANCA and antiphospholipid antibodies have been associated with various forms of necrotizing vasculitis [29]. ANCA have been detected in patients with microscopic polyangiitis and cutaneous vasculitis associated with hepatitis C virus infection [30]. The most common vascular cutaneous feature in patients with ANCA is palpable purpura. Microscopic polyangiitis is associated with small-vessel systemic vasculitis that also involves the skin, in which venules and arterioles are involved [31]. It is associated with necrotizing and crescentic glomerulonephritis and peripheral ANCA with antimyeloperoxidase specificity [3,31–33].

Antiphospholipid antibodies, either anticardiolipin antibodies and/or lupus anticoagulant, occur in patients with necrotizing vasculitis and associated autoimmune and connective tissue diseases and as an idiopathic disorder [34–36]. Livedo reticularis is the most frequently recognized cutaneous finding [37,38].

## B. Infections and Drugs

Infections [39] and drugs are known to precipitate episodes of cutaneous necrotizing venulitis. The most commonly recognized infectious agents are group A β-hemolytic streptococci, *Staphylococcus aureus*, and hepatitis B virus. Limited episodes of urticarial vasculitis may occur early in the course of hepatitis B virus infection [25]. Cutaneous vasculitis was identified in patients with hepatitis A and C virus infections [40–47] and cryoglobulins. Human immunodeficiency virus (HIV) infection has been recognized in a limited number of individuals with cutaneous vasculitis [48,49].

Erythema nodosum leprosum, which appears as cutaneous nodular lesions in lepromatous leprosy, is a form of necrotizing vasculitis involving capillaries, venules, arterioles, small- to medium-sized arteries, and veins [50]. The vascular lesions occur spontaneously or are precipitated by the administration of chemotherapeutic agents, and they may be accompanied by fever, malaise, arthralgias, lymphadenopathy, and polyneuritis.

Cutaneous necrotizing vasculitis caused by the direct invasion of the blood vessel walls occurs with a variety of microorganisms, such as in *Neisseria meningitidis* bacteremia, in Rocky Mountain spotted fever, and in infections localized at the site of a catheter.

In serum sickness, urticaria occurs in about 70% of patients. Skin biopsy specimens often show necrotizing venulitis. Inasmuch as cutaneous vasculitis is an infrequent form of drug reaction, the evidence consists of case reports rather than prospective or retrospective studies. The most frequently incriminated therapeutic agents are penicillin, sulfonamides, thiazides, allopurinol, hydantoins, and nonsteroidal anti-inflammatory agents. Propylthiouracil and hydralazine may cause vasculitis in association with ANCA. Cutaneous vasculitis has occurred after the administration of streptokinase [51], radiocontrast media, monoclonal antibodies, granulocyte colony-stimulating factor [52,53], staphylococcal protein A column immunoabsorption therapy [54], drug additives [55], and exposure to fumes released from photocopy paper.

## C. Idiopathic Disorders

The most widely recognized subgroup of idiopathic cutaneous necrotizing venulitis is the Henoch-Schönlein syndrome, formerly known as anaphylactoid purpura. Although it occurs predominantly in children, it may also occur in adults [56]. A history of recent upper respiratory tract infection is obtained in up to 75% of individuals. The syndrome includes involvement of the skin, synovia, gastrointestinal tract, and kidneys.

Acute hemorrhagic edema of childhood is an uncommon disorder that affects infants and children less than 2 years of age [57–59]. The lesions appear as painful, edematous petechiae and ecchymoses that affect the head and distal portions of the extremities [60]. The skin lesions may be associated with a target-like appearance. Infections, drugs, or immunizations may be triggering factors. Features that distinguish acute hemorrhagic edema of childhood from Henoch-Schönlein syndrome, with which it has been confused, include the observations that it occurs in younger children aged 4 months to 2 years, has no systemic features, and resolves within 1–3 weeks without sequelae.

Episodes of recurrent urticaria and angioedema may be a clinical manifestation of cutaneous necrotizing venulitis [19,61,62]. Known as urticarial vasculitis, this edematous form of necrotizing venulitis occurs in patients with serum sickness; connective tissue disorders; an $IgM_KM$ component (Schnitzler's syndrome); infections; physical urticarias; after the administration of potassium iodide, nonsteroidal antiflammatory agents, and fluoxetine [63]; colon carcinoma; and as an idiopathic disorder. Infections include hepatitis B and C [64] viruses and infectious mononucleosis. A plethora of diagnostic appellations, such as atypical erythema multiforme, unusual SLE-like syndrome, hypocomplementemic vasculitis, and hypocomplementemic-urticaria-vasculitis syndrome, have been given to the idiopathic disorder.

The skin lesions appear as erythematous, occasionally indurated, wheals. Foci of purpura in the wheals are an important distinctive feature. Other skin manifestations include angioedema, macular erythema, livedo reticularis, nodules, and rarely bullae. Although the individual urticarial lesions may last for fewer than 24 hours, they often persist for 3–5 days, which is an important historic clue. The lesions are pruritic or possess a burning or painful quality; they usually resolve without residua, although certain individuals may develop transient contusions and hyperpigmentation. The episodes of urticaria are chronic, range in duration from months to years, and vary in frequency. Approximately 70% of the afflicted individuals are women. The prevalence of this disorder remains unknown. General features include fever, malaise, and myalgia; enlargement of the lymph nodes, liver, and spleen may occur (Table 2).

Episodic arthralgias with associated stiffness are a major clinical manifestation. Arthritis occasionally develops, and this syndrome has been associated with Jaccoud's syndrome [65]. Renal involvement occurs as a diffuse glomerulitis or glomerulonephritis;

---

**Table 2** Extracutaneous Manifestations of Urticarial Vasculitis

General features
  Pyrexia
  Malaise
  Myalgia
Specific organ involvement
  Lymphadenopathy
  Hepatosplenomegaly
  Synovia (arthralgia, arthritis)
  Kidneys (diffuse glomerulitis or glomerulonephritis)
  Gastrointestinal tract (nausea, vomiting, pain, diarrhea)
  Respiratory tract (laryngeal edema, shortness of breath, chronic
    obstructive and interstitial pulmonary disease)
  Eyes (conjunctivitis, episcleritis, uveitis)
  Central nervous system (headache, benign intracranial
    hypertension)

however, progression to severe impairment of renal function is rare. Gastrointestinal tract manifestations include nausea, vomiting, diarrhea, and pain. Laryngeal edema may occur. Chronic obstructive pulmonary manifestations and interstitial lung disease may develop [64]. Conjunctivitis, episcleritis, and uveitis occur in some individuals. There is one report of an individual becoming blind. Central nervous system involvement occurs as headaches and pseudotumor cerebri (benign intracranial hypertension).

Knowledge of the natural history of urticarial vasculitis is limited. In one series with a follow-up for one year, 40% of patients experienced resolution of skin lesions; in another series of individuals followed for 14 years, resolution occurred in only one patient. The development of Sjögren's syndrome and of SLE has been noted. Deaths have been reported mainly from obstructive pulmonary disease.

Necrotizing vasculitis of cutaneous venules has been described in isolated instances of dermographism, cold urticaria [66], delayed-pressure urticaria, solar urticaria, and exercise-induced urticaria [67]. However, the prevalence of necrotizing vasculitis in patients with physical urticarias is unknown, and the importance of this histological finding for prognosis and therapy remains to be elucidated. However, individuals with physical urticarias have provided experimental models for time-course studies of the evolution of cutaneous necrotizing venulitis [68].

Schnitzler's syndrome [69,70] consists of episodes of urticarial vasculitis that occur in association with a monoclonal $IgM_K$ M component. Other manifestations include fever, lymphadenopathy, hepatosplenomegaly, bone pain, and a sensorimotor neuropathy.

Erythema elevatum diutinum [71–73] appears as symmetrical, persistent, red-purple or red-brown plaques that are predominantly disposed over the joints of extensor surfaces and over the gluteal area. Although arthralgia of the associated joints may be a feature, systemic manifestations are lacking. A history of recurrent streptococcal infections of the pharynx and sinuses is often obtained. This condition may be associated with IgA monoclonal gammopathy, multiple myeloma, myelodysplasia [74], celiac disease [75], relapsing polychondritis [76], and HIV infection [77–79].

Nodular vasculitis appears as tender, red, subcutaneous nodules that occur over the lower extremities, especially the calves, without systemic manifestations. At times, the nodules may ulcerate. This disorder is more common in women and has a peak incidence in individuals between 30 and 40 years of age. Recurrent episodes are common. Erythema induratum represents a form of nodular vasculitis, which has been associated with *Mycobacterium tuberculosis* as demonstrated by PCR amplification for *M. tuberculosis* DNA in skin biopsy specimens [80–82].

Livedoid vasculitis, also known as livedo reticularis with summer/winter ulcerations, segmental hyalinizing vasculitis, and atrophie blanche, is a disorder that occurs more frequently in women as recurrent, painful ulcers of the lower extremities in association with a persistent livedo reticularis (livedo racemosa) that has a deep purple color. Healing results in sclerotic pale areas surrounded by telangiectases that are known as atrophie blanche. Many patients have arteriosclerosis or stasis of the lower extremities. Livedoid vasculitis also may occur in patients with SLE who develop central nervous system features. Atrophie blanche, however, probably represents the end stage of a variety of forms of vascular damage in the skin. Pathogenesis has focused on the fibrin thrombi in the lumens of the superficial blood vessels. Some consider this condition a thrombogenic vasculopathy rather than a primary small-vessel vasculitis [83]. Antiphospholipid antibodies have been detected in a few individuals [84].

Sneddon's syndrome [85–87] is a condition in which livedo reticularis and livedoid vasculitis have been associated with ischemic cerebrovascular lesions, hypotension, and extracerebral arterial and venous thromboses. Antiendothelial cell antibodies were detected in 35% of individuals [16], and antiphospholipid antibodies were detected in some patients.

Genetic complement deficiencies have been noted in a few patients with cutaneous necrotizing venulitis [88].

Eosinophilic vasculitis has been described in some individuals with connective tissue disorders or as an idiopathic syndrome [89,90]. The skin lesions consist of recurrent, pruritic and purpuric, papules, angioedema, urticaria, and palpable purpura.

## IV. LABORATORY FINDINGS

The laboratory evaluation of patients with cutaneous necrotizing venulitis should depend on information obtained from the history and physical examination (Table 3). An elevated erythrocyte sedimentation rate is the most consistent abnormal laboratory. The platelet count is normal. Other abnormalities reflect either a coexistent underlying disorder or the involvement of additional organ systems. Serum complement levels are usually normal. Acquired hypocomplementemia may develop in patients with concomitant connective tissue diseases or cryoglobulinemia. Hypocomplementemia also occurs in some individuals with idiopathic cutaneous necrotizing venulitis and in 40% of individuals with urticarial vasculitis.

In a few patients with urticarial vasculitis and hypocomplementemia, a low molecular weight 7s C1q precipitin identified as an IgG autoantibody against the collagen-like region of C1q was detected [91]. In the Henoch-Schönlein syndrome, increased levels of serum $IgA_1$ may occur [92]. IgG autoantibodies against IgE also have been identified in four of eight patients with urticarial vasculitis.

**Table 3** Laboratory Evaluation of Cutaneous Necrotizing Venulitis

---

Erythrocyte sedimentation rate
White-cell count with differential analysis
Platelet count
Urinalysis
24-Hour urine protein and creatinine clearance
Blood chemistry profile
Serum protein electrophoresis
Hepatitis B antigens and hepatitis A and C antibodies
Cryoglobulins
CH 50
Antinuclear antibody
Rheumatoid factor
Antineutrophil cytoplasmic antibodies
antiphospholipid antibodies
Circulating immune complexes
Skin biopsy

---

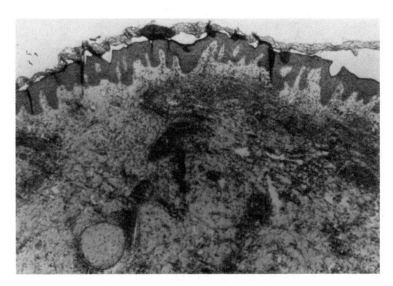

**Figure 2** Superficial and deep perivenular infiltrate of neutrophils with some mononuclear cells and with fibrin deposition. (H&E $\times$ 50 in the original magnification.)

## V. PATHOLOGY

In routinely prepared skin biopsy specimens (Fig. 2), the diagnostic histological criteria for the diagnosis of cutaneous necrotizing venulitis include necrosis of the blood vessels with the deposition of fibrinoid material and dermal cellular infiltrates that consist of various numbers of neutrophils with nuclear debris, mononuclear cells, and extravasated erythrocytes. The fibrinoid material consists predominantly of fibrin but also contains necrotic endothelial cells and deposited immunoreactants.

In 1-μm sections, two cellular patterns were recognized; one pattern is rich in neutrophils and the other in lymphocytes. These two patterns of cell infiltration do not appear to be the result of the evolution of the inflammatory infiltrate. Other features in both cell patterns include hypogranulated mast cells, macrophages containing debris, and the perivenular and interstitial deposition of fibrin. Venular alterations in both cell patterns consist of endothelial cell swelling, necrosis, and basement-membrane reduplication and thickening.

By direct immunofluorescence techniques, fibrin deposition in venules has been identified routinely in biopsy specimens. IgG is the most commonly deposited immunoglobulin, although IgM and IgA have also been detected. IgA is deposited about blood vessels in the skin, intestine, and kidney in the Henoch-Schönlein syndrome and has become an immunopathological diagnostic feature of this condition [93].

## VI. TREATMENT

Therapeutic approaches may be divided into removal of the antigen, treatment of an underlying disease, and treatment of cutaneous necrotizing venulitis. Treatment of necrotizing vasculitis consists of prevention of the deposition of immune complexes, suppression of the inflammatory response, and modulation of underlying immunopathological mechanisms. When the eruption is associated with a precipitating event, withdrawal of the medication or treatment of an infection results in resolution of the cutaneous lesions. If a coexistent chronic disease is present, treatment of the underlying disease often is associated with improvement in the cutaneous vascular lesions.

The treatment of cutaneous necrotizing venulitis can be divided into two phases, each of which depends on an analysis of the cutaneous disability as well as on the toxicity and side effects of the therapeutic agents. $H_1$ antihistamines may be used to alleviate pruritus and perhaps to prevent tissue deposition of circulating immune complexes. Nonsteroidal anti-inflammatory agents are combined with the $H_1$ antihistamine. Depending on the therapeutic response, colchicine or hydroxychloroquine sulfate can be added to or substituted for these agents. If there is still no benefit, dapsone should be used. If there is no therapeutic response, a major therapeutic decision occurs since the medications to be considered in the second phase are associated with a more serious side-effect profile. These agents are systemic glucocorticosteroids [94], azathioprine, cyclophosphamide, methotrexate [95], intramuscular gold, plasmapheresis, cyclosporin [96], and high-dose immunoglobulin therapy [97]. Although these therapeutic agents have been reported to be of benefit in some patients, controlled clinical trials are not available. Colchicine, however, was shown to have no significant therapeutic effect in a prospective, randomized controlled trial [98].

In patients with erythema elevatum diutinum, dapsone is the drug of choice [71]. The treatment of nodular vasculitis consists of empirical trials of a saturated solution of potassium iodide, nonsteroidal anti-inflammatory agents, colchicine, and systemic glucocorticosteroids. Thalidomide is the treatment of choice for erythema nodosum leprosum.

In the treatment of livedoid vasculitis, empiric trials of aspirin and dipyridamole, colchicine, low-dose heparin, systemic glucocorticoids, nicotinic acid, low molecular weight dextran, phenphormin and ethylestranol, nifedipine, and pentoxifylline are used [99]. Low-dose recombinant tissue plasminogen activator therapy was reported to be successful in one therapeutic trial [100] but not in another study [101].

## VII. CONCLUSIONS

Vasculitis in the skin involves predominantly venules and may be associated with an underlying chronic disease, may be precipitated by infections or drugs, or may be idiopathic. Pathogenic mechanisms include the participation of immune complexes, neutrophils, lymphocytes, mast cells, endothelial cells, and adhesion molecules. The signature clinical sign is palpable purpura. The laboratory evaluation should depend on information obtained from the history and physical examination. Histopathological changes in skin biopsy specimens include fibrinoid necrosis of venules, an infiltrate of neutrophils with leukocytoclasis and lymphocytes, and extravasated erythrocytes. Therapy consists of removal of the antigen (infection or medication) or treatment of the underlying chronic disease and/or cutaneous vasculitis. The information on the use of therapeutic agents in cutaneous vasculitis is not based on controlled clinical trials with measured outcomes but rather on anecdotal case reports and open studies with small numbers of patients. The agents employed are $H_1$ antihistamines, nonsteroidal anti-inflammatory agents, colchicine, hydroxychloroquine, dapsone, glucocorticoids, various chemotherapeutic agents, and cyclosporine.

## REFERENCES

1. Sanchez NP, Van Hale HM, Su WPD. Clinical and histopathologic spectrum of necrotizing vasculitis: report of findings in 101 cases. Arch Dermatol 1985; 121:220–224.
2. Soter NA. Cutaneous necrotizing venulitis. In: Freedberg IM, Eizen AZ, Wolff K, Austen KF, Goldsmith LA, Katz SI, Fitzpatrick TB, eds. Fitzpatrick's Dermatology in General Medicine, 5th ed. New York: McGraw-Hill, 1999:2044–2053.
3. Jeanette JC, Falk RJ, Andrassay K, Bacon PA, Churg J, Gross WL, Hagen EC, Hoffman GS, Hunder GG, Kallenberg CGM, McCluskey RT, Sinico A, Russ AJ, van Es LA, Waldherr R, Wilk A. Nomenclature of systemic vasculitides: proposal of an international consensus conference. Arthritis Rheum 1994; 37:187–192.
4. Leavitt RY, Fauci AS. Polyangiitis overlap syndrome: classification and prospective experience. Am J Med 1986; 81:79–85.
5. Carmichael A, Marsden JR. Urticarial vasculitis: a presentation of C3 nephritic factor. Br J Dermatol 1993; 128:589.
6. Durand JM, Kaplanski G, Richard MA, Lefevre P, Quiles N, Trepo C, Soubeyrand J. Cutaneous vasculitis in a patient infected with hepatitis C virus: detection of hepatitis C virus RNA in the skin by polymerase chain reaction. Br J Dermatol 1993; 128:359–360.
7. Ghersetich I, Campanile G, Comacchi C, Lotti T. $\gamma/\delta$ TCR lymphocytes in cutaneous necrotizing vasculitis (CNV): a clue to the infective etiology. J Invest Dermatol 1993; 100:465.
8. Ghersetich I, Campanile G, Comacchi C, Romagnoli P, Lotti T. Immunohistochemical and ultrastructural aspects of leukocytoclastic cutaneous necrotizing vasculitis (CNV). J Invest Dermatol 1993; 100:545.
9. Wedi B, Elsner J. Czech W, Butterfield JH, Kapp A. Modulation of intercellular adhesion molecule 1 (ICAM-1) expression on the human mast-cell line (HMC)-1 by inflammatory mediators. Allergy 1996; 51:676–684.
10. Rohde D, Schlüter-Wigger W, Mielke V, von den Driesch P, von Gaudecker B, Sterry W. Infiltration of both T cells and neutrophils in the skin is accompanied by the expression of endothelial leukocyte adhesion molecule-1 (ELAM-1): an immunohistochemical and ultrastructural study. J Invest Dermatol 1992; 98:794–799.
11. Sais G, Vidaller A, Jucglá A, Condom E, Peyri J. Adhesion molecule expression and endothelial cell activation in cutaneous leukocytoclastic vasculitis: an immunohistologic and clinical study of 42 patients. Arch Dermatol 1997; 133: 443–450.
12. Jurd KM, Stephens CJM, Black MM, Hunt BJ. Endothelial cell activation in cutaneous vasculitis. Clin Exp Dermatol 1996; 21:28–32.
13. Jeanette C, Ewert BH, Falk RJ: Do antineutrophil cytoplasmic autoantibodies cause Wegner's granulomatosis and other forms of necrotizing vasculitis? Rheumat Dis Clin North Am 1993; 19:1–14.
14. Damianovich M, Gilburd B, George J, Del Papa N, Afek A, Goldberg I, Kopolovic Y, Roth D, Barkai G, Meroni P-L, Shoenfeld Y. Pathogenic role of anti-endothelial cell antibodies in vasculitis: an idiotypic experimental model. J Immunol 1996; 156:4946–4951.
15. Chan TM, Frampton G, Jayne DRW, Perry GJ, Lockwood CM, Cameron JS. Clinical significance of anti-endothelial cell antibodies in systemic vasculitis: a longitudinal study comparing anti-endothelial cell antibodies and anti-neutrophil cytoplasm antibodies. Am J Kidney Dis 1993; 22:387–392.
16. Francès C, Le Tonquèze M, Salohzin KV, Kalashnikova LA, Piette JC, Godeau P, Nasonov EL, Youinou P. Prevalence of anti-endothelial cell antibodies in patients with Sneddon's syndrome. J Am Acad Dermatol 1995; 33:64–68.
17. Diaz-Perez JL, Winkelmann RK. Cutaneous periarteritis nodosa. Arch Dermatol 1974; 110:407–414.
18. Francès C, Du LTH, Piette J-C, Saada V, Boisnic S, Wechsler B, Biétry O, Godeau P. Wegen-

er's granulomatosis: dermatological manifestations in 75 cases with clinicopathologic correlation. Arch Dermatol 1994; 130:861–867.

19. Soter NA. Chronic urticaria as a manifestation of necrotizing venulitis. N Engl J Med 1977; 296:1440–1442.

20. Sanchez-Perez J, Fernandez-Herrera J, Sols M, Jones M, Diez AG. Leukocytoclastic vasculitis in subacute cutaneous lupus erythematosus. Br J Dermatol 1993; 128:469–470.

21. Waltuck J, Buyon JP. Autoantibody-associated congenital heart block: outcome in mothers and children. Ann Intern Med 1994; 120:544–551.

22. DeArgila D, Ravenga F, Llmas R, Iglesias L. Cutaneous vasculitis with anti-Ro SSA antibodies not associated to connective-tissue disease. Actas Derm—Sifiliog 1995; 86:499–505.

23. Borrego L, Rodríguez J, Soler E, Jiménez A, Hernández B. Neonatal lupus erythematosus related to maternal leukocytoclastic vasculitis. Pediatr Dermatol 1997; 14:221–225.

24. Cohen SJ, Pittlekow MR, Su WPD. Cutaneous manifestations of cryoglobulinemia: clinical and histopathologic study of seventy-two patients. J Am Acad Dermatol 1991; 25:21–27.

25. Dienstag JL, Rhodes AR, Bhan AK, Dvorak AM, Mihm MC Jr, Wands JR. Urticaria associated with acute viral hepatitis type B: studies of pathogenesis. Ann Intern Med 1978; 89: 34–40.

26. Inman RD, Hodge M, Johnston MEA, Wright J, Heathcote J. Arthritis, vasculitis, and cryoglobulinemia associated with relapsing hepatitis A virus infection. Ann Intern Med 1986; 105:700–703.

27. Hearth-Holmes M, Zahradka SL, Baethge BA, Wolfe RE. Leukocytoclastic vasculitis associated with hepatitis C. Am J Med 1991; 90:765–766.

28. Chen K-R, Kawahara Y, Miyakawa S, Nishikawa T. Cutaneous vasculitis in Behçet's disease: a clinical and histopathologic study of 20 patients. J Am Acad Dermatol 1997; 36:689–696.

29. Burrows NP, Lockwood CM. Antineutrophil cytoplasmic antibodies and their relevance to the dermatologist. Br J Dermatol 1995; 132:173–181.

30. Romani J, Puig L, de Moragas JM. Detection of antineutrophil cytoplasmic antibodies in patients with hepatitis C virus-induced cutaneous vasculitis with mixed cryoglobulinemia. Arch Dermatol 1996; 132:974–975.

31. Homas PB, David-Bajar KM, Fitzpatrick JE, West SG, Tribelhorn DR. Microscopic polyarteritis: report of a case with cutaneous involvement and antimyeloperoxidase antibodies. Arch Dermatol 1992; 128:1223–1228.

32. Peñas PF, Porras JI, Fraga J, Bernis C, Sarriá C, Daudén E. Microscopic polyangiitis: a systemic vasculitis with a positive P-ANCA. Br J Dermatol 1996; 134:542–547.

33. Irvine AD, Bruce IN, Walsh MY, Bingham EA. Microscopic polyangiitis: delineation of a cutaneous-limited variant associated with antimyeloperoxidase autoantibody. Arch Dermatol 1997; 133:474–477.

34. Burden AD, Tillman DM, Foley P, Holme E. IgA class anticardiolipin antibodies in cutaneous leukocytoclastic vasculitis. J Am Acad Dermatol 1996; 35:411–415.

35. Stephansson EA, Scheynius A. Immunological studies of cutaneous vasculitis and primary antiphospholipid syndrome. Eur J Dermatol 1993; 3:289–293.

36. Renfro L, Franks Jr AG, Grodberg M, Kamino H. Painful nodules in a young female. Arch Dermatol 1992; 128:847–852.

37. Naldi L, Locati F, Marchesi L, Cortelazzo S, Finazzi G, Galli M, Brevi A, Cainelli T, Barbui T. Cutaneous manifestations associated with antiphospholipid antibodies in patients with suspected primary antiphospholipid syndrome: a case-control study. Ann Rheum Dis 1993; 52: 219–222.

38. Nahaas GT. Antiphospholipid antibodies and the antiphospholipid syndrome. J Am Acad Dermatol 1997; 36:149–168.

39. Somer T, Finegold SM. Vasculitides associated with infections, immunization, and antimicrobial drugs. Clin Infect Dis 1995; 20:1010–1036.

40. Marcellin P, Descamps V, Martinot-Peignoux M, Larzul D, Xu L, Boyer N, Pham B-N,

Crickx B, Guillevin L, Belaich S, Erlinger S, Benhamou J-P. Cryoglobulinemia with vasculitis associated with hepatitis C infection. Gastroenterology 1993; 104:272–277.

41. Pakula AS, Garden JM, Roth SI. Cryoglobulinemia and cutaneous leukocytoclastic vasculitis associated with hepatitis C virus infection. J Am Acad Dermatol 1993; 28:850–853.

42. Revenga Arranz F, Diáz R, Iglesias Díez L, Cassis Herce B, Sánchez Gómez F, Fuertes Ortiz A. Cryoglobulinemic vasculitis associated with hepatitis C infection: a report of eight cases. Acta Derm Venereol (Stockh) 1995; 75:234–236.

43. Karlsberg PL, Lee WM, Casey DL, Cockerell CJ, Cruz Jr PD. Cutaneous vasculitis and rheumatoid factor positivity as presenting signs of hepatitis C virus-induced mixed cryoglobulinemia. Arch Dermatol 1995; 131:1119–1123.

44. Dupin N, Chosidow O, Lunel F, Cacoub P, Musset L, Cresta P, Franguel L, Piette J-C, Godeau P, Opolon P, Francès C. Essential mixed cryoglobulinemia: a comparative study of dermatologic manifestations in patients infected or noninfected with hepatitis C virus. Arch Dermatol 1995; 131:1124–1127.

45. Pawlotsky J-M, Dhumeaux D, Bagot M. Hepatitis C virus in dermatology: a review. Arch Dermatol 1995; 131:1185–1193.

46. Daoud MS, el-Azhary RA, Gibson LE, Lutz ME, Daoud S. Chronic hepatitis C, cryoglobulinemia, and cutaneous necrotizing vasculitis: clinical, pathologic, and immunopathologic study of twelve patients. J Am Acad Dermatol 1996; 34:219–223.

47. Abe Y, Tanaka Y, Tanenaka M, Yoshida H, Yatsuhashi H, Yano M. Leukocytoclastic vasculitis associated with mixed cryoglobulinaemia and hepatitis C infection. Br J Dermatol 1997; 136:272–274.

48. Weimer CE Jr, Sahn EE. Follicular accentuation of leukocytoclastic vasculitis in an HIV-seropositive man: report of a case and review of the literature. J Am Acad Dermatol 1991; 24:898–902.

49. Watkins KV, Ittman MM. Necrotizing vasculitis in a patient with acquired immunodeficiency syndrome. J Oral Maxillofac Surg 1992; 50:1000–1003.

50. Murphy GF, Sanchez NP, Flynn TC, Sanchez JL, Mihm MC Jr, Soter NA. Erythema nodosum leprosum: nature and extent of the cutaneous microvascular alterations. J Am Acad Dermatol 1986; 14:59–69.

51. Lantin JP, Gattesco S, Duclos A, Zanchi A, Schaller MD, Pecoud A, Aubert V. Anaphylactoid purpura like vasculitis following fibrinolytic therapy: role of the immune response to streptokinase. Clin Exp Rheumatol 1994; 12:429–433.

52. Jain KK. Cutaneous vasculitis associated with granulocyte colony-stimulating factor. J Am Acad Dermatol 1994; 31:213–215.

53. Johnson ML, Grimwood RE. Leukocyte colony-stimulating factors: a review of associated neutrophilic dermatoses and vasculitides. Arch Dermatol 1994; 130:77–81.

54. Arbiser JL, Dzieczkowski JS, Harmon JV, Duncan LM. Leukocytoclastic vasculitis following staphylococcal protein A column immunoabsorption therapy: two cases and a review of the literature. Arch Dermatol 1995; 131:707–709.

55. Lowry MD, Hudson CF, Callen JP. Leukocytoclastic vasculitis caused by drug additives. J Am Acad Dermatol 1994; 30:854–855.

56. Tancrede-Bohin E, Ochonisky S, Vignon-Pennamen M-D, Flageu B, Morel P, Rybojad M. Schönlein-Henoch purpura in adult patients: predictive factors for IgA glomerulonephritis in a retrospective study of 57 cases. Arch Dermatol 1997; 133:438–442.

57. Legrain V, Lejean S, Taïeb A, Guillard J-M, Battin J, Maleville J. Infantile acute hemorrhagic edema of the skin: study of ten cases. J Am Acad Dermatol 1991; 24:17–22.

58. Cribier B, Asch PH, Heid E, Grosshans E. Cutaneous vasculitis with edema: acute hemorrhagic edema of the skin in an adult? Eur J Dermatol 1996; 5:286–289.

59. Tomaç N, Saraçlar Y, Turktas I, Kalayci Ö. Acute haemorrhagic oedema of infancy: a case report. Clin Exp Dermatol 1996; 21:217–219.

60. Ince E, Mumcu Y, Suskan E, Yaleinkaya F, Tümer N, Cin S. Infantile acute hemor-

rhagic edema: a variant of leukocytoclastic vasculitis. Pediatr Dermatol 1995; 12:224–227.

61. Mehregan DR, Hall MJ, Gibson LE. Urticarial vasculitis: a histopathologic and clinical review of 72 cases. J Am Acad Dermatol 1992; 26:441–448.
62. O'Donnell B, Black AK. Urticarial vasculitis. Int Angiol 1995; 14:166–174.
63. Roger D, Rollé F, Mausett J, Lavignac C, Bonnetblanc JM. Urticarial vasculitis induced by fluoxetine. Dermatology 1995; 191:164.
64. Lin RY, Caren CB, Menikoff H. Hypocomplementaemic urticarial vasculitis, interstitial lung disease and hepatitis C. Br J Dermatol 1995; 132:821–823.
65. Ishikawa O, Miyachi Y, Watanabe H. Hypocomplementaemic urticarial vasculitis associated with Jaccoud's syndrome. Br J Dermatol 1997; 137:804–807.
66. Demierre M-F, Winkelman WJ. Idiopathic cold-induced urticarial vasculitis and monoclonal IgG gammopathy. Int J Dermatol 1996; 35:151–152.
67. Kano Y, Orihara M, Shiohara T. Cellular and molecular dynamics in exercise-induced urticarial vasculitis lesions. Arch Dermatol 1998; 134:62–67.
68. Soter NA, Mihm Jr MC, Dvorak HF, Austen KF. Cutaneous necrotizing venulitis: a sequential analysis of the morphological alterations occurring after mast cell degranulation in a patient with a unique syndrome. Clin Exp Immunol 1978; 32:46–58.
69. Baty V, Hoen B, Hudziak H, Aghassian C, Jeandel C, Canton P. Schnitzler's syndrome: two case reports and review of the literature. Mayo Clin Proc 1995; 70:570–572.
70. Lebbe C, Rybojad M, Klein F, Oksenhendler E, Catala M, Danon F, Morel P. Schnitzler's syndrome associated with sensorimotor neuropathy. J Am Acad Dermatol 1994; 30:316–318.
71. Katz SI, Gallin JI, Hertz KC, Fauci AS, Lawley TJ. Erythema elevatum diutinum: skin and systemic manifestations, immunologic studies, and successful treatment with dapsone. Medicine 1977; 56:443–455.
72. Yiannias JA, El-Azhary RA, Gibson LE. Erythema elevatum diutinum: a clinical and histopathologic study of 13 patients. J Am Acad Dermatol 1992; 26:38–44.
73. Wilkinson SM, English JSC, Smith NP, Wilson-Jones E, Winkelmann RK. Erythema elevatum diutinum: a clinicopathological study. Clin Exp Dermatol 1992; 17:87–93.
74. Queipo de Llano MP, Yebra M, Cabrera R, Suarez E. Myelodysplastic syndrome in association with erythema elevatum diutinum. J Rheumatol 1992; 19:1005.
75. Rodriguez-Serna M, Fortea J-M, Perez A, Febrer I, Ribes C, Aliaga A. Erythema elevatum diutinum associated with celiac disease: response to a gluten-free diet. Pediatr Dermatol 1993; 10:125–128.
76. Bernard P, Bedane C, Delrous J-L, Catanzano G, Bonnetblanc J-M. Erythema elevatum diutinum in a patient with relapsing polychronditis. J Am Acad Dermatol 1992; 26:312–315.
77. Sangüeza OP, Pilcher B, Sangüeza JM. Erythema elevatum diutinum: a clinicopathological study of eight cases. Am J Dermatopathol 1997; 19:214–222.
78. LeBoit PE, Cockerell CJ. Nodular lesions of erythema elavatum diutinum in patients infected with human immunodeficiency virus. J Am Acad Dermatol 1993; 28:919–922.
79. Dronda F, Gonzales-López A, Lecona M, Barros C. Erythema elevatum diutinum in human immunodeficiency virus-infected patients: report of a case and review of the literature. Clin Exp Dermatol 1996; 21:222–225.
80. Schneider JW, Jordaan HF, Geiger DH, Victor T, Van Helden PD, Rossouw DJ. Erythema induratum of Bazin: a clinicopathological study of 20 cases and detection of *Mycobacterium tuberculosis* DNA in skin lesions by polymerase chain reaction. Am J Dermatopathol 1995; 17:350–356.
81. Baselga E, Margall N, Barnadas MA, Coll P, de Moragas JM. Detection of *Mycobacterium tuberculosis* DNA in lobular granulomatous panniculitis (erythema induratum-nodular vasculitis). Arch Dermatol 1997; 133:457–462.
82. Schneider JW, Jordaan HF. The histopathologic spectrum of erythema induratum of Bazin. Am J Dermatopathol 1997; 19:323–333.

83. McCalmont CS, McCalmont TH, Jorizzo JL, White WL, Leshin B, Rothberger H. Livedo vasculitis: vasculitis or thrombotic vasculopathy? Clin Exp Dermatol 1992; 17:4–8.
84. Acland KM, Darvay A, Wakelin SH, Russell-Jones R. Livedoid vasculitis: a manifestation of the antiphospholipid syndrome? Br J Dermatol 1999; 140:131–135.
85. Grattan CE, Burton JL, Boon AP. Sneddon's syndrome (livedo reticularis and cerebral thrombosis) with livedo vasculitis and anticardiolipin antibodies. Br J Dermatol 1989; 120:441–447.
86. Zelger B, Sepp N, Schmid KW, Hintner H, Klein G, Fritsch PO. Life history of cutaneous vascular lesions in Sneddon's syndrome. Hum Pathol 1992; 23:668–675.
87. Zelger B, Sepp N, Stockhammer G, Dosch E, Hilty E, Öfner D, Aichner F, Fritsch PO. Sneddon's syndrome: a long-term follow-up of 21 patients. Arch Dermatol 1993; 129:437–447.
88. Lilic D, Charmichael AJ. Cutaneous vasculitis with partial C4 deficiency responsive to dapsone. Br J Dermatol 1997; 137:476.
89. Chen K-R, Pittelkow MR, Su WPD, Gleich GJ, Newman W, Leiferman KM. Recurrent cutaneous eosinophilic vasculitis: a novel eosinophil-mediated syndrome. Arch Dermatol 1994; 130:1159–1166.
90. Chen K-R, Su WPD, Pittelkow MR, Conn DL, George T, Leiferman KM. Eosinophilic vasculitis in connective tissue disease. J Am Acad Dermatol 1996; 35:173–182.
91. Wisnieski JJ, Jones SM. IgG autoantibody to the collagen-like region of C1q in hypocomplementemic urticarial vasculitis syndrome, systemic lupus erythematosus, and 6 other musculoskeletal or rheumatic diseases. J Rheumatol 1992; 19:884–888.
92. Saulsbury FT. Heavy and light chain composition of serum IgA and IgA rheumatoid factor in Henoch-Schönlein purpura. Arthritis Rheum 1992; 35:1377–1380.
93. Helander SD, De Castro FR, Gibson LE. Henoch-Schönlein purpura: clinicopathologic correlation of cutaneous vascular IgA deposits and the relationship to leukocytoclastic vasculitis. Acta Derm Venereol (Stockh) 1995; 75:125–129.
94. Cupps TR, Springer RM, Fauci AS. Chronic, recurrent small-vessel cutaneous vasculitis: clinical experience in 13 patients. JAMA 1982; 247:1994–1998.
95. Stack PS. Methotrexate for urticarial vasculitis. Ann Allergy 1994; 72:36–38.
96. Tosca AD, Ioannidou DJ, Katsantonis JC, Kyriakis KP. Cyclosporin A in the treatment of cutaneous vasculitis: clinical and cellular effects. J Eur Acad Dermatol Venereol 1996; 6:135–141.
97. Rostoker G, Desvaux-Belghiti D, Pilatte Y, Petit-Phar M, Philippon C, Deforges L, Terzidis H, Intrator L, André C, Adnot S, Bonin P, Bierling P, Rémy P, Lagrue G, Lang P, Weil B. High-dose immunoglobulin therapy for severe IgA nephropathy and Henoch-Schönlein purpura. Ann Intern Med 1994; 120:476–484.
98. Sais G, Vidaller A, Jucglà A, Gallardo F, Peyrí J. Colchicine in the treatment of cutaneous leukocytoclastic vasculitis: results of a prospective, randomized controlled trial. Arch Dermatol 1995; 131:1399–1402.
99. Nikolova K, Popov J, Obreshkova E. Leg ulcerations due to livedo vasculitis: successful combined therapy with pentoxifylline and nifedipine. J Eur Acad Dermatol Venereol 1995; 5:54–58.
100. Klein KL, Pittelkow MR. Tissue plasminogen activator for treatment of livedoid vasculitis. Mayo Clin Proc 1992; 67:923–933.
101. Murrell DF, Jensen J, O'Keefe EJ. Failure of livedoid vasculitis to respond to tissue plasminogen activator. Arch Dermatol 1995; 131:231–232.

# 15
## Drug-Induced Cutaneous Reactions

**Rebecca S. Gruchalla**
*University of Texas Southwestern Medical Center, Dallas, Texas*

**Vincent S. Beltrani**
*College of Physicians and Surgeons, Columbia University, New York, New York;*
*University of Medicine and Dentistry of New Jersey, Newark, New Jersey*

## I. INTRODUCTION

Any dermatological condition that involves the skin, hair, nails, or mucous membranes and that appears within 2 weeks of the initiation of a medication is, very likely, drug-induced. Adverse cutaneous reactions to drugs are a common problem, and they are a source of much frustration for the practicing clinician. Often it is not only difficult to determine if a reaction is drug-induced, but morphological classification of the skin lesions themselves and identification of the culprit agent responsible for a reaction can be challenging tasks as well. Drug reactions may occur to any drug, including prescribed medications, over-the-counter medications, and herbal concoctions, and, in many cases, a single agent may elicit more than one type of eruption. Adding to this complexity is the fact that the mechanisms responsible for drug reactions are numerous and that, at times, more than one mechanism may be operative.

Understandably, clinicians commonly are frustrated when confronted with patients who have presumed drug-induced skin eruptions. However, recent data is allowing us to better elucidate the various mechanisms underlying drug-induced reactions and, because of this information, we are beginning to be able to develop more optimal treatment plans for our patients. In this chapter, we will discuss the mechanisms responsible for drug-induced skin reactions and the diagnostic tools that may be useful in their evaluation. A practical management algorithm, based upon this information and that incorporates these tools, will be outlined.

## II. EPIDEMIOLOGY OF ADVERSE CUTANEOUS DRUG ERUPTIONS

Epidemiology is the study of the factors determining and influencing the frequency and distribution of disease, injury, and other health-related events and their causes in a defined population for the purpose of establishing programs to prevent and control their development and spread [1]. Both the prevalence and incidence of adverse drug reactions, as well as the natural history of these reactions, are important epidemiological issues. However, due to the complexities involved in evaluating these reactions and the fact that they many times are not reported, their incidence is difficult to determine.

An adverse drug reaction (ADR), as defined by the World Health Organization (WHO) [2], is any noxious, unintended, and undesired effect of a drug that occurs at doses used in humans for prevention, diagnosis, or treatment. Currently, the incidence of ADRs only can be estimated since the intensive monitoring and documenting that is required to make this determination does not exist at most hospitals and clinics. Despite these limitations, an attempt to estimate this incidence has been made by several groups, and their collective results are presented in Table 1. Lazarou and colleagues [3] estimated the incidence of serious and fatal ADRs in hospitalized patients by conducting a meta-analysis. They evaluated 39 studies, done in the United States from 1966 to 1996, that prospectively monitored and recorded all ADR occurrences in hospitalized patients. The patients evaluated were of two types: those who were admitted to the hospital because of an ADR and those who experienced an ADR while in the hospital. Drug-related events, such as errors in drug administration, noncompliance, overdose, drug abuse, therapeutic failures, and possible ADRs, were not included in the analysis.

It was found that the overall incidence of serious ADRs was 6.7% of hospitalized patients and that the overall incidence of fatal ADRs was 0.32%. When both serious and nonserious ADRs were considered together, the percentage of ADRs more than doubled, to 15.1% of hospitalized patients. In addition, using available statistics, the authors estimated that, in 1994 alone, 2,216,000 hospitalized patients had serious ADRs and 106,000 had fatal ADRs. Thus, it is apparent from these data that ADRs contribute importantly to increased lengths of stay and increased hospital costs.

While most cutaneous ADRs are not associated with serious morbidity, they are very important since these reactions are the most commonly encountered ADRs and they are frequently the reason for discontinuation of drug therapy. However, as for ADRs in general, the incidence of cutaneous ADRs is difficult to determine since information sources that are used to gather the data are diverse and often not complete or accurate. However, studies do exist that report the estimated incidence. The Boston Collaborative Drug Surveillance Program, the most extensive study performed to date in the United States, evaluated data from over 37,000 patients to determine the frequency of cutaneous

**Table 1**  Adverse Drug Reaction Incidence

| Study | ADR incidence | Comments |
|-------|---------------|----------|
| Lazarou et al. [3] (serious and fatal ADRs) | 7% of hospitalized patients | Meta-analysis of 39 studies (1966–1996) |
| Boston Collaborative Study (cutaneous ADRs) | 2% of hospitalized patients | Over 37,000 patients evaluated; most common drugs are ampicillin/amoxicillin, trimethoprim/sulfamethoxazole |
| Hunziker et al. [6] (cutaneous ADRs) | 2.7% of hospitalized patients | 20-year period evaluated; most common drugs are penicillins/sulfonamides; most common rxns are maculopapular (91%), urticarial (6%) |

drug reactions to agents commonly used in the hospital [4,5]. The data were evaluated in two series, and the overall cutaneous reaction rate (number of reactions per exposed patient) was slightly more than 2% for both series. Reaction rates were highest for ampicillin/amoxicillin (51/52 per 1000 exposed patients) and for trimethoprim-sulfamethoxazole (34 per 1000 exposed patients). Other drugs that caused reaction rates greater than 10 per 1000 exposed patients were penicillin, cephalosporins, semisynthetic penicillins, and quinidine. Most reactions occurred within a week of the initiation of therapy, and the predominant reaction types were generalized pruritus, morbilliform rashes (drug exanthems), and urticaria.

More recently, Hunziker et al. [6] determined the number of drug-induced adverse skin reactions that occurred in three hospitals in Switzerland over a 20-year period from 1974 to 1993. These data were available and accessible since each of these hospitals had comprehensive hospital drug-monitoring systems in place during this time period. Of 48,005 drug-exposed individuals, a total of 1317 had drug-induced adverse skin reactions that were recorded (reaction rate of 2.7%). Similar to the Boston Collaborative Drug Surveillance Program, the most common culprit drugs were penicillins and sulfonamides and the most common reactions were maculopapular exanthems (91.2%) and urticaria (5.9%).

Fortunately, severe cutaneous reactions to drugs occur rarely. However, when they do occur, death or disability may result. Studies aimed at determining the incidence of severe drug-induced skin reactions typically focus upon two particular reactions: Stevens-Johnson syndrome and toxic epidermal necrolysis. Attempts to determine the incidence of Stevens-Johnson syndrome and toxic epidermal necrolysis have been hampered by the lack of a consensus definition of these disorders, by the rare occurrence of these disorders, and by the limited availability of data. Despite these difficulties, some data regarding incidence do exist (Table 2).

In the 1980s, population-based retrospective studies conducted in France and Germany over a 5-year period revealed the incidence rate of toxic epidermal necrolysis to be 1.2 per 1 million inhabitants per year in France [7] and 0.93 per 1 million per year in Germany [8]. More recently, prospective epidemiological studies are being conducted that use standardized definitional criteria and standardized methods of case selection and information collection. These studies include the ongoing population-based registry on

**Table 2** Incidence of Severe Cutaneous Adverse Drug Reactions

| Study [Ref.] | ADR incidence |
| --- | --- |
| Roujeau et al. (retrospective study) [7] | TEN: 1.2 cases per million in France |
| Schof et al. (retrospective study) [8] | TEN: 0.93 cases per million in Germany |
| Rzany et al. (prospective study) [10] | SJS, SJS/TEN overlap, TEN: 1.53 cases per million in Germany |
| Chan et al. (based on insurance billing data) [12] | EM, SJS, TEN: 1.8 cases per million (ages 20–64); 7 cases per million (<20 years old); 9 cases per million (>65 years old) |
| Strom et al. (based on Medicaid billing data) [13] | SJS: 7.1 cases per million (Michigan); 2.6 cases per million (Minnesota), 6.8 cases per million (Florida) |

TEN = Toxic epidermal necrolysis; SJS = Stevens-Johnson syndrome; EM = erythema multiforme.

severe skin reactions in Germany and the International Collaborative Case-Control Study of Severe Cutaneous Adverse Reactions (SCAR) [9].

A population-based registry was established in 1990 in Germany to determine the number of severe cutaneous reactions that occur in hospitalized patients. Initially, the registry was limited to former West Germany and Berlin. However, in 1996, case assessment was extended to the new federal states in former East Germany. Using data gathered from this registry, an incidence of 1.53 per 1 million inhabitants was calculated for Stevens-Johnson syndrome, Stevens-Johnson syndrome/toxic epidermal necrolysis overlap, and toxic epidermal necrolysis all together for the year 1991 [10].

At the same time that Germany began its registry, an international collaborative case-control study of severe cutaneous adverse reactions was initiated in France, Italy, Portugal, as well as in Germany. The aims of this study were severalfold: "a) to evaluate and quantify the role of drugs and other factors in the development of Stevens-Johnson syndrome and toxic epidermal necrolysis; b) to explore and quantify the etiologic role of various potentially predisposing factors, such as HIV infection, history of cancer, and tobacco and alcohol consumption; and c) to develop standardized clinical definitions of these diseases suitable for use in epidemiologic studies and, using epidemiologic methods, to evaluate whether the etiology of the diseases shows any variability according to disease classification" [9]. Data from phase I (up until June 1993) of this study have been analyzed and published. A total of 245 hospitalized patients with Stevens-Johnson syndrome, Stevens-Johnson syndrome/toxic epidermal necrolysis overlap, and toxic epidermal necrolysis, along with 1147 controls were compared in regards to drug use prior to the development of their disease [11]. Drugs were grouped into two different categories: those taken for short periods of time and those taken for longer periods of time such as months or years. Of drugs usually taken for short time periods, increased risk was noted for co-trimoxazole, other sulfonamides, aminopenicillins, quinolones, cephalosporins, and chlormezanone. Of drugs taken for longer time periods, an increased relative risk was found for carbamazepine, phenobarbital, phenytoin, valproic acid, oxicam-NSAIDS, allopurinol, and corticosteroids. For this latter group of drugs, the risk of the development of severe cutaneous reactions was found to be higher during the first 2 months of treatment. No increased risk was found for many other agents including thiazide diuretics, oral hypoglycemic agents, beta blockers, calcium channel blockers, and other antihypertensive agents.

While most of the epidemiological studies examining the incidence of severe cutaneous drug reactions have been performed in Europe, several have been conducted in the United States as well. A population-based study was conducted by Chan et al. [12] in 1990 that investigated reaction rates in hospitalized patients from 1972 to 1986 using data obtained from the Group Health Cooperative of Puget Sound, Seattle, Washington. The incidence of erythema multiforme, Stevens-Johnson syndrome, and toxic epidermal necrolysis was estimated to be 1.8 cases per million person-years for patients between 20 and 64 years of age. For individuals less than 20 years and 65 or older the incidence increased to 7 and 9 cases per million person-years, respectively. The most commonly implicated drugs were phenobarbital, nitrofurantoin, co-trimoxazole, and ampicillin and amoxicillin. A second study, based on computerized Medicaid billing data for 1980–84 from the states of Michigan, Minnesota, and Florida, estimated the incidence of Stevens-Johnson syndrome to be 7.1, 2.6, and 6.8 per million per year, respectively. In this study, aminopenicillins were the most common culprit drugs [13].

More recently, the European community has again banded together to investigate the epidemiology of severe cutaneous drug reactions. In 1997, a European case-control surveillance of severe cutaneous adverse reactions, termed EuroSCAR, was initiated. The participating countries include those who participated in the original SCAR study: France, Germany, and Italy along with three additional countries—Austria, Israel, and the Netherlands. It is hoped that as a result of these intensive efforts, both the etiology and epidemiology of severe cutaneous drug reactions will be further elucidated [14]. Also, a study such as this should help determine the reasons underlying the differences seen in reaction rates and causative agents of Stevens-Johnson syndrome and toxic epidermal necrolysis in different countries.

## III. CLASSIFICATION OF DRUG REACTIONS

While most ADRs are called "allergic," more commonly they are mediated by nonimmunologic mechanisms. Unlike immunologically mediated reactions, the majority of adverse drug reactions are dose-related, they often are related to the known pharmacological actions of the drug, and they potentially may occur in all individuals (Type A, predictable reactions). In contrast, true allergic or immunological reactions fall into the category of Type B reactions, which are not predictable. They are not dose-dependent, they are not related to the pharmacological actions of the drug, and they occur only in susceptible patients. Type B reactions include drug intolerance (tinnitus due to aspirin), idiosyncratic reactions (coumadin-induced skin necrosis in patients with protein C deficiency), and hypersensitivity reactions. Hypersensitivity or allergic reactions demonstrate features that are common to immunological reactions in general: (1) a period of sensitization is required before they are elicited; (2) they may be triggered by a drug (antigen) amount that is far below the therapeutic range; and (3) they are restricted to a limited number of syndromes that have a known or a presumed immunopathological basis.

Attempts often are made to classify immunological drug reactions, including those that are manifested in the skin, into one of the four hypersensitivity types described by Gell and Coombs [15]: Type I, immediate-hypersensitivity reactions (urticaria, angioedema); Type II, cytotoxic reactions (pemphigus-like); Type III, immune complex reactions (urticarial vasculitis); or Type IV, delayed-type hypersensitivity reactions (allergic contact dermatitis). The first three reaction types are mediated by drug-specific antibodies, while Type IV reactions are caused by drug-specific T lymphocytes. Hypersensitivity drug reactions pose a major problem to physicians because they are unpredictable and potentially fatal.

In some instances, drug-induced cutaneous reactions fit nicely into one of the above categories. Urticaria, caused by mast cell mediator release resulting from the cross-linking of penicillin-specific IgE antibodies on the mast cell surface, is a classic example of a cutaneous drug-induced immediate hypersensitivity reaction. Drug-induced eczematous eruptions and contact dermatitis are classic examples of T-cell–mediated skin disease. In most instances, unfortunately cutaneous drug reactions are difficult to classify since the mechanism or mechanisms responsible for their elicitation often are not known. In addition, since these reactions are uncommon and unpredictable, they usually cannot be reproduced in animal models [16]. The next part of this chapter will focus on recently published exciting information that is allowing us to have better insight into the pathophysiology of drug-induced cutaneous reactions.

## IV. DRUG HYPERSENSITIVITY: THE HAPTEN HYPOTHESIS AND THE ROLE OF DRUG METABOLISM

The term "hypersensitivity" is used commonly in the adverse drug reaction literature. However, often it is used loosely. While many drug reactions are placed in the hypersensitivity category, for the majority of drugs the mechanisms responsible for the reactions they produce have not been elucidated. As the hapten hypothesis of drug hypersensitivity is discussed, keep in mind that the term "hypersensitivity," while commonly used, is often poorly defined.

In order to understand the types of "hypersensitivity" reactions that drugs may produce, it is critical to understand their chemical properties as well as how they are metabolized. It is now well established that, in order for hypersensitivity reactions to occur, most drugs must be "bioactivated" or metabolized to chemically reactive products [17]. Generally, drug metabolism is regarded as a type of detoxification process, whereby drugs are converted from lipid-soluble, nonpolar compounds to more polar, hydrophilic compounds that are easily excreted. Two steps usually are required. The first is either oxidation, reduction, or hydrolysis (phase I reactions) and the second is conjugation (phase II reactions). Oxidation reactions frequently involve cytochrome P450 enzymes, flavin-containing monooxygenases, prostaglandin synthetase, and various tissue peroxidases. Phase II reactions are mediated by enzymes such as epoxide hydrolase, glutathione S-transferase (GST), and N-acetyltransferase (NAT) [18].

In most instances, when drug-metabolizing enzymes convert a drug that was previously inactive into a chemically reactive metabolite, prompt detoxification occurs (bioinactivation). In certain circumstances, however, if the metabolite is not adequately detoxified, it may cause direct toxicity or immune-mediated hypersensitivity (Fig. 1) [19]. When direct toxicity occurs, chemically reactive metabolites bind to proteins or nucleic acids and cause cellular necrosis or the production of an altered gene product, respectively. Alternatively, reactive metabolites may act as haptens that may initiate an immune response after covalent binding with cellular macromolecules (hapten hypothesis [20]). The immune response may be directed towards the hapten, the hapten-carrier complex, or new antigenic determinants (neoantigen) that are created through the combination of the drug with the protein. The response that is elicited may be antibody-mediated, T-cell–mediated, or both. While reactions of this type occur rarely, they are of major concern because they are not detected by routine animal toxicology studies, and they often are not detected in early clinical trials due to the limited number of individuals who are exposed to the drug in these trials.

The development of an adverse drug reaction mediated by reactive drug metabolites and the clinical manifestations of that reaction are dependent upon several factors: the chemical nature of the drug, interindividual differences in drug metabolism, and the nature of the target cellular macromolecule [17]. Whether or not a chemically reactive metabolite will cause direct toxicity or immune-mediated hypersensitivity often cannot be determined. However, clinical manifestations of drug eruption, fever, lymphadenopathy, and eosinophilia all are suggestive of a hypersensitivity reaction. In addition, by using the knowledge we are gathering regarding drug metabolism along with select immunochemical assays, we are beginning to further understand some of the mystery surrounding the reactions caused by chemically reactive drug species.

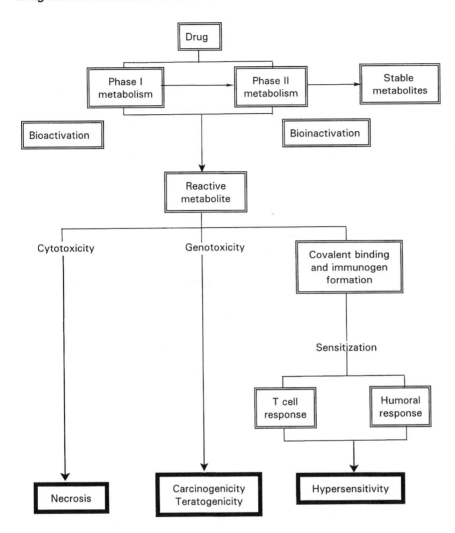

**Figure 1** The role of drug-metabolizing enzymes in the bioactivation and bioinactivation of drugs. Adapted from Ref. 19.

## V. THE IMPORTANCE OF THE SKIN IN DRUG METABOLISM

The skin, which is the largest organ in the body, is metabolically active, containing cells that possess both phase I and phase II drug-metabolizing enzymes [21,22]. Neutrophils, monocytes, and keratinocytes, in particular, have enzymes that potentially can oxidize drugs to reactive metabolites. The skin also is an active immunological organ containing both Langerhans cells and dendritic cells that may play a role in antigen presentation of allergenic drug determinants [18]. It has been hypothesized that this combination of metabolic activity along with immunological responsiveness may account for why the skin is the organ most frequently affected by adverse drug reactions [18].

## VI. PATTERNS OF DRUG-INDUCED CUTANEOUS REACTIONS

It is not possible to discuss in a single chapter all of the various kinds of skin reactions produced by systemically administered drugs (Table 3) [23]. Adding to the complexity of this dermatological problem is the fact that one drug may produce several types of eruptions and, in addition, similar skin reactions may be produced by many different drugs. For a complete review of drug-induced skin reactions, we refer the reader to several recent, very comprehensive texts devoted to this topic [23,24]. In addition, a just-published text entitled *Drug Hypersensitivity* [25] describes in great detail the immune mechanisms of drug allergy, diagnostic testing for drug hypersensitivity, and types of systemic reactions produced by particular drugs. For this chapter, we have chosen to discuss in depth several common cutaneous drug reactions (morbilliform eruptions, urticaria/angioedema, fixed drug eruption) and some that are the most severe (Stevens-Johnson syndrome, toxic epidermal necrolysis, hypersensitivity syndrome). Another reason we have chosen to focus on these particular drug-induced skin reactions is that exciting data regarding the pathogenesis of each of these are being published at a rapid rate. We will present these data and provide the latest information regarding diagnosis and treatment options.

### A. Maculopapular or Morbilliform Eruptions

#### 1. Clinical Features

Maculopapular or morbilliform eruptions are the most common of the drug-induced cutaneous reactions, and they can be induced by almost any drug. Often these eruptions are generalized and symmetrical, and they consist of erythematous, confluent macules

**Table 3** Common Drug-Induced Cutaneous Reaction Patterns

| | |
|---|---|
| Maculopapular eruptions | Eczematous eruptions |
| Purpura | Bullous eruptions |
| Annular erythema | Porphyria and pseudoporphyria |
| Pityriasis rosea–like eruptions | Drug-induced bullous pemphigoid |
| Psoriasiform eruptions | Drug-induced pemphigus |
| Erythroderma | Vasculitis |
| Exfoliative dermatitis | Lupus erythematosus–like |
| Urticaria/Angioedema | syndrome |
| Serum sickness | Drug-induced dermatomyositis |
| Erythema multiforme | Scleroderma-like reactions |
| Stevens-Johnson syndrome | Eosinophilia-myalgia syndrome |
| Toxic epidermal necrolysis | Erythema nodosum |
| Fixed drug eruptions | Pseudolymphomatous eruptions |
| Lichenoid eruptions | Erythromelalgia |
| Photosensitivity | Drug-induced alopecia |
| Pigmentary abnormalities | Drug-induced hypertrichosis |
| Acneiform and pustular eruptions | Drug-induced nail abnormalities |
| Hypersensitivity syndrome | Drug-induced oral conditions |

*Source*: Ref. 23.

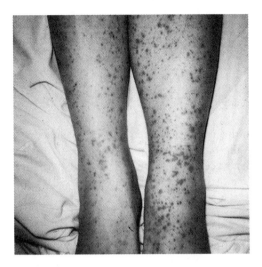

**Figure 2** Amoxicillin-induced maculopapular eruption in a 32-year-old woman that occurred on the eighth day of a course of therapy for an upper respiratory infection. The patient had been previously exposed to penicillin. The eruption was very pruritic, but within 48 hours after drug discontinuation the pruritus had lessened, and the rash completely resolved by the tenth day. Treatment consisted of topical 0.1% triamcinalone cream.

and/or papules that spare the face, palms, and soles (Fig. 2). However, the lesions can be pleomorphic and may vary in appearance on a single patient. The trunk and extremities usually are involved, with more pronounced involvement of the intertriginous areas. The lesions usually arise within a week to 2 weeks after the initiation of drug therapy, but occasionally the eruption may appear after therapy has been terminated (within days). The lesions may be accompanied by pruritus, fever, facial/eyelid edema, malaise, and joint aches, and they usually fade within several days to a week after the incriminating drug has been stopped. In rare instances, the eruption actually may resolve despite continued administration of the drug. On the other hand, the rash also may progress to generalized erythroderma or exfoliative dermatitis with continued drug administration.

### 2. Causative Agents

While maculopapular eruptions may occur with the administration of any drug, they most frequently are associated with the use of ampicillin, other penicillins, NSAIDs, sulfonamides, anticonvulsants, and allopurinol. Also, it must be remembered that not all morbilliform or maculopapular exanthams are drug-induced. Certain infections, especially viral infections, may induce exanthams that are difficult to differentiate from those induced by drugs.

### 3. Pathophysiology

The mechanism responsible for drug-associated maculopapular eruptions is not clearly known, and it is likely that more than one mechanism is operative. Since in most instances these reactions occur after several days of therapy and typically do not occur after the first dose, it could be said that a period of "sensitization" is required before the reaction is elicited. However, despite this "immunological feature," few data exist that clearly elucidate the role of the immune response in these reactions. Recently, there has been some evidence generated supporting the involvement of CD8+ T cells in both morbilliform and bullous drug eruptions. By using limiting dilution analysis, Kalish et al. [26] detected lymphocytes that proliferated in response to sulfamethoxazole (SMX) in the peripheral blood of three patients with SMX-induced drug eruptions. In addition to these findings, CD8+ lymphocytes reactive with both sulfonamides [27,28] and penicillin [29,30] have been isolated from bullous eruptions.

Further evidence is accumulating supporting the involvement of CD8+ lymphocytes in drug eruptions, and this may result from the bioactivation of drugs to their reactive intermediates [31–34]. It is hypothesized that once formed, these intracellular reactive intermediates covalently link to cytoplasmic proteins, which then are processed by the "endogenous pathway" of presentation (by major histocompatibility complex (MHC) class I molecules) to CD8+ T cells. While data supporting this role for T lymphocytes in the etiology of morbilliform and other drug eruptions remain sparse at this time, they continue to accumulate and offer an exciting new hypothesis regarding a potential mechanism responsible for these drug-induced eruptions.

## 4. Diagnosis and Treatment

At this time, there is no reliable test available that can be used to determine the etiology of maculopapular eruptions. While the histology of the lesions is nonspecific, a skin biopsy may be of value in ruling out other clinically similar eruptions. Unlike drug-induced urticaria, prick skin testing has little usefulness as a diagnostic method in drug-induced maculopapular and morbilliform eruptions since it is not thought that these reactions are IgE mediated. On the other hand, patch testing may prove to be useful in some instances. However, as expected, positive patch tests are elicited more often in eczematous reactions compared to maculopapular reactions. Osawa et al. [35] skin tested 242 patients with various delayed-type skin eruptions. Patch tests were positive in 52.9% of those individuals who had eczematous eruptions and in 13.9% of those individuals who had maculopapular eruptions. Thus, these results support the hypothesis that at least some maculopapular eruptions may be T-cell–mediated. Recently, Bruynzeel and Maibach [36] discussed the role of patch testing in systemic drug eruptions. In this review, they outlined when it may be useful to perform patch testing, with which drugs it may be performed, and how the procedure is done.

Treatment is directed towards symptomatic relief once the offending agent is discontinued. Typically the reaction subsides within a few days. Cool compresses and topical corticosteroid creams and ointments may be helpful with the discomfort. However, systemic corticosteroid therapy may be justified if the eruption is extensive or pruritus is severe. Antihistamines usually are not helpful, since there is no evidence of mast cell involvement in reactions of this type.

It remains unclear whether or not a patient who has experienced a maculopapular eruption to a drug can safely receive the same or similar drug at a future time. Since the mechanism is not presumed to be IgE-mediated, a graded challenge may be considered. Graded challenge involves administering a small amount of the drug, such as one milligram, and then progressing at relatively large incremental increases to full-dose therapy within hours to days [37]. Graded challenges should not be performed sooner than 2–3 months after resolution of the eruption, and it is absolutely contraindicated in those patients who have experienced anaphylaxis, toxic epidermal necrolysis, erythema multiforme, Stevens-Johnson syndrome, exfoliative dermatitis, or erythroderma.

## B. Urticaria/Angioedema

### 1. Clinical Features

Urticaria and its ''deeper counterpart,'' angioedema, are the second-most common reactions induced by drugs. Urticarial lesions are generalized, symmetrical, and characterized by pruritic, erythematous wheals. They vary in size and shape, and each wheal is evanescent, lasting only a few hours and rarely more than 24 hours (Fig. 3). The epidermis remains intact, and there is never any scaling or vesiculo-bullous formation. Histology of both urticaria and angioedema reveal marked dermal edema with a sparse perivascular infiltrate of lymphocytes and eosinophils. In the case of angioedema, the edema and inflammation is deeper, often extending into the subcutaneous fat [38].

### 2. Pathophysiology and Causative Agents

Drug-induced urticaria may be caused by one of several mechanisms. The best understood mechanism involves drug-specific IgE antibodies that bind to the high-affinity IgE receptor on the surface of mast cells and basophils. Subsequently, when the drug is reintroduced, IgE cross-linking occurs, causing the release of a multitude of mediators and resulting in the appearance of urticaria, angioedema, or systemic anaphylaxis if mast cell activation

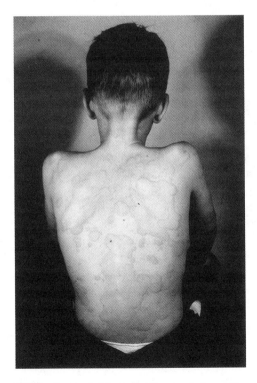

**Figure 3** Penicillin-induced urticaria in an 11-year-old boy that appeared 15–20 minutes following an intramuscular penicillin injection for streptococcal pharyngitis. The rapidly appearing, generalized, intensely pruritic eruption was accompanied by diaphoresis and a slight decrease in blood pressure. The patient was treated with and responded to 0.2 ml subcutaneous epinephrine (1:1000) and 25 mg oral diphenhydramine. Six weeks after the reaction, the patient was skin-tested and found to be skin test positive to Pre-Pen (penicilloyl-poly-L-lysine).

is widespread. In addition to this Type I immediate-type hypersensitivity mechanism, urticaria also may be seen as part of Type III, drug-induced immune complex reactions such as vasculitis and serum sickness. In these cases, circulating immune complexes, consisting of drug-specific IgG/IgM antibodies and the drug, are formed and are deposited on the vascular endothelium. Subsequently, complement is activated and the anaphylatoxins, C3a and C5a, are formed. These can trigger mast cell and basophil release directly and can lead to the development of urticaria or angioedema in the absence of drug-specific IgE antibodies. Certain agents, such as NSAIDs, angiotensin-converting enzyme inhibitors, and hyperosmolar solutions may cause mast cell and basophil degranulation by yet another not-yet-determined mechanism.

While urticaria caused by most antibiotics is thought to be IgE-mediated, some of these agents may cause mast cell mediator release by a direct, nonimmunological mechanism. Vancomycin causes a dose-dependent reaction characterized by erythema and pruritus that appears not to be IgE mediated and that may be caused by nonimmunological histamine release [39,40]. Like vancomycin, ciprofloxacin-induced urticaria also may result from direct histamine release [41]. For both of these agents, reactions may occur with the first dose, unlike reactions that are immunologically mediated. Other drugs that may cause urticaria by direct mast cell/basophil degranulation include opiates and the various muscle relaxants that are used in the induction of anesthesia: succinylcholine, alcuronium, vecuronium, pancuronium, d-tubocurarine, and gallamine. Determining the mechanism responsible for urticarial reactions to the muscle relaxants is especially difficult since, in addition to causing nonimmunological histamine release, these agents also may induce the formation of drug-specific IgE antibodies [42–44].

## 3. Diagnosis and Treatment

Virtually any drug may elicit urticaria or angioedema. However, often it is not possible to determine the mechanism responsible for every urticarial reaction. For urticarial lesions that persist for more then 24 hours, vasculitis should be considered and a biopsy is warranted. Typically, however, a biopsy is not useful.

In some instances, the presence of IgE antibodies can be assessed by the prick skin test. Not only is it useful to detect IgE antibodies to various aeroallergens, but it may be and has been used to determine the presence of IgE antibodies to those drugs that are multivalent and of large molecular weight. Drugs such as foreign antisera, hormones, enzymes, and toxoids are immunogenic in their native form. Thus, they, in the absence of metabolism or degradation, can induce the production of IgE antibodies, can cross-link them on the surface of mast cells and basophils, and can cause a localized wheal and flare reaction when they are used as prick skin test reagents. In contrast, for urticaria that is induced by antibiotics and that is thought to be IgE-mediated, there are a few standardized skin tests that allow us to determine if drug-specific IgE antibodies are present and, thus, possibly playing a role in the reaction demonstrated. To date, since the immunochemistry of penicillin and its degradation products have been determined, it is the only antibiotic for which reliable skin test reagents have been developed. Using these reagents, numerous studies have documented the presence of penicillin-specific IgE antibodies in those individuals who have experienced penicillin-induced urticaria or angioedema [45–63]. In contrast to penicillin, IgE antibodies to other antibiotics have not been demonstrated routinely in patients who have experienced an antibiotic-induced urticaria or angioedema. While it is possible that these reactions are not IgE-mediated, it is more likely that the IgE antibodies have not been detected due to the absence of reliable diagnostic testing reagents.

Despite the fact that no validated diagnostic reagents exist for most antibiotics, skin testing performed with nonirritative doses of the native drug may provide useful information. Bernstein et al. [37] suggest that allergists familiar with drug allergy skin testing techniques may want to try this diagnostic approach. If the skin test is positive, it is likely that drug-specific IgE antibodies are present. Therefore, if the patient requires this antibiotic, he or she should receive an alternative antibiotic or should undergo drug desensitization. On the other hand, if the skin test is negative, it cannot be ascertained that drug-specific IgE antibodies are absent; it is possible that drug-specific IgE antibodies exist but that they are directed to a relevant drug metabolite not used in the testing. A negative skin test does provide some useful information, however. The amount of drug used for intradermal skin testing can be calculated, and this amount may be used as the initial starting dose for a drug-desensitization procedure if this drug is required for therapy [37].

Skin tests to other nonantibiotic agents such as those used during anesthesia may be difficult to interpret since many of these drugs cause nonimmunological histamine release. Despite this difficulty, certain reactions have been shown to be IgE mediated, and drug-specific IgE antibodies have been detected by skin testing. Skin testing may be of value in the evaluation of allergy to muscle relaxants [64,65], barbiturates [64,66], chymopapain [67], streptokinase [68], latex [69], and miscellaneous other agents.

Treatment of drug-induced urticaria is fairly simple. The etiological agent should be identified, if possible, and then discontinued. In addition, while the lesions are resolving, patients should avoid acetylsalicylic acid, nonsteroidal anti-inflammatory drugs (NSAIDs), and known mast cell degranulators as well. For the pruritus, the mainstay of treatment continues to be antihistamines. Both classical first-generation antihistamines, as well as the newer second-generation agents that have little or no sedative or anticholinergic side effects, can be used. Medications in this latter category include astemizole, loratadine, fexofenadine, and cetirizine. These agents may be used alone or in combination with a first-generation antihistamine. $H_2$-receptor antihistamines may be beneficial in the presence of dermographism [70], angioedema or when systemic symptoms accompany the urticaria [71]. Because of the various side effects, corticosteroids should be avoided, if possible.

If urticaria occurs during a course of drug therapy, the reaction may be suppressed with continuous, ''round-the-clock'' antihistamines, alone or in combination with low-dose corticosteroids, in patients in whom an alternative drug is not available. The decision to continue a drug in the face of a cutaneous reaction must be made by a physician with extensive experience in the management of drug reactions. Anaphylaxis has not been reported to occur after the first hours of uninterrupted therapy with beta-lactam antibiotics and has not been observed during sustained therapy in the presence of urticaria. However, anaphylactic reactions may be induced by a dose that is administered 24–48 hours after discontinuation of the drug [72]. Also, if the choice is made to continue therapy, the patient must be observed closely and the drug stopped immediately if the cutaneous eruption progresses. Evidence of the development of severe reactions, presumed not to be IgE-mediated, such as erythroderma, erythema multiforme, Stevens-Johnson syndrome, toxic epidermal necrolysis, or exfoliative dermatitis warrants immediate drug discontinuation.

## C. Fixed Drug Eruptions

### 1. Clinical Features and Causative Agents

Fixed drug eruption (FDE) is the only drug-induced skin reaction that is provoked solely by drugs or chemicals. No other etiological factors can cause its elicitation. FDE consists of circumscribed, well-demarcated red or brown macules and sometimes blisters or bullous lesions (most severe form) that have a predilection for the distal parts of the body (hands, feet, genitalia), but lesions may be seen more centrally as well (Fig. 4). The lesions may be pruritic or burning. With initial drug administration, a solitary lesion alone may form. However, with readministration of the offending drug, lesions recur not only at the original site, but also at other sites as well. Numerous drugs are capable of producing fixed eruptions, the most common culprits being analgesics, sulfonamides, tetracyclines, barbiturates, and phenazones [23,38].

## 2. Pathophysiology

Histologically, in the acute stage, the epidermal changes are very similar to those seen in erythema multiforme. Epidermal basal cells undergo hydropic degeneration, and scattered dyskeratotic keratinocytes with pycnotic nuclei are found within the epidermis. Increased melanin is seen in epidermal macrophages and within melanocytes in the dermis. There also are increased numbers of T lymphocytes, both of the helper and suppressor phenotypes, seen in the epidermis and upper dermis [73–75]. Epidermal suppressor/cytotoxic T lymphocytes have been found adjacent to necrotic keratinocytes [73], and it has been postulated that the persistence of T lymphocytes in lesional skin may contribute to immunological memory and, thus, the recurrence of lesions at identical sites [76]. Lesional keratinocytes have been found to have increased expression of both intercellular adhesion molecule-1 (ICAM-1) and HLA-DR [77–80], and it is thought that this increased keratinocyte expression of ICAM-1 may, in part, explain the migration of T lymphocytes into the epidermis.

## 3. Diagnosis and Treatment

In most cases, the causative agent can be identified from the patient history, and, in some instances, patch testing on the previously affected site may be positive [81]. Currently,

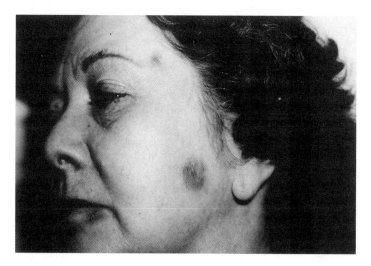

**Figure 4**  Phenophthalein-induced fixed drug eruption in a 55-year-old woman. The patient had been taking phenophthalein-containing Ex-lax at least weekly "for years." After discontinuing the medication, a brownish-gray pigmentation remained at the lesion site for over 4 weeks. The patient was instructed to avoid foods containing phenophthalein dyes (maraschino cherries) in the future.

the most reliable method of determining the causative agent is the oral challenge test. Usually, one tenth to one fourth of a single dose of the causative agent is sufficient to provoke a reaction, and provocation typically occurs within a few hours [38].

Treatment consists of drug discontinuation. Lesions usually fade within one week, but increased pigmentation may remain for months. Typically, corticosteroid treatment is not required. However, in the generalized bullous form of the disease, topical corticosteroids, systemic antimicrobial agents, and sedatives may be necessary.

## D. Erythema Multiforme, Stevens-Johnson Syndrome, and Toxic Epidermal Necrolysis

### 1. Clinical Features

These clinical entities can be the most severe of the drug-induced eruptions, and, while they are discussed in the same section, much controversy continues to exist regarding the diagnostic criteria for each and their classification. While the specific diagnostic criteria for these disorders remain controversial, many clinicians believe that Stevens-Johnson syndrome and toxic epidermal necrolysis are disorders of different severity within the spectrum of erythema multiforme. Based upon this belief, a classification scheme of these disorders, which is frequently used in clinical practice, was outlined by Bastuji-Garin and colleagues [82] in 1993. According to this classification scheme, both disorders have mucosal involvement, bullous lesions, and skin detachment. However, in the case of Stevens-Johnson syndrome, skin detachment is usually below 10% of the body surface area (BSA), whereas in toxic epidermal necrolysis it is greater than 30% of BSA. Other features that help to distinguish these disorders include the characteristics and distribution of skin lesions and associated signs and symptoms.

Patterson et al. [83] also consider these syndromes to be severity variants of the same disease process, whereas Roujeau [84] considers erythema multiforme to be distinct from both Stevens-Johnson syndrome and toxic epidermal necrolysis. Despite the fact that there is no consensus regarding the diagnostic criteria for or definitions of these conditions, these syndromes do have certain features in common, and, for that reason, they will be discussed together.

Erythema multiforme is an erythematous, polymorphic eruption, as its name suggests. While the classical lesion is a target lesion that is most predominant on the extremities, other types of lesions may be present including macules, papules, vesicles, and bullae (Fig. 5). Typically, the lesions are symmetrical and a mucous membrane may or may not be involved. Drugs are responsible for approximately 10% of the erythema multiforme cases, while infections and other disease processes are responsible for the remainder.

Eighty percent of erythema multiforme is classified as ''minor'' since most cases are mild, self-limited conditions of the skin and involve no more than one mucosal surface. However, in 20% of cases there is more extensive and severe cutaneous and mucosal membrane involvement. The form of erythema multiforme is termed erythema multiforme major, and most dermatologists consider this disease process to be identical to Stevens-Johnson syndrome, a clinical condition described in 1922 by Stevens and Johnson [85] and characterized by erosive stomatitis, severe ocular involvement, and a widespread cutaneous eruption of dark red, often necrotic, macules (Fig. 6). Roujeau and Stern [84,86], on the other hand, consider erythema multiforme major and Stevens-Johnson syndrome to be distinct entities for several reasons. Unlike Stevens-Johnson syndrome, erythema

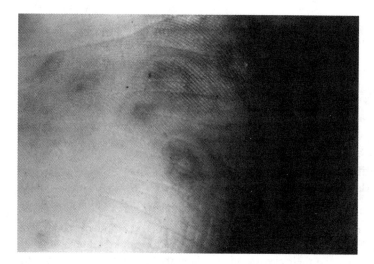

**Figure 5** Trimethoprim/sulfamethoxazole-induced erythema multiforme in a 27-year-old woman who was being treated for a urinary tract infection. The eruption occurred on the tenth day of therapy and was accompanied by malaise, fatigue, fever, and muscle and joint aches. The drug was discontinued, and because of the systemic symptoms the patient was treated with a course of oral corticosteroid therapy.

multiforme major usually is not drug-induced. More often, it occurs after infections (especially herpes simplex and mycoplasma). Also, the lesions of erythema multiforme major are typical target lesions with few blisters, whereas in Stevens-Johnson syndrome there is widespread blistering with the blisters occurring on purple macules or on "flat atypical targets" [84,87]. The controversy regarding whether Stevens-Johnson syndrome and erythema multiforme major are one and the same disease remains unresolved.

The remainder of this section will focus upon the clinical features and pathogenesis of drug-induced Stevens-Johnson syndrome and toxic epidermal necrolysis. Here too, while most dermatologists agree that the latter is a more severe form of the former, others believe that these are distinct entities [88]. Although the precise diagnostic boundaries between these two diseases have not been established, there continues to be many similarities between these two syndromes. For that reason, we are choosing to discuss them as though they are different severity classifications of the same disease process.

Approximately 50% of cases of Stevens-Johnson syndrome are related to the use of therapeutic agents. However, infections too may be causative with the more well-established infectious causes being *Mycoplasma pneumoniae*, herpes simplex virus, and streptococcal species [89–91]. The syndrome itself often is characterized by a prodromal period that mimics an upper respiratory infection. Frequently, patients will have fever, cough, and malaise for several days prior to the development of mucocutaneous lesions. When the eruption develops, it is symmetrically distributed on the face and upper trunk and later extends to the entire body. The lesions develop over a few days or even hours, and they consist of erythematous plaques and papules that rapidly develop a dusky center ("target" lesion) or a bullous center ("iris" lesion) [89–92]. In addition to skin lesions, there must be involvement of at least two mucous membranes. The most frequently involved mucous membranes are the oropharyngeal mucosa and the ocular mucosa [89,91,93]. However, the genitourinary, gastrointestinal, and tracheobronchial mucous membranes also may be

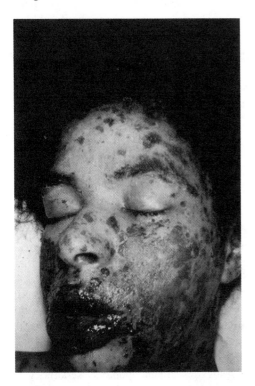

**Figure 6** Trimethoprim/sulfamethoxazole-induced Stevens-Johnson syndrome in a 24-year-old woman. The patient developed extensive bullae and crusted erosions and had oral, ocular, and anal mucosal membrane involvement. She also experienced fever, malaise, and volume depletion and required care in the intensive care unit where she was treated with cephalosporins and corticosteroids. The patient recovered and was discharged after 10 days.

affected. If the erosions are widespread, impaired alimentation, photophobia, and difficult micturition can result. Laboratory abnormalities are not uncommon and include leukocytosis, uremia, elevated sedimentation rate, and electrolyte disturbances. On histological analysis, perivascular mononuclear cells, dermal edema, and necrotic keratinocytes are found, and, in the areas most severely affected, subepidermal bullae may be seen [94].

If Stevens-Johnson syndrome progresses, it may evolve into an even more severe disease, toxic epidermal necrolysis. There is a large amount of overlap between these two syndromes, and the same drugs can induce both. In the case of toxic epidermal necrolysis, over 80% of the reactions are drug-induced. Typically, toxic epidermal necrolysis presents with a prodromal period characterized by fever, rhinitis, and conjunctivitis that lasts for a few days up to a few weeks. Subsequently, skin lesions develop and progress rapidly, usually within 3 days. Initially, the patient may develop an initial burning or painful maculopapular, urticarial, or erythema-multiforme–like eruption that rapidly becomes confluent. Widespread blistering and sloughing of large areas of the skin then occur, leading to an often-positive Nikolsky's sign (extension of the area of sloughing by lateral pressure).

## 2. Causative Agents

While some drugs may be more associated with causing Stevens-Johnson syndrome and others with causing toxic epidermal necrolysis, often the same type of drugs can induce both reactions. Many drugs have been implicated in these syndromes [7,11,12,86,95], with the most frequent offenders being sulfonamides, aromatic anticonvulsants, aminopenicillins, some NSAIDs, chlormezanone, and allopurinol. Luckily, with all of these agents, the reaction rates typically are low [86]. The number of cases related to a particular drug is dependent upon two factors: the level of risk associated with that drug and the number of patients exposed to that drug [96]. In the past, reactions to sulfadiazine and sulfadoxine were quite low. However, more recently, with the advent of AIDS, there has been an increase in the sales of these drugs, and with this increase in drug exposure, the incidence of severe drug-induced cutaneous disease has risen as well [97].

## 3. Pathophysiology

The immunopathology underlying both Stevens-Johnson syndrome and toxic epidermal necrolysis is thought to be due to an alteration in the detoxification of reactive drug metabolites [98–101]. In some instances, direct cellular toxicity may be occurring. However, in addition, there are several arguments that support the involvement of an immunological mechanism as well [96]: (1) the timing of the reaction (it usually occurs 12–14 days after the initiation of therapy), (2) the linkage of toxic epidermal necrolysis to particular HLA genotypes [102], and (3) the demonstration of positive patch tests to the culprit drug, in some instances [102]. In addition, fever, lymphadenopathy, and eosinophilia, if present, also support the involvement of a hypersensitivity mechanism.

Recently, Paul et al. [103] provided some exciting data supporting the role of apoptosis as the final mechanism of the extensive cell death that is seen in toxic epidermal necrolysis. Using several methods, these investigators found apoptotic keratinocytes throughout the epidermis of five patients who had either toxic epidermal necrolysis or overlap toxic epidermal necrolysis/Stevens-Johnson syndrome. The authors were unable to determine the exact stimulus responsible for the extensive apoptosis, but they hypothesized that an immune mechanism was involved for several reasons. First, immunohistochemical studies demonstrated a predominance of CD8+ T lymphocytes and macrophages in the epidermis of toxic epidermal necrolysis lesions [104,105], and, in addition, abundant amounts of tumor necrosis factor (TNF) were found in the epidermis of patients with toxic epidermal necrolysis [106]. Both TNF and cytotoxic T lymphocytes are known to induce apoptosis in target cells [107]. While much remains unknown about the mechanisms that promote apoptosis in toxic epidermal necrolysis, research is in progress to identify antiapoptotic molecules that may be useful clinically [108].

## 4. Diagnosis and Treatment

Stevens-Johnson syndrome and toxic epidermal necrolysis both are clinical diagnoses. At this time, there are no diagnostic tests available to help confirm the diagnosis of any of these disorders. It has been suggested that both skin biopsies and direct immunofluorescence studies be performed to exclude any bullous diseases that are not related to drug therapy [109]. Typically, the pathological lesions reveal full-thickness epidermal necrosis with little dermal changes. Importantly, immunofluorescence studies are negative.

Treatment of Stevens-Johnson syndrome and toxic epidermal necrolysis have been discussed in great detail in a recent publication by Roujeau [110]. Since these reactions are thought to be immunological in nature, a rationale is provided for the use of corticosteroids, immunosuppressive agents, or anticytokines in the halting of disease progression. However, to date, the use of these agents remains controversial. Other treatments aimed at accelerating the regrowth of the epidermis, using growth factors such as EGF, have been suggested but never studied [110]. Thus, what remains is symptomatic treatment that is directed at close monitoring, fluid replacement, anti-infective therapy, nutrition, warming, and skin, eye, and mucous membrane care [110].

## E. Hypersensitivity Syndrome

### 1. Clinical Features and Causative Agents

Drug-induced hypersensitivity syndrome is characterized by a mucocutaneous eruption and fever, and it is often associated with lymphadenopathy, hepatitis, and eosinophilia. The rash, which usually begins as a benign morbilliform eruption, may become indurated and infiltrated, and it may progress to an exfoliative dermatitis. In 30% of cases, eosinophilia and atypical lymphocytosis occurs and hepatitis occurs in approximately 50% of cases [109]. Unlike most other drug reactions, the drug-induced hypersensitivity syndrome usually appears 4 or more weeks after the initiation of therapy with the offending agent [111]. The drugs most commonly implicated in the induction of this syndrome include dapsone and other sulfonamides [112], phenytoin and other anticonvulsants [113], allopurinol [114], and minocycline [115].

### 2. Pathophysiology

The presence of a long latency period before the development of the reaction and the resemblance of the reaction to infectious mononucleosis suggest that underlying viral infections may trigger and may activate the disease in susceptible individuals. Recently, two groups have provided evidence that supports the hypothesis that underlying viral infections may predispose patients to develop drug-induced hypersensitivity syndrome. Suzuki et al. [111] found that a patient who developed an allopurinol-induced hypersensitivity syndrome had titers of human herpesvirus 6 (HHV-6) IgG antibodies that increased dramatically as the eruption progressed. In addition, HHV-6 was detected in the skin lesions using both polymerase chain reaction methodology and in situ hybridization. In addition, Tohyama and colleagues [116] described two cases of sulfasalazine-induced hypersensitivity syndrome that were associated with reactivation of HHV-6. While HHV-6 has been shown previously to induce severe infectious mononucleosis [117], graft-versus-host disease [118], and interstitial pneumonitis [119], these two groups together have provided the first evidence for a possible association between drug-induced hypersensitivity syndrome and reactivation of HHV-6. While HHV-6 reactivation may be an epiphenomenon only and not related to the clinical manifestations of the hypersensitivity syndrome, it also is possible that HHV-6 reactivation may be facilitated by the immunological events that are associated with adverse drug reactions. Alternatively, HHV-6 reactivation may modify drug metabolism and thus lead to the development of a drug reaction.

For sulfonamides and anticonvulsants, the development of the hypersensitivity syndrome may be related to individual genetic polymorphisms in the enzymes that metabolize these drugs [99,120]. Reactive sulfonamide metabolites generated by oxidative metabolism have been shown to be directly cytotoxic to lymphocytes [99]. In addition, these metabolites can bind to human proteins, and it has been hypothesized that, upon covalent binding, immunogenic complexes may be produced that lead to the elicitation of an immune response [121,122]. Supporting this hypothesis is the demonstration by Mauri-Hellweg and colleagues [123] of drug-induced activation and proliferation of peripheral blood mononuclear cells in patients with hypersensitivity syndrome. However, despite this demonstration, the mechanisms responsible for the actual clinical manifestations of the disease are unknown. In light of the fact that T-cell activation has been shown to be required for reactivation of HHV-6 [124], Tohyama et al. [116] hypothesized that drug-induced hypersensitivity syndrome may result from a two-stage process: first, T-cell activation occurs in response to covalent binding of reactive drug metabolites to tissue proteins, and second, HHV-6 becomes reactivated by activated T cells and then produces mononucleosis-like symptoms. While an intriguing hypothesis, other factors must be involved as well, since many drugs can cause T-cell activation but only a limited few induce the hypersensitivity syndrome.

### 3. Diagnosis and Treatment

There are no particular laboratory tests that are helpful in making the diagnosis of hypersensitivity syndrome. While lymphocytes from patients experiencing sulfonamide-induced hypersensitivity syndrome have been shown to be more susceptible to the cytotoxic effects of in vitro–generated drug metabolites [99], this lymphocyte assay is a research tool only, and it is not available to practicing clinicians. Typically, the diagnosis is made when a patient develops characteristic symptoms following the administration of a drug commonly implicated in this disease process. Treatment usually consists of systemic corticosteroid therapy, and improvement has been noted with this therapy despite no confirmation in controlled studies [109]. Tohyama et al. [116] hypothesized that corticosteroids may be acting to suppress an excessive immune response to drug metabolites and/or they may inhibit the production of cytokines caused by HHV-6 replicating viruses. These authors also suggest that antiviral drugs such as ganciclovir may be another treatment option. To date, however, studies evaluating the effectiveness of antiviral drugs in treating hypersensitivity syndrome have not yet been performed.

Patients who have experienced drug-induced hypersensitivity syndrome should avoid other drugs in the same chemical class. Thus, if a patient has a reaction to one aromatic anticonvulsant, he or she should avoid all three main aromatic anticonvulsants in the future: phenytoin, carbamazepine, and phenobarbital. In addition, patients who react to a particular sulfonamide should avoid other sulfonamides as well as other drugs that may have an aromatic amine structure [125].

### F. Other Drug-Induced Eruptions

While we have chosen to discuss the most common as well as the most severe of the drug-induced eruptions, it is important to understand that there are numerous other types of eruptions that may be elicited by drugs. Cutaneous vasculitis [126], purpura [127], photodermatoses [128], lichenoid eruptions [129], acneiform eruptions, and numerous other types of eruptions have been associated with drug therapy. In addition, drugs may also trigger or exacerbate existing dermatological conditions. Viral infections (i.e., herpes, verrucca, molluscum) may be triggered by prolonged corticosteroid or other immunosuppressant therapies. Psoriasis and acne may flare with lithium and/or fluoxetine therapy, and porphyria cutanea tarda may be exacerbated when therapy is initiated with estrogen, androgens, methotrexate, griseofulvin, quinidine, or colchicine. Finally, it must be remembered that pruritus alone may be the only manifestation of an adverse drug reaction. As stated previously, we refer the reader to several recent, very comprehensive texts for further information and for a complete review of drug-induced skin reactions [23,24].

## VII. APPROACH TO MANAGEMENT OF PATIENTS WITH DRUG-INDUCED CUTANEOUS DISEASE

Evaluating patients with cutaneous reactions that are possibly drug-induced can be a challenging task for the physician. As Shear [130] has pointed out, one of the first questions the physician must ask is: Did a drug cause this patient's skin condition, and, if so, what drug is responsible? When the type of reaction that develops is a known adverse cutaneous effect of the particular drug administered and if the reaction occurs within 1–2 weeks after initiation of therapy, the diagnosis may be obvious. Alternatively, when the patient is taking multiple medications and when other co-existing disease processes are present, such as a coexistent viral infection, the diagnosis can be more challenging. Is it a drug that is causing the eruption? Is it a systemic disease process that is causing the eruption? Possibly the drug is exacerbating or triggering an already-existing dermatological condition [127].

The simplest clinical approach is the ''better-safe-than-sorry'' tactic [130]. This strategy involves assuming the patient had an adverse reaction to a particular drug or at least telling the patient that he or she might be sensitive to a particular drug and should not receive that drug again. While this solution may seem practical, its consequences are not always desirable. First, the patient may needlessly be deprived of important drugs and others in the same class forever. Second, patients may be erroneously labeled as having multiple ''drug allergies,'' thus limiting their future therapeutic options if that particular drug therapy is again required.

We feel that a systematic approach, as outlined in Figure 7 [131], is more scientifically rational than the ''better-safe-than-sorry'' approach when evaluating a patient for a suspected adverse cutaneous drug reaction. First of all, as stated previously, the correct diagnosis must be made! This may require a consultation from either a qualified allergist or qualified dermatologist. These individuals should be able to determine if a skin biopsy would be helpful in categorizing an eruption and should be able to direct the attending physician to appropriate laboratory tests that may help elucidate the disease process.

Once it has been decided that a reaction is drug-induced, all administered drugs should be assessed for their propensity to cause the reaction demonstrated. An excellent resource that may help the physician in this task is the *Drug Eruption Reference Manual* [132]. This manual describes and catalogues the adverse cutaneous effects of over 370 commonly used medications, and the drugs are listed and indexed both by their generic as well as by their trade names. Once it is determined which drug or drugs may be responsible for causing the reaction, a decision must be made as to whether or not the drug(s) should be discontinued. Before this decision is made, the type of adverse reaction that is occurring should be determined, if possible. If the reaction is a predictable, Type A reaction and is caused by drug overdosage, then a dosing modification only may be required. However, since in most instances it is difficult to classify the reaction type, the suspected culprit drug(s) typically are discontinued and the patient is treated supportively until the reactions resolves. If an alternative drug is needed, then an agent that is chemically unrelated to the suspect drug should be administered.

Some physicians may choose to ''treat through'' a cutaneous reaction, especially if an alternative treatment does not exist. For those patients who develop drug-induced urticaria, the reaction may be suppressed with antihistamines alone or in combination with low-dose corticosteroids if no alternative drug is available [72]. However, it is critical to understand that the decision to continue a drug in the face of a cutaneous reaction must

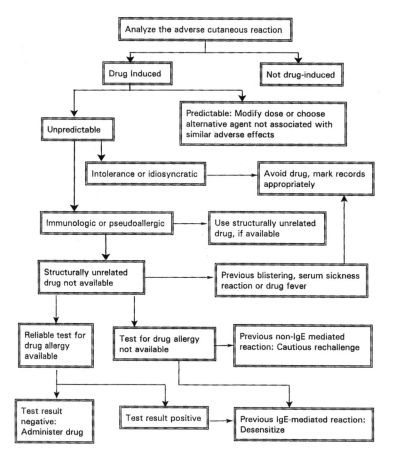

**Figure 7**  Approach to the patient with a suspected cutaneous drug reaction. Adapted from Ref. 131.

be made by a physician who has extensive experience with the management of drug reactions. If the drug is continued, the patient must be monitored very carefully. The drug should be discontinued immediately if the eruption progresses since other severe immunological complications such as erythroderma, erythema multiforme, Stevens-Johnson syndrome, toxic epidermal necrolysis, or exfoliative dermatitis may result from continued treatment.

For those patients who present with a history of a previous drug-induced cutaneous reaction, it is imperative to try to confirm the drug-disease connection. Imperative to this process is accurate historical information. Unfortunately, however, patients often cannot remember information, such as timing of the reaction after initiation of therapy, drug dosage, previous exposure history, and lesion characteristics, that may be critical in making the diagnosis.

Although there are several diagnostic tests for drug hypersensitivity, the positive and negative predictive values of most of these tests are not known. Weiss and Adkinson [133] recently reviewed the diagnostic tests that are currently available, and these are outlined in Table 4 [133]. It must be realized, however, that not all of these tests are commercially available, and, in addition, the clinical utility of many of them has not yet

**Table 4** Diagnostic Tests for Drug Hypersensitivity

Skin testing for immediate hypersensitivity
Skin biopsy
Patch testing
Provocative drug challenge
Radioallergosorbent test
Measurement of drug-specific IgG or IgM antibodies
Assays to measure complement activation
Release of histamine and other mediators by basophils
Measurement of mediators
Lymphocyte blast transformation
Leukocyte toxicity assay
Computer-assisted evaluation of adverse events

*Source*: Ref. 133.

been confirmed. In order to have more reliable and useful diagnostic tests, there must be further research that is focused on understanding the immunochemistry of allergenic drugs as well as on improving the sensitivity and specificity of currently available assays.

If a patient has experienced a previous drug-induced cutaneous reaction and the drug is required again, the physician faces a difficult dilemma. For many clinical situations, alternative drugs are available. However, in some instances, a particular drug cannot be avoided. In these instances, the physician must determine whether or not the patient should undergo a graded drug challenge or a true immunological desensitization procedure. This decision should be made by an allergist knowledgeable in the area of drug allergy and challenge/desensitization procedures. Recently, Greenberger [134] comprehensively discussed the issues surrounding drug challenge and drug desensitization. Typically, drug desensitization is performed in those individuals in whom drug-specific IgE antibodies may exist. The procedure itself involves the conversion of a drug-allergic individual from a highly sensitive state into a "tolerant" state, and it is accomplished by the administration of gradually increasing doses of the drug over a period of hours to days. In contrast, graded drug challenge is reserved for those individuals whose drug allergy history is not consistent with an IgE-mediated mechanism. This procedure involves first administering a small amount of the drug initially and then progressing, by large increments, to full-dose therapy within an hour or two. For those individuals who previously experienced severe cutaneous reactions such as Stevens-Johnson syndrome, erythroderma, exfoliative dermatitis, or toxic epidermal necrolysis, no type of rechallenge or desensitization procedure should be performed.

## VIII. CONCLUSIONS

Adverse reactions to drugs always will be an undesired consequence of all medical therapy, because few, if any, therapeutic agents can produce beneficial effects without having the potential for causing adverse effects as well. The diagnosis of adverse drug-induced cutaneous reactions will continue to be an intellectual challenge for all physicians. However, by knowing the appropriate questions to ask, by properly interpreting drug-induced skin manifestations, by performing select immunodiagnostic tests, if they are available, and by determining the propensity each drug has for causing particular reactions, the clinician is better able to identify the culprit drug. At present, management strategies are limited to drug avoidance, drug rechallenge (if appropriate), and/or drug desensitization. However, as research progresses in the areas of drug immunochemistry and drug metabolism, we should become better able to diagnose, classify, and manage drug-induced adverse reactions.

Importantly, in addition to managing the patient who has had a drug-induced reaction, it is the responsibility of the physician to curtail the frequency of future adverse drug events in that patient as well as in those individuals who have had no reaction history. We must all remember that any therapeutic agent can elicit a drug reaction. Therefore, prior to the administration of any drug, risk/benefit factors should be seriously evaluated.

## REFERENCES

1. Dorland's Illustrated Medical Dictionary. In: Dorland WAN, ed. Philadelphia: W.B. Saunders Co., 1988.
2. International Drug Monitoring: The Role of the Hospital. Geneva: World Health Organization, 1966.
3. Lazarou J, Pomeranz B, Corey P. Incidence of adverse drug reactions in hospitalized patients—a meta-analysis of prospective studies. JAMA 1998; 279:1200–1205.
4. Arndt K, Jick H. Rates of cutaneous reactions to drugs. A report from the Boston Collaborative Drug Surveillance Program. JAMA 1976; 235:918–922.
5. Bigby M, Jick S, Jick H, Arndt K. Drug-induced cutaneous reactions. A report from the Boston Collaborative Drug Surveillance Program on 15,238 consecutive inpatients, 1975 to 1982. JAMA 1986; 256:3358–3363.
6. Hunziker T, Kunzi U, Braunschweig S, Zehnder D, Hoigne R. Comprehensive hospital drug monitoring (CHDM): adverse skin reactions, a 20-year survey. Allergy 1997; 52:388–393.
7. Roujeau J, Guillaume J, Fabre J, Penso D, Flechet M, Girre J. Toxic epidermal necrolysis (Lyell's syndrome): Incidence and drug etiology in France, 1981–1985. Arch Dermatol 1990; 126:37–42.
8. Schof E, Stuhmer A, Rzany B, Victor N, Zentgraf R, Kapp J. Toxic epidermal necrolysis and Stevens-Johnson syndrome. An epidemiologic study from West Germany. Arch Dermatol 1991; 127:839–842.
9. Kelly J, Auquier A, Rzany B, Naldi L, Bastuji-Garin S, Correia O, Shapiro S, Kaufman D. An international collaborative case-control study of severe cutaneous adverse reactions (SCAR). Design and methods. J Clin Epidemiol 1995; 48:1099–1108.
10. Rzany B, Mockenhaupt M, Baur S, Schroder W, Stocker U, Mueller J, Hollander N, Bruppacher R, Schopf E. Epidemiology of erythema exsudativum multiforme majus (EEMM), Stevens-Johnson syndrome (SJS) and toxic epidermal necrolysis (TEN) in Germany (1990–1992). Structure and results of a population-based registry. J Clin Epidemiol 1996; 49:769–773.
11. Roujeau J, Kelly J, Naldi L, Rzany B, Stern R, Anderson T, Auquier A, Bastuji-Garin S, Correia O, Locati F, Mockenhaupt M, Paoletti C, Shapiro S, Shear N, Schopf E, Kaufman D. Medication use and risk of Stevens-Johnson syndrome or toxic epidermal necrolysis. N Engl J Med 1995; 333:1600–1607.
12. Chan H, Stern R, Arndt K, Langlois J, Jick S, Jick H, Walker A. The incidence of erythema multiforme, Stevens-Johnson syndrome, and toxic epidermal necrolysis: A population-based study with particular reference to reactions caused by drugs among outpatients. Arch Dermatol 1990; 126:43–47.

13. Strom B, Carson J, Halpern A, Schinnar R, Snyder E, Shaw M, Tilson H, Joseph M, Dai W, Chen D, Stern R, Bergmann U, Stolley P. A population-based study of Stevens-Johnson syndrome: Incidence and antecedent drug exposures. Arch Dermatol 1991; 127:831–838.

14. Mockenhaupt M, Schopf E. Epidemiology of severe cutaneous drug reactions. In: Kauppinen K, Alanko K, Hannuksela M, Maibach H, eds. Skin Reactions to Drugs. Boca Raton, FL: CRC Press, 1998:3–15.

15. Coombs R, Gell, PGH. Classification of allergic reactions responsible for clinical hypersensitivity and disease. In: Gell P, Coombs, RRA, Lachman, PJ, eds. Clinical Aspects of Immunology. Oxford: Blackwell Scientific Publications, 1975:761.

16. Park B, Pirmohamed M, Kitteringham N. Idiosyncratic drug reactions: a mechanistic evaluation of risk factors. Br J Clin Pharmacol 1992; 34:377–395.

17. Riley R, Leeder J. In vitro analysis of metabolic predisposition to drug hypersensitivity reactions. Clin Exp Immunol 1995; 99:1–6.

18. Shapiro L, Shear N. Mechanisms of drug reactions: the metabolic track. Sem Cut Med Surg 1996; 15:217–227.

19. Pirmohamed M, Madden S, Park K. Idiosyncratic drug reactions: metabolic bioactivation as a pathogenic mechanism. Clin Pharmacokinet 1996; 32:215–230.

20. Park B, Coleman J, Kitteringham N. Drug disposition and drug hypersensitivity. Biochem Pharmacol 1987; 36:581–590.

21. Kao J. Estimating the contribution by skin to systemic metabolism. Ann NY Acad Sci 1988; 548:90–96.

22. Mukhtar H, Khan W. Cutaneous cytochrome P-450. Drug Metab Rev 1989; 20:657–673.

23. Breathnack S, Hintner H. Adverse Drug Reactions and the Skin. Oxford: Blackwell Scientific Publications, 1992:394.

24. Kauppinen K, Alanko K, Hannuksela M, Maibach H. Skin Reactions to Drugs. Boca Raton, FL: CRC Press, 1998:178.

25. Tilles S. Immunology and allergy clinics of North America. In: Tilles S, ed. Drug Hypersensitivity. Vol. 18. Philadelphia: WB Saunders Co, 1998:934.

26. Kalish R, LaPorte A, Wood J, Johnson K. Sulfonamide-reactive lymphocytes detected at very low frequency in the peripheral blood of patients with drug-induced eruptions. J Allergy Clin Immunol 1994; 94:465–472.

27. Boecker C, Hertl M, Merk H. Dermal T lymphocytes from sulfamethoxazole-induced bullous exanthem are stimulated by allergen-modified microsomes (abstr). J Invest Dermatol 1993; 100:540.

28. Hertl M, Jugert F, Merk H. CD8$^+$ dermal T cells from a sulphamethoxazole-induced bullous exanthem proliferate in response to drug-modified liver microsomes. Br J Dermatol 1995; 132:215–220.

29. Hertl M, Geisel J, Boecker C, Merk H. Selective generation of CD8$^+$ T-cell clones from the peripheral blood of patients with cutaneous reactions to beta-lactam antibiotics. Br J Dermatol 1993; 128:619–626.

30. Hertl M, Bohlen H, Jugert F, Boecker C, Knaup R, Merck H. Predominance of epidermal CD8+ T lymphocytes in bullous cutaneous reactions caused by beta-lactam antibiotics. J Invest Dermatol 1993; 101:794–799.

31. Spielberg S. In vitro assessment of pharmacogenetic susceptibility to toxic drug metabolites in humans. Fed Proc 1984; 43:2308–2313.

32. Shear N, Spielberg S. An in vitro lymphocytotoxicity assay for studying adverse reactions to sulfonamides. Br J Dermatol 1985; 28:S112–S113.

33. Rieder M, Uetrecht J, Shear N, Cannon M, Miller M, Spielberg S. Diagnosis of sulfonamide hypersensitivity reactions by in vitro rechallenge with hydroxylamine metabolites of sulfonamides. Ann Intern Med 1989; 110:286–289.

34. Kalish R. Antigen processing: the gateway to the immune response. J Am Acad Dermatol 1995; 32:640–652.

35. Osawa J, Naito S, Aihara M, Kitamura K, Ikezawa Z, Nakajima H. Evaluation of skin reactions in patients with non-immediate type drug eruptions. J Dermatol 1990; 17:235–239.

36. Bruynzeel D, Maibach H. Patch testing in systemic drug eruptions. In: Kauppinen K, Alanko K, Hannuksela M, Maibach H, eds. Skin reactions to drugs. Boca Raton: CRC Press, 1998: 97–109.

37. Bernstein IL, Gruchalla RS, Lee RE, Nicklas RA, Dykewicz MS. Disease management of drug hypersensitivity: a practice parameter. Ann Allergy Immunol (In press.)

38. Kauppinen K, Kariniemi A-L. Clinical manifestations and histological characteristics. In: Kauppinen K, Alanko K, Hannuksela M, Maiback H, eds. Skin Reactions to Drugs. Boca Raton, FL: CRC Press, 1998:25–50.

39. Levy J, Kettlekamp N, Goertz P, Hermens J, Hirshman CA. Histamine release by vancomycin: a mechanism for hypotension in man. Anesthesiology 1987; 67:122–125.

40. Polk R. Anaphylactoid reactions to glycopeptide antibiotics. J Antimicrobial Chemother 1991; 27:17–29.

41. Landor M, Lashinsky A, Waxman J. Quinolone allergy? Ann Allergy Asthma Immunol 1996; 77:273–276.

42. Baldo B, Fisher MM. Detection of serum IgE antibodies that react with alcuronium and tubocurarine after life threatening reactions to muscle-relaxant drugs. Anaesth Intensive Care 1983; 11:194–197.

43. Baldo B, Fisher MM. Anaphylaxis to muscle relaxant drugs: cross-reactivity and molecular basis of binding of IgE antibodies detected by radioimmunoassay. Mol Immunol 1983; 20: 1393–1400.

44. Baldo B, Fisher MM. Mechanisms in IgE-dependent anaphylaxis to anaesthetic drugs. Ann Fr Anesth Reanim 1993; 12:131–140.

45. Parker C, Shapiro J, Kern M, Eisen H. Hypersensitivity to penicillenic acid derivatives in human beings with penicillin allergy. J Exp Medicine 1962; 115:821–838.

46. Rytel M, Klion F, Arlander T, Miller L. Detection of penicillin hypersensitivity with penicilloyl-polylysine. JAMA 1963; 186:894–898.

47. Brown B, Price E, Moore M. Penicilloyl-polylysine as an intradermal test of penicillin sensitivity. JAMA 1964; 189:599–604.

48. Budd M, Parker C, Norden C. Evaluation of intradermal skin tests in penicillin hypersensitivity. JAMA 1964; 190:203–205.

49. deWeck A, Blum G. Recent clinical and immunological aspects of penicillin allergy. Int Arch Allergy 1965; 27:221–256.

50. Finke S, Grieco M, Connell J, Smith E, Sherman W. Results of comparative skin tests with penicilloyl-polylysine and penicillin in patients with penicillin allergy. Amer J Med 1965; 38:71–82.

51. Levine B, Redmond A, Fellner M, Voss H, Levytska V. Penicillin allergy and the heterogenous immune responses of man to benzylpenicillin. J Clin Invest 1966; 45:1895–1906.

52. Levine B, Zolov D. Prediction of penicillin allergy by immunological tests. J Allergy 1969; 43:231–244.

53. Van Dellen R, Gleich G. Penicillin skin tests as predictive and diagnostic aides in penicillin allergy. Med Clin North Am 1970; 54: 997–1007.

54. Adkinson N, Thompson W, Maddrey W, Lichtenstein L. Routine use of penicillin skin testing on an inpatient service. N Engl J Med 1971; 285:22–24.

55. Green G, Rosenblum A. Report of the penicillin study group—American Academy of Allergy. J Allergy Clin Immunol 1971; 48:331–343.

56. Green G, Rosenblum R, Sweet L. Evaluation of penicillin hypersensitivity value of clinical history and skin testing with penicilloyl-polylysine and penicillin G. A cooperative prospective study of the penicillin study group of the American Academy of Allergy. J Allergy Clin Immunol 1977; 60:339–345.

57. Chandra R, Joglekar S, Tomas E. Penicillin allergy: anti-penicillin IgE antibodies and immediate hypersensitivity skin reactions employing major and minor determinants of penicillin. Arch Dis Childhood 1980; 55:857–860.

58. Sullivan T, Wedner H, Shatz G, Yecies L, Parker C. Skin testing to detect penicillin allergy. J Allergy Clin Immunol 1981; 68:171–180.

59. Solley G, Gleich G, VanDellen R. Penicillin allergy: clinical experience with a battery of skin test reagents. J Allergy Clin Immunol 1982; 69:238–244.

60. Sogn D, Evans RE, Shepherd G, Casale T, Condemi J, Greenberger P, Kohler P, Saxon A, Summers R, VanArsdel P, Massicot J, Blackwelder W, Levine B. Results of the National Institute of Allergy and Infectious Diseases collaborative clinical trial to test the predictive value of skin testing with major and minor penicillin derivatives in hospitalized adults. Arch Intern Med 1992; 152:1025–1032.

61. Gadde J, Spence M, Wheeler B, Adkinson N. Clinical experience with penicillin skin testing in large inner-city STD clinic. JAMA 1993; 270:2456–2463.

62. Silviu-Dan F, McPhillips S, Warrington R. The frequency of skin test reactions to side-chain penicillin determinants. J Allergy Clin Immunol 1993; 91:694–701.

63. Macy E, Richter P, Falkoff R, Zeiger R. Skin testing with penicilloate and penilloate prepared by an improved method: amoxicillin oral challenge in patients with negative skin test responses to penicillin reagents. J Allergy Clin Immunol 1997; 100:586–591.

64. Fisher M. Intradermal testing in the diagnosis of acute anaphylaxis during anesthesia-results of five years experience. Anaesth Inten Care 1979; 7:58–61.

65. Vervloet D, Nizankowska M, Arnaud A, Senft M, Alazi M, Charpin J. Adverse reactions to suxamethonium and other muscle relaxants under general anaesthesia. J Allergy Clin Immunol 1983; 71:552–558.

66. Moscicki R, Sockin SM, Corsello BF, Ostro MG, Bloch KJ. Anaphylaxis during induction of general anesthesia: subsequent evaluation and management. J Allergy Clin Immunol 1990; 86:325–332.

67. Grammer L, Patterson R. Proteins: chymopapain and insulin. J Allergy Clin Immunol 1984; 74:635–640.

68. Dykewicz M, McGrath KG, Davison R, Kaplan KJ, Patterson R. Identification of patients at risk for anaphylaxis due to streptokinase. Arch Int Med 1986; 146:305–307.

69. Hamilton R, Adkinson N Jr. MultiCenter Latex Skin Testing Study Task Force. Diagnosis of natural rubber latex allergy: multicenter latex skin testing efficacy study. J Allergy Clin Immunol 1998; 102:482–490.

70. Mansfield L, Smith J, Nelson H. Greater inhibition of dermographia with a combination of H1 and H2 antagonists. Ann Allergy 1983; 50:264–270.

71. Bleehen S, Thomas S, Greaves M, Newton J, Kennedy C, Hindley F, Marks R, Hazell M, Rowell N, Fairiss G, et al. Cimetidine and chlorpheneramine in the treatment of chronic idiopathic urticaria: a multicenter randomized double-blind study. Br J Dermatol 1987; 117:81–91.

72. Sullivan T. Drug allergy. In: Middleton E, Jr., Reed CE, Ellis EF, Adkinson NF, Jr., Yunginger JW, Busse WW, ed. Allergy: Principles and Practice. St. Louis: Mosby, 1993:1726–1746.

73. Murphy G, Guillen F, Flynn T. Cytotoxic T lymphocytes and phenotypically abnormal epidermal dendritic cells in fixed cutaneous eruption. Hum Pathol 1985; 16:1264–1271.

74. Hindsen M, Christensen O, Gruic V, Lofberg H. Fixed drug eruption: an immunohistochemical investigation of the acute and healing phase. Br J Dermatol 1987; 116:351–356.

75. Smoller B, Luster A, Krane J, Krueger J, Gray M, McNutt N, Hsu A, Gottlieb A. Fixed drug eruptions: evidence for a cytokine-mediated process. J Cutan Pathol 1991; 18:13–19.

76. Scheper R, Von Blomberg M, Boerrigter G, Bruynzeel D, Van Dinther A, Vos A. Induction of immunological memory in the skin. Role of local T cell retention. Clin Exp Immunol 1983; 51:141–148.

77. Nickoloff B, Basham T, Merigan T, Morhenn V. Keratinocyte class II histocompatibility antigen expression. Br J Dermatol 1985; 112:373–374.

78. Dustin M, Singer K, Tuck D, Springer T. Adhesion of T lymphoblasts to epidermal keratinocytes is regulated by interferon gamma and is mediated by ICAM-1. J Exp Med 1988; 167: 1323–1340.

79. Shiohara T, Nickoloff B, Sagawa Y, Gomi T, Nagashima M. Fixed drug eruption. Expression of epidermal keratinocyte intercellular adhesion molecule-1 (ICAM-1). Arch Dermatol 1989; 125:1371–1376.

80. Teraki Y, Moriya N, Shiohara T. Drug-induced expression of intercellular adhesion molecule-1 on lesional keratinocytes in fixed drug eruption. Am J Pathol 1994; 145:550–560.

81. Alanko K, Stubb S, Reitamo S. Topical provocation of fixed drug eruption. Br J Dermatol 1987; 116:561–567.

82. Bastuji-Garin S, Rzany B, Stern R, Shear N, Naldi L, Roujeau J-C. Clinical classification of cases of toxic epidermal necrolysis, Stevens-Johnson syndrome, and erythema multiforme. Arch Dermatol 1993; 129:92–96.

83. Patterson R, Dykewicz M, Gonzales A, Grammer L, Green D, Greenberger P, McGrath K, Walker C. Erythema multiforme and Stevens-Johnson syndrome: descriptive and therapeutic controversy. Chest 1990; 98:331–336.

84. Roujeau J-C. Stevens-Johnson syndrome and toxic epidermal necrolysis are severity variants of the same disease which differs from erythema multiforme. J Dermatol 1997; 24:726–729.

85. Stevens A, Johnson F. A new eruptive fever associated with stomatitis and ophthalmia: report of two cases in children. Am J Dis Child 1922; 24:526–533.

86. Roujeau J, Stern R. Severe adverse cutaneous reactions to drugs. N Engl J Med 1994; 19: 1272–1285.

87. Huff J, Weston W, Tonnesen M. Erythema multiforme; a critical review of characteristics, diagnostic criteria, and causes. J Am Acad Dermatol 1983; 8:763–775.

88. Goldstein S, Wintroub B, Elias P, Wuepper K. Toxic epidermal necrolysis. Unmuddying the waters. Arch Dermatol 1987; 123:1153–1156.

89. Araujo O, Flowers F. Stevens-Johnson syndrome. J Emerg Med 1984; 2:129–135.

90. Stitt VJ. Stevens-Johnson syndrome: a review of the literature. J Natl Med Assoc 1988; 80: 106–108.

91. Levy M, Shear N. *Mycoplasma pneumoniae* infections and Stevens-Johnson syndrome. Report of eight cases and review of the literature. Clin Pediatr 1991; 30:42–49.

92. Manders S. Serious and life-threatening drug eruptions. Am Fam Physician 1995; 51:1865–1872.

93. Edell D, Davidson J, Muelenaer A, Majure M. Unusual manifestation of Stevens-Johnson syndrome involving the respiratory and gastrointestinal tract. Pediatrics 1992; 89:429–432.

94. Lever W, Schaumburg-Lever G. Noninfectious vesicular and bullous diseases. In: Lever W, Schaumburg-Lever G, eds. Histopathology of the Skin. Philadelphia: Lippincott, 1990:135–138.

95. Revuz J, Penso D, Roujeau J, Guillaume J, Payne C, Wechsler J, Touraine R. Toxic epidermal necrolysis. Clinical findings and prognosis factors in 87 patients. Arch Dermatol 1987; 122: 1160–1165.

96. Revuz J, Roujeau J. Advances in toxic epidermal necrolysis. Sem Cut Med Surg 1996; 15: 258–266.

97. Correia O, Chosidow O, Saiag P, Bastuji-Garin S, Revuz J, Roujeau J. Evolving pattern of drug-induced toxic epidermal necrolysis. Dermatology 1993; 186:32–37.

98. Spielberg S, Gordon G, Blake D, Goldstein D, Herlong H. Predisposition to phenytoin hepatotoxicity assessed in vitro. N Engl J Med 1981; 305:722–727.

99. Shear N, Speilberg S, Grant D, Tang B, Kalow W. Differences in metabolism of sulfonamides predisposing to idiosyncratic toxicity. Ann Intern Med 1986; 105:179–184.

100. Wolkenstein P, Charue D, Laurent P, Revuz J, Roujeau J-C, Bagot M. Metabolic predisposi-

tion to cutaneous drug reactions: role in toxic epidermal necrolysis caused by sulfonamides and anticonvulsants. Arch Dermatol 1995; 131:544–551.

101. Merk H, Hertl M. Immunologic mechanisms of cutaneous drug reactions. Sem Cut Med Surg 1996; 15:228–235.

102. Roujeau J-C, Huynh TN, Bracq C, Guillaume J, Revuz J, Touraine R. Genetic susceptibility to toxic epidermal necrolysis. Arch Dermatol 1987; 123:171.

103. Paul C, Wolkenstein P, Adle H, Wechsler J, Garchon H, Revuz J, Roujeau J. Apoptosis as a mechanism of keratinocyte death in toxic epidermal necrolysis. Br J Dermatol 1996; 134: 710–714.

104. Villada G, Roujeau J, Clerici T, Bourgault I, Revuz J. Immunopathology of toxic epidermal necrolysis: keratinocytes, HLA-DR expression, Langerhans cells, and mononuclear cells: an immunopathologic study of five cases. Arch Dermatol 1992; 128:50–53.

105. Correia O, Delgado L, Ramos J, Resende C, Torrinha J. Cutaneous T-cell recruitment in toxic epidermal necrolysis: further evidence of CD8+ lymphocyte involvement. Arch Dermatol 1993; 129:466–468.

106. Paquet P, Nikkels A, Arrese J, Vanderkelen A, Pierard G. Macrophage and tumor necrosis factor in toxic epidermal necrolysis. Arch Dermatol 1994; 130:627–628.

107. Cohen J, Duke R. Apoptosis and programmed cell death in immunity. Annu Rev Immunol 1992; 10:267–293.

108. Kroemer G, Martinez A. Pharmacological inhibition of programmed lymphocyte death. Immunol Today 1994; 15:235–242.

109. Wolkenstein P, Revuz P. Drug-induced severe skin reactions: incidence, management and prevention. Drug Safety 1995; 13:56–68.

110. Roujeau J-C. Treatment of SJS and TEN. In: Kauppinen K, Alanko K, Hannuksela M, Maibach H, eds. Skin Reactions to Drugs. Boca Raton, FL: CRC Press, 1998:141–150.

111. Suzuki Y, Inagi R, Aono T, Yamanishi K, Shiohara T. Human herpesvirus 6 infection as a risk factor for the development of severe drug-induced hypersensitivity syndrome. Arch Dermatol 1998; 134:1108–1112.

112. Prussick P, Shear N. Dapsone hypersensitivity syndrome. J Am Acad Dermatol 1996;35: 346–349.

113. Chopra S, Levell N, Cowley G, Gilkes J. Systemic corticosteroids in the phentoin hypersensitivity syndrome. Br J Dermatol 1996; 134:1109–1112.

114. Singer J, Wallace S. The allopurinol hypersensitivity syndrome: unnecessary morbidity and mortality. Arthritis Rheum 1986; 29:82–87.

115. MacNeil M, Haase D, Tremaine R, Marrie T. Fever, lymphodenopathy, eosinophilia, lymphocytosis, hepatitis, and dermatitis: a severe adverse reaction to minocycline. J Am Acad Dermatol 1997; 36:347–350.

116. Tohyama M, Yahata Y, Yasukawa M, Inagi R, Urano Y, Yamanishi K, Hashimoto K. Severe hypersensitivity syndrome due to sulfasalazine associated with reactivation of human herpesvirus 6. Arch Dermatol 1998; 134:1113–1117.

117. Akashi K, Eizuru Y, Sumiyoshi Y, Minematsu T, Hara S, Harada M, Kikuchi M, Niho Y, Minamishima Y. Severe infectious mononucleosis-like syndrome and primary human herpesvirus 6 in an adult. N Engl J Med 1993; 329:168–171.

118. Appleton A, Peiris J, Taylor C, Sviland L, Cant A. Human herpesvirus 6 DNA in skin biopsy tissue from marrow graft recipients with severe combined immunodeficiency. Lancet 1994; 344:1361–1362.

119. Carrigan D, Drobyski W, Russler S, Tapper M, Knox K, Ash R. Interstitial pneumonitis associated with human herpesvirus-6 infection after marrow transplantation. Lancet 1991; 338:147–149.

120. Shear N, Spielberg SP. Anticonvulsant hypersensitivity syndrome: In vitro assessment of risk. J Clin Invest 1988; 82:1826.

121. Meekens C, Sullivan T, Gruchalla R. Immunochemical analysis of sulfonamide drug allergy:

Identification of sulfamethoxazole-substituted human serum proteins. J Allergy Clin Immunol 1994;94:1017–1024.

122. Gruchalla R, Pesenko RD, Do TT, Skiest DJ. Sulfonamide-induced reactions in patients with AIDS—role of covalent protein haptenation. J Allergy Clin Immunol 1998;101:371–378.

123. Mauri-Hellweg D, Bettens F, Mauri D, Brander C, Hunziker T, Pichler W. Activation of drug-specific CD4$^+$ and CD8$^+$ T cells in individuals allergic to sulfonamides, phenytoin and carbamazepine. J Immunol 1995; 155:462–472.

124. Frenkel N, Schirmer E, Katsafanas G, June C. T-cell activation is required for efficient replication of human herpesvirus 6. J Virol 1990; 64:4598–4602.

125. Shapiro L, Knowles S, Shear N. Sulfonamide allergies-management in the nineties. Allergy Clin Immunol Int 1996;8:5–8.

126. Calabrese L, Duna G. Drug-induced vasculitis. Curr Opin Rheumatol 1996; 8:34–40.

127. Beltrani V. Cutaneous manifestations of adverse drug reactions. In: Tilles S, ed. Immunology and Allergy Clinics of North America: Drug Hypersensitivity. Vol. 18. Philadelphia: WB Saunders, 1998;867–896.

128. Marks J, DeLeo V. Photoallergens. In: Marks J, DeLeo V, eds. Contact and Occupational Dermatology. St. Louis: Mosby Yearbook, 1992:173–176.

129. Bork K. Lichenoid eruptions. In: Bork K, ed. Cutaneous Side Effects of Drugs. Philadelphia: WB Saunders Co., 1985:170–171.

130. Shear N. Diagnosing cutaneous adverse reactions to drugs. Arch Dermatol 1990; 126:94–97.

131. DeShazo RD, Kemp, SF. Allergic reactions to drugs and biologic agents. JAMA 1997; 278:1895–1906.

132. Litt J, Pawlak WA, Jr., eds. Drug Eruption Reference Manual. Cleveland: Wal-Zac Enterprises, 1995.

133. Weiss M, Adkinson F. Diagnostic testing for drug hypersensitivity. In: Tilles S, ed. Immunology and Allergy Clinics of North America: Drug Hypersensitivity. Vol. 18. Philadelphia: WB Saunders, 1998:731–744.

134. Greenberger P. Drug challenge and desensitization protocols. In: Tilles S, ed. Immunology and Allergy Clinics of North America: Drug Hypersensitivity. Vol. 18. Philadelphia: WB Saunders, 1998:759–772.

# 16

## Mastocytosis

**Cem Akin and Dean D. Metcalfe**

*National Institute of Allergy and Infectious Diseases, National Institutes of Health, Bethesda, Maryland*

Mastocytosis is a disease characterized by the presence of excessive numbers of mast cells in skin and internal organs such as the bone marrow, gastrointestinal tract, lymph nodes, liver, and spleen. Although the disease can occur at any age, a pediatric and an adult form can be distinguished based on the age of onset of symptoms. Pediatric disease, which constitutes approximately 55% of all cases, usually starts before 6 months of age, whereas adult-onset disease has a peak around the fourth and fifth decades of life. It has been reported that the disease has a slight male-to-female predominance (1.5:1.0). The prevalence of this rare disease is unknown, but it is reported that one in every 1000–2500 patients seen in a dermatology practice carried this diagnosis [1]. Although most cases are sporadic, the disease rarely presents in more than one individual in the same family [2]. We have evaluated two such families at the Clinical Center in NIH, in whom two siblings were involved.

## I. ETIOLOGY

Mast cell precursors originate in the bone marrow from the CD34+ pluripotent hematopoietic stem cells [3]. They then enter the blood and lymphatic circulation and migrate into tissues, where they undergo terminal differentiation under the influence of local growth factors. This migration process is believed to be regulated by sequential expression of adhesion molecules on the mast cells [4]. Mature mast cells are in part located along the endothelial and epithelial basement membrane, along nerves, and around glandular structures. These structures are rich in laminin and other structural proteins, which may help to target the mast cells into these sites. Tissues such as the skin and gastrointestinal tract, which interface the external and internal environments, are rich in mast cells.

Mast cell growth and differentiation are influenced by cytokines produced in the bone marrow as well as lymphoid and connective tissues. Interleukins 3, 4, 5, 6, 9, 10, and 15 have been shown to modulate mast cell growth and maturation [5–12]; however, the principal growth factor for mast cell differentiation is stem cell factor (SCF), also known as mast cell growth factor or kit ligand [13,14]. This growth factor cytokine is produced by fibroblasts, endothelial cells, and bone marrow stromal cells and is critical for mast cell growth, differentiation, survival, and chemotaxis. It is present as a soluble and a membrane-bound form. The soluble form of SCF may be measured in blood [15,16]. Altered metabolism of SCF has been suggested in mastocytosis, leading to a local increase in soluble SCF in skin [17].

Stem cell factor binds to its receptor, c-kit. C-kit belongs to the family of type III receptor tyrosine kinases together with the receptors for monocyte colony-stimulating factor, platelet-derived growth factor, and fms-like tyrosine kinase3/fetal liver kinase 2 (flt3/flk2) [18]. The proto-oncogene c-kit is also expressed on a variety of hematopoietic and nonhematopoietic cells [19–22]. This receptor is found on the surface of hematopoietic progenitor cells and is downregulated as they differentiate into their mature progeny. Subcutaneous administration of recombinant SCF results in a wheal-and-flare reaction and accumulation of mast cells at injection sites [23]. Among the nonhematopoietic cells that express c-kit are melanocytes, germ cells, and neural tissue. It is apparently critical for the migration of melanocytes, as loss of function mutations in this receptor are associated with the pigmentation disorder piebaldism [24].

A number of point mutations have been described in the intracellular tyrosine kinase and juxtamembrane domains of c-kit in patients with mastocytosis (Fig. 1). The most

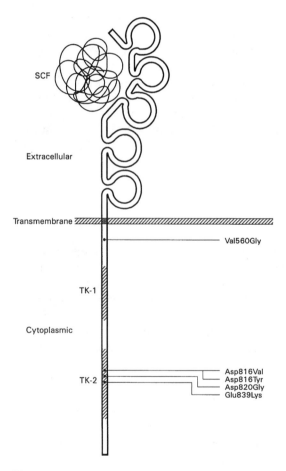

**Figure 1** Reported mutations in the c-kit gene in human mastocytosis. SCF, Stem cell factor; TK, tyrosine kinase.

frequent of these mutations involves a transition of adenine to thymine, which leads to the replacement of an aspartic acid residue by a valine at the amino acid position 816 (Asp816Val). This mutation results in ligand independent activation of c-kit and confers tumorigenicity when introduced into growth factor–dependent murine cell lines [25,26]. The Asp816Val mutation has been demonstrated in the lesional skin as well as peripheral white blood cells of patients with mastocytosis [27,28]. The level of the intensity of the expression of the mutation in the peripheral blood appears to correlate with the severity of the disease, as it is found in all adult patients with an associated hematological disorder and some patients with extensive forms of the indolent disease [29]. The mutation is usually undetectable in most pediatric patients, although it has been reported in cases of severe disease [30]. It therefore appears that there may be different molecular mechanisms involved in the etiology of adult and some forms of pediatric-onset mastocytosis.

## II. CLINICAL MANIFESTATIONS

The clinical presentation of mastocytosis is due to the excessive presence of mast cells and their mediators or defective hematopoiesis accompanying the disease. Mast cell derived mediators and their contribution to the symptoms of the disease are listed in Table 1. The incidence of atopy is believed to be the same as in the general population; however, the presence of increased mast cells may augment the magnitude of preexisting allergic responses.

The current classification of mastocytosis is shown in Table 2 [31]. The four categories of disease have distinct presentations, pathological findings, and prognosis. Most mastocytosis patients present with indolent disease. Patients in this category may have one or more of the following findings: syncope, cutaneous disease, ulcer disease, malabsorption, bone marrow mast cell aggregates, skeletal disease, hepatosplenomegaly, and lymphadenopathy. The second most common form of mastocytosis is that associated with a

**Table 1** Selected Mast Cell Mediators and Their Possible Contribution to Pathogenesis

| | |
|---|---|
| Granule associated | |
| Histamine | Pruritus, increased vascular permeability, gastric hypersecretion, bronchoconstriction |
| Heparin | Local anticoagulation |
| Tryptase, proteases | Degradation of local connective tissues, bone lesions |
| Lipid-derived | |
| Sulfidopeptide leukotrienes | Increased vascular permeability, bronchoconstriction, vasoconstriction ($LTC_4$); increased vascular permeability, bronchoconstriction, vasodilation ($LTD_4$ and $LTE_4$) |
| Prostaglandin $D_2$ | Vasodilation, bronchoconstriction |
| Platelet-activating factor | Increased vascular permeability, vasodilation, bronchoconstriction |
| Cytokines | |
| TNF-$\alpha$ | Activation of vascular endothelial cells, cachexia, fatigue |
| TGF-$\beta$ | Fibrosis |
| IL-3 | Stimulation of hematopoiesis |
| IL-5 | Eosinophilia |
| IL-16 | Lymphocyte accumulation |

**Table 2** Consensus Revised Classification of
Mastocytosis

| |
|---|
| Indolent |
|   Syncope |
|   Cutaneous disease |
|   Ulcer disease |
|   Malabsorption |
|   Bone marrow mast cell aggregates |
|   Skeletal disease |
|   Hepatosplenomegaly |
|   Lymphadenopathy |
| Hematological disorder |
|   Myeloproliferative |
|   Myelodysplastic |
| Aggressive |
|   Lymphadenopathic mastocytosis and eosinophilia |
| Mast cell leukemia |

hematological disorder. Approximately one third of the patients referred to NIH fall within this category of disease. These patients appear to have increased genomic instability as evidenced by frequent chromosomal aberrations in routine karyotyping, although no consistent pattern has been demonstrated [32]. Progression from category I to category II is unusual. A third category of patients with aggressive mastocytosis present with enlarged lymph nodes and peripheral eosinophilia. This disease has a more rapid course. The fourth category, mast cell leukemia, is rare and is characterized by the presence of malignant mast cells in the peripheral blood, which by definition must constitute greater than 10% of the nucleated cells [33]. Small numbers of mast cells may be seen in the peripheral blood in category II and III disease.

## A. Cutaneous Mastocytosis

The most common skin manifestation of mastocytosis is urticaria pigmentosa (UP). It is seen in more than 90% of patients with indolent disease and less than 50% of those with an associated hematological disorder or other aggressive forms of the disease. The lesions of UP appear as scattered small, red-brown macules or papules (Figs. 2 and 3). They usually spare the areas exposed to sun or are more subtle in these areas. Darier's sign is the elicitation of urtication and erythema around the individual lesions by scratching or rubbing. The lesions are associated with pruritus, which may be exacerbated by heat, skin irritation, alcohol, or spicy foods and certain medications such as narcotic analgesics. Biopsy of an urticaria pigmentosa lesion reveals extensive dermal mast cell infiltrates and accumulation of the melanin pigment in the epidermis and in macrophages (Fig. 4) [34]. Biopsy of normal-appearing skin in patients with mastocytosis also reveals a slight increase in mast cell numbers [35]. Flushing of the face and upper chest area is a common complaint in mastocytosis.

Other less frequent patterns of skin involvement in mastocytosis include diffuse cutaneous mastocytosis, telangiectasia macularis eruptiva perstans (TMEP), and mastocytomas. Diffuse cutaneous mastocytosis is characterized by a uniform increase in mast cell

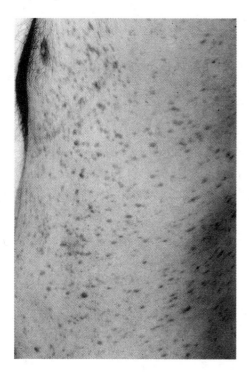

**Figure 2**  Urticaria pigmentosa in an adult patient with indolent mastocytosis.

numbers in the entire skin [36,37]. This presentation is seen in pediatric-onset disease. Children affected with this form of disease may have thickened skin and coarse facial features. The skin may have a peau d'orange appearance. Fortunately, most children experience improvement in the skin texture with time as the disease regresses, although this cutaneous form may persist into adulthood.

TMEP affects mainly adults and presents with generalized telangiectasia [34]. The disease is usually localized to skin but may occasionally be associated with systemic symptoms. The biopsy reveals increased numbers of perivascular mast cells. TMEP should be

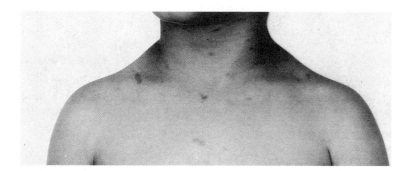

**Figure 3**  Urticaria pigmentosa in a child. The lesions in this child are somewhat larger than the adult form.

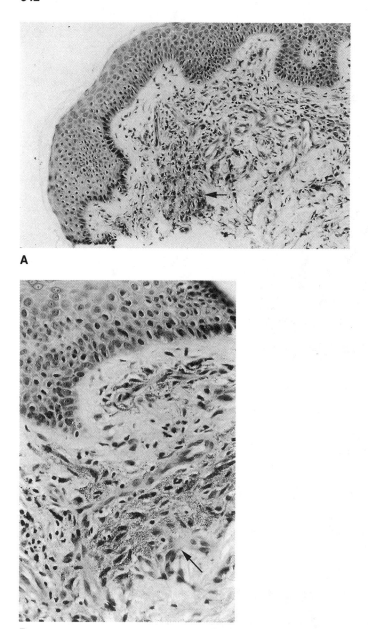

A

B

**Figure 4** (A) Histological appearance of urticaria pigmentosa. Toluidine blue staining. Arrow denotes an area of mast cell infiltration. (B) Higher magnification of another region from the same lesion. Arrow denotes an area of mast cell infiltration with their granules positively stained for toluidine blue.

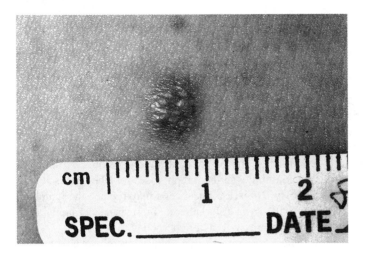

**Figure 5** Mastocytoma in an infant.

differentiated from UP with telangiectasia or scattered telangiectasia associated with other clinical conditions such as liver disease. Biopsies in such cases may appear similar.

Mastocytomas consist of collections of mature mast cells and may appear as macules, plaques, or nodules (Fig. 5). They can be solitary or multiple. Irritation of the mastocytoma lesion may cause systemic symptoms such as flushing. Solitary mastocytomas have been known to be identified before the onset of generalized UP.

Infants and young children with cutaneous mastocytosis may experience idiopathic bullous eruptions or have such bullous eruptions in association with infections or following routine immunizations [38,39]. These may be accompanied by hemorrhage into the bullae. Although the precise mechanism of bulla formation is not known, it is suspected that the mast cell–associated proteases may play a role. Although the bullae are sterile, superinfection may occur as they break down. Such bullae should be differentiated from other bullous diseases of the childhood such as scalded disease syndrome or erythema multiforme.

## B. Extracutaneous Manifestations

Patients with mastocytosis often develop gastrointestinal symptoms. Gastritis and peptic ulcer disease due to histamine-induced gastric hypersecretion and associated abdominal pain are the most common problems [40]. Diarrhea is also common and may be associated with malabsorption in some patients. Radiographic examination may, in addition, reveal abnormal mucosal patterns, multiple polyps, and motility disturbances. Histological sections of jejunal biopsies have shown moderate blunting of the villi, although significant mast cell hyperplasia is unusual. Hepatic involvement appears fairly common, as one study found 61% of patients had evidence of liver disease [41]. Hepatomegaly is seen in approximately one third of the patients and is more common in categories II and III. The most common biochemical abnormality is elevated alkaline phosphatase, and this should be differentiated from bone-derived alkaline phosphatase. Ascites and portal hypertension may develop in patients with more aggressive forms of the disease [42]. Increased portal fibrosis accompanied by portal mast cell infiltrates is seen frequently in biopsy specimens, although cirrhosis is uncommon. Venopathy is observed in association with category II disease.

An enlarged spleen is found in more than 90% of patients with category II or III disease and in 30–40% of those in category I [41,43]. Mast cell infiltrates are usually found in paratrabecular areas. Splenectomy may be considered if there is evidence for hypersplenism but does not appear to change the course of mastocytosis [44]. Peripheral and central lymphadenopathy was encountered in 26% and 19% of the patients, respectively, in one study and was also more common in patients with an associated hematological disorder or aggressive disease [43]. Mast cell infiltrates are most commonly seen in paracortical areas followed by the follicles, medullary cords, and the sinuses. The histopathological appearance of mast cell infiltrates in the lymph nodes may be confused with that of a T-cell lymphoma. In category III disease, mast cells may replace the lymphoid follicles, thus resembling follicular hyperplasia or lymphoma. Fibrosis is commonly associated with mast cell infiltration in spleen as well as lymph nodes [45].

The most common hematological abnormality in systemic mastocytosis is anemia [46]. This is followed by thrombocytopenia, eosinophilia, monocytosis, and leukopenia. Circulating mast cells are unusual. Examination of bone marrow biopsies reveals characteristic lesions consisting of paratrabecular spindle-shaped focal mast cell aggregates mixed with lymphocytes, eosinophils, and occasional plasma cells, histiocytes, and fibroblasts (Fig. 6) [47–49]. These lesions may resemble granulomas. They rarely occur in children [50]. A diffuse increase in mast cell numbers and fibrosis may be seen in advanced disease. Patients who present with category II disease have evidence of malignant or premalignant hematopoiesis in bone marrow biopsies. This includes evidence of myelodysplastic syndromes and myeloproliferative states such as chronic myelomonocytic leukemia. Secondary acute leukemias may also develop. A recent study found that 15 out of 16 patients with such bone marrow pathology also had abnormal bone marrow MRI findings [51]. Bone marrow infiltration with mast cells may induce bone changes that cause radiographically detectable lesions in up to 70% of patients [52]. These lesions may present as patchy areas of osteosclerosis on an osteoporotic background. The pathophysiology of these bone changes is not well understood but is probably related to mast cell mediators such as histamine, heparin, TNF-$\alpha$, and prostaglandins. The proximal long bones are most often affected, followed by the pelvis, ribs, and skull. Bone pain is a common symptom. It is present in 19–28% of the patients but must be distinguished from superficial muscular

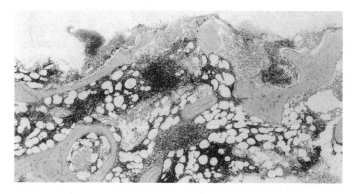

**Figure 6**    Toluidine blue staining of a plastic embedded bone marrow biopsy section from a patient with mastocytosis.

discomfort. Bone scans are more sensitive than radiographic surveys in detecting active lesions [53]. These may show generalized or focal uptake of radiotracer. Pathological fractures may occur in advanced disease. Patients in categories II and III with bone pain refractory to pharmacological management may benefit from localized irradiation therapy to the site of the lesion [54].

Patients in every category of mastocytosis sometimes experience flushing or systemic anaphylaxis [46]. In some patients, reactions may be provoked by alcohol, certain medications like aspirin or nonsteroidal anti-inflammatory drugs, exercise, iodinated contrast material, infections, or hymenoptera stings. Neuropsychiatric problems have been reported and may include a decreased attention span, imparied memory, irritability, and depression [55,56].

## III. DIAGNOSIS

The diagnosis of mastocytosis is suspected on clinical grounds and confirmed by histology [57]. Biochemical and radiographic tests provide supportive evidence. Most patients with indolent mastocytosis have urticaria pigmentosa, which is diagnosed on physical examination. The diagnosis should be confirmed by skin biopsy (Fig. 4). The most useful stains for mast cells include metachromatic stains such as toluidine blue and Giemsa, enzymatic stains such as chloroacetate esterase and aminocaproate esterase, and avidin, which binds to heparin. In urticaria pigmentosa, mast cells are found in increased numbers, usually more than 10-fold, in the dermal papillae, particularly near blood vessels [35,58–60]. Although the greatest numbers are found beneath the urticaria pigmentosa lesions, unaffected skin may also show a mild increase in mast cells. Occasional patients may show only two- to fourfold increases. Similar slight increases in dermal mast cell numbers can be seen in other conditions such as idiopathic flushing and anaphylaxis [35], scleroderma [61], chronic urticaria [62], or following chronic house dust mite exposure [63]; this underscores the need to correlate the gross skin examination with the biopsy findings. Histopathology of diffuse cutaneous mastocytosis shows prominent band-like infiltrates in the papillary dermis. Dermal mast cells from patients with urticaria pigmentosa are positive for both chymase and tryptase [64]. Electron microscopic analysis of the lesional mast cells reveals larger mean cytoplasmic area, nuclear size, and granular diameter than mast cells from healthy skin [60].

Bone marrow examination is useful in the diagnostic work-up and has prognostic implications. Bone marrow biopsy is more informative than an aspirate, but care must be taken during the processing of the biopsy specimen since decalcification of the bone marrow interferes with mast cell staining. This procedure should be performed in patients suspected of having mastocytosis without skin lesions or in patients with peripheral blood abnormalities, hepatomegaly, splenomegaly or lymphadenopathy to determine if they have an associated hematological disorder. Observation of characteristic mast cell aggregates and the condition of the normal hematopoietic marrow should be noted. Other tissue specimens from gastrointestinal mucosa, liver, spleen, or lymph nodes are generally obtained only if there is a clinical indication. Again, it should be remembered that up to fourfold increases in mast cell number is observed in other conditions such as inflammatory bowel disease.

Mastocytosis should be considered in the differential diagnosis of patients without skin lesions if they have one or more of the following: unexplained ulcer disease or malabsorption, radiographic or bone scan abnormalities, hepatomegaly, splenomegaly, lymphadenopathy, peripheral blood abnormalities, or unexplained flushing or anaphylaxis. For patients in the latter group, carcinoid syndrome or pheochromocytoma must be eliminated from consideration based on clinical picture and by measurements of 24-hour urine 5-hydroxyindoleacetic acid (5-HIAA) or metanephrines, respectively.

Elevated levels of urinary metabolites of histamine and prostaglandin $D_2$ are frequently seen in mastocytosis but are not diagnostic of the disease [65,66]. Plasma mast cell tryptase measurements are helpful if found elevated [67]. It has recently been shown that the predominant form of tryptase in plasma under baseline conditions is antigenically different than the form stored in mast cell granules [68]. These are termed alpha- and beta-tryptase, respectively. The amount of alpha-tryptase in plasma appears to correlate with the total body mast cell burden, as this form is constantly secreted from the mast cell as opposed to being targeted to the granules. The test, however, may reveal normal results in patients without systemic involvement.

## IV. TREATMENT

The primary objective of treatment in all categories of mastocytosis is to control mast cell mediator-induced signs and symptoms such as vascular collapse, gastric hypersecretion, gastrointestinal cramping, and pruritus. H1 receptor antagonists such as hydroxizine and doxepin are helpful in reducing pruritus, flushing, and tachycardia. Nonsedating H1 antagonists such as loratadine or cetirizine may also be considered. If insufficient relief occurs, the addition of an H2 antagonist such as ranitidine may be helpful. However, many patients continue to complain of musculo-skeletal pain, headaches, and flushing, resulting in part from the inability to block the effects of high levels of histamine with histamine antagonists and the presence of other mast cell mediators.

Cromolyn sodium is known to inhibit degranulation of mast cells and may have some efficacy in the treatment of mastocytosis in relieving gastrointestinal complaints [56,69,70]. Cromolyn sodium is poorly absorbed and thus does not prevent flushing, anaphylaxis, or skin responses, nor does it lower plasma or urinary histamine levels in patients with mastocytosis.

Epinephrine is used to treat episodes of vascular collapse [71]. Patients should be prepared to self-administer this drug. If subcutaneous epinephrine is insufficient, intensive therapy for vascular collapse should be instituted. Such episodes may be spontaneous but also have been observed after stings from insects, following administration of iodinated radiocontrast materials and nonsteroidal anti-inflammatory medications such as ketorolac.

Methoxalen with long-wave ultraviolet radiation (PUVA) has been shown to relieve pruritus and whealing after 1–2 months of treatment [72–75]. Improvement is associated with a temporary decrease in dermal mast cells. Pruritus recurs within 3–6 months after stopping treatment. Photochemotherapy should be used only in instances of extensive cutaneous disease unresponsive to other forms of therapy. Some patients report a diminution in the number or intensity of cutaneous lesions after exposure to natural sunlight.

Topical corticosteroids such as 0.05% betamethasone diproprionate ointment under plastic film occlusion for 8 hours per day over 8–12 weeks can be used to treat extensive urticaria pigmentosa or diffuse cutaneous mastocytosis. Mast cell numbers decrease as the lesions clear. These lesions eventually recur after discontinuation of therapy, although the treatment may lead to improvement in the cutaneous lesions for up to 1 year [76,77].

Adrenal suppression occurs especially if large areas of skin are treated. Repeated applications may leave the skin thin and atrophic.

Treatment of gastrointestinal disease is directed at controlling peptic symptoms, diarrhea, and malabsorption. Gastric acid hypersecretion leading to peptic symptoms and ulceration is controlled by H2 antagonists and proton pump inhibitors. Diarrhea is difficult to manage, and H2 antagonists are generally not effective at reducing cramping and stool frequency. Anticholinergics may give partial relief. In patients with severe malabsorption, systemic corticosteroids have been effective. Ascites is also difficult to control. Portal hypertension in one patient was successfully managed with portacaval shunt [78]. Another patient with exudative ascites was treated successfully with systemic corticosteroid therapy [79].

Patients with mastocytosis and an associated hematological disorder are managed as dictated by the specific hematological abnormality. In patients with mast cell leukemia, chemotherapy has not yet been shown to produce remission or to prolong survival. Chemotherapy has no place in the treatment of indolent mastocytosis. Such disappointing results are because tissue mast cells are not in division. Thus, bone marrow suppression occurs before substantial mast cell death may be induced.

Interferon alpha-2b has been used with mixed success in patients with advanced mastocytosis. In one study, three patients with systemic mastocytosis (one from each of categories I, II, and III) were administered interferon alpha-2b at a dose of 4–5 million units per square meter of body surface area for at least 12 months. All patients demonstrated continued progression of disease at one year of therapy [80].

Bone marrow transplantation may provide a hope for those patients who harbor a somatic mutation in their hematopoietic cells and have advanced disease or bone marrow failure. Limited experience is reported in the literature. One patient who had mastocytosis with an associated myeloproliferative disorder was free of disease at 2-year follow-up [81]. Two other patients with mastocytosis and myelodysplastic syndrome (MDS) who received bone marrow transplantation for the myelodysplasia were cured of their MDS but not of mastocytosis [82,83]. New onset cutaneous mastocytosis has been reported after an autologous bone marrow transplantation [84].

## V. PROGNOSIS

The prognosis is different for each category of disease. Patients with indolent mastocytosis and skin involvement alone have the best prognosis. Among children with isolated urticaria pigmentosa, at least half of the cases resolve by adulthood [39]. Adults with urticaria pigmentosa usually progress gradually to systemic disease, as defined by bone marrow involvement, and rarely may develop a hematological disorder. The survival of the patients in this category is rarely affected by the disease. Diffuse cutaneous mastocytosis is usually associated with indolent systemic disease. Patients with an associated hematological disorder have a variable course dependent on the prognosis of their hematological disorder. One study found that, in addition to an associated hematological disorder, six other variables were strongly associated with poor survival: constitutional symptoms, anemia, thrombocytopenia, abnormal liver function tests, a lobated mast cell nucleus, and a low percentage of fat cells in the bone marrow biopsy [46]. Other poor prognostic variables may include absence of urticaria pigmentosa, male sex, absence of skin and bone symptoms, hepatomegaly, splenomegaly, and normal bone x-ray findings. Average survival with lymphadenopathic mastocytosis with eosinophilia is approximately 1–2 years without therapy. Mast cell leukemia has a mean survival of less than 6 months.

## REFERENCES

1.  Metcalfe DD, Austen, KF. Mastocytosis. In: Frank MM, Austen KM, Claman HN, Unanue ER, eds. Samter's Immunologic Diseases. Boston: Little, Brown and Co., 1995:599–606.
2.  Fowler JF, Jr., Parsley WM, Cotter PG. Familial urticaria pigmentosa. Arch Dermatol 1986; 122:80–81.
3.  Kirshenbaum AS, Kessler SW, Goff JP, Metcalfe DD. Demonstration of the origin of human mast cells from CD34+ bone marrow progenitor cells. J Immunol 1991; 146:1410–1415.
4.  Thompson HL, Burbelo PD, Segui-Real B, Yamada Y, Metcalfe DD. Laminin promotes mast cell attachment. J Immunol 1989; 143:2323–2327.
5.  Kirshenbaum AS, Goff JP, Kessler SW, Mican JM, Zsebo KM, Metcalfe DD. Effect of IL-3 and stem cell factor on the appearance of human basophils and mast cells from CD34+ pluripotent progenitor cells. J Immunol 1992; 148:772–777.
6.  Dvorak AM, Seder RA, Paul WE, Morgan ES, Galli SJ. Effects of interleukin-3 with or without the c-kit ligand, stem cell factor, on the survival and cytoplasmic granule formation of mouse basophils and mast cells in vitro. Am J Pathol 1994; 144:160–170.
7.  Rottem M, Kirshenbaum AS, Metcalfe DD. Early development of mast cells. Int Arch Allergy Appl Immunol 1991; 94:104–109.
8.  Yanagida M, Fukamachi H, Ohgami K, Kuwaki T, Ishii H, Uzumaki H, Amano K, Tokiwa T, Mitsui H, Saito H, Iikura Y, Ishizaka T, Nakahata T. Effects of T-helper 2-type cytokines, interleukin-3 (IL-3), IL-4, IL-5, and IL-6 on the survival of cultured human mast cells. Blood 1995; 86:3705–3714.
9.  Godfraind C, Louahed J, Faulkner H, Vink A, Warnier G, Grencis R, Renauld JC. Intraepithelial infiltration by mast cells with both connective tissue-type and mucosal-type characteristics in gut, trachea, and kidneys of IL-9 transgenic mice. J Immunol 1998; 160:3989–3996.
10. Renauld JC, Kermouni A, Vink A, Louahed J, Van Snick J. Interleukin-9 and its receptor: involvement in mast cell differentiation and T cell oncogenesis. J Leukoc Biol 1995; 57:353–360.
11. Thompson-Snipes L, Dhar V, Bond MW, Mosmann TR, Moore KW, Rennick DM. Interleukin 10: a novel stimulatory factor for mast cells and their progenitors. J Exp Med 1991; 173:507–510.
12. Tagaya Y, Burton JD, Miyamoto Y, Waldmann TA. Identification of a novel receptor/signal transduction pathway for IL-15/T in mast cells. Embo J 1996; 15:4928–4939.
13. Galli SJ, Tsai M, Wershil BK, Tam SY, Costa JJ. Regulation of mouse and human mast cell development, survival and function by stem cell factor, the ligand for the c-kit receptor. Int Arch Allergy Immunol 1995; 107:51–53.
14. Valent P, Spanblochl E, Sperr WR, Sillaber C, Zsebo KM, Agis H, Strobl H, Geissler K, Bettelheim P, Lechner K. Induction of differentiation of human mast cells from bone marrow and peripheral blood mononuclear cells by recombinant human stem cell factor/kit-ligand in long-term culture. Blood 1992; 80:2237–2245.
15. Langley KE, Bennett LG, Wypych J, Yancik SA, Liu XD, Westcott KR, Chang DG, Smith KA, Zsebo KM. Soluble stem cell factor in human serum. Blood 1993; 81:656–660.
16. Topar G, Staudacher C, Geisen F, Gabl C, Fend F, Herold M, Greil R, Fritsch P, Sepp N. Urticaria pigmentosa: a clinical, hematopathologic, and serologic study of 30 adults. Am J Clin Pathol 1998; 109:279–285.
17. Longley BJ, Jr., Morganroth GS, Tyrell L, Ding TG, Anderson DM, Williams DE, Halaban R. Altered metabolism of mast-cell growth factor (c-kit ligand) in cutaneous mastocytosis. N Engl J Med 1993; 328:1302–1307.

18. O'Farrell A, Kinoshita T, Miyajima A. The hematopoietic cytokine receptors. In: Whetton AD, Gordon J, eds. Blood Cell Biochemistry. Vol. 7. New York: Plenum Press, 1996:1–40.

19. Ashman LK, Cambareri AC, To LB, Levinsky RJ, Juttner CA. Expression of the YB5.B8 antigen (c-kit proto-oncogene product) in normal human bone marrow. Blood 1991; 78:30–37.

20. Funasaka Y, Boulton T, Cobb M, Yarden Y, Fan B, Lyman SD, Williams DE, Anderson DM, Zakut R, Mishima Y, Haloban R. c-Kit-kinase induces a cascade of protein tyrosine phosphorylation in normal human melanocytes in response to mast cell growth factor and stimulates mitogen-activated protein kinase but is down-regulated in melanomas. Mol Biol Cell 1992; 3:197–204.

21. Manova K, Bachvarova RF. Expression of c-kit encoded at the W locus of mice in developing embryonic germ cells and presumptive melanoblasts. Dev Biol 1991; 146:312–324.

22. Zhang SC, Fedoroff S. Cellular localization of stem cell factor and c-kit receptor in the mouse nervous system. J Neurosci Res 1997; 47:1–15.

23. Dvorak AM, Costa JJ, Monahan-Earley RA, Fox P, Galli SJ. Ultrastructural analysis of human skin biopsy specimens from patients receiving recombinant human stem cell factor: subcutaneous injection of rhSCF induces dermal mast cell degranulation and granulocyte recruitment at the injection site. J Allergy Clin Immunol 1998; 101:793–806.

24. Spritz RA, Hearing VJ, Jr. Genetic disorders of pigmentation. Adv Hum Genet 1994; 22:1–45.

25. Hashimoto K, Tsujimura T, Moriyama Y, Yamatodani A, Kimura M, Tohya K, Morimoto M, Kitayama H, Kanakura Y, Kitamura Y. Transforming and differentiation-inducing potential of constitutively activated c-kit mutant genes in the IC-2 murine interleukin-3-dependent mast cell line. Am J Pathol 1996; 148:189–200.

26. Kitayama H, Kanakura Y, Furitsu T, Tsujimura T, Oritani K, Ikeda H, Sugahara H, Mitsui H, Kanayama Y, Kitamura Y, Matsuzawa Y. Constitutively activating mutations of c-kit receptor tyrosine kinase confer factor-independent growth and tumorigenicity of factor-dependent hematopoietic cell lines. Blood 1995; 85:790–798.

27. Nagata H, Worobec AS, Oh CK, Chowdhury BA, Tannenbaum S, Suzuki Y, Metcalfe DD. Identification of a point mutation in the catalytic domain of the protooncogene c-kit in peripheral blood mononuclear cells of patients who have mastocytosis with an associated hematologic disorder. Proc Natl Acad Sci USA 1995; 92:10560–10564.

28. Longley BJ, Tyrrell L, Lu SZ, Ma YS, Langley K, Ding TG, Duffy T, Jacobs P, Tang LH, Modlin I. Somatic c-KIT activating mutation in urticaria pigmentosa and aggressive mastocytosis: establishment of clonality in a human mast cell neoplasm. Nat Genet 1996; 12:312–314.

29. Worobec AS, Semere T, Nagata H, Metcalfe DD. Clinical correlates of the presence of the c-kit mutation in the peripheral blood of mastocytosis patients. Cancer 1998; 83:2120–2129.

30. Shah PY, Sharma V, Worobec AS, Metcalfe DD, Zwick DC. Congenital bullous mastocytosis with myeloproliferative disorder and c- kit mutation. J Am Acad Dermatol 1998; 39:119–121.

31. Metcalfe DD. Classification and diagnosis of mastocytosis: current status. J Invest Dermatol 1991; 96:2S–4S.

32. Worobec AS, Akin C, Scott LM, Metcalfe DD. Cytogenetic abnormalities and their lack of relationship to the Asp816Val c-kit mutation in the pathogenesis of mastocytosis. J Allergy Clin Immunol 1998; 102:523–524.

33. Travis WD, Li CY, Hoagland HC, Travis LB, Banks PM. Mast cell leukemia: report of a case and review of the literature. Mayo Clin Proc 1986; 61:957–966.

34. Soter NA. The skin in mastocytosis. J Invest Dermatol 1991; 96:32S–38S, 38S–39S.

35. Garriga MM, Friedman MM, Metcalfe DD. A survey of the number and distribution of mast cells in the skin of patients with mast cell disorders. J Allergy Clin Immunol 1988; 82:425–432.

36. Findlay GH, Schulz EJ, Pepler WJ. Diffuse cutaneous mastocytosis. S Afr Med J 1960; 34: 353.

37. Orkin M, Good RA, Clawson CC, Fisher I, Windhorst DB. Bullous mastocytosis. Arch Dermatol 1970; 101:547–564.

38. Golitz LE, Weston WL, Lane AT. Bullous mastocytosis: diffuse cutaneous mastocytosis with extensive blisters mimicking scalded skin syndrome or erythema multiforme. Pediatr Dermatol 1984; 1:288–294.

39. Kettelhut BV, Metcalfe DD. Pediatric mastocytosis. J Invest Dermatol 1991; 96:15S–18S.

40. Cherner JA, Jensen RT, Dubois A, O'Dorisio TM, Gardner JD, Metcalfe DD. Gastrointestinal dysfunction in systemic mastocytosis. A prospective study. Gastroenterology 1988; 95:657–667.

41. Mican JM, Di Bisceglie AM, Fong TL, Travis WD, Kleiner DE, Baker B, Metcalfe DD. Hepatic involvement in mastocytosis: clinicopathologic correlations in 41 cases. Hepatology 1995; 22:1163–1170.

42. Horny HP, Kaiserling E, Campbell M, Parwaresch MR, Lennert K. Liver findings in generalized mastocytosis. A clinicopathologic study. Cancer 1989; 63:532–538.

43. Travis WD, Li CY. Pathology of the lymph node and spleen in systemic mast cell disease. Mod Pathol 1988; 1:4–14.

44. Friedman B, Darling G, Norton J, Hamby L, Metcalfe D. Splenectomy in the management of systemic mast cell disease. Surgery 1990; 107:94–100.

45. Metcalfe DD. The liver, spleen, and lymph nodes in mastocytosis. J Invest Dermatol 1991; 96:45S–46S.

46. Travis WD, Li CY, Bergstralh EJ, Yam LT, Swee RG. Systemic mast cell disease. Analysis of 58 cases and literature review [published erratum appears in Medicine (Baltimore) 1990; 69(1):34]. Medicine (Baltimore) 1988; 67:345–368.

47. Webb TA, Li CY, Yam LT. Systemic mast cell disease: a clinical and hematopathologic study of 26 cases. Cancer 1982; 49:927–938.

48. Horny HP, Parwaresch MR, Lennert K. Bone marrow findings in systemic mastocytosis. Hum Pathol 1985; 16:808–814.

49. Travis WD, Li CY, Yam LT, Bergstralh EJ, Swee RG. Significance of systemic mast cell disease with associated hematologic disorders. Cancer 1988; 62:965–972.

50. Kettelhut BV, Parker RI, Travis WD, Metcalfe DD. Hematopathology of the bone marrow in pediatric cutaneous mastocytosis. A study of 17 patients. Am J Clin Pathol 1989; 91:558–562.

51. Avila NA, Ling A, Metcalfe DD, Worobec AS. Mastocytosis: magnetic resonance imaging patterns of marrow disease. Skeletal Radiol 1998; 27:119–126.

52. de Gennes C, Kuntz D, de Vernejoul MC. Bone mastocytosis. A report of nine cases with a bone histomorphometric study. Clin Orthop 1992:281–291.

53. Rosenbaum RC, Frieri M, Metcalfe DD. Patterns of skeletal scintigraphy and their relationship to plasma and urinary histamine levels in systemic mastocytosis. J Nucl Med 1984; 25:859–864.

54. Johnstone PA, Mican JM, Metcalfe DD, DeLaney TF. Radiotherapy of refractory bone pain due to systemic mast cell disease. Am J Clin Oncol 1994; 17:328–330.

55. Rogers MP, Bloomingdale K, Murawski BJ, Soter NA, Reich P, Austen KF. Mixed organic brain syndrome as a manifestation of systematic mastocytosis. Psychosom Med 1986; 48:437–447.

56. Soter NA, Austen KF, Wasserman SI. Oral disodium cromoglycate in the treatment of systemic mastocytosis. N Engl J Med 1979; 301:465–469.

57. Metcalfe DD. Conclusions. J Invest Dermatol 1991; 96:64S.

58. Kasper CS, Tharp MD. Quantification of cutaneous mast cells using morphometric point counting and a conjugated avidin stain. J Am Acad Dermatol 1987; 16:326–331.

59. Mihm MC, Clark WH, Reed RJ, Caruso MG. Mast cell infiltrates of the skin and the masto-cytosis syndrome. Hum Pathol 1973; 4:231–239.

60. Tharp MD, Glass MJ, Seelig LL, Jr. Ultrastructural morphometric analysis of lesional skin: mast cells from patients with systemic and nonsystemic mastocytosis. J Am Acad Dermatol 1988; 18:298–306.

61. Nishioka K, Kobayashi Y, Katayama I, Takijiri C. Mast cell numbers in diffuse scleroderma. Arch Dermatol 1987; 123:205–208.

62. Elias J, Boss E, Kaplan AP. Studies of the cellular infiltrate of chronic idiopathic urticaria: prominence of T-lymphocytes, monocytes, and mast cells. J Allergy Clin Immunol 1986; 78: 914–918.

63. Mitchell EB, Crow J, Williams G, Platts-Mills TA. Increase in skin mast cells following chronic house dust mite exposure. Br J Dermatol 1986; 114:65–73.

64. Irani AA, Garriga MM, Metcalfe DD, Schwartz LB. Mast cells in cutaneous mastocytosis: accumulation of the MCTC type. Clin Exp Allergy 1990;20:53–58.

65. Keyzer JJ, de Monchy JG, van Doormaal JJ, van Voorst Vader PC. Improved diagnosis of mastocytosis by measurement of urinary histamine metabolites. N Engl J Med 1983; 309: 1603–1605.

66. Roberts LJD, Sweetman BJ, Lewis RA, Austen KF, Oates JA. Increased production of prostaglandin D2 in patients with systemic mastocytosis. N Engl J Med 1980; 303:1400–1404.

67. Schwartz LB, Metcalfe DD, Miller JS, Earl H, Sullivan T. Tryptase levels as an indicator of mast-cell activation in systemic anaphylaxis and mastocytosis. N Engl J Med 1987; 316:1622–1626.

68. Schwartz LB, Sakai K, Bradford TR, Ren S, Zweiman B, Worobec AS, Metcalfe DD. The alpha form of human tryptase is the predominant type present in blood at baseline in normal subjects and is elevated in those with systemic mastocytosis. J Clin Invest 1995; 96:2702–2710.

69. Frieri M, Alling DW, Metcalfe DD. Comparison of the therapeutic efficacy of cromolyn so-dium with that of combined chlorpheniramine and cimetidine in systemic mastocytosis. Results of a double-blind clinical trial. Am J Med 1985; 78:9–14.

70. Horan RF, Sheffer AL, Austen KF. Cromolyn sodium in the management of systemic masto-cytosis. J Allergy Clin Immunol 1990; 85:852–855.

71. Turk J, Oates JA, Roberts LJ. Intervention with epinephrine in hypotension associated with mastocytosis. J Allergy Clin Immunol 1983; 71:189–192.

72. Christophers E, Honigsmann H, Wolff K, Langner A. PUVA-treatment of urticaria pig-mentosa. Br J Dermatol 1978; 98:701–702.

73. Granerus G, Roupe G, Swanbeck G. Decreased urinary histamine metabolite after successful PUVA treatment of urticaria pigmentosa. J Invest Dermatol 1981; 76:1–3.

74. Vella Briffa D, Eady RA, James MP, Gatti S, Bleehen SS. Photochemotherapy (PUVA) in the treatment of urticaria pigmentosa. Br J Dermatol 1983; 109:67–75.

75. Czarnetzki BM, Rosenbach T, Kolde G, Frosch PJ. Phototherapy of urticaria pigmentosa: clinical response and changes of cutaneous reactivity, histamine and chemotactic leukotrienes. Arch Dermatol Res 1985; 277:105–113.

76. Barton J, Lavker RM, Schechter NM, Lazarus GS. Treatment of urticaria pigmentosa with corticosteroids. Arch Dermatol 1985; 121:1516–1523.

77. Lavker RM, Schechter NM. Cutaneous mast cell depletion results from topical corticosteroid usage. J Immunol 1985; 135:2368–2373.

78. Bonnet P, Smadja C, Szekely AM, Delage Y, Calmus Y, Poupon R, Franco D. Intractable ascites in systemic mastocytosis treated by portal diversion. Dig Dis Sci 1987; 32:209–213.

79. Reisberg IR, Oyakawa S. Mastocytosis with malabsorption, myelofibrosis, and massive as-cites. Am J Gastroenterol 1987; 82:54–60.

80. Worobec AS, Kirshenbaum AS, Schwartz LB, Metcalfe DD. Treatment of three patients with systemic mastocytosis with interferon alpha-2b. Leuk Lymphoma 1996; 22:501–508.

81. Przepiorka D, Giralt S, Khouri I, Champlin R, Bueso-Ramos C. Allogeneic marrow transplantation for myeloproliferative disorders other than chronic myelogenous leukemia: review of forty cases. Am J Hematol 1998; 57:24–28.

82. Ronnov-Jessen D, Lovgreen Nielsen P, Horn T. Persistence of systemic mastocytosis after allogeneic bone marrow transplantation in spite of complete remission of the associated myelodysplastic syndrome. Bone Marrow Transplant 1991; 8:413–415.

83. Fodinger M, Fritsch G, Winkler K, Emminger W, Mitterbauer G, Gadner H, Valent P, Mannhalter C. Origin of human mast cells: development from transplanted hematopoietic stem cells after allogeneic bone marrow transplantation. Blood 1994; 84:2954–2959.

84. Van Hoof A, Criel A, Louwagie A, Vanvuchelen J. Cutaneous mastocytosis after autologous bone marrow transplantation. Bone Marrow Transplant 1991; 8:151–153.

# 17

## Pathophysiology and Management of "Sensitive Skin"

**Mary Steidl Matsui**
*The Estee Lauder Companies, and Columbia University, New York, New York*

**Kenneth D. Marenus and Daniel H. Maes**
*The Estee Lauder Companies, New York, New York*

Routine testing of cosmetic and skin treatment formulations for skin irritancy and allergic sensitization potential has been the standard practice of reputable cosmetic firms for some time. However, two decades ago investigators became aware that there is a category of response to topical agents that cannot be categorized as either irritancy or allergy in the conventional sense. This response is purely subjective, neurosensory in nature, and usually described as "sting." Having noticed a discrepancy between primary irritancy and capacity to induce a stinging response, Laden [1] in 1973 reported the results of a series of experiments in which he attempted to find predictive characteristics to evaluate the stinging potential of various solutions. In the mid-1970s, interest in a phenomenon called "sensitive skin" arose, possibly resulting from a substantial number of reports by individuals who experienced a peculiar stinging sensation from sunscreens containing *p*-aminobenzoic acid (PABA), particularly in the absence of erythema, dermatitis, or urticaria.

Eventually, attention turned from identifying agents most likely to cause stinging in the general population to identifying individuals most likely to react to certain chemicals with a sting response. In 1977, Frosch and Kligman [2] developed the prototype for the traditional, or standard, methodology used to identify those individuals most likely to react with this subjective neurosensory response to topically applied substances. This assay became known as the "sting test." This sting test is predictive for a narrowly defined subset of individuals with a specific type of cutaneous reaction to certain topical agents and will be discussed below. In addition, the following topics will also be covered: a definition of sensitive skin, the history of research on sensitive skin, a discussion of theories of sensitive skin etiology, other clinical assays used to distinguish either sensitive-skin individuals or chemicals most likely to cause stinging in sensitive skin, its occurrence in different populations (based on skin type, gender, age), and recent studies designed to develop treatment therapies to reduce skin reactivity of those individuals identified as having sensitive skin.

## I. CAN THE TERM "SENSITIVE SKIN" HAVE A UNIVERSALLY MEANINGFUL DEFINITION?

In 1980 Fisher [3] coined the phrase "status cosmeticus" and defined it as "a condition . . . in which every cosmetic or soap that is applied to the face produces itching, burning, or stinging sensations." He observed further that these subjective reactions were localized to the face, present with an unremarkable clinical picture (no erythema, rash, etc.), and that patch test results as performed on the arms or back were negative. He concluded that it is a nonallergic, primarily neurosensory irritant-type response that occurs in certain persons in whom a susceptibility to stinging can usually be demonstrated by exposure to 5–10% lactic acid on the nasolabial fold. Even using this relatively narrow definition, there probably exist two populations of individuals who experience this intolerance for topical agents. As described by Berardesca and Maibach, "primarily, sensitive skin seems to be caused by a constitutional anomaly, whereas, secondarily sensitive skin may be caused by skin disease, aging or occupational exposure to irritants" [4]. For the cosmetic and toiletries industry, sensitive skin is a useful "diagnosis" to isolate a population of individuals with a reproducible sensory response [5–7]. These individuals can then be used as a test population for product formulation to eliminate materials with potential to cause facial stinging that have already passed standard irritancy and allergy screening tests.

It has been somewhat difficult, however, to achieve a consensus among dermatologists and cosmetic and skin treatment groups regarding a clinical definition, reproducible assay, and pathophysiological basis for the subpopulation of people who self-identify as having sensitive skin. Self-identified sensitive skin individuals define themselves with a wide variety of adverse responses. Draelos [8] noted that approximately 40% of the population believes that it has sensitive skin based on reactions such as stinging, burning, pruritus, erythema and desquamation. Amin et al. state that "consumer studies in all races and continents identify a complex entity involving from one-quarter to one-half of the adult population" [9]. In addition to cosmetically induced facial stinging, some of the symptoms described by self-identified sensitive skin individuals include dry skin, acne, erythema due to diet or alcohol or stress and reddening, scaling, and tightness associated with cold, wind, cosmetics, soap, water. Clearly, the percent of "self-reporters" is going to depend on how inclusive their definition of "sensitive skin" is, whether the questioner applies any specific words or definitions to the category, and whether the questioner asks if they have ever experienced, currently experience, or often experience the symptoms. For example, how should individuals with seasonal sensitive skin be categorized? Is the etiology of their sensitivity the same as those with year-round sensitive skin?

One of the most encompassing definitions of sensitive skin was developed by the C.E.R.I.E.S. skin research center in France [10]. As opposed to the more narrow definition of sensitive skin as status cosmeticus (primarily a stinging phenotype), they have created four classifications of sensitive skin: (1) redness associated with diet, alcohol, stress, or rapid temperature changes; (2) redness, scaling, and tightness associated with cold weather, wind, and air conditioning; (3) redness, tightness, stinging, and blemishes associated with certain cosmetics, soap, and water; and (4) blemishes associated with the menstrual cycle.

At present, the use of the term "sensitive skin" is imprecise and its meaning and implications are extremely variable. A listing of the various conditions that do not fit the most limited definition is helpful, because the use of the term sensitive skin is most instru-

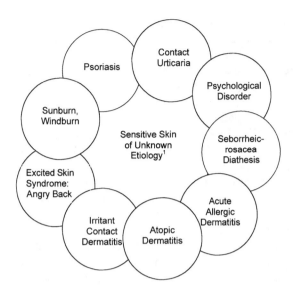

**Figure 1** This figure illustrates the many skin conditions that can confuse the perception of "sensitive skin" by either being identified as the problem (perhaps erroneously), or being the undiagnosed underlying cause for the symptoms. Not all those with these conditions report having sensitive skin. [1] This category also includes those individuals identified with cosmetic intolerance syndrome by Maibach and Engasser and status cosmeticus by Fisher. In at least two studies, these individuals generally had a history of symptomology after application of cosmetics, but they were not more likely to have a history of dermatological disease [22,24].

mental when used as an exclusionary term. Figure 1 is an attempt to carve out a niche for the term "sensitive skin" that describes a unique skin condition that cannot also be categorized as one of the others shown in the diagram. One example is a phenomenon called "the excited skin syndrome" or the "angry back," a condition of hyperreactivity that occurs when patients with active eczema or dermatitis have false-positive reactions to molecules that would not otherwise be contact irritants or allergens [11–13]. The hyper-irritability is caused by a preexisting inflammation, which decreases the threshold for nonspecific irritant reactions. This occurs in a clinical patch testing situation and is not what this chapter will regard as "sensitive skin," although it may provide some clues to the etiology of sensitive skin. It has been suggested that cosmetic intolerance syndrome and "sensitive skin" cover the same range of pathophysiology, but that the sensitive skin category is less severe [9].

There are many additional examples of unrestrained use of the term "sensitive skin." In a recent patent application for a lotion to be used on "sensitive skin," the product was supposed to address "hyperreactive skin conditions and more generally allergic-type reactions and/or intolerance phenomena, whether they are caused by external factors or factors intrinsic to the individual." Use was also made of the terms "reactive skin" and "intolerant skin." In another application, sensitive skin was described as easily subject to sensations of stabbing pain, itching or pricking, sensations of heat, biting, or burning. According to this use of the sensitive skin term, objective reactions such as reddening, desquamation, xerosis, seborrheic dermatitis, edema, vesicles, or even telangiectasia may occasionally be observed. Marketing text designed for sensitive skin may include the terms "allergy-tested, dermatologist tested, clinically tested, nonirritating, nonsensitizing, fragrance-free, preservative-free, and all natural" [3].

Mills and Berger [14] suggested that self-identified sensitive-skin individuals can be classified into four categories. The first group includes those with actual dermatological disease, including atopic dermatitis, seborrheic dermatitis, rosacea, ichthyosis, and others. Not all those with these conditions report having sensitive skin. The second group of individuals would be those who identify themselves as having sensitive skin, but in reality have undiagnosed disease because the clinical signs for the disease are minimal or atypical. Included in this second group would be those patients with atopic dermatitis or atypical rosaceae. The third group includes those individuals who have a history of severe skin damage from sunburn, contact irritancy, or contact allergy but at present appear normal. Their skin retains what is apparently memory with accompanying increased sensitivity to subsequent environmental insults. The fourth group described by Mills and Berger would be those individuals not included in the groups above who have clinically normal appearing skin but who consistently report specific negative sensations in response to topically applied materials. Further, there are those individuals who find it fashionable to describe their skin as sensitive.

The fourth group would fall into the center of the diagram in Figure 1 and would also most likely be "diagnosed" by the classic lactic acid sting test. It is this group, and possibly the third as well, who were the subject of studies designed to recognize "chemically vulnerable and delicate skin" that took place in the late 1970s and early 1980s [5]. Much of this initial work attempted to define a relatively safe and accurate predictive test that would distinguish individuals with a high susceptibility to irritants. Although it was assumed at first that materials identified as skin irritants would be the same materials that stimulated a reaction in sensitive-skin individuals, that was later found not to be the case.

An interesting use of the "sensitive skin" category of consumer complaints has arisen in a number of studies from Sweden and Norway, in which a correlation has been observed between skin "symptoms" and visual display units (VDU) [15–18]. In a number of epidemiological studies, no physiological changes were associated with the complaints and in controlled studies the patients were not able to distinguish when the electromagnetic fields were turned off or on. However, one study [16] compared a group of noncomplaining control individuals with patients who attributed their subjective symptoms (itching, burning, stinging, prickling, or tingling) to their VDUs and found that 19% of control versus 43% of the patients could be classified as stingers according to the lactic acid sting test developed by Frosch and Kligman [5].

Finally, a further expansion of the term "sensitive skin" relates to jewelry so marketed. These items are designed to avoid nickel in earrings by using stainless steel or surgical steel (thereby presumably avoiding allergic dermatitis).

## II. AN HISTORICAL REVIEW OF SENSITIVE SKIN RESEARCH: DEVELOPMENT OF A RELIABLE DIAGNOSTIC INSTRUMENT

The research history of what this chapter considers to be sensitive skin can be examined in several somewhat overlapping phases: the development of assays used to distinguish sensitive-skin individuals, the search for predictive characterization properties to identify molecules likely to cause stinging in susceptible individuals, the search to determine the biophysical defect/condition in sensitive skin, and the efforts toward developing products to avoid the stinging response and to treat or remediate the susceptible skin so that it is no longer sensitive. In addition, the question of whether the lactic acid sting test can also be used to predict increased susceptibility to classic irritants elsewhere on the body will be addressed.

Reasonably reliable predictive assays are in place for assessing the likelihood of toxicity from irritants, contact sensitizers and photosensitizers, and potential allergens [19]. Products that pass these tests may still be unacceptable, however, if they induce unpleasant sensations in a susceptible population of consumers. Maes et al. stated in 1990 [20] that products that have been thoroughly tested and found to be nonirritant via accepted protocols have been shown to induce occasional stinging, burning, and other unpleasant sensations in subjects of varying skin types, showing that in a real usage situation, stinging and burning are not always correlated to the classical definition of skin irritancy. In addition, the very phenomenon of sensitive skin is difficult to document because of a lack of objective physical or histological measures [21].

Laden also reported that stinging potential and primary irritancy are unrelated [1]. When subjects were asked to rank the applied solutions for pain level, citric and acetic acids repeatedly proved to be the most painful in stinging experiments but frequently scored low when compared to other acids for irritancy. Even within the acidic compound category, the stinging potential of a range of acidic solutions could not be accurately ranked based on characteristics such as hydrogen ion concentration, tonicity, or the nature of the anion.

As mentioned above, the classic studies of "chemically vulnerable and delicate skin" took place in the late 1970s and early 1980s, primarily by Frosch, Kligman, and others [1–3,5]. This work attempted to develop a relatively safe and accurate in vivo skin test that would distinguish individuals with high susceptibility to irritants. At that time, it was believed that these individuals would be more sensitive to classic irritants, and therefore the following tests were devised to assay skin responsiveness: the ammonium hydroxide blistering time (believed to be a function of the number of cell layers of the stratum corneum and measures the permeability of the barrier), the ability of DMSO to provoke whealing (also believed to be a function of the diffusional resistance of the barrier), the sodium lauryl sulfate (SLS) response (believed to correlate with barrier function and skin "reactivity"), the chloroform-methanol pain threshold (primarily subjective), and finally, the lactic acid sting test. This last test does not correlate with most primary irritants, has a characteristic development and resolution, and can be used to assess the likelihood of "disagreeable sensations" as opposed to toxic irritation, contact sensitization, photosensitization, or allergenicity. The lactic acid sting test is, however, subjective rather than objective, and it is primarily a facial phenomenon.

The lactic acid sting test is commonly performed [7,22–26] by placing a 5–10% lactic acid in water solution on the nasolabial grooves of subjects with cotton stick applicators. Ideally, the test is performed in a double-blind manner with water as the control vehicle, which is placed on the contralateral nasolabial groove. The qualitative aspect of sting itself has been described as a "sting" or "burn" arising within a minute or two after application of the lactic acid. "The discomfort intensifies over the next 5 to 10 minutes and may become so severe that frenetic attempts are made at removal. Intense stinging generally abates within about 15 minutes. Signs of irritation—redness, scaling, edema—do not develop'' [2]. Subject reactions can be recorded at intervals of 2–2.5 minutes for 10–15 minutes. A mild, transient erythema may appear in unusually suscepti- ble persons. Immediately after the test area is washed and rinsed, the stinging stops.

Recently a modified version of the lactic acid sting test was published in response to sharp criticism regarding the irreproducibility of the original version [7]. The modified version requires a 10-minute exposure of the cheek to 10% racemic lactic acid in a Hilltop chamber. Two values are obtained: (1) the time required for stinging to be perceived and (2) the intensity of peak stinging on a 0-to-3 interval scale. The authors claimed that identical results were obtained when the test was repeated on the same group of individuals after an interval of one year. They also reported that increasing the concentration of lactic acid to 20% or higher increased the incidence of visible irritation without significantly increasing peak intensity scores. Interestingly, two other observations were also noted: (1) deliberately damaging the skin by repeated washing with a harsh soap neither decreased the time to onset of stinging nor converted ''nonstingers'' to ''stingers,'' and [2] sub- stances cannot be tested simultaneously on both sides of the face because strong stinging on one side enhances the perception of stinging on the opposite side. In this study, as with others, the chemical structure of the test agent was not a predictor of stinging potential. At present, despite the drawbacks of the lactic acid sting test, its most useful attribute is its correlation with those individuals who experience unpleasant neurosensory responses dur- ing actual cosmetic and skin care product use [8].

Because of the subjective nature of the lactic acid sting test and its inherent bias and lack of quantification, efforts have been made to develop more objective measurements of this sensory phenomena. It has been suggested that the sensory response is actually due to a low level irritation that is not visible. Unfortunately, convincing biochemical evidence has not yet been presented to show that stinging is due to suberythemal irritation. Indeed, it has been stated that ''subjective irritation is not merely a mild form of objective irrita- tion'' [9]. It has also, however, been observed that early in the course of contact dermatitis, irritants are more likely to produce burning or stinging, whereas allergens produce itching [19].

There have been few studies that have employed objective, physiologically based instruments to distinguish stingers from nonstingers. Those that have, have focused pri- marily on determining the physiological anomaly responsible for the phenotype of ''sensi- tive skin with unknown etiology'' and have focused on the question of whether individuals with sensitive skin as defined by the lactic acid sting test are also more reactive to standard skin irritants. That topic—the pathophysiology of sensitive skin—is addressed below.

Maibach and others have claimed that stingers react more vigorously to vasodila- tors than control subjects [27,28]. If this response could be shown to be at least semi- quantitative and reliably reproducible, then laser Doppler velocimetry would be a reason- able technique to screen sensitive skin individuals as well as product formulations in a more objective manner. Unfortunately, most researchers have attempted to correlate ery- thema and edema with the stinging phenotype by applying the irritants to body sites other than the face, such as the back and volar forearms. If the sensory response is due to the peculiar characteristics of facial skin, such as the larger number of appendages and more easily compromised barrier function, leading to increased permeability of test substances, then agents applied to the back and forearm will not necessarily elicit the same magnitude or type of response.

## III. DOES A SENSITIVE SKIN PHENOTYPE BASED ON THE LACTIC ACID STING TEST CORRELATE WITH AN INCREASED RESPONSIVENESS TO PRIMARY IRRITANTS?

The next question that arises in this field pertains to the usefulness or applications of a sensitive skin "diagnosis." Are sensitive-skin individuals subject to heightened responsiveness to other irritants or an increased propensity to certain reactions such as urticaria, erythema, pruritus, or other nonimmunological reactions? This question has been addressed by several investigators, and in general the answer appears to indicate that a positive lactic acid sting test does not correlate well with increased reactivity in patch test–type protocols. The converse is also true. For example, sodium lauryl sulfate is a strong objective irritant but does not routinely cause stinging [13]. This absence of a relationship may be another indicator that a stinging response, as defined by the lactic acid sting test, is primarily a neurosensory response rather than suberythemal irritation. This question clearly overlaps with and relates to the development of a reliable objective assay for sensitive skin and subsequent use of that assay to prescreen topical agents. It also has important implications regarding the pathophysiology of sensitive skin and mechanisms of the sting response.

If the definition of sensitive skin is restricted to include only those individuals who report facial stinging, and perhaps some itching, upon cutaneous exposure to common topical agents, it will probably include those individuals with very dry skin but exclude many individuals who react to common irritants or allergens with clinically significant erythema, rash, hyperpigmentation or hypopigmentation, urticaria, or acne. Therefore, it is important to ascertain to what extent the individuals fitting the narrow definition of sensitive skin (positive lactic acid stingers) overlap with individuals who appear to have a heightened responsiveness to general irritants or, perhaps even more important, a heightened responsiveness to specific irritants. For example, it has been suggested that the class of chemicals most likely to be troublesome for sensitive-skin populations are surfactants [8]. If this is the case, then more attention should be paid to uncover possible correlations between inducers of sting and their performance in surfactant-based safety assays such as the collagen swelling test, pH rise test, and the zein test (listed in Table 1).

A series of reports by Lammintausta, Basketter, and others have examined the degree of overlap between sensitive skin as defined by the facial neurosensory sting response and hyperreactive skin as defined by a propensity to react to known irritant molecules either more frequently or more vigorously [24,25,28,29]. In one of the first studies, Lammintausta et al. reported that "stingers" had a greater likelihood of responding to sorbic acid and benzoic acid with higher scores of erythema and edema [28]. However, except for one comparison, that between stingers and nonstingers for erythema from 0.5% sorbic acid, the differences were not statistically significant due to very high standard deviations within the groups. In the same study, stingers did not have a higher rate of reaction to SLS-induced irritation.

Basketter and Griffiths compared 25 stingers to 25 nonstingers and asked if there was also a difference in their responses to a sodium dodecyl sulfate (SDS) patch test performed on the upper arm [25]. To identify stingers, they performed four repeat tests (one per week) of individual applications of 10% w/v aqueous lactic acid versus dH$_2$O to nasolabial folds using a cotton stick applicator. Sting or other reactions were recorded

**Table 1** Testing Methodologies for Sensitive Skin

Tests for the development of sensitive skin panels
    Lactic acid facial sting test
    Chloroform:Methanol (20:80) test
    Dimethyl sulfoxide (DMSO) test
    Erythema after sodium lauryl sulfate occlusion test
    Nicotinate test
Bioengineering tests to measure skin response
    Evaporimetry
    Polysulfide rubber replicas
    Squametry
    Chromametry
    Laser doppler flowmetry
    A-scan ultrasound
In vivo testing on sensitive-skin population
    Patch testing
    Modified soap chamber test
    Forearm controlled-application technique
In vitro tests to demonstrate irritancy
    Collagen swelling test
    PH rise test
    Zein test

*Source*: Ref. 8.

at 2.5, 5, and 8 minutes after application. Sting was classified arbitrarily with scores of 0–3 (nothing to severe). "Stingers" experienced stinging on three or four occasions, "inconsistent stingers" experienced stinging on two occasions, and "nonstingers" experienced stinging no more than once.

The patch test was performed by placing 0.3% SDS versus distilled water on filter paper discs taped to the upper outer arm. Patches were removed at 24 hours, wiped, and reapplied for another 24 hours. Application sites were assessed for erythema and dryness 1 and 23 hours later.

There was no significant difference between the groups in either the pattern or strength of the irritant response when assessed by subjective erythema and dryness scores. They concluded that the stinging response is unlikely to be a reliable indicator of a more generally reactive skin type. They further indicated that stinging is a phenomenon that occurs primarily, but not uniquely, on the face and more particularly on the nasolabial folds. The sensitivity of this region appears to be qualitatively as well as quantitatively different from the rest of the body and "is a reflection of its microanatomy, including a more permeable horny layer, a high density of sweat glands and hair follicles, and an elaborate network of sensory nerves" [25]. The neurosensory response, unlike the more classic irritant or allergic response, tends to be transient and mild, with little or no objectively perceivable effects.

In a later study, Coverly et al. [24] divided volunteers into stingers or nonstingers based on the results of a 10% lactic acid sting test. They then examined the erythema response to five irritants, which were placed on the volar forearm. An effort was made to test a variety of materials that had different chemical structures and mechanisms of action. They showed that there was no difference in the mean intensity and spread of erythema between stingers and nonstingers for methyl nicotinate, cinnamic aldehyde, and DMSO. The response of stingers to benzoic acid and *trans*-cinnamic acid was statistically greater in terms of both mean intensity and spread of erythema. These findings confirmed the earlier observations of Lammintausta et al. [28].

Although as a group stingers had an enhanced reactivity to those two materials, there was not a correlation within the stinger group between sting scores and degree of reaction to benzoic acid and *trans*-cinnamic acid. They concluded that strong reactivity to one nonimmunological urticant is not necessarily predictive of the degree of response to other urticants and that it is unlikely that susceptibility to lactic acid stinging would correlate generally with urticant susceptibility. They suggested that the difference in response between the first three compounds (cinnamaldehyde, methyl nicotinate, and DMSO) and the last two (benzoic acid and *trans*-cinnamic acid) is due to differences in mechanism of action. The theory that stingers represent a subpopulation with a more general tendency to have skin reactions was clearly not supported, but the possibility that they have increased sensitivity to specific molecules may have some merit.

This last idea is indirectly reinforced by work describing a potential therapeutic treatment regime for alleviating the symptoms of sensitive skin. Muizzuddin et al. [22] published a study in which correlations were made at three points important to the question of general reactivity of sensitive skin: first, individuals self-reporting as having sensitive or reactive skin exhibited significantly stronger responses to lactic acid than self-reporting nonsensitive skin individuals; second, a higher proportion of self-reported sensitive-skin individuals took less time to develop balsam of Peru (*trans*-cinnamic acid)–induced increased blood flow when compared to the non–sensitive-skin panelists; and third, this same group of reactive individuals appeared to have a more easily damaged barrier as assessed by trans-epidermal water loss (TEWL). The study supports the observations made by Coverly et al. [24] and by Lammintausta et al. [28]. The third correlation also addresses the question of possible etiological roots or mechanisms of sensitive skin.

## IV. THE PHYSIOLOGICAL BASIS FOR SENSITIVE SKIN

The possible causes of "sensitive skin of unknown etiology" will be discussed next, because a logical approach toward the remediation of symptoms should take into account the physiological basis for such symptoms. There is currently some agreement that sensitive skin, as defined by the propensity for facial stinging, is dependent at least in part on a defective or more easily disrupted barrier function. Over 10 years ago, in a review of what was referred to as sensitive, or hyperirritable, skin, Frosch observed that "individuals with dry or hyperirritable skin, particulary atopics, are prone to develop a cumulative insult dermatitis. Subjects with hyperirritable skin have a thin and/or permeable stratum corneum with a small surface area of corneocytes. The effects or irritants on cutaneous targets are extremely variable and depend on the type of chemical, concentration, and mode of exposure" [29]. Added to this list of variables should probably also be the body site of exposure, previous dermatological history, and other factors not yet completely characterized. The latter variables may not just modulate the likelihood of response, but also the qualitative aspects of response-elicitation of sting rather than burn or itch, with no visible change as opposed to erythema, edema, desquamation, or vesiculation.

A survey of the research designed to determine why some individuals react to common, generally nonirritating nonallergenic materials with an acute unpleasant sensation

**Table 2** Causes of Sensitive Skin Symptoms

Exogenous
    Subjective irritation (burn, sting, itch)
    Objective irritation
    Allergic contact dermatitis/Photoallergic contact
      dermatitis
    Contact urticaria
Endogenous
    Seborrheic diathesis, psoriasis
    Rosacea and perioral dermatitis
    Atopic dermatitis
    Status eczematous
    Status cosmeticus
    Dysmorphophobia

*Source*: Ref. 9.

characterized as stinging would find evidence in several categories. Summarized in Table 2 are a number of possible factors that may contribute to the condition of sensitive skin. Defective barrier function has been the most examined, with several approaches to measuring the contribution of this factor. In addition, other possible differences between sensitive-skin individuals and nonsensitive ones may involve an increased neurosensory input, enhanced immune responsiveness (unlikely), abnormal dermal vasodilation, an abnormal pH-buffering capacity, a higher incidence of *Demodex folliculorum* colonization, and increased penetration of topical agents due to differences in appendages such as sweat ducts and hair follicles. Some individuals may have sensitive skin due to underlying disease, as indicated by Figure 1, in which case the symptoms of sensitive skin should be ameliorated by successful treatment of the disease. Skin properties of those in this category tend to support the theory that sensitive skin is due primarily to a defective barrier.

In 1977 Frosch and Kligman interpreted their data to suggest that stingers have a lower threshold for the stinging stimulus and that the mechanism for the neurosensory response without any other signs of irritation or inflammation was due to direct excitation of nerve endings by acids below pH 2.0 and bases above pH11 [2]. They stated that the sensitive-skin population possesses skin that is more ''delicate'' and vulnerable to such direct excitation because they have a ''thinner,'' more permeable barrier. Most researchers attempting to determine the accuracy of this theory have used other irritants that cause visible, objectively measurable reactions in order to compare the rate of reaction and the extent of reaction and, in general, have examined these parameters using sites on the forearm or back. These techniques, as mentioned above, failed to establish a clear relationship between sensitive skin and a more reactive skin, and thus did not support the theory that sensitive skin is the result of a nonspecific defective barrier function.

As late as 1997, Issachar et al. complained that the phenomenon of sensitive skin is hard to document because of a lack of physical or histological objective signs [21]. They attempted to find an objective sign by examining ''normal'' versus ''sensitive'' skin in terms of differences in baseline skin pH and change in pH due to challenge and recovery. Baseline pH values were not different for the sensitive-skin group compared to the control group when measured either on the nasolabial fold or on the forearm. On the forearm, the kinetics of the pH change after application of lactic acid were also no different between the sensitive and control groups. However, somewhat surprisingly, after application of lactic acid to the nasolabial fold, the sensitive-skin group returned to baseline values faster than the control group, and in general the pH went back to normal much faster on the face than it did on the forearm. The authors' interpretation of these results was based on the assumption that lactic acid directly stimulates the sensory nerves to trigger the perception of stinging. They concluded that their data suggested that sensitive-skin individuals have a more permeable stratum corneum barrier, allowing the lactic acid to penetrate faster and more completely.

In the most recent large-scale investigation reported, researchers recruited approximately 1000 Caucasian women at diverse locations in North America who answered a questionnaire and participated in a study of facial reactivity to three probes: 10% lactic acid, 10% balsam of Peru, and a 10:90 chloroform methanol solution [30]. For each of the probes, the time to onset of burning/stinging and the peak grade of burning/stinging was recorded. As a group, the self-assessed sensitive-skin population had a shorter response time to all three probes and a higher peak grade for the sensations of burning and stinging. Although there was a statistically significant difference in response parameters between the self-identified sensitive-skin group versus the self-identified non–sensitive-skin group, it was observed that there was a relatively large number of nonresponders in the sensitive-skin group as well as a number of strong responders in the self-assessed nonsensitive group. Their conclusion was that individual consumer perception of sensitive skin was not a good predictor of heightened reactivity to the probes used. In addition, they reported that the results were not climatically dependent and that balsam of Peru reactions decreased with age.

The relationship between a disrupted barrier (as expressed by an elevated TEWL) and skin reactivity is obviously not straightforward. Increased penetration of irritants due to defective barrier function has been cited as an important component of sensitive skin [8], although a recent review of over 20 citations relating to the topic of defective barrier and irritant contact dermatitis noted that no general conclusion could be made from the accumulated data [31]. Patients with atopic dermatitis are considered to have defective skin barrier function and to therefore be at greater risk of developing acute irritant contact dermatitis. Atopics are often considered to be the prototype group in which to study effects of barrier damage and its contribution to skin reactivity to topically applied chemicals. However, even in this group there is not a general or universal increase in reactions to all irritants. For example, one study showed that atopic skin had a higher rate of reaction to 20% SDS when compared to controls, but was not different in terms of irritation provoked by 35% cocotrimethyl ammonium chloride or 10% hydrochloric acid [32]. This limited hyperreactivity of atopic skin to a surfactant was supported by Nassif et al. [33] using concentrations of SLS from 0.06 to 4.0% [33]. In addition, using TEWL as a tool to assess barrier function and atopic patients as a study group, no consistent correlation could be found between higher TEWL values and irritancy even though baseline TEWL in atopics is usually higher than in nonatopics. The reviewers noted the numerous parameters that may lead to inconsistent results between studies, including methods of patch testing (open or occluded, body site of patch), type of chemicals used, and measurement tools (visual erythema, TEWL). Finally, there is no indication that sensitive skin as defined by the subjective sting response correlates with positive irritancy response, as discussed above.

Muizzuddin et al. assessed barrier function by dynamic TEWL measurements and asked if there were differences between sensitive-skin individuals and a control population [6,22]. They reported that the sensitive-skin individuals, on average, required fewer tape strippings to significantly increase the TEWL values when compared to normal skin. They concluded that the sensitive-skin population had a more easily damaged barrier. However, simple interpretation of the data to reach a conclusion that sensitive-skin individuals have a defective barrier is not possible. After an 8-week therapeutic regime, which brought dynamic TEWL values of sensitive skin individuals to normal and significantly reduced facial skin reactivity to balsam of Peru, the perception of lactic acid sting was reduced by 40%, but the change was not statistically significantly different due to high variability. Another important piece of evidence that sensitive skin is not purely determined by barrier function is the observation noted earlier that nonstingers were not converted to stingers by washing with a harsh detergent [7].

Because the sting response is such a qualitatively different phenomenon than visible dermatitis, it seems likely that these individuals might have a qualitative difference in cytokine signaling, neuropeptide signaling, receptor activation, etc. If a more permeable barrier were the sole defect in sensitive-skin individuals, then the rate (time to perception) or intensity of sting would be expected to differ from control individuals, but not the entire response itself. Itch is one description of the sensation sensitive-skin individuals occasionally give, and the mechanism for itch is somewhat better understood than sting. Several comments regarding itch in a recent review of the topic by Greaves may have relevance to the sensation of sting as well, if both phenomena are the result of neuropeptide release and subsequent stimulation of sensory but not vascular responses [34]. He states that "the molecular and physiological basis of pruritus associated with clinically normal skin in the absence of underlying systemic disease is in most instances uncertain. . . . it is also conceivable that localized . . . itching without physical signs may be a manifestation of mild urticaria. In such cases levels of histamine and other mediators could be subthreshold with regard to vascular but not sensory effects'' [34]. No specific receptors have been identified for itch, but they are probably members of the polymodal nociceptor class with unspecialized free nerve endings located close to the dermo-epidermal junction. Differentiation of itch from pain probably occurs within the central nervous system. Itch does have specific endogenous molecular mediators, such as histamine, Il-2, and substance P, that can be shown to reliably reproduce the sensation, even though the sensation may not be a direct effect of any one of them, but rather may also require other intervening second messenger neuropeptides. Based on the example of itch, it may prove productive to examine sensitive-skin facial skin for neuropeptide release and expression of neuropeptide receptors. It has been suggested that agents causing subjective irritation unaccompanied by visible inflammation act via a mechanism similar to that of pyrethroids by interfering with the neuronal gating channel and impulse firing [33]. It may be the case that very low levels of histamine or Il-2, for example, may initiate the sensation of sting under certain circumstances, whereas higher levels would induce itch and/or inflammation.

Draelos, in a recent review, discussed the possibility that sensitive-skin individuals may have altered nerve endings, inappropriate neurotransmitter release, unique central information processing, chronic nerve-ending trauma, or slower neurotransmitter removal [8]. She cited examples in other anatomical areas of sensory responses known to occur in the absence of objective evidence. For example, in patients with "acid-sensitive esophagus," the classic symptoms of acid reflux occur in the absence of demonstrable endoscopic or histological esophageal damage, despite documented abnormal acid reflux by 24-hour pH determination. Draelos suggested that the acid-sensitive esophagus may be analogous to the sensitive-skin individual who has no clinical signs of cutaneous irritation. She further went on to suggest that a defective barrier function may be a critical component of sensitive skin, in that "lack of an intact barrier can result in heightened neurosensory input by inadequately protecting nerve endings and also . . . through altered percutaneous absorption." Interestingly, there are two references in the literature to unpublished data which indicate that local anesthetics block the sting response [35,36]. These data along with a more thorough investigation into the characterization of neurotransmitters involved in the perception of sting would be of great value.

In reviewing the physiological, contributions to sensitive skin Draelos included enhanced immune responsiveness. Altered percutaneous absorption due to a defective barrier function would provide increased antigen access to the dermal vasculature and antigen-presenting cells. This situation may be relevant in patients with allergic dermatitis, but there is no evidence to suggest that an antigenic response is consistent with the phenomenon of sensitive skin as defined by "facial stinging in the absence of clinical signs of irritation" (and the self-reported chronic nature of the complaints). It is, however, possible for a patient to experience an allergic reaction on the face despite a negative patch test elsewhere on the body due to the higher permeability of the facial skin [19].

One group of researchers has reported that they have observed a higher incidence and density of the mite *Demodex folliculorum* on the faces of sensitive-skin individuals by follicular biopsy sampling techniques [14]. Although they felt that the mite could play a role in the skin condition of some of these patients, no data have been published on this potential factor as of this date.

## V. GENDER, AGE, RACIAL, AND ETHNIC FACTORS IN SENSITIVE SKIN

The concept of sensitive skin itself is fraught with ambiguity and inconsistency, and the effects of such factors as gender, age, race, or ethnicity are even less well studied and characterized. In general, women, older individuals, and lighter-skinned people are assumed to have more "delicate" skin with a greater "sensitivity" to reactions induced by cosmetics and skin care products. This assumption is based on little, if any, experimental or epidemiological data, although it is accepted to be the case that the elderly and very young are more likely to develop irritant responses and less likely to develop allergic ones [19].

Although the North American Contact Dermatitis Group surveys from 1973 and 1977 published epidemiological data, which showed no significant differences in the black/white ratio of either allergic contact dermatitis or irritant contact dermatitis, respectively, experimental racial differences in cutaneous irritation (primarily surfactant induced) have been reported [4,9,32,38,39]. In the first study by Berardesca and Maibach, which compared "black" versus "white" skin, no definition was given for the skin type—presumably the subjects self-identified with one group or the other. There were no baseline differences in TEWL, laser doppler velocimetry readings, or capacitance between the two groups, but the data seemed to indicate that black skin was more responsive in terms of SLS-induced increased TEWL. A later study by the same group addressed the somewhat popular notion that black skin is more resistant to chemical and environmental damage and concluded that "the statement that black skin is tougher than white cannot be accepted." Nevertheless, Kligman maintains that a higher stinging response is found in light-completed persons of Celtic ancestry who sunburn easily [2,5]. Seasonal variations in intensity of the sting response have also been reported, with higher values occurring during the winter months, presumably to winter xerosis [40].

Racial differences in the structure of the stratum corneum have been proposed, although there are no differences in average thickness [4,39]. Organizational/structural differences were described following observations that more tape strippings were required to remove the stratum corneum in blacks due to a greater number of cell layers. This difference in corneocyte size and organization may affect penetration of exogenous molecules, and it has been shown that stripped skin tends to give equal responses between groups [4].

Again, it should be noted that the classic irritant response, measured by increased TEWL or erythema (visual grading, chromameter, or laser doppler velocimetry readings), is not a completely satisfactory analog or model of the subjective neurosensory sting reaction. Sensitive-skin individuals are identified through self-reporting, and the lactic acid sting response is subjective. Therefore, cultural and societal factors are likely to play an important part in the interaction between the epidemiologist/dermatologist/researcher and the members of a study population/patient/subject.

## VI. MANAGEMENT OF SENSITIVE-SKIN PATIENTS

If the mechanism behind sensitive skin could be identified, products could be designed to ameliorate the defect or exclude specific problem molecules. But even if the etiological factors are not definitively characterized, it is possible that agents that improve the barrier will decrease symptoms by inhibiting the penetration of offending molecules. Another approach to solving the cosmetic intolerance of sensitive skin consumers is to include in products anything that might work to diminish the adverse response, including antioxidants, anti-inflammatory agents, and inhibitors of neuromediators such as VIP, CGRP, neuropeptide Y, and somatostatin. A product designed for the sensitive-skin consumer might contain agents to reduce the inflammatory response, reduce the neuronal response, and improve the barrier function.

Sensitive skin, as it is addressed in this review, is a chronic nonallergic, subjective response to commonly used cosmetic and skin care products, accompanied by few or no visual signs of inflammation. Individual assessment can be made with the use of the lactic acid sting test and a patient history.

Management of cosmetic intolerant patients has been reviewed by both Maibach and Draelos [8,36,37]. Essentially, an attempt is made to obtain a medical diagnosis and the patient thoroughly screened for endogenous and exogenous causes of symptoms. If conditions such as seborrheic dermatitis, rosacea, atopic dermatitis, or psoriasis are determined to exist, the underlying disease is treated. All products used by the patient are examined for known irritants and sensitizers, and, if indicated, patch testing and photopatch testing of specific agents is performed. Any possible psychological contributions to the situation should be recognized and considered.

Both Maibach and Draelos would require the patient to eliminate all cosmetics, over-the-counter treatments products, cleansers, and, if possible, topical prescription medications for a period of 2 weeks to 6 months or more, if possible. Skin care routine should be limited to washing with water only or a synthetic detergent and the use of a bland moisturizer. Selected cosmetic items including skin care products designed for leave-on use can be individually provocative use-tested, and after the period of analysis, the patient can begin to use any nonoffending products, adding them one at a time. Both Maibach and Draelos offer additional details concerning selection criteria for use by the patient and dermatologist in the evaluation of cosmetics intended to be used by sensitive-skin individuals. A more thorough review of the theory and practice of evaluating patients with contact and occupational dermatoses, lists of known irritants and allergens (including alternative nomenclature), and sources of patch test kits and related products can be found in Ref. [19].

The identification and use of sensitive-skin individuals can be an important factor in skin care product formulation. As early as 1990, panels comprised of "sunscreen stingers" were used in product testing [20]. Products passing chronic tests by individuals in these panels were much less likely to induce skin reactions such as irritation, stinging, and burning once they were sold on the market. Currently, a few cosmetic and personal care product companies have a practice of assembling specific sensitive-skin panels for use in testing products designed for that market. Criteria for inclusion in the panel are primarily based on a positive lactic acid sting test but also may include assessments of subclinical erythema using a chromameter or changes in capillary blood flow as measured by laser doppler or thermography.

## VII. SUMMARY

In conclusion, the term "sensitive skin" is a consumer-driven expression that refers to a neurosensory response characterized primarily as "sting" unaccompanied by significant visual signs of irritation. It is a phenomenon important to the cosmetic and skin care industry, but which has been somewhat difficult to address because of its subjective nature. As commonly used, it does not refer to either the sensitization phase of an allergic response or molecules that are sensitizers, rather it is regarded as a nonallergic response characterized by the propensity to facial stinging in response to commonly used topical products. It is not necessarily related to skin that shows extensive or chronic dermatitis or that seems to be highly reactive to true irritants or allergens. In medical practice it is a term best used when all other diagnoses have been excluded or treated.

"Sensitive skin" is an important concept to understand and define. The value of reaching a consensus regarding the use of the term is in the improvement in communication both between consumers and the skin care industry and between patient and dermatologist. Use of a term with a universally accepted definition increases the precision and utility of communication.

The most predictive diagnostic and predictive clinical assay for sensitive skin is the lactic acid sting test in which 5–10% lactic acid placed on the nasolabial fold elicits a reproducible characteristic subjective sting response. The sting is immediate and lasts for only 15–30 minutes.

The physiological factors that are present in individuals who are classified as "stingers" are not yet clearly and unambiguously defined. As a primarily facial phenomenon, a compromised barrier function and increased permeability to small molecules seems to be a component of the etiology. However, as a qualitatively unique response in a subset of individuals, it is also likely that there is a genetically or environmentally determined alteration in neuropeptide signaling.

Treatment of sensitive-skin individuals may include a program in which topical product use is eliminated for a period of time, after which products are added back one at a time. It should be remembered that it is possible to have a negative patch test reaction to a contact irritant if there is a significant permeability difference between the test site (usually the back or arm) and the use site (particularly the face). It may also prove helpful to use products that are designed to increase barrier function and that contain anti-inflammatory agents or ingredients that inhibit neurotransmission.

## REFERENCES

1. Laden K. Studies on irritancy and stinging potential. J Soc Cosmet Chem 1973; 24:385–393.
2. Frosch PJ, Kligman AM. A method for appraising the stinging capacity of topically applied substances J Soc Cosmet Chem 1977; 28:197–209.
3. Fisher A. Cosmetic actions and reactions: therapeutic, irritant, and allergic. Cutis 1980; 26: 22–29.
4. Berardesca E, Maibach HI. Sensitive and ethnic skin. A need for special skin-care agents? Dermatol Clin 1991; 1:89–92.
5. Frosch PJ, Kligman AM. Recognition of chemically vulnerable and delicate skin. In: Frost P, Horwitz SN, eds. Principles of Cosmetics for the Dermatologist. St. Louis: CV Mosby, 1982:287–296.
6. Maes D, Marenus K, Muizzuddin N, Goyarts E, Fthenakis C, McKeever M. Evaluation and treatment of sensitive skin: a multi-faceted approach J Cosmet Sci 1998; 49:52–53.
7. Christensen M, Kligman AM. An improved procedure for conducting lactic acid stinging tests on facial skin. J Soc Cosmet Chem 1996; 47:1–11.
8. Draelos ZD. Sensitive skin: perceptions, evaluation, and treatment Am J Contact Dermatitis 1997; 8:67–78.
9. Amin S, Engasser P, Maibach HI. Sensitive skin: What is it? In: Baran R, Maibach HI, eds. Textbook of Cosmetic Dermatology. London: Martin Dunitz, 1998:343–349.
10. CE.R.I.E.S. Studies sensitive skin. HAPPI 1998; 35(11):130.
11. Mitchell J, Maibach HI. Managing the excited skin syndrome: patch testing hyperirritable skin. Contact Dermatitis 1997; 37:193–199.
12. Rietschel RL. Physiologic response of chronically inflamed and accommodated human skin. Curr Probl Dermatol 1995; 23:104–107.
13. Rietschel RL. Stochastic resonance and angry back syndrome: noisy skin. Am J Contact Dermat 1996; 7:152–154.
14. Mills OH, Berger RS. Defining the susceptibility of acne-prone and sensitive skin populations to extrinsic factors. Dermatol Clin 1991; 9:93–98.
15. Oftedal G, Vistnes AL, Rygge K. Skin symptoms after the reduction of electric fields from visual display units Scand J Work Environ Health 1995; 21:335–344.
16. Berg M, Lonne-Rahm S-B, Fischer T. Patients with visual display unit-related facial symptoms are stingers. Acta Derm Venereol 1998; 78:44–45.
17. Swanbeck G, Bleeker T. Skin problems from visual display units. Acta Derm Venereol 1989; 69:46–51.
18. Berg M. Facial skin complaints and work at visual display units. Epidemiological, clinical and histopathological studies. Acta Derm Venereol Suppl 1989; 150:1–40.
19. Marks JG, Jr, and DeLeo VA. Contact and Occupational Dermatology. 2d ed. St. Louis: Mosby, 1997.
20. Maes D, Marenus K, Smith WP. Invisible irritation: a new look at product safety. Cosmet Toilet 1990; 105:43–50.
21. Issachar N, Gall Y, Borell MT, Poelman MC. pH measurements during lactic acid stinging test in normal and sensitive skin. Contact Dermatitis 1997; 36:152–155.

22. Muizzuddin, N, Marenus K, Maes DH. Factors defining sensitive skin and its treatment. Am J Cont Dermat 1998; 9:170–175.

23. Jenkins HL, Adams MG. Progressive evaluation of skin irritancy of cosmetics using human volunteers. Int J Cosmet Sci 1989; 11:141–149.

24. Coverly J, Peters L, Whittle E, Basketter DA. Susceptibility to skin stinging, non-immunologic contact urticaria and acute skin irritation; Is there a relationship? Contact Dermatitis 1998; 38(2):90–95.

25. Basketter DA, Griffiths HA. A study of the relationship between susceptibility to skin stinging and skin irritation. Contact Dermatitis 1993; 29(4):185–188.

26. Grove G, Soschin D, Kligman AM. Guidelines for performing facial stinging tests. Proc. 12th Congress Internat. Fed. Soc. of Cosmet. Chem., Paris, Sept. 13–17, 1982.

27. Maibach HI, Lammintausta K, Berardesca E, Freeman S. Tendency to irritation: sensitive skin. J Am Acad Dermatol 1989; 21:833–835.

28. Lammintausta K, Maibach H, Wilson DP. Mechanisms of subjective (sensory) irritation: propensity to non-immunologic contact urticaria and objective irritation in stingers. Dermatozen 1988; 36:45–49.

29. Frosch PJ. Irritant contact dermatitis. In: Frosch PJ, Dooms-Goossens A, Lachapelle, J-M, Rycroft RJG, Scheper RJ, eds. Current Topics in Contact Dermatitis. Berlin: Springer-Verlag, 1989, pp. 385–398.

30. Bowman JP, Floyd AK, Kligman AM, Stoudemayer T, Mills OH. An evaluation of sensory-inducing chemical probes comparing women's self-perception of sensitive skin. Proceedings of the Society of Cosmetic Chemists Annual Scientific Meeting and Technology Showcase, New York, 1998, pp. 39–40.

31. Gallacher G, Maibach HI. Is atopic dermatitis a predisposing factor for experimental acute irritant contact dermatitis? Contact Dermatitis 1998; 38:1–4.

32. Basketter DA, Griffiths HA, Wang XM, Wilhelm K-P, McFadden J. Individual, ethnic and seasonal variability in irritant susceptibility of skin: the implications for a predictive human patch test. Contact Dermatitis 1996; 35:208–213.

33. Nassif A, Chan SC, Storr FJ, Hanifin JM. Abnormal skin irritancy in atopic dermatitis and in atopy without dermatitis. Arch Dermatol 1994; 130:1402–1407.

34. Draelos ZD, Rietschel RL. Hypoallergenicity and the dermatologist's perception J Am Acad Dermatol 1996; 35:248–251.

35. Greaves MW. Pruritus. In: Champion RH, Burton JL, Ebling FJG, eds. Textbook of Dermatology. London: Blackwell Scientific Publications, 1992:527–536.

36. Amin S, Engasser P, Maibach HI. Adverse cosmetic reactions. In: Baran R, Maibach HI, eds. Textbook of Cosmetic Dermatology. London: Martin Dunitz Ltd, 1998:709–746.

37. Amin S, Maibach HI. Cosmetic intolerance syndrome: pathophysiology and management. Cosmetic Dermatol. 1996; 9:34–42.

38. Berardesca E, Maibach HI. Racial differences in sodium lauryl sulphate induced cutaneous irritation: black and white. Contact Dermatitis 1988; 18:65–70.

39. Hamami I, Marks R. Structural determinants of the response of the skin to chemical irritants. Contact Dermatitis 1988; 18:71–75.

40. Leyden JJ. Risk assessment of products used on the skin. Am J Contact Dermatitis 1993; 4:158–161.

# 18

## Differential Diagnosis of Allergic Skin Disease

**Werner Aberer**
*University of Graz Medical School, Graz, Austria*

**Klaus Wolff**
*University of Vienna, Vienna, Austria*

## I. INTRODUCTION

Urticaria, contact dermatitis, and atopic dermatitis represent disease entities that are commonly termed "allergic skin disease." But whereas allergic contact dermatitis by definition always represents an allergic disease (i.e., type IV allergy) and immediate as well as delayed-type reactions play an important role in atopic dermatitis, true allergic reactions, such as immediate-type allergic reactions, are much less frequently the cause of urticaria than commonly believed. Although all three entities are easily identified clinically when presenting with classical manifestations, diagnosis may often be difficult: clinical appearance may differ depending on the provoking conditions (internal or exogenous exposure), pathomechanisms (type of allergy, intolerance), and severity, concomitant or underlying disease, constitutional, and other factors. Atopic dermatitis not only manifests differently in children and adults, but clinical disease expression in the individual case may be considerably influenced by exogenous factors like food allergy, contact allergy, or wool intolerance. Importantly, other disease entities may resemble allergic skin disease. The differential diagnosis is thus as important for allergic skin disease as it is for many other disease entities and requires in-depth dermatological training.

Differential diagnostic assessment rests on the clinical presentation, history, and, if required, laboratory and other tests, and the sequence of evaluational steps should be in this order. Of these, the clinical presentation is the most important because allergic skin diseases in general have a characteristic morphology. This will permit the physician to elicit, in a second step, a focused history, which provides a rational approach to the patient's condition. Since skin disease is visible to the patient, he or she may consult the physician with a history that is already the result of interpretation and may thus be misleading. For example, patients may link contact dermatitis with ingested foodstuffs or drugs, and much time is lost if the patient is permitted to ramble on with a historical account that may be irrelevant. Laboratory and other tests should be performed only as a third step and should aim at a verification of the clinical diagnosis or, as is the case for

*371*

patch testing, the identification of individual, noxious agents. Again, to give an example, individuals with nickel sensitivity may have urticaria and will thus have a positive patch test to nickel without this being of any relevance to the urticarial eruption. To employ the whole battery of laboratory and other tests available for allergic skin disease without a focused approach is therefore inappropriate because it is costly, a burden to the patient, and time-consuming. The general rule is therefore to (1) examine the patient carefully and to arrive at a provisional diagnosis on purely clinical grounds, (2) take a careful but focused history in order to confirm or exclude the clinical impression, and (3) employ laboratory tests, again in a focused manner.

Allergic skin disease may clinically present as either urticarial or eczematous eruptions, and we will therefore discuss the differential diagnosis in this order.

## II. URTICARIAL ERUPTIONS

### A. Clinical Manifestations

Urticaria (and angioedema) are easily recognizable disorders (see Chapters 3 and 9). Urticarial eruptions are episodic and evanescent, with multiple lesions occurring in various stages of evolution and resolution. Seldom do individual urticarial or angioedematous lesions persist for more than 48 hours, but they may continue to recur for indefinite periods; wheals can be seen as an allergic response to innumerable agents such as drugs, food, or insect bites but may also be the result of nonallergic mechanisms.

The wheal as the basic skin lesion is easily identified on clinical grounds. It represents a usually sharply demarcated, slightly elevated pruritic plaque that is transient in nature and reflects vasodilatation and edema of the papillary body. Diagnostic problems may arise if the duration of the single lesion cannot be determined during the first visit or if the characteristic pruritus is missing. Uncertainty also arises when wheals occur simultaneously with other skin lesions or when they persist for prolonged time periods such as in urticarial vasculitis. The diagnosis of urticaria may also be missed if the patient does not present with typical urticarial lesions but with an eczematous picture as in protein contact dermatitis, latex hypersensitivity reactions (see Chapter 12), or atopic contact dermatitis (see Chapter 7).

In a patient with an urticarial eruption, the first decision that has to be made is whether the rash is purely urticarial or whether it is a polymorphic eruption where urticarial lesions are only part of a more mixed clinical picture. In the purely urticarial eruptions the next step determines whether the condition is urticaria associated with angioedema (often but not always IgE-dependent, related to alimentary agents, parasites, penicillin, or complement-mediated in serum thickness–like reactions) and whether the urticarial lesions are large wheals (usually again IgE-dependent and complement-mediated but also nonallergic intolerance reactions), medium-sized wheals (usually in chronic, idiopathic urticaria), or small papular wheals as is the case in cholinergic urticaria or in papular urticaria inflicted by insect bites (see Chapter 9). It is also important to establish whether urticarial lesions occur anywhere on the body in a generalized fashion or are localized, for instance, to exposed sites (cold urticaria, solar urticaria).

### B. History

The patient's history will first have to determine whether the eruption is the first episode or recurring, whereby acute urticaria is defined as an eruption lasting less than 60 days (see Chapter 24). Acute urticaria associated with large wheals and with or without angioedema is usually IgE dependent or complement mediated. Urticaria due to mast cell–releasing agents, often associated with angioedema and anaphylaxis-like syndromes, may occur with radiocontrast media and may be a consequence of intolerance to salicylates, azo dyes, or benzoates. History should therefore include an evaluation of medications like those mentioned, penicillin, and nonsteroidal anti-inflammatory drugs. Acute urticaria, however, is also a consequence of alimentary agents (fish, shellfish, peanuts, strawberries, etc.) and parasites (e.g., nematodes) and may be the first episode of chronic idiopathic urticaria.

Chronic urticaria is rarely IgE dependent and is in 80% of cases idiopathic. It is often associated with intolerance to salicylates or benzoates or may be a presenting sign of other, usually systemic diseases. As for the duration of individual lesions, it should be noted that with lesions that do not disappear within 1 or 2 days, pure urticaria has to be questioned and additional procedures have to be performed to exclude urticarial vasculitis (see Chapter 14).

As for constitutional symptoms, fever may be present in serum sickness and the angioedema-urticaria-eosinophilia syndrome [1], and in angioedema there may be stridor and dyspnea. Arthralgia may be present in urticaria with serum sickness. Pruritus and pain on walking suggest penicillin or food involvement; flushing, burning, and wheezing may be found in cholinergic urticaria where papular urticarial eruption occurs after exertion (see Chapter 9). Solar urticaria occurs after response to visible light or UV radiation and is initially confined to exposed body regions (see Chapter 11), as is cold urticaria following contact with a cold object or exposure to cold ambiance. Pressure urticaria (usually manifesting as subcutaneous swelling) is confined to pressure sites and accompanied by an appropriate history, as is vibration urticaria (see Chapter 9). Hereditary angioedema (which may show urticarial rashes) has a positive family history and is characterized by angioedema following trauma and accompanied by constitutional symptoms (such as abdominal pain) [2]. The angioedema-urticaria-eosinophilia syndrome has high fever and a striking increase of body weight due to the retention of water and occurs in a cyclic pattern [1].

## C. Diagnostic Procedures

Clinical and laboratory procedures that help to diagnose and differentiate different forms of urticaria include systematic review to detect infestation with parasites, foci of chronic bacterial infection, pathogenic microbial flora (including helicobacter and candida) in the gastrointestinal tract, eosinophilia from reactions to foods, parasites, and drugs. A check for hepatitis-associated antigens, assessment of complement and of specific IgE antibodies by RAST, as well as a search for autoantibodies against FcεRI may be helpful in chronic idiopathic urticaria (see Chapter 8). High levels of eosinophilia are found in the angioedema-urticaria-eosinophilia syndrome. Dermatohistopathology including immunopathology will detect urticarial vasculitis or in mixed eruptions rule out other dermatological diseases, and specific complement studies will detect the absence or a functionally inactive C1 esterase inhibitor. Finally, it should be kept in mind that urticarial lesions that are not urticarial vasculitis may also be a symptom of connective tissue disease. Systems review should therefore exclude lupus erythematosus, Sjögren's syndrome, Schnitzler's syndrome [3], and rheumatic fever.

If physical urticaria is suspected this should be assessed by appropriate challenge testing (see Chapter 9). Cholinergic urticaria can best be diagnosed by exercise, response to sweating, and intracutaneous injections of acetylcholine or mecholyl. Solar urticaria is verified by testing with UVB, UVA, and visible light, cold urticaria by the application to the skin of an ice cube, and pressure urticaria by pressure tests.

Dermographism is one of the physical urticarias, where stroking of the skin may produce wheals in normal persons. When this is associated with significant itching, it is called symptomatic dermographism.

Table 1 shows the differential diagnosis of the most common types of chronic urticaria.

## D.  Disorders that Resemble Urticaria

Papular urticaria consists of small wheals inflicted by insect bites, usually in children, which are symmetrically distributed and may involve any area of the body; the mechanism of these reactions, whether toxic or allergic, was hitherto unknown. Recent studies from Finland, where almost all children show delayed papular reactions and/or immediate whealing to Aedes mosquito bites, revealed a positive correlation between the size of the 15-minute wheal and mosquito saliva–specific IgE; children with small/papular wheals

**Table 1**   Features of Common Types of Chronic Urticaria

| Type of urticaria | Age, range of patients (yr) | Principal clinical features | Associated angioedema | Diagnostic test |
|---|---|---|---|---|
| Chronic idiopathic | 20–50 | Profuse or sparse generalized, pink or pale edematous papules or wheals, often annular with itching | Yes | — |
| Symptomatic dermographism | 20–50 | Itchy, linear wheals with a surrounding bright-red flare at sites of scratching or rubbing | No | Light stroking of skin causes an immediate wheal with itching |
| Other physical urticarias | | | | |
| Cold | 10–40 | Itchy pale or red swelling at sites of contact with cold surfaces or fluids | Yes | Ten-minute application of an ice cube, wheal within 5 minutes of the removal of ice |
| Pressure | 20–50 | Large painful or itchy red swelling at sites of pressure | No | Application of pressure perpendicular to skin produces persistent red swelling after a latent period of 1–4 hours |
| Solar | 20–50 | Itchy pale or red swelling at site of exposure to UV or visible light | Yes | Irradiation by a 2.5 kW solar simulator (290–690 nm) for 30–120 seconds causes wheals in 30 minutes |
| Cholinergic | 10–50 | Itchy, small (<5 mm), monomorphic pale or pink wheals on trunk, neck, and limbs | Yes | Exercise or a hot shower elicits an eruption, acute stressful situation |

*Source*: Ref. 19.

revealed less intense bands in IgE immunoblots. Papular urticaria may thus represent an allergic reaction pattern occurring after a mild antigenic stimulus but is not a distinct disease entity [4]. Papular urticarial eruptions are, however, also a manifestation of cholinergic urticaria (see above).

Urticarial vasculitis is characterized by urticarial lesions that persist for longer than 24 or 48 hours, change their shape slowly, and may exhibit intralesional purpura as well as hyperpigmentation after resolution and are often associated with vascular/connective tissue autoimmune diseases such as lupus erythematosus (see Chapter 14). They are often associated with hypocomplementemia and renal disease. It should be noted, however, that classical chronic urticaria (without urticarial vasculitis) may also be associated with Sjögren's syndrome and SLE.

Contact urticaria is a wheal-and-flare skin reaction that occurs following contact with antigens or as a reaction to urticariogenic agents that cause a nonallergic urticaria. It comprises a heterogeneous group of inflammatory reactions, which include not only wheals and flares but also transient eczematous lesions. Contact nonimmunological urticaria that occurs on normal skin can be caused by sorbic acid, benzoic acid, insect stings, and moths. On the other hand, contact immunological urticaria occurs in preexisting eczematous skin and may be caused by topical antibiotics, miscellaneous topical medications like benzocaine, lindane, menthol, or polyethylenglycol, polysorbate 16, and metals like nickel and platinum, or animal keratins such as guinea pig hairs.

There has been much confusion in the use of such terms as "contact urticaria," "immediate contact reaction," "atopic contact dermatitis," and "protein contact dermatitis" [5]. Depending on the mechanisms underlying contact reactions, they are divided into two main types: immunological (IgE-mediated) and nonimmunological. Hundreds of substances have been reported to cause immediate reactions; they include chemicals in medications, industrial contactants, and components of cosmetic products, foods, and drinks, as well as many chemically undefined environmental agents [6]. Special awareness arose when during the latex allergy epidemic patients presented with a picture clinically typical for contact dermatitis and a type IV reaction against rubber additives was suspected [7]. We now know that latex gloves may induce contact urticaria in sensitized patients with symptoms ranging from local erythema/urticaria/eczema to systemic anaphylactic reactions [8].

## E. Other Conditions in Which Urticaria Is Associated with Other Lesions (Mixed Eruptions) or in Which Lesions Mimic Urticaria

Papulovesicular or bullous eruptions with mucosal involvement and typical target lesions characterize erythema multiforme; the differentiation might be difficult if mucosal lesions are missing and if iris lesions are absent. Maculopapulous drug eruptions or viral disease can sometimes be distinguished only due to their typical persistence and the purpuric residues upon vanishing. Numerous annular erythemas and exanthems may be difficult to differentiate on purely clinical grounds: annular lesions that may be macular or slightly raised can occur in erythema marginatum and other figurate erythemas (erythema annulare centrifugum, erythema gyratum repens, familial annular erythemas, erythema chronicum migrans/Lyme disease, necrolytic migratory erythema, etc.), drug eruptions, mycosis fungoides, secondary syphilis, or lupus erythematosus. Annular papules might be produced by secondary syphilis, erythema multiforme, lichen planus, lupus erythematosus, dermato-phytosis, and the figurate erythemas.

The wheals of creeping eruptions (larva migrans) form a serpiginous arrangement of lesions and are not as transient as in urticaria. Wheal-like lesions occur in dermatitis herpetiformis and bullous pemphigoid; the latter may resemble an urticarial reaction before the first blisters develop.

Sweet's syndrome [9] may mimic urticaria, particularly since some forms of urti-caria (i.e., urticaria in association with macroglobulinemia, delayed-pressure urticaria, cold urticaria) may be accompanied by fever and leukocytosis. Tinea corporis may resemble urticaria when the typical scaling is masked by topical treatment. The wheal produced in response to the stroking of a reddish or brown macule (Darier's sign) is pathognomonic of urticaria pigmentosa (mastocytosis).

## III.  ECZEMATOUS DERMATITIS

### A.  Clinical Manifestations

Allergic skin diseases falling into this group are allergic contact dermatitis, photoallergic contact dermatitis, and atopic dermatitis, which must be differentiated from toxic (irritant) contact dermatitis and a number of other types of eczema and noneczematous dermatoses that may have clinical features similar to those of contact dermatitis. The clinical features of an eczematous reaction are erythema, papules, and vesicles that may be followed by scaling and crusting (see Chapter 10). In subacute and chronic eruptions there may be associated lichenification and hyperkeratosis; these are features that are found in allergic contact dermatitis, irritant dermatitis, both acute and chronic, in phototoxic and photoaller-gic dermatitis (see Chapter 11), in atopic dermatitis (see Chapter 7), and in a number of other nonallergic eczematoid eruptions. Localization and distribution are therefore impor-tant, and it has to be determined whether the condition is confined to exposed body sites, whether the condition is localized and remains confined to the involved area, or whether it spreads, even becoming generalized, and whether there are predilection sites for the eruption such as the neck area and large flexures in patients with atopic dermatitis.

Toxic irritant contact dermatitis usually manifests as dull, nonglistening erythema that may be followed by vesiculation, erosion, crusting, and scaling. In severe reactions there may be necrosis, like in scalding. When toxic irritant contact dermatitis becomes chronic there will be inflammatory thickening of skin with scaling, hyperkeratosis, fissures, and crusting. A previously sharp margination will give way to an ill-defined border and lichenification. In contrast, allergic contact dermatitis in the acute eruption presents with erythema and, in contrast to irritant dermatitis, with papules accompanied by vesicles, erosions, crusts, and scaling. In the chronic form the papules will lead to lichenification, scaling, and also excoriations.

Contact dermatitis, both toxic and allergic, is always confined to the site of exposure to the noxious agent. Margination is originally sharp in both types of contact dermatitis, but in allergic contact dermatitis it may later spread peripherally beyond the actual site of exposure and when strong sensitization has occurred, spreading to other parts of the body and resulting in a generalized rash. The main differences between toxic irritant and allergic contact dermatitis are summarized in Table 2, and a practically identical differen-tial diagnostic outline can be given for the difference between phototoxic and photoallergic dermatitis where the distinguishing feature is the fact that the eruptions are confined to

**Table 2** Differences Between Toxic Irritant and Allergic Contact Dermatitis

| | | Toxic irritant | Allergic CD |
|---|---|---|---|
| Lesions | Acute | Erythema → vesicle → erosion → crust → scaling | Erythema → papules → vesicles → erosions → crusts → scaling |
| | Chronic | Papules, plaques, fissures, scaling, crusts | Papules, plaques, scaling, crusts |
| Margination and site | Acute | Sharp, strictly confined to site of exposure | Sharp, confined to site of exposure but spreading. In the periphery, usually tiny papules, may become generalized |
| | Chronic | Ill-defined | Ill-defined, spreads |
| Evolution | Acute | Rapid (few hours after exposure) | Not so rapid (12–72 hours after exposure) |
| | Chronic | Months to years of repeated exposure | Months or longer; exacerbation after every reexposure |
| Causative agent | | Dependent on concentration of agent; occurs only above threshold level | Relatively independent of amount applied—usually very low concentrations sufficient, but depends on degree of sensitization |
| Incidence | | May occur in practically everyone | Occurs only in the sensitized |

*Source*: Ref. 20.

areas exposed to light. Subtle clinical observation may often be a decisive factor in distinguishing allergic contact dermatitis from photoallergic dermatitis. Both may occur in the face and look alike. But in allergic photodermatitis the upper lids or the area under the nose or under the chin are often spared because they are shielded from light, whereas these areas are involved in classical contact dermatitis, particularly to airborne allergens. Allergic contact dermatitis can therefore be diagnosed only after careful consideration of many variables.

Atopic dermatitis is a chronically relapsing eczematous dermatitis that is frequently associated with elevated serum IgE levels and a personal or family history of atopic dermatitis, allergic rhinitis, and asthma (see Chapter 8). Atopic dermatitis has a number of features in common with allergic contact dermatitis, which may be superimposed on atopic dermatitis. Distribution, predilection sites, other features of atopic dermatitis such as Morgan folds and lateral eyebrow alopecia together with xerosis of the skin are therefore as important for diagnosis of atopic dermatitis as is the history (see below).

Irritant hand dermatitis in atopic persons may be impossible to differentiate from atopic hand eczema [10]. And atopic persons are not less prone to develop allergic contact dermatitis to common allergens—a topic that was long hotly debated in the literature [11,12]. Worsening of atopic dermatitis due to *Pityrosporum ovale* has been described as a contact urticaria reaction [13], and staphylococcal infections were reported to elicit eczematous immediate-type reactions in the skin of atopic patients [14].

Since there are no single distinguishing features, the clinical diagnosis is based on a combination of historical and morphological findings. Still, the diagnosis is most often primarily based on clinical criteria, and if a certain number of Hanifin and Rajka's [15] diagnostic criteria (see Chapter 8) are present, the diagnosis is not too difficult to make.

In the individual patient, one must consider a number of other conditions. Seborrheic dermatitis might be difficult to differentiate from infantile atopic dermatitis in the first few months of life [16] or in the adult when facial and anogenital involvement is seen. Immunodeficiency states should be considered in infants, in whom the disease is unusually severe, when there are recurrent systemic or ear infections and when there is failure to thrive, malabsorption, or petechiae. Thus, an eruption resembling atopic dermatitis, with or without other atopic manifestations, and sometimes with raised IgE levels may be found in several syndromes: agammaglobulinemia, anhidrotic ectodermal defect, ataxia-telangiectasia, celiac disease, cystic fibrosis (heterozygote), genetic hearing loss, Hurler syndrome, Jung's disease, nephrotic syndrome, Netherton's syndrome, phenylketonuria, Wiskott-Aldrich syndrome, and C5 dysfunction (Leiner's disease) [17].

## B. History

The history is of considerable importance in eczematous dermatitis. It involves a personal history with regard to the exposure to potentially sensitizing or irritant (toxic) substances, the time lapse since exposure and eruption, and occupational and recreational factors. It often involves efforts that are reminiscent of a detective's work. For instance, contact dermatitis of the lips may be due to nickel sensitivity, to coloring agents in lipsticks, or to topical medications for herpes; it may also represent irritant dermatitis in an atopic dermatitis or be the result of compulsive licking and sucking in patients with emotional instability. Family history is important in atopic dermatitis and includes a history of rhinitis and asthma. In phototoxic and photoallergic dermatitis a relevant historical issue is the exposure to (long-wave) UV light and includes sun exposure through window glass.

## C. Clinical and Laboratory Investigations

Laboratory and clinical testing that may help in the differentiation of eczematous dermatitis are mainly patch or photopatch tests that will reveal an allergic or photoallergic reaction. So are the determination of total IgE and IgE to specific allergens in atopic dermatitis by RAST and skin testing (Prick test) for immediate-type allergy in atopic dermatitis or hypersensitivity to latex, food allergens, or atopic (protein) contact dermatitis [18]. It should be noted that a positive patch test does not necessarily prove the nature of a particular eczematous reaction. For instance, hypersensitivity to chromates, verified by a patch test, may be present in a patient who has irritant contact dermatitis, and it is only the synopsis of the clinical appearance, the localization of an eruption, and the history that may indicate exposure to a sensitizing agent together with the positive patch test to this specific agent that will definitely rule out other conditions.

Also, a negative patch test does not exclude an allergic mechanism. Irritant contact dermatitis is not an exclusion diagnosis (wrong conclusion: negative test, thus nonallergic but irritant dermatitis), but the result of a careful case history, investigations into the sources of exposure to irritants, and a negative patch test result.

A diagnosis of allergic contact dermatitis cannot be made by means of histological examination of a biopsy specimen, but a biopsy may be useful in excluding a number of eczematous dermatitis-like conditions (see below).

Infestations that may become eczematous like scabies, particularly in children, and tinea or candida infections or viral infections (herpes, molluscum contagiosum, etc.) have to be excluded using adequate techniques.

## D. Other Forms of Eczema-Like Eruptions

Pityriasis alba is morphologically characteristic with dry patches of eczema on the cheeks and/or upper arms and may be mistaken for contact dermatitis. Lichen simplex chronicus is eczematous dermatitis that is lichenified and aggravated by rubbing, and nummular eczema occurs as oozing and crusted plaques of eczematous dermatitis associated with bacterial infections/overgrowth. Both may or may not be associated with atopic dermatitis.

Seborrheic dermatitis may be difficult to distinguish from contact dermatitis when there is facial and anogenital involvement. And low-humidity dermatoses may have clinical features similar to those of seborrheic dermatitis of the face. Asteatotic eczema is seen mainly in elderly persons due to xerosis of the skin.

Most cases of psoriasis and hyperkeratotic eczema are easily recognized as distinct entities, but psoriasis of the hands may be difficult to distinguish from chronic allergic or irritant contact dermatitis. And Koebner-induced psoriasis at the site of nickel contact dermatitis in a nickel-sensitive person is another difficult differential diagnosis. Acrodermatitis of Hallopeau and palmoplantar pustulosis may have clinical features similar to those of pustular contact dermatitis. And palmar lichen planus can have a striking resemblance to hand eczema.

Intertrigo as well as Hailey-Hailey disease may mimic contact dermatitis, and chronic cutaneous lupus erythematosus of the palms and soles may have eczematous features. Rare metabolic diseases such as acrodermatitis enteropathica, acquired zinc deficiency, phenylketonuria, or pellagra may also look like contact dermatitis but have other distinguishing features such as localization, distribution, mucosal involvement, or associated systemic symptoms.

Infectious processes and infestations, especially of the palms, can resemble contact dermatitis; Norwegian scabies and dermatophytosis call for a high degree of suspicion. Vesicular eruptions on the fingers in children after inappropriate topical treatment with steroids are clinically indistinguishable from vesicles associated with systemically induced contact dermatitis. Even erysipelas may at times be difficult to differentiate from acute contact dermatitis; fever and serological signs of systemic inflammation are helpful.

Bowen's disease and Paget's disease may have certain features in common with small patches of circumscribed chronic contact dermatitis. A single lesion of patch stage mycosis fungoides may also have eczematoid features and be misdiagnosed as contact dermatitis.

## IV. CONCLUSION

What the nonexpert may casually diagnose as an ''allergic'' skin disease frequently does not deserve this designation. Urticaria, allergic contact dermatitis, and atopic dermatitis can vary in their clinical expression and may thus be misdiagnosed. Careful examination of the patient and his or her entire skin and a detailed case history usually suffice to diagnose most patients, but in some, additional clinical and laboratory tests may be necessary to arrive at the correct diagnosis. The leading feature is the clinical appearance of the condition, and only the trained dermatologist is capable of putting this into a proper perspective using the patient's history and other investigations.

## REFERENCES

1. Gleich GJ, Schroeter AL, Marcoux P, Sachs M, O'Connell EJ, Kohler PF. Episodic angio-edema associated with eosinophilia. N Engl J Med 1984; 310:1621–1626.
2. Gigli I, Rosen FS. Urticaria and angioedema. In: Freedberg IM, Eisen AZ, Wolff K, et al., eds. Fitzpatrick's Dermatology in General Medicine. 5th ed. New York: McGraw-Hill, 1999: 1419–1425.
3. Berdy SS, Bloch K. Schnitzler's syndrome: a broader clinical spectrum. J Allergy Clin Immunol 1991; 87:849–854.
4. Brummer-Korvenkontio H, Palosuo K, Palosuo T, Brummer-Korvenkontio M, Leinikki P, Reunala T. Detection of mosquito saliva-specific IgE antibodies by capture ELISA. Allergy 1997; 52:342–345.
5. Hjorth N, Roed-Petersen J. Occupational protein contact dermatitis in foodhandlers. Contact Dermatitis 1976; 2:28–42.
6. Lahti A, Maibach HI. Immediate contact reactions: contact urticaria syndrome. Semin Dermatol 1987; 6:313–320.
7. Estlander T, Jolanki R, Kanerva L. Dermatitis and urticaria from rubber and plastic gloves. Contact Dermatitis 1986; 14:20–25.
8. Van der Meeren HLM, Van Erp PEJ. Life-threatening contact urticaria from glove powder. Contact Dermatitis 1986; 14:190–191.
9. Hönigsmann H, Cohn PR, Wolff K. Acute febrile neurophilic dermatosis (Sweet's syndrome). In: Freedberg IM, Eisen AZ, Wolff K, et al., eds. Fitzpatrick's Dermatology in General Medicine. 5th ed. New York: McGraw-Hill, 1999:1117–1123.
10. Meding B. Epidemiology of hand eczema in an industrial city. Acta Derm Venereol 1990; Suppl 153.
11. Christophersen J, Menné T, Tanghøj P, Andersen KE, Brandrup F, Kaaber K, Osmundsen PE, Thestrup-Pedersen K, Veien NK. Clinical patch test data evaluated by multivariate analysis. Contact Dermatitis 1989; 21:291–299.
12. Cronin E, McFadden JP. Patients with atopic eczema do become sensitised to contact allergens. Contact Dermatitis 1993; 28:225–228.
13. Jensen-Jarolim E, Poulsen LK, With H, Kieffer M, Ottevanger V, Stahl Skov P. Atopic dermatitis of the face, scalp, and neck: Type I reaction to the yeast Pityrosporum ovale? J Allergy Clin Immunol 1992; 89:44–51.
14. McFadden JP, Noble WC, Camp RDR. Superantigenic exotoxin-secreting potential of staphylococci isolated from atopic eczematous skin. Br J Dermatol 1993; 128:631–632.
15. Hanifin JM, Rajka RG. Diagnostic features of atopic dermatitis. Acta Derm Venereol 1980; 92(suppl 144):44–47.
16. Yates VM, Kerr REI, MacKie RM. Early diagnosis of infantile seborrhoic dermatitis and atopic dermatitis. I. Clinical features; "total" and specific IgE levels. Br J Dermatol 1983; 108:633–639.
17. Leung DYM, Tharp M, Boguniewicz M. Atopic dermatitis (atopic eczema). In: Freedberg IM, Eisen AZ, Wolff K, et al., eds. Fitzpatrick's Dermatology in General Medicine. 5th ed. New York: McGraw-Hill, 1999:1464–1480.
18. Hamann CP. Natural rubber latex protein sensitivity in review. Am J Contact Dermatitis 1993; 4:4–21.
19. Greaves MW. Chronic urticaria: a review. N Engl J Med 1995; 332:1767.
20. Fitzpatrick TB, Johnson A, Wolff K, et al. Color Atlas and Synopsis of Clinical Dermatology. New York: McGraw-Hill, 1997.

# 19

## Assessing Health-Related Quality of Life in Patients with Allergic Skin Diseases

**Roger T. Anderson and Jeffery S. McBride**
*Wake Forest University School of Medicine,*
*Winston-Salem, North Carolina*

**Rukmini Rajagopalan**
*Glaxo Wellcome, Inc.,*
*Research Triangle Park, North Carolina*

## I. INTRODUCTION

Like many concepts drawn from daily life experiences common to people, the term "quality of life," like the term "stress," has entered our lexicon and is now in widespread use. Perhaps the ease with which this concept has been embraced by the professional and lay person alike reflects an absence of a more traditional phrase in the English language capable of describing the opposite of illness: conveying a richness or enjoyment from living that originates with health. Many health researchers point to the World Health Organization (WHO) as the midwife of this concept, providing in their 1947 document an expanded definition of "health" as including social and emotional well-being in addition to physical components of health [1]. Today we use the more polished term "health-related quality of life," or HRQL, to refer to impacts (positive and negative) upon "core" areas of life including, at least, physical, social, and emotional well-being and satisfaction with life attributed to health states or health care (both prevention and restoration) [2]. Another unique feature of the concept of HRQL is that it refers solely to the patient's perspective. This important criterion requires that the desired information be obtained from patient self-report rather than clinician judgment. Much like judging the comfort and quality of last night's sleep, the individual's own assessment is indispensable and inherently valid.

It is from this vantage point that we apply HRQL to the context of dermatology, focusing on HRQL assessment and issues of measurement in allergic contact dermatitis patients, citing examples obtained from our research. The reader will see that HRQL as-

---

The data reported in this chapter originate from research studies supported by Glaxo Wellcome, Inc., Research Triangle Park, North Carolina.

sessment resembles what is already performed in a focused patient interview by the dermatologist to obtain the patient's perspective. This useful tradition allows the clinician to understand the level of suffering experienced from the disease condition and to form qualitative appraisals about how much the patient has benefited from treatment. The value added from taking a formal approach to collecting this information is that the set of HRQL measures used have been tested and are sensitive to clinically important changes and that the scores can be compared within the scientific literature.

## II. HRQL ASSESSMENT IN DERMATOLOGY

The need to consider outcomes other than morbidity and mortality as a basis for comparing or evaluating therapies has pushed the development of HRQL from a ''soft'' outcome measure in clinical trials to a secondary or primary outcome of treatment. In dermatology, HRQL is a natural primary goal of treatment: the patient's perspective is valued because of the complexity that skin diseases may have on people's lives and not assessed in measures of skin disease severity. While the nature and extent of HRQL impairment from skin disease has not been systematically observed, it is known anecdotally from patients' comments that some may be profoundly affected involving physical discomfort, restricted movement, and weariness and distress, which, over time or with increased intensity may cascade as significant decrements in overall emotional well-being, social functioning, productivity at work or school, and sleep habits. Altered appearance may become a catalyst for further embarrassment or stigma.

    Another valuable role of HRQL assessment is to document benefits from treatment in terms of the patient's daily life. For example, what benefits may the patient realize from early identification and avoidance of the contact allergen that produces a skin rash? How can these benefits be described, and what treatments produce the largest momentum toward improved well-being in the shortest time period? These are only a few of the types of questions that HRQL assessment is designed to answer.

    Whether HRQL information is collected to examine treatment effectiveness among groups, perhaps in a clinical trial, or to assess individual patients' experiences for the purpose of planning treatment, the advantages of modern HRQL assessment are considerable.

1. The items have been chosen to cover aspects of day-to-day functioning that most patients care about relevant to their skin condition.
2. The items or scales in the instrument are useful in describing different dimensions of life impact from skin disease.
3. HRQL assessment supplements traditional disease severity measures, providing the clinician reliable data across patients from which patterns of impact from disease or benefits from treatment can be discerned over time.
4. HRQL assessment tools provide a systematic and scientific basis for evaluating the benefits of treatment.

## A. Advantage 1: Patient Relevance

While there exist several well-validated generic measures of HRQL developed expressly for use across diverse disease or illness groups (i.e., the MOS SF-36 [3] and the Sickness Impact Profile [4]), these instruments do not include many of the salient factors known to be associated with skin disease and which may respond to medical treatment. In order to identify and refine item content relevant to skin diseases, developers often begin with focus groups of patients and conduct several pretests of the items to remove rare or highly skewed items that provide little or no useful information. This first step is crucial to the subsequent testing steps and ensures that the end result—the data—are applicable to patients rather than to a ''generic'' model of HRQL. Table 1 displays the abbreviated item content of the Dermatology Specific Quality of Life (DSQL) questionnaire developed by the authors using the focus groups of dermatology patients as a starting point [5,6]. Later, the items were refined and tested for their applicability to specific dermatology disease groups (e.g., acne, contact dermatitis) in pilot studies.

## 1. Physical Symptoms

A common core of symptom items was identified, including sensations of soreness or tenderness, pain, itching, burning, and dry skin. A nonspecific item was included to capture other symptoms of physical discomfort.

**Table 1**  Selected Items from the Dermatology-Specific Quality-of-Life (DSQL) Questionnaire

---

I. Scale Items (item number)
  A. Symptoms. How often did the affected area(s) of your skin . . .
    (1) feel dryer than nonaffected areas, (2) feel sore/tender, (3) feel more oily,
    (4) feel painful, (5) feel itchy, (6) cause burning sensation, (7) cause other symptoms?
    How often did you (8) experience intervals of discomfort?
    How often did your discomfort cause you (9) to lose sleep or sleep badly?
  B. ADL. Because of your *skin condition*, how often did you limit yourself in . . .
    (11) participating in vigorous physical activity, (12) shaving/wearing makeup,
    (13) choice of clothes worn, (14) choice of hairstyle, (15) choice of food/beverage?
  C. Social functioning. How often did you feel that your *skin condition* limited your:
    (17) chances for making friends, (18) being comfortable in group activities,
    (19) freedom to do things you enjoy, (20) desire to be with friends, (21) desire to date,
    (22) extent of satisfaction with personal relationships,
    (23) readiness to go shopping/browsing, (24) dating habits/plans,
    (25) planned social activities, (26) time spent in the community?
  D. Work/school performance.
    (37) getting ahead at work/school, (38) getting a better job,
    (39) talking to coworkers/classmates, (40) being effective in meetings,
    (41) being effective in giving directions,
    (42) being punctual because of doctors appts,
    (43) being punctual due to physical or emotional discomfort?
  E. Personal perceptions. To what extent has your *skin condition* caused you to . . .
    (45) lack self-confidence, (46) feel frustrated, (47) feel embarrassed about appearance,
    (48) feel angry, (49) worry about what others think of you?
II. Global items (item number)
  On scale of 1 to 10 . . .
    (10) how bothered were you by any physical symptoms due to your *skin condition*?
    (16) how much did your *skin condition* interfere with grooming/styling?
    (27) how much did your *skin condition* interfere with your social activities?
    (44) how satisfied have you been with how others respond to you at work/school?
    (40) how satisfied have you been with your social life?
    (51) how satisfied have you been with your skin appearance?
    (50) how severe is your *skin condition* today?
    (53) how severe has your *skin condition* been in the last month?

---

## 2. Activities of Daily Living

Items included under this category involve self-care, such as grooming and physical appearance (hair style and clothes style) and participation in physical activity, which may affect skin (e.g., sweating).

## 3. Social Activities and Functioning

Core items in this scale pertain to disruptions of normal or desired social activities, time spent out in the community, chances for making new friends, and feeling comfortable in social settings.

## 4. Work/School

An additional aspect of social functioning affected by skin disease identified by patients was participation and interaction at work and/or school.

## 5. Self-Perceptions

Perhaps the most prominent HRQL impact reported by patients with skin disease is self-perception. Several studies have documented the effect of acne on attitudes about appearance and its profound effects on self-esteem. Item content developed for the DSQL instruments includes frustration about appearance, anger, embarrassment, and low self-confidence.

## 6. Global Items

Global items capture information about intensity of the HRQL impact that may not be captured in the clusters of scale items concerning frequency. Global ratings were developed for severity of distress from physical symptoms, interference with personal care and appearance, social activities, and behaviors at work or school. Overall ratings of satisfaction with skin appearance and severity of the skin problem today and in the last month were developed to assess self-rated HRQL associated with the skin condition.

## B. Advantage 2: More Than One Dimension of Health

Allergic skin diseases, from their potential to produce considerable physical discomfort through chronic irritation, soreness or tender skin, and itching, may affect various aspects of living. A sensitive HRQL instrument should be capable of describing which areas of life quality are affected and the intensity of the impact. It should monitor the complex benefits of treatment as well as address areas of HRQL limitations specifically in the treatment plan. Similarly, a medical treatment may benefit some aspects of HRQL more than others. This could occur if the treatment is not completely effective in controlling or curing the disease, or it could occur with a medication that produces unwanted effects such as discomfort or features that make compliance difficult or complex to achieve.

## C. Advantage 3: A Supplement to Disease Severity Measures

HRQL status, though correlated with disease severity, is capable of providing unique information about the patient's status. For example, if nearly all patients with severe skin disease also had high scores on a depression screener, such a measure of severity could reliably be further used to also indicate need for follow-up of the patient's probable psychological distress. In this case, although establishing the link with depression is an important result of HRQL assessment, routine use of the depression screener would add little new knowledge. However, because HRQL is a subjective phenomenon, reflecting factors unique to the individual, such high correspondence with severity measures is unlikely, and in practice only modest correlation coefficients (r = 0.20–0.40) are obtained [8,9].

## D.  Advantage 4: Reflects Improvements from Treatment

In addition to describing or characterizing life quality, another use of HRQL assessment is to detect changes in well-being resulting from treatment. This is referred to as the "responsiveness" of the measure. Though the validity of a measure may appear sound in cross-sectional analyses, it still may not perform well at detecting small but clinically meaningful changes over time. Thus, claims about the responsiveness of an HRQL measure should be based upon empirical data. In order to show responsiveness, quality-of-life changes can be compared to change in clinical status, intervening health events, interventions of known or expected efficacy, and direct reports of change by patients or providers. With sensitive and responsive measures, clinicians and researchers may draw conclusions about variations in treatment effectiveness and improved life quality among alternative treatments or identify practice characteristics that promote improved functioning. Such issues, for example, could include clinical treatment pathways, diagnostic skill, follow-up care, and patient self-management skills.

## III.  QUALITY OF LIFE IN ATOPIC DERMATITIS AND URTICARIA

The effect of urticaria and atopic dermatitis on a patient's quality of life may be more important than the pain and annoyance of having abnormal skin. While most clinicians assess the impact of skin disorders on the patient's life when making clinical decisions, not all incorporate the formal measurement of life quality into their decision-making process. This is unfortunate, because it has been shown by a number of studies [10–13] that distinct measures of life quality are necessary to adequately reflect a patient's state of well-being.

Atopic dermatitis is characterized as causing erythema, exudation, excoriation, dryness, cracking, and lichenification to appear on the head, neck, hands, elbows, feet, legs, and trunk of the body [11]. In addition to the physical discomfort exhibited by atopic dermatitis patients, considerable psychosocial disturbances are also known to occur [14]. Although the disease begins in infancy and can gradually improve throughout adolescence, some patients remain affected throughout their adult life. Despite the high incidence of this disease and the apparent psychosocial impact of atopic dermatitis, very little has been done to assess the life quality impairment.

Finlay and colleagues [11–13] have conducted much of the work in the area of life quality and atopic dermatitis. In the most comprehensive study, a multicenter, randomized, double-blind, controlled crossover clinical trial, Berth-Jones et al. [11] used the United Kingdom Sickness Impact Profile (UKSIP) and the Eczema Disability Index [15] to examine quality-of-life benefits from treatment of atopic dermatitis with cyclosporin. Results demonstrated significant improvement in life quality with cyclosporin, however, equally important, there was a lack of a relationship between the level of patients' health-related quality of life and clinical assessments of atopic dermatitis. This result demonstrated that objective clinical assessments may not adequately reflect a patient's state of well-being or the precise outcome of the intervention. Similar results were also found in an open and uncontrolled study [12] assessing the effect of cyclosporin on the life quality of both children stricken with atopic dermatitis and their parents. Significant improvements were found in terms of itching, soreness, pain, sleep, and extent of teasing for both children with atopic dermatitis and the parent's assessment of their child's life quality. Furthermore, the drug was also found to reduce the impact of the disease on the family as a whole.

Urticaria is characterized by short-lived, erythematous, cutaneous swellings due to transient dermal edema and vasodilation [16]. The wheals exhibited by this disorder are typically itchy and last less than 24 hours. However, among those with delayed-pressure urticaria, cutaneous erythema and subcutaneous edema occur between 30 minutes and 9 hours after the application of pressure to the skin [16]. The lesions, which can be provoked by walking, standing, sitting, or wearing tight clothing are itchy, painful, or burning and may last up to 48 hours. Urticaria patients often suffer considerable loss of energy and sleep and can be emotionally upset. Despite this fact, the impact of urticaria on the quality of life has been documented in the recent literature by only one study. O'Donnel and colleagues [10] assessed quality of life in patients with chronic urticaria and delayed-pressure urticaria. Using the Nottingham Health Profile [17] and an investigator-created disease-specific questionnaire, they found that urticaria patients suffered considerable loss of energy and sleep and were emotionally upset. Greater problems were found to be experienced by patients suffering from delayed-pressure urticaria compared with those having chronic urticaria solely, particularly in the areas of mobility, clothing, gardening, employment, hobbies, and pain. These results highlight the deprivation suffered by patients with chronic urticaria and delayed-pressure urticaria.

These studies suggest the necessity of assessing quality of life in patients with atopic dermatitis and urticaria. Quality-of-life measures, however, may be either general or specific. Measures such as the United Kingdom Sickness Impact Profile and SF-36 [3] were not designed to assess these diseases directly. However, generalized measures do allow researchers the advantage of providing data that can be compared with other skin diseases. Specific measures, such as the Eczema Disability Index (EDI) [15], the Dermatology Life Quality Index (DLQI) [18], and the Dermatology Specific Quality of Life (DSQL) instrument [5] have been used to describe the unique profile of quality of life with skin diseases.

## IV. QUALITY OF LIFE IN ALLERGIC CONTACT DERMATITIS

We have reported on the impact on allergic contact dermatitis on life quality and subsequent benefits from its timely treatment using patch-testing to make an early diagnosis of the allergen. The data were collected in an observational study of 565 patients with contact dermatitis recruited from 10 clinical centers in the United States. Patients who enrolled in the study had a suspicion of contact allergy and exhibited at least moderate disease activity (described in Refs. 6 and 7). The DSQL questionnaire for contact dermatitis was administered to all participants at baseline and during the scheduled 6- and 12-month follow-up assessments.

Figure 1 displays baseline means for the DSQL scale scores, categorized by level of frequency of bother or limitation in life quality. The items for ADL, Social, Work and

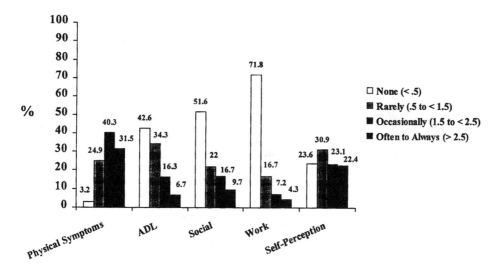

**Figure 1** Distribution of DSQL scale means in patients with allergic contact dermatitis (n = 565).

Self-Perceptions scales are scored on a Likert scale of 0–4, ranging from never bothered or limited (0) to always or constantly bothered or limited (4) during the last month. Mean scale scores are taken so that the scales may be compared. Results for the Symptoms scale, which asks about the frequency symptoms experienced, show that symptom burden is considerable in this sample, with approximately 31% reporting, on average, multiple symptoms at least "often" within the last month.

A full picture of the "severity" of this disease in terms of its impact on the patient's day-to-day life is evident by looking at the other DSQL scales (ADL Social, Work/School, and Self-Perceptions). Nearly one quarter (22.4%) of the study participants were afflicted with negative self-perceptions (e.g., embarrassment, lack of self-confidence, and frustration) at least often; social functioning was reported as often limited in 1 in 10 patients (9.7%). Performance of daily activities such as grooming, dressing, and bathing were limited in about 7%, attributed to contact dermatitis. For each scale content area, mild or intermittent limitations were common. Beyond its role in characterizing the impact of allergic skin disease on well-being, this information could help identify thresholds for clinically significant changes in disease condition by expressing change in terms of percent reduction in limitations in daily life and to examine the rate of improvement once treatment is initiated.

Figure 2 presents percentages of persons reporting being at least often limited or bothered in the DSQL instrument content areas by degree of symptom distress (intensity of symptoms) from ACD. Among patients reporting severe distress from symptoms (score > 7 on a scale of 1–10), a substantial proportion (23.7–64.4%) have frequent limitations in daily activities (ADL), social functioning, work, or school activities and negative self-perceptions. A clear gradient is evident for the level of distress and impairment in life quality from ACD. These data show that many ACD patients in our sample suffered from negative self-appraisals, and for some their skin disease has led to reductions in social functioning, daily activities, and work. The toll of these limitations in terms of lost wages,

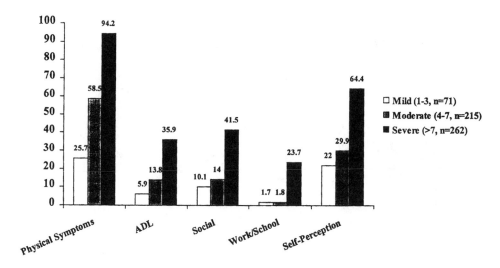

**Figure 2**  Percentage of persons with ACD reporting often or usually limited in HRQL, by level of symptom distress.

productivity, and satisfaction is untold but likely to be considerable. Clearing or controlling skin disease would potentially not only improve satisfaction with skin appearance and reduce bothersome symptoms, but would also improve functioning and well-being for many. Certainly, the benefit side of the ledger for the treatment of allergic skin disease should include societal value for improvements made in these important areas in addition to wage recovery and productivity issues.

Figure 3 presents the distribution of DSQL mean scores for participants who were

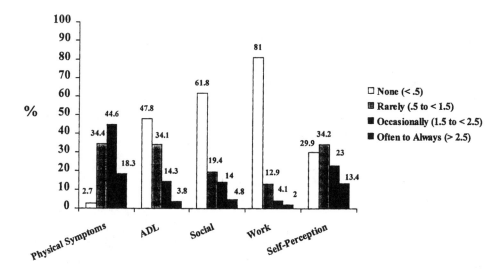

**Figure 3**  Distribution of DSQL scale means in patients with moderate to severe allergic contact dermatitis (n = 190).

classified as having moderate allergic skin disease. This determination of disease severity (as mild, moderate, or severe) was made based upon (1) percent of disease activity, (2) number of dermatitis-related physician visits, and (3) subject perceived severity. These data demonstrate the considerable heterogeneity in HRQL distress within this rather narrowly defined patient group. Although a large proportion have either no or only a modest level of distress on any one DSQL domain, appreciable proportions also experience more severe HRQL distress.

Table 2 presents DSQL mean change scores for patients with a history of chronic ACD who were not patch-tested with those who were patch-tested from the observational study of patch-testing with contact dermatitis described above. The decision to patch-test and choice of patch-test product or series were left entirely to the discretion of the dermatologist. After 6 months of study observation time, the DSQL was readministered to examine changes from the baseline period. The results show that patch-testing followed by relevant avoidance and appropriate treatment resulted in significantly greater improvement in quality of life described by the DSQL domains (except the test for Work/School scale, which was not statistically significant) than not patch-testing. This finding was obtained despite the fact that patients who were not patch-tested had, as a group, less severe ACD than those patch-tested. The magnitude of these changes range from 10 to 30% of the baseline means. The pathway to improved HRQL with patch testing was revealed in an additional analysis showing that patch-testing produced a shorter time to a confirmed diagnosis [7] than not patch-testing. The benefits in life quality, then, can be viewed in terms of the number of days, weeks, or months saved from diminished well-being.

Finally, DSQL mean change scores 12 months postbaseline are presented in Table 3. It is evident that, over the longer course, the patch-tested group has not experienced additional gains in life quality than were realized without patch-testing. Gains in quality of life among the non–patch-tested group, which were negligible at 6 months, have now caught up with the patch-tested group, who have largely maintained their HRQL improvements since the 6-month assessment. Since the added value of patch-testing was shown to be an earlier time to confirmed diagnoses [7], with the passage of time such an advantage from testing would predictably fade. This example illustrates the importance of considering both the time course of changes in life quality from treatment and the utility of valuing time averted from impaired life quality as a treatment outcome, similar to how we look at survival with life-threatening diseases. Relying solely on a 12-month outcome would

**Table 2** Comparison of Mean 6-Month Change (Δ) Score in DSQL Scales Between Patch-Tested and Non–Patch-Tested Groups with Chronic ACD

| DSQL scales | Non–patch-tested | | | Patch-tested | | | |
| --- | --- | --- | --- | --- | --- | --- | --- |
| | *n* | mean Δ | SE | *n* | mean Δ | SE | *p*-value |
| Physical symptoms | 74 | −0.71 | 0.11 | 62 | −0.98 | 0.16 | 0.157 |
| ADLs[a] | 72 | −0.18 | 0.10 | 56 | −0.56 | 0.11 | 0.009 |
| Social functioning | 75 | −0.19 | 0.09 | 60 | −0.54 | 0.14 | 0.034 |
| Work/School | 47 | −0.01 | 0.05 | 30 | −0.44 | 0.12 | 0.001 |
| Self-perceptions | 74 | −0.21 | 0.12 | 56 | −0.86 | 0.17 | 0.002 |
| Perceived severity[b] | 75 | −2.09 | 0.37 | 61 | −3.18 | 0.44 | 0.050 |

[a] Daily self-care activities.
[b] Self-reported severity on a scale of 1 to 10.

**Table 3** Comparison of Mean 12-Month Change (Δ) Score in DSQL Scales Between Patch-Tested and Non–Patch-Tested Groups with Chronic ACD

| DSQL scales | Non–patch-tested | | | Patch-tested | | | |
|---|---|---|---|---|---|---|---|
| | n | mean Δ | SE | n | mean Δ | SE | p-value |
| Physical symptoms | 52 | −0.71 | 0.14 | 53 | −0.82 | 0.14 | 0.536 |
| ADLs[a] | 50 | −0.30 | 0.10 | 53 | −0.38 | 0.12 | 0.586 |
| Social functioning | 51 | −0.32 | 0.09 | 52 | −0.38 | 0.14 | 0.700 |
| Work/School | 26 | −0.11 | 0.05 | 32 | −0.39 | 0.15 | 0.144 |
| Self-perceptions | 49 | −0.39 | 0.15 | 51 | −0.57 | 0.16 | 0.426 |
| Perceived severity[b] | 52 | −1.98 | 0.43 | 53 | −2.98 | 0.40 | 0.090 |

[a] Daily self-care activities.
[b] Self-reported severity on a scale of 1 to 10.

have completely missed the important gains in life quality among the patch-tested group. Adding up, as the utility scientists do, all of the quality-adjusted life-years added (assuming that a treatment produces an average 6-month gain) would result in many years of quality of life gained. Of course, the economic value of these gains will depend upon the cost differential between treatments and what society is willing to pay to achieve these gains; without HRQL assessment, many of these treatment benefits will be hidden, without valuation. Assessing HRQL aids the clinician in determining the most beneficial treatment in terms of patient outcomes, providing a mechanism for valuing the patient's subjective experiences in the treatment decision process.

## V. HOW TO SELECT AN HRQL INSTRUMENT FOR CLINICAL PRACTICE OR RESEARCH

Generally, clinical uses of HRQL in office practice require briefer measures. They are self-administered and include information familiar to health-care providers demonstrated to predict level or duration of need for health services. In contrast, research uses, such as for clinical trials, often have different emphases, including discriminability of relatively small treatment differences relative to a comparison group. When selecting an HRQL measure for allergic dermatitis sample of patients, it is best to look for instruments that have been used in similar samples. It is not always clear whether an instrument validated for one skin disease will demonstrate its original psychometric properties in another disease, age, or even ethnic group. Perhaps a term in popular usage no less abused than "quality of life" is the one "validated." An instrument is not "validated" as if a trait, rather evidence about the validity of an instrument is collected and evaluated by the scientist as to its adequacy for a specific use and purpose. An instrument that is suitable for psoriasis may be completely unsuitable for acne or contact dermatitis.

### A. Standards for Reliability

A reliability level of 0.90 was advocated as a minimum standard for measurement designed for interpretation of scores at the individual level [19]. This recommendation stems from the fact that the standard error of measurement is about one third of the measure's standard deviation if it has a reliability of 0.90 (standard error of measurement is estimated by the product of the measure's standard deviation and the square root of the difference between 1.0 and the reliability of the measure). Although the confidence interval around an individual patient's score is wider than one might like, the interval is still tighter than that based on no information at all [20]. Clinicians need to be aware of the extent of unreliability in all of their measures and interpret them with appropriate caution. For group comparisons, in randomized clinical trials and other clinical studies, reliabilities exceeding 0.70 are acceptable. The standard for reliability of measures is less stringent than it is for individual assessment because different groups of people (e.g., patients who receive or do not receive patch-testing after unsuccessful treatment for contact dermatitis) are compared rather than individuals [20]. Ideally, test-retest and internal consistency reliability testing should be considered in evaluating an instrument.

## B. Validity

Validity of a scale reflects how well it measures what it is intended to measure. The distinction between reliability and validity is important because a measure may be reliable (i.e., always yield the same score for the same patient), but it may be consistently measuring the wrong thing (i.e., not what it is supposed to measure). While demonstrating reliability in measurement is essentially accumulating evidence of the existence of a stable property over repeated measurement, validity is an estimation of the extent to which an instrument measures what it was intended to measure. The key question for validity evidence is whether the scale is valid for a particular application and a specific population.

The assessment of validity normally begins with an assessment of content validity and then proceeds with an evaluation of construct validity and responsiveness of the scale to clinically meaningful changes in HRQL.

An optimal instrument covers a range of content within the core concept area of physical, emotional, and social well-being. Next, the instrument should combine the information in a way that is meaningful to the user. A central issue is whether only negative components of HRQL should be assessed. Do the hypotheses about HRQL effects from treatment include more than just the absence of negative effects? Could positive experiences result from treatment?

Construct validity and responsiveness are key psychometric criteria for measures used in clinical trials. Construct validity is essentially evidence that the concept of interest is being measured according to our preformed notions about what life quality is—and isn't. This means that we define quality of life and then suggest hypotheses that would provide evidence of whether or not our assumptions are correct. For example, since we expect that disease severity drives HRQL, we expect that an HRQL instrument should be capable of differentiating between mild and moderate disease activity. We also might expect that certain features of life quality may be affected more than others (e.g., physical functioning vs. psychological distress). We also need to say what our HRQL instrument should *not* be a measure of—such as personality traits or social standing, etc. Sometimes hypotheses are made about the structure of the items (one scale vs. several subscales) that can be tested using factor analysis. The user of a quality-of-life scale should carefully review the validity evidence of an instrument to determine whether it demonstrates adequate validity according to what the developer intended or how it has been used in practice.

## VI. DISCUSSION

The effects of skin diseases on people's lives are complex, such as psychological stress, embarrassment, stigma, and physical discomfort. If it is worthwhile to have this information in patient care or research, it is critical to employ valid and reliable measures. These states are not measurable by any known objective clinical indicator. Since successful treatment in terms of total alleviation of all or even some of the disease effects on life quality for many conditions is difficult, a key advance in developing a matrix for quality of life is that information can be integrated across domains of functioning and used to understand how manipulation of one aspect of life quality from treatment would affect other aspects. For each problem area, specific treatment strategies may be developed with the patient in a care-management plan.

This brief chapter describes a rationale for assessing life quality outcomes and provides examples that illustrate the effects that allergic skin disease can have upon its sufferers. Data presented from the DSQL were not intended as much to highlight the benefits of patch-testing as they are to highlight the complexity of changes in life quality that are brought about from effective treatment. The concept of "cascading benefits" apply to managing ACD. Much more than reducing frequency of symptoms, treatment effectiveness can be described in terms of better social functioning, easier self-care, and less psychological distress. In the data reported above, the gains in life quality were quite noticeable for some persons, while others seemed less affected by their disease. The nature of life quality is that it is subjective and varies uniquely on an individual basis. Despite this fact, those with severe disease activity have more decrements in life quality from their skin disease than those with mild disease; those who received an effective diagnostic procedure had larger improvements in quality of life than their counterparts. Another benefit of HRQL assessment is to monitor any untoward, unwanted side effects from medications. If the application of more intensive medical interventions could produce unwanted side effects, this probability must be weighed against the known probability of any gains in life quality from clinical trials. Obviously, the more information there is about the magnitude of improvement in life quality and which patient groups respond most favorably, the more precision there will be in selecting an effective therapy that can deliver the treatment goals valued by the patient. In clinical studies, it is important to profile both the effectiveness and time course of HRQL outcomes in order to value the benefits for treatment against costs. Without HRQL analyses, a treatment may be undervalued by society or become discounted.

## VII. CONCLUSION

Only in the past decade or so has HRQL been used as a major outcome in clinical trials of therapeutic interventions to differentiate among medications, dosages, or regimens in terms of costs and benefits to the patient and the value added to society. In dermatology, it is only recently that HRQL has been broadly included in clinical studies and descriptive research. There are still too few studies describing the impact of allergic skin disease on HRQL, and it will be beneficial to devote more studies to both the impact of skin diseases on life quality and the application of this knowledge to improving care.

# REFERENCES

1. World Health Organization. Constitution of the World Health Organisation. Geneva: WHO, 1947.
2. Berzon R, Shumaker S. International use, application and performance of health-related quality of life instruments. In: Shumaker S, Anderson RT, eds. International Use Application and Performance of Health-Related Quality of Life Instruments. J Qual Life Res (special issue).
3. Ware JE, Sherbourne C. The MOS 36-Item Short-form Health Survey (SF-36): I. Conceptual framework and item selection. Med Care 1992; 30:473–483.
4. Bergner M, Bobbitt RA, Carter WB, et al. The Sickness Impact Profile: Development and final revision of a health status measure. Med Care 1981; 19:787–805.
5. Anderson RT, Rajagopalan R. Development and validation of a quality of life instrument for cutaneous diseases. J Am Acad Dermatol 1997; 37:41–50.
6. Rajagopalan R, Anderson RT. A profile of patients with contact dermatitis with suspected allergy (history, physical characteristics and quality of life). Am J Contact Dermatitis 1997; 8(4):215–212.
7. Rajagopalan R, Anderson RT, Sarma S, Retchin C, Jones J. The use of decision-analytical modeling in economic evaluation of patch testing in allergic contact dermatitis. Pharmacoeconomics 1998; 14(1):79–95.
8. Finlay AY. The Dermatology Life Quality Index. Initial experience with a practical measure. In: Rajagopalan R, Sherertz E, Anderson RT, eds. Care Management of Skin Diseases: Life Quality and Economic Impact. New York: Marcel Dekker, 1998; pp. 85–94.
9. Anderson RT, Rajagopalan R. Responsiveness of the DSQL instrument to treatment for acne vulgaris in a placebo-controlled clinical trial. J Qual Life Res 1998; 723–734.
10. O'Donnel BF, Lawlor F, Simpson J, Morgan M, Greaves MW. The impact of chronic urticaria on the quality of life. Br J Dermatol 1997; 136:197–201.
11. Berth-Jones J, Finlay AY, Zaki I, Tan B, Goodyear H, Lewis Jones S, Cork MJ, Bleehen SS. Cyclosporin in severe childhood dermatitis: a multicenter study. J Am Acad Dermatol 1996; 34(6):1016–1021.
12. Salek MS, Finlay AY, Luscombe DK, Allen B, Berth-Jones J, Camp RDR, Graham-Brown RAC, Khan G, Marks R, Motley RJ. Cyclosporin greatly improves the quality of life of adults with severe atopic dermatitis. A randomized, double-blind, placebo-controlled trial. Br J Dermatol 1993; 129:422–430.
13. Finlay AY. Measurement of disease activity and outcome in atopic dermatitis. Br J Dermatol 1996; 135:509–515.
14. Shuster S, Fisher GH, Harris E, Binnell D. The effect of skin disease on self image. Br J Dermatol 1978; 99(suppl. 16):18–19.
15. Eun HC, Finlay AY. Measurement of atopic dermatitis disability. Ann Dermatol 1990; 2:9–12.
16. Greaves MW. Chronic urticaria. N Engl J Med 1995; 332(26):1767–1772.
17. Hunt S, McKenna SP, Williams J. Reliability of a population survey tool for measuring perceived health problems: a study of patients with osteoarthritis. J Epidemiol Commun Health 1981; 35:297–300.
18. Finlay AY, Kahn G. Dermatology Life Quality Index (DLQI)—a simple practical measure for routine clinical use. Clin Exp Dermatol 1994; 19:210–216.
19. Nunnally J. Psychometric Theory. 2d ed. New York: McGraw-Hill, 1978.
20. Hays RD, Anderson R, Revicki D. Psychometric considerations in evaluating health-related quality of life measures. J Qual Life Res 1993; 2:441–450.

# 20

## Evaluation of Allergic Contact Dermatitis

**Yung-Hian Leow**
*National Skin Centre,*
*Singapore, Singapore*

**Howard I. Maibach**
*University of California School of Medicine,*
*San Francisco, California*

## I. INTRODUCTION

Allergic contact dermatitis is the prototype clinical manifestation of a type IV delayed-type inflammatory reaction arising from percutaneous contact with putative allergens. It should be differentiated from sensitization, which refers to the immunological response upon first contact with the allergen. It is not clinically apparent and is considered as the afferent pathway of the contact reaction.

In most clinical circumstances, allergic contact dermatitis can be easily recognized by both patient and physician. Classical features of eczema, namely itch, erythema, blisters, and swelling after direct contact with the incriminating agent on the affected site, are clues to an overt allergy. Good examples would be allergic contact dermatitis to Rhus or poison ivy and nickel in costume jewelry. The clinical diagnosis is straightforward, and testing is thus rarely required.

However, occult or covert allergic contact dermatitis to an assortment of environmental allergens may not be clinically apparent, as when the circumstances in which the rash appears do not point to an apparent specific inciting agent. This is true in circumstances when the person is later found to be allergic to a specific ingredient that has been added to a complex product. Good examples would be fragrances, preservatives, or sunscreens that have been incorporated into cosmetics/skin care products; or rubber chemicals, like accelerators, that can be found in occupational-related personal protective equipment, like rubber gloves. Another clinical illustration where the source of the putative allergen is unclear would be an airborne contact dermatitis. Thus the logarithmic and systemic approach to solving a clinical problem of suspected contact dermatitis requires detailed history taking, meticulous physical examination, a high index of suspicion, and relevant investigation.

## II. TESTING METHODS

Good clinical skills, namely, detailed history taking and thorough physical examination, are imperative in the initial assessment and evaluation in approaching a clinical case of possible allergic contact dermatitis.

### A. Clinical Presentation

A selective and probing history is a prerequisite in arriving at the final diagnosis. Detailed questioning should include contact history, occupational history, hobbies, effects of vacation, topical medications, cosmetics, drugs, previous atopic skin disorders, known allergies, and family history of skin disease. The temporal relationship between the initial contact with the putative allergen, onset of rash, and the site of the dermatitis are important clues to establish a provisional working diagnosis that facilitates the investigative process.

Distribution and the appearance of the skin lesions are leading clues to the cause or possible cause for the rash. Classical sites of skin involvement that may suggest an endogenous or compounding endogenous dermatitis should be looked for in the general physical examination, like the presence of flexural eczema. Nonetheless, history and physical examination do not supersede the investigation, but provide the necessary basic framework for the physician to plan the investigative approach to solving the clinical problem.

### B. Patch-Testing

Patch testing is the time-tested investigative tool that has been studied for more than 100 years since Jadassohn first introduced this testing method in 1895 [1]. It is at present the only practical test for demonstrating suspected contact allergy. The procedure basically attempts to reproduce an acute eczema by applying the suspected allergens onto the skin to ascertain the clinical suspicion.

### C. Indications

Some of the indications for patch-testing include the following: confirmation of clinically diagnosed case of contact dermatitis, determination of the exact allergen to which the patient is clinically suspected to be allergic, detection of relevant but clinically unsuspected contact sensitizers, predictive testing for materials that the patient is able to tolerate, and need to unravel a perplexing clinical problem.

### D. The Procedure

The current system of patch-testing in use in most dermatological institutions has largely been standardized by experts in the field through numerous years of experiment and discussion. In the classical closed patch-testing, it involves the epicutaneous application of suspected allergens incorporated in a suitable vehicle, which are then placed in position with the aid of a suitable device and adhesive tape on intact skin for 48 hours [2–4]. The reaction is evaluated after 48, 72, or 96 hours or 1 week later. The midportion of the upper back is the preferred site, though the upper outer arm may be used in some circumstances. The patch test unit that is in use in most clinical circumstances is the Finn Chamber, which is essentially a shallow aluminum cup holding the test material. The virtually nonsensitizing and low-irritancy Scanpor® tape (Norgesplaster A/S Norway) is a popular choice as the occluding tape. For the convenience of patch testers, there are commercially available allergens dispersed in an appropriate vehicle. Petrolatum is the preferred and most often used diluent because most materials are soluble, stable, nonirritating, and well dispersed in it. Other vehicles also in use include alcohol, olive oil, acetone, and water. Information on appropriate dilutions of different chemicals can be found in referenced textbooks [2–6]. However in situations where the patch test concentration of a ''new'' material is encountered, the lowest concentration that does not irritate or sensitize will be appropriate. Concentrations of 0.1–1.0% are preferred. Serial dilutions and testing in adequate controls may be required to establish the validity of testing with such unfamiliar materials.

## E. Patch-Test Materials

Over the past millennium, eminent patch-testers from different parts of the world have contributed the experience through scientific publication. They have identified and compiled the most commonly occurring allergens into a list of standard series. Obviously, the standard series of allergens may not be entirely applicable for physicians practicing in different parts of the world where social and cultural differences contribute to minor differences in the exposure pattern to environmental agents. A shortened ''minimal international standard series'' has been recently proposed by the International Contact Dermatitis Research Group (ICDRG) [7] (Table 1).

**Table 1** Proposed Allergens for a Modified International Standard Series[a]

| Allergen | % |
| --- | --- |
| 1. Potassium dichromate | 0.5 |
| 2. Neomycin sulfate | 20 |
| 3. Thiuram mix | 1 |
| 4. *p*-Phenylenediamine base (PPD) | 1 |
| 5. Formaldehyde | 1 (aq.) |
| 6. Colophony | 20 |
| 7. Balsam of Peru | 25 |
| 8. Wool (lanolin) alcohols | 30 |
| 9. Mercapto mix | 1 |
| 10. Epoxy resin | 1 |
| 11. *p-tert*-Butylphenol-formaldehyde (BPF) resin | 1 |
| 12. Fragrance mix | 8 |
| 13. Nickel sulfate ($NiSO_4.6H_2O$) | 2.5 |
| 14. Mercaptobenzothiazole (MBT) | 1 |
| 15. Budesonide | 0.1 |
| 16. Quaternium 15 | 2 |
| 17. Cl + Me-isothiazolinone | 0.01(aq.) |
| 18. Imidazolidinyl urea | 2 (aq.) |
| 19. Tixocortol pivalate | 1 |
| 20. Dibromodicyanobutane | 0.1 |

[a] Concentrations refer to petrolatum unless otherwise stated.
*Source*: Adapted from Ref. 7.

**Table 2** Sources of Patch Test Materials
and Related Items

---

Hermal Pharmaceutical Laboratories, Inc.
Route 145
Oak Hill, NY 12460
OmniDerm Inc/Pharmascience
8400 Ch. Darnley Rd
Montreal, Quebec H4T 1M4
Canada
Dormer Laboratories Inc.
6600 Trans Highway
Suite 750
Pointe Claire, Quebec H9R 4S2
Canada
Chemotechnique Diagnostics AB
Ringugnsgatan 7
S-216 16 Malmo
Sweden
Hermal Kurt Herrmann
Patch Test Allergens
PO Box 1228
D-2057 Reinbeck bei Hamburg
Germany
TRUE Test™
Glaxo Dermatology
Five Moore Drive
PO Box 134
Research Triangle Park, NC 27709

---

Additional special series listing the key allergens prepared in the appropriate concentration and vehicle are commercially available for different clinical situations and for evaluation for contact dermatitis occurring in different occupations (Table 2).

## F.  Pitfalls of the Conventional Patch-Test System

Patch-testing is not perfect. The patch-tester should be aware of the frequent encounters with possible false-positive and false-negative results [8].

   False-positive irritant results can arise in the following situations: excessively high test concentration, excessive amount of test material, uneven dispersion of test material in the vehicle, presence of active dermatitis, excited skin without visible dermatitis, and pressure artifact from test material or irritation from the tape or test unit. Excited skin syndrome or angry back syndrome refer to the peculiar situation where in testing with various test materials, nonspecific cutaneous hyperirritability arises as a result of multiple false-positive test reactions [9].

   False-negative reactions occur in the following situations: negligible test concentra-

**Table 3** Assessment of Clinical Relevance

1. History of exposure to the sensitizer
   Occupational exposure
   Nonoccupational exposure (homework, hobbies)
   Use of pharmaceutical products (over-the-counter and prescription), cosmetics, clothing,
      jewerly, bandages (especially when intolerance is referred)
   Type of exposure: dose, frequency, site
   Environmental conditions: humidity, temperature, occlusion, vapors, powders, photo-
      exposure
2. Clinical characteristics of the dermatitis
   Dermatitis area corresponding to the exposure site
   Some morphologies suggest specific allergens
   Clinical course (caused or aggravated by the exposure)
3. Correlation with other tests
   Positive patch test to a product
   Positive patch test to a product's extract
   Positive provocation use test (PUT) or repeated open application test (ROAT): twice daily
      application to small test area for 7 days
   Positive use test (typical product use)
4. Reproduction or aggravation of dermatitis by the patch test or use tests

*Source*: Adapted from Ref. 10.

tion or amount of test material, inappropriate vehicle, missed delayed patch-test reaction, refractory clinical state of the skin, and inappropriate test for photo-contact allergy.

## G. Relevance of Patch-Test Reactions

Interpretation of a positive patch-test requires sound judgment, as it may not be relevant to the patient's clinical problem. Generally, the reaction will be scored as being of present relevance (complete or partial), past relevance, or unknown or no relevance. Very often, the clinical relevance of a positive patch-test reaction may become clinically apparent in the course of exploring possible occult source of allergen exposure during the follow-up visits. Strict criteria may be required for accurate interpretation of patch test reactions [10,11] (Tables 3–5).

**Table 4** Suggested Guidelines for the Assessment of Relevance

Requestion the patient in light of the test results.
Show the patient a list of products containing the allergen (sometimes, he/she
   will be able to recognize the source of exposure).
Seek cross-reacting substances.
Consider concomitant and simultaneous sensitization.
Repeat the patch test with dilution, test with extracts, Use test, PUT, ROAT, test
   in vitro.
Use "lists" of allergens for specific occupations.
Obtain information from the product's manufacturer.
Perform chemical analysis of products.

*Source*: Adapted from Ref. 10.

**Table 5** Operational Definition of Allergic Contact Dermatitis

1. Appropriate morphology
2. Positive patch test
3. Repatch test—when appropriate—to rule out excited skin syndrome and "rogue" reactions
4. Provocative use test (PUT), repeated open application test (ROAT), or use test
5. Serial dilution patch testing (when indicated)
6. Review reliability of irritant control for not commonly utilized allergens

*Source*: Adapted from Ref. 11.

## H. Provocative Usage Test (Repeated Open Application Test)

The provocative usage test (PUT) is sometimes required in certain clinical situations to confirm the relevance of a particular positive or negative reaction. It basically requires the patient to apply the product twice daily to a small test site of the antecubital fossa or forearm for 7 days [12]. It is also known as repeated open application test (ROAT). It is particularly useful in the evaluation of allergy to cosmetic products.

## I. TRUE Test™

Patch-testing is currently the most established method to verify a suspected case of allergic contact dermatitis. However, it is fraught with technical inadequacy, especially the rather unsatisfactory pharmaceutical preparation of the test material. The TRUE test (thin-layer rapid use epicutaneous test) is a standardized, ready-to-use patch-test system that overcomes some of the inconsistencies of the traditional patch-test system [13,14]. The allergens are incorporated in hydrophilic gels, which are then coated on water-impermeable sheets of polyester. They are mounted on nonwoven cellulose tape with acrylic adhesive, covered with siliconized plastic, and encased in an air-tight and light-impermeable envelope. Upon direct contact with the skin, perspiration hydrates the film and transforms it into a gel, which then releases the allergens. The advantages of this test system are multiple, namely the ease of handling by physicians, comfort to the patients, exact dosage, stability of the test substances, consistent panel-to-panel location, and reproducibility of test results. Studies have verified the high accuracy and high quality of the TRUE test system [15,16]. The commercial preparation of this new test system probably serves the general purpose of patch-testing to the standard series of allergens. However, this test system does not replace the conventional patch-test system with Finn Chamber and Scanpor® tape, as the latter is still the benchmark by which investigative work is measured, not withstanding the more competitive cost of the conventional patch-test system. Furthermore, clinical investigation that involves testing with a multitude of additional and unusual patch test allergens still requires the conventional patch-test system. TRUE test probably serves as a screening tool and remains as an adjunct to the conventional patch-test system.

## III. CONCLUSION

Over the past decade, noninvasive bioengineering methods offer an alternative method to "read" the skin in turmoil. However, a traditional systematic logarithmic approach to a clinical problem, which involves history, physical examination, and investigation is pertinent, crucial, and probably irreplaceable in the management of allergic contact dermatitis.

Patch-testing will survive as the investigative tool for the study of delayed-type IV hypersensitivity to topically applied materials for the next millennium, though there may be a need to further refine and explore newer methods of detecting contact allergy.

## REFERENCES

1. Foussereau J. History of epicutaneous testing. The blotting paper and other methods. Contact Dermatitis 1984; 11:219–223.
2. Cronin E. Contact Dermatitis. Edinburgh: Churchill Livingstone, 1980.
3. Adams RM. Occupational Skin Disease. 2d ed. Philadelphia: Saunders, 1990.
4. Rietschel RL, Fowler JF, Jr. Fisher's Contact Dermatitis. 4th ed. Baltimore: Williams & Wilkins, 1995.
5. Foussereau J, Benezra C, Maibach HI. Chemical and Clinical Aspects of Occupational Dermatology. Copenhagen: Munksgaard, 1982.
6. De Groot AC. Patch Testing. Test Concentrations for 3700 Chemicals. Netherland: Elsevier, 1994.
7. Lachapelle J-M, Ale SI, Freeman S, Frosch PJ, Goh CL, Hannusela M, Hayakawa R, Maibach HI, Wahlberg JE. Proposal for a revised international standard series of patch tests. Contact Dermatitis 1997; 36:121–123.
8. Fregert S. Manual of Contact Dermatitis. 2d ed. Copenhagen: Munksgaard, 1981.
9. Bruynzeel DP, Maibach HI. Excited skin syndrome (angry back). Arch Dermatol 1986; 122: 323–328.
10. Ale SI, Maibach HI. Clinical relevance in allergic contact dermatitis. An algorithmic approach. Derm Beruf Umwelt 1995; 43:119–121.
11. Marrakchi S, Maibach HI. What is occupational contact dermatitis? An operational definition. Clin Dermatol 1994; 12:477–483.
12. Hannuksela M. Sensitivity of various skin sites in the repeated open application test. Am J Contact Dermatitis 1991; 2:102–104.
13. Fischer T, Maibach HI. The thin layer rapid use epicutaneous test (TRUE-test), a new patch test method with high accuracy. Br J Dermatol 1985; 112:63–68.
14. Fischer T, Maibach HI. Easier patch testing with TRUE test. J Am Acad Dermatol 1989; 20: 447–453.
15. Lachapelle JM, Bruynzeel DP, Ducombs G, Hannuksela M, Ring J, White R, Wilkinson J, Rischer T, Billberg K. European multicenter study of the TRUE Test™. Contact Dermatitis 1988; 19:91–97.
16. Ruhnek-Forsbeck M, Fischer T, Meding B, Pettersson L, Stenberg B, Strand A, Sunberg K, Svensson L, Wahlberg JE, Widstrom L, Wrangsjo K, Billberg K. Comparative multi-center study with TRUE test™ and Finn chamber® patch test methods in eight Swedish hospitals. Acta Derm Venereol (Stockh) 1988; 68:123–128.

# 21

## Role of Food Allergens

**Scott H. Sicherer and Hugh A. Sampson**
*Mount Sinai School of Medicine,*
*New York, New York*

## I. INTRODUCTION

A number of acute and chronic skin disorders result from an immunological response to specific proteins in foods. These immunological responses are termed ''allergies'' [1], and the resulting skin manifestations include urticaria, atopic dermatitis (AD), contact dermatitis, and dermatitis herpetiformis. In contrast to food-allergic responses, adverse skin reactions to foods can occur on a nonimmunological basis. Examples of these adverse reactions (intolerances) include erythema from skin contact with irritants in citrus and tomatoes [2], urticaria caused by ingestion of histamine elaborated from ''spoiled'' dark meat fish (scombroid fish poisoning), urticaria resulting from direct mast cell histamine release following ingestion of certain food dyes or additives, and vasodilatation from neurogenic reflexes induced by tart foods [3]. These latter reactions will not be discussed in detail here, but must be maintained on the differential diagnosis for food-related skin disorders.

Allergic hypersensitivity responses to food can be divided into IgE-mediated and non–IgE-mediated reactions. The role of IgE-mediated skin reactions to foods is well established [4,5]. Individuals who are genetically predisposed to allergies make increased amounts of specific IgE antibody to particular food proteins to which they are exposed [6]. These antibodies bind to high-affinity IgE receptors on mast cells found in body tissues, basophils circulating in the bloodstream, and Langerhans cells in the skin [7]. Following ingestion of a causal food protein, IgE antibodies specific for allergenic epitopes on the protein are cross-linked, resulting in release of mediators (histamine) and cytokines from mast cells and basophils. Following the ingestion of causal food proteins, acute urticaria and pruritis may occur; while continued, frequent ingestion in sensitized individuals may result in AD or chronic urticaria. The pathophysiology of non–IgE-mediated immunological responses to food proteins is not completely understood, but involves mechanisms mediated by T cells. Non–IgE-mediated skin disorders include dermatitis herpetiformis [8] and a subset of patients with food-sensitive AD [9]. This chapter will describe the allergic skin diseases in which food allergy plays a role and will review the modes of diagnosis, treatment, and natural history of food allergies as they apply to skin disease.

## II.  ATOPIC DERMATITIS

The causal link between food allergy and AD has been the focus of controversy [2]. However, a large and increasing body of evidence indicates that food allergy plays a pathogenic role in AD for at least a subset of patients, particularly children. A large number of studies implicate immunological mechanisms in the pathogenesis of AD. Most studies support the role of IgE-mediated reactions with food-induced responses apparent within 2 hours after oral challenge following a period of dietary elimination [4,5,10,12]. Other studies have reported delayed eczematous responses after such food challenges [9], implying non–IgE-mediated mechanisms [13,14]. The following discussion will explore the evidence for, and methods employed in evaluating, the role of food allergy in AD.

### A.  Historical Evidence

By the turn of the twentieth century, physicians were suggesting that reactions to food proteins could cause eczematous skin rashes. In 1915, Schloss [15] presented several case reports of patients who experienced improvement in their eczema after avoiding specific foods. Shortly thereafter, Talbot [16] and then Blackfan [17] each described a series of patients who had positive allergic skin tests to certain foods and experienced clearing of their skin when the foods were removed from their diets. In a series of experiments, Walzer and colleagues [18,19] demonstrated that ingested food antigens penetrate the gastrointestinal barrier and are transported in the circulation to mast cells in the skin. To demonstrate this, 65 normal adults were passively sensitized by intracutaneous injection of serum from a patient with severe fish allergy and from a normal control [18]. The following day, the volunteers were fed fish: 61 of 65 developed a wheal and flare reaction within 90 minutes at the sensitized site but not the control site. In 1936, Engman et al. [20] reported a child with AD and allergy to wheat. To demonstrate the role of scratching and rubbing in the development of eczema, they admitted the patient to the hospital when his skin was clear and wrapped one arm and leg in a thick bandage. The child was given two wheat crackers, and within 2 hours he experienced pruritus and began scratching. The following morning the boy had typical eczematous lesions, except under the bandages where the skin remained clear. Taken together, these studies conducted over 60 years ago clearly showed that ingested food allergens were readily accessible to cutaneous mast cells and the "skin-associated lymphoid tissue" and that in the sensitized host they could produce intense pruritus, scratching, and rubbing which led to typical eczematous lesions.

### B.  Challenge Studies

Over the past 25 years, researchers have performed oral food challenges to characterize the relationship of food allergy and AD. In the late 1970s, Hammar reported the induction of eczematous skin lesions in 15 of 81 hospitalized children less than 5 years of age after 2–3 days of ingesting 100 ml of milk daily [21]. The significance of these findings was questioned, however, because the challenges were done openly and a repeat challenge 18 months later produced similar symptoms in only 4 of 15 patients [22]. In their studies of children primarily with suspected food hypersensitivity and respiratory allergy, May and Bock et al. [23] reported that 4 of 7 children with a history of eczematous reactions to foods developed skin rashes within 2 hours of administration of a double-blind, placebo-controlled oral food challenge (DBPCFC). The DBPCFC has become the "gold standard" for the diagnosis of food allergy. Patients undergoing DBPCFCs are tested while not taking antihistamines, after their skin has undergone intensive therapy to induce a stable baseline in the hospital, and after they have strictly eliminated the food to be tested from their diet for over 7 days. Using DBPCFCs, the author (H. A. Sampson) has systematically studied 470 patients referred for evaluation of AD, as reviewed below. Burks et al. [4] also employed the DBPCFC to study 165 children with mild to severe AD presenting to a university allergy clinic. As seen in other controlled oral challenge studies, positive DBPCFCs resulted in cutaneous, respiratory, and gastrointestinal symptoms. Sixty percent of the patients with AD had a positive prick skin test to at least one of seven foods tested (milk, egg, peanut, soy, wheat, codfish, cashew). The patients underwent a total of 266 DBPCFCs and 64 (38.7% of the total group with AD) were food allergic. There was no correlation between the likelihood of having a positive food challenge and the severity of the AD.

In the past 18 years, the author's studies have addressed the etiological role of IgE-mediated food hypersensitivity in AD by utilizing DBPCFCs [5,24–27]. In the initial evaluation of 470 children with AD fulfilling the criteria of Hanifin and Rajka [28], a total of 1776 DBPCFCs were conducted. DBPCFCs were not conducted in 193 instances because clinical history indicated a "convincing" account of a major anaphylactic reaction (mostly to peanuts and nuts). History was considered "convincing" when a patient experienced severe respiratory symptoms (laryngeal edema and/or wheezing) and/or hypotension within minutes of ingesting an isolated food and requiring emergency care by a physician. In each case where the challenge was not performed, the patients had a markedly positive prick skin test to the food in question. No patient experienced a severe anaphylactic reaction during DBPCFC, although about one half of the patients required oral diphenhydramine for severe pruritus and several patients required subcutaneous epinephrine for respiratory symptoms. Subjects ranged in age from 3 months to 24 years with a median age of 4.1 years. Family history was positive for atopic disease in 91% of subjects. One hundred and fifty-seven patients (39%) had allergic rhinitis and asthma at the time of initial evaluation, and only 94 (20%) had neither allergic rhinitis nor asthma. Serum total IgE concentration was elevated in 376 (80%) patients with a median of 3410 IU/ml and a range of 1.5–45,000 IU/ml.

Of the 1776 DBPCFCs performed, 714 were positive and 1062 were interpreted as negative. Cutaneous reactions developed in 529 cases (74%) and consisted of a pruritic, erythematous, macular, or morbilliform rash primarily in previous predilection sites for AD. Symptoms confined exclusively to the skin occurred in 30% of the reactions. Typical urticarial lesions were rarely seen and generally consisted of only a few lesions. Intense pruritus and scratching frequently resulted in superficial excoriations and occasionally bleeding. Gastrointestinal symptoms (abdominal pain, vomiting, diarrhea) were seen in 358 of the reactions (50%) even though a history of gastrointestinal symptoms was rarely elicited from the patients. Respiratory symptoms (nasal congestion/rhinorrhea, sneezing, throat tightness, wheezing) most frequently involved the upper respiratory tract and were seen in 322 of the positive DBPCFCs (45%).

Symptoms during DBPCFCs generally developed between 5 minutes to 2 hours of initiating the challenge. Symptoms associated with the immediate response were generally abrupt in onset and lasted 1–2 hours. Several patients experienced a second episode of increased cutaneous pruritus and transient morbilliform rash 6–10 hours after the initial positive challenge. Symptoms associated with the late response were less prominent than the immediate symptoms and tended to last for several hours. Only one child (3 years of age) developed an isolated "delayed" reaction; a pruritic, erythematous rash developed approximately 4 hours after the child ingested egg. Such "delayed" reactions have been reported by others [9,13]. These blinded studies and others [4,12,29], along with previous unblinded studies, have established that cutaneous symptoms are invoked by ingestion of causal food proteins in children with AD. It is important to note that positive challenges often induced a morbilliform rash rather than a typical eczematous lesion. This morbilliform eruption likely represents the early phase of AD and is induced in these challenges by acute ingestion of a food previously causing symptoms on a chronic basis.

## C.  Studies of Dietary Elimination

The therapeutic effect of removing foods to which children with AD are allergic has been addressed in a number of studies. Atherton et al. [30] reported that two thirds of children with AD between the ages of 2 and 8 years showed marked improvement during a double-blind crossover trial of egg and milk exclusion. The trial was conducted over a 12-week period in the patients' homes. In this study, 45% of the patients enrolled dropped out or were excluded from analysis, environmental and other triggers of AD were not controlled for, and a significant order effect was found, all raising some question about the authors' conclusions. Utilizing a similar trial design, Neild et al. [31] were able to demonstrate improvement in some patients during the milk and egg exclusion phase, but overall no significant difference was seen in 40 patients completing the crossover trial. Juto and colleagues [32] reported that 7 of 20 infants with eczema healed and 12 of 20 improved on a highly restricted elimination diet. Nonblinded challenges to cow's milk reportedly resulted in increased itching and rash in 12 of 20 infants. Hill and Lynch [33] treated 8 children with severe AD with an elemental formula for 2 weeks followed by the addition of two vegetables and two fruits for 3 months. All patients experienced improvement in their eczema while on the diet and relapsed within weeks of discontinuing it. While supporting a role for food allergy in the exacerbation of AD, most of these studies fail to control for other trigger factors, placebo effect, or observer bias.

In a prospective follow-up study [11] of 34 patients with AD, 17 children with food allergy who were appropriately diagnosed and placed on an allergen-elimination diet experienced a marked and significantly greater improvement in their eczematous rash at 1–2 and 3–4 year follow-up than 12 similar patients who did not have food allergy and 5 children with food allergy who did not adhere to the diet. In a blinded, prospective study, Lever and colleagues [34] performed a randomized controlled trial of egg elimination in young children with AD and positive RAST to egg (majority under age 2 years) who presented to a dermatology clinic. At the close of the study, egg allergy was confirmed by oral challenge, and 55 egg-allergic children were ultimately identified. A physician blinded to the dietary instructions evaluated the children. There was a significant decrease in area affected (19.6% to 10.9%, $p = 0.02$) and symptom scores (33.9 to 24.0, $p = 0.04$) in the children avoiding egg compared to controls (percent involved 21.9% to 18.9%; symptom score 36.7 to 33.5). Further studies utilizing blinded diet protocols are in progress.

The potential therapeutic effect of dietary avoidance in infants at risk to develop AD and other atopic diseases has also been the focus of study. Several investigators have evaluated the effect of eliminating certain foods from the maternal diet during lactation [35–38]. In two series, infants from atopic families whose mothers excluded egg, milk, and fish from their diets during lactation (prophylaxis group) had significantly less AD and food allergy at 18 months compared to infants whose mothers' diets were unrestricted

[38,39]. Follow-up at 4 years showed that the prophylaxis group had less AD, but there was no difference in food allergy or respiratory allergy [39]. In a prospective nonrandomized study of 1265 unselected neonates, the effect of solid food introduction was evaluated over a 10-year period [40,41]. A significant linear relationship was found between the number of solid foods introduced into the diet by 4 months of age and subsequent AD, with a threefold increase in recurrent eczema at 10 years of age in infants receiving four or more solid foods compared to infants receiving no solid foods prior to 4 months of age. A prospective, nonrandomized study comparing breast-fed infants who first received solid foods at 3 months or 6 months of age, revealed reduced AD and food allergy at 1 year of age in the group avoiding solids for the 6-month period [42] but no significant difference in these parameters at 5 years [43]. Since neither series randomized patients, these studies must be considered suggestive until an appropriate randomized trial confirms the benefit of delaying solid food introduction.

In a comprehensive, prospective, randomized allergy-prevention trial, Zeiger and colleagues compared the benefits of maternal and infant food allergen avoidance on the prevention of allergic disease in infants at high risk for allergic disease [44–47]. Breast feeding was encouraged in both prophylaxis and control groups. In the prophylaxis group, the diets of lactating mothers were restricted of egg, cow milk, and peanut, a casein hydrolysate formula was utilized for supplementation or weaning, and solid food introduction was delayed. The control infants received cow's milk formula for supplementation, and the American Academy of Pediatrics' recommendations for infant feeding were followed (peanuts, nuts, and fish are not recommended in the first 2 years). The prevalence of AD and food allergy in the prophylaxis group was reduced significantly during the first 2 years compared to the control group. However, the period prevalence of AD was no longer significantly different beyond 2 years. These investigators concluded that maternal and infant food allergen avoidance reduce food allergy and AD in the first 2 years but fail to modify allergic disease after 2 years of age. Consequently these investigators felt that the benefits of food allergy preventative measures are of limited duration because of the frequent remission of food allergy in early childhood [45]. As a group, these studies clearly show the link between dietary allergens and the clinical manifestations of AD.

## D. Laboratory Investigations/Pathophysiology

Laboratory evaluations of patients with AD have provided further evidence for the role of IgE-mediated hypersensitivity and immunological responses to food proteins in the pathogenesis of this illness. Although the histological appearance of eczematous lesions has suggested a classical type IV, cell-mediated hypersensitivity reaction in the pathogenesis of AD [48], further studies of the "late-phase" IgE response following allergen-induced mast cell activation have shown that the terminal stages of IgE-mediated hypersensitivity reactions are characterized by infiltration of lymphocytes and monocytes [49,50]. Approximately 4–8 hours after initial cutaneous mast cell activation, neutrophils and eosinophils infiltrate the dermis in subjects without AD. Biopsies obtained 8 hours after initiation of the reaction revealed 48% lymphocytes, 27% eosinophils, 9% neutrophils, and 7% monocytes while lymphocytes predominate at 1–2 days [49]. Although histological studies initially suggested that the eosinophil (the cell type typically seen at the site of chronic allergic inflammation) was not present in AD lesions, immunocytochemical studies have demonstrated extensive deposition of eosinophil-derived extracellular major basic protein (MBP) in AD lesions but not in normal-appearing skin from affected patients or in lesions of contact dermatitis [51]. In addition, increased numbers of activated eosino-phils have been demonstrated in chronic AD lesions but not in acute lesions or normal-appearing skin [52]. One explanation for the development of this infiltrate is that it represents the chronic stages of a "late-phase" response in eczematous skin following the "immediate-phase" allergic response characterized by the IgE-mediated release of cutane-ous mast cell mediators that recruit and activate these cells.

The pattern of cytokine expression found in lymphocytes infiltrating skin lesions in AD has been studied using in situ hybridization and also represents an allergic immunolog-ical milieu. Infiltrating T lymphocytes in acute AD lesions express predominantly the Th2 cytokines, IL-4, IL-5, and IL-13, while T cells in chronic lesions express predominantly IL-5 and IL-13 [52,53]. This is in contrast to classic type IV cellular responses, where cells express primarily IFN-$\gamma$ (Th-1 cells) [54]. This Th2 profile of cytokines promotes chronic allergic inflammation by upregulating adhesion molecules on vascular endothelial cells, upregulating high-affinity receptors for IgE antibodies on Langerhans cells and other antigen-presenting cells, recruiting eosinophils and other inflammatory cells to the site, and promoting local synthesis of IgE antibodies. High-affinity receptors for IgE on Langer-hans cells, through bound IgE, play a special role as "nontraditional" receptors on these antigen-presenting cells [55]. These IgE-bearing Langerhans cells are 100- to 1000-fold more efficient at presenting allergen to T cells (primarily Th2 cells) and activating T-cell proliferation [7,56].

A number of lines of evidence support the role of food allergy in these immunologi-cal responses. Patients with AD generally have elevated levels of total [57] and food protein–specific IgE [25]. Positive oral food challenges are accompanied by sharp in-creases in plasma histamine concentrations [58], activation of plasma eosinophils [59], and elaboration of eosinophil products [60]. In addition, patients with IgE-mediated milk-induced skin symptoms possess allergen-specific, cutaneous lymphocytes antigen (CLA)–bearing T cells in their circulation, which are not present in patients with milk-induced gastrointestinal disease [61] or asthma. Food-antigen specific [62] (and aeroallergen-spe-cific [63]) T cells have been cloned from active skin lesions of AD. Food antigen–specific T cells have been routinely identified from peripheral blood in subjects with relevant food protein–induced AD [61,64,65]. Some workers have correlated specific food-induced, late-onset (increased rash developing at least 2 hours after oral challenge) AD with in vitro lymphocyte proliferative responses to the implicated food [66]. However, other work-ers have found an increased lymphocyte proliferative response to relevant food proteins also in patients with immediate reactions [64], and the use of this test as a diagnostic modality is limited since there is great overlap in individual proliferative responses [67].

Mechanisms involving IgE molecules, other than direct IgE allergen activation of cutaneous mast cells, also may be involved in the inflammation of eczematous skin. Chil-dren with AD and food hypersensitivity who were chronically ingesting foods to which they were allergic were found to have high "spontaneous" basophil histamine release (SBHR) from peripheral blood basophils in vitro compared to patients with AD without food allergy or to normal controls (mean: 35.1 $\pm$ 3.9% vs. 1.8 $\pm$ 0.2% vs. 2.3 $\pm$ 0.2%; $p < 0.001$) [68]. When the food-allergic children were placed on an appropriate elimina-tion diet for at least one year, they experienced good clearing of their eczema and a signifi-cant fall in SBHR (38.0 $\pm$ 9.6% to 4.3 $\pm$ 2.1%; $p < 0.01$). Peripheral blood mononuclear cells from food-allergic subjects with high SBHR were found to elaborate cytokines termed histamine-releasing factors (HRFs) that could activate basophils from food-sensitive, but not food-insensitive, children. It has been established that several isoforms of IgE are secreted [69]. It has been postulated that some isoforms of IgE interact with HRFs. Passive sensitization experiments using basophils from nonatopic donors and IgE from food-allergic patients revealed that these basophils could be rendered sensitive to HRF [68]. Passive transfer of IgE from nonallergic individuals did not render the basophils sensitive to HRF.

## E.  Prevalence of Food Allergy in Atopic Dermatitis

The prevalence of food allergy in patients with AD varies with the age of the patient and the severity of the rash. Using DBPCFCs, Sampson and McCaskill implicated food allergy in 60% of a selected population of children with AD referred for the evaluation of food allergy [5]. Burks and colleagues [29], also utilizing DBPCFCs, diagnosed food allergy in 33% of 46 children with mild to severe AD from a population enrolled in part from a dermatology clinic (15 patients) and the remainder from referrals to the allergy clinic. In a larger study of 165 children with AD referred to the allergy clinic, Burks and colleagues diagnosed food allergy in 38.7% [4]. Because of a possible bias in ascertainment of these patients referred to the allergist, Eigenmann and colleagues [27] evaluated 63 unselected children with moderate to severe AD (median age 2.8 years; range, 0.4–19.4 years) who were referred to a university dermatologist. These children were evaluated with oral food challenges, and 37% were diagnosed with food allergy (95% confidence interval, 25–50%). The above studies did not stratify patients by severity [27,29] or demonstrate a direct relationship between severity of AD and the presence of food allergy [4]. However, Guillet and Guillet [70] evaluated 250 children with AD and noted that increased severity of AD and younger age of patients were directly correlated with the presence of food allergy. Most childhood food allergies are outgrown [71], although children with moderate to severe AD tend to have more persistent food allergy. Studies in adults with severe AD are very limited and have not shown a significant role for food allergy [72] or success in reducing symptoms during trials of antigen-free diets [73].

## III.  URTICARIA

Urticaria is characterized by pruritic, transient, erythematous raised lesions with central clearing, sometimes accompanied by localized swelling (angioedema). Urticaria is arbitrarily defined as chronic, as opposed to acute, when the lesions continue to appear for over 6 weeks [74]. Food allergy accounts for 20% [75] to 57% [76] of acute urticaria and is mediated by specific IgE to food protein. Lesions usually occur within minutes and rarely beyond an hour of ingestion of, or contact with, the causal food [77,78]. In some cases, the acute urticaria is a part of a more dramatic multiorgan system reaction that may include respiratory, gastrointestinal, and even cardiac manifestations. In contrast to acute urticaria, food allergy plays a very limited role in patients with chronic urticaria, only 1.4% [79] to 2.2% [80] of patients. In a study limited to children with chronic urticaria, the cause was attributed to food in 4% and food dyes in 2.6% [81] of 226 children studied. Thus, a rigorous search for a causative food in the initial evaluation of chronic urticaria is not generally recommended.

## IV. CHRONIC HAND DERMATITIS

Chronic allergic hand dermatitis due to direct, prolonged skin contact with foods is primarily an occupational disorder among food handlers [82,83]. Skin edema, erythema, vesiculation, and lichenification characterize this disorder. The pathophysiology of the disorder is not completely understood. In general terms, contact dermatitis is considered to be a T-cell–mediated immune reaction. However, in chronic hand dermatitis caused by foods, patch tests with causal foods are often negative while prick skin tests are positive [82–84]. Thus, the disorder may represent an immediate-type hypersensitivity response in most patients. Both skin prick and patch tests may be needed to help identify the causal food. Eliminating contact with the food, usually with barriers such as latex-free gloves or the use of utensils, allows resolution of the rash.

## V. DERMATITIS HERPETIFORMIS

Dermatitis herpetiformis is an uncommon, chronic papulovesicular skin disorder in which lesions are distributed symmetrically over the extensor surfaces of the elbows, knees, and buttocks [85]. Biopsy of perilesional skin reveals granular IgA deposits in the basement membrane and neutrophilic microabscesses at the dermal papillary tips. The disorder is associated with a specific immune sensitivity to gluten [86] but is not an IgE-mediated sensitivity. Although the disorder is associated with small intestinal villous atrophy (celiac disease, gluten-sensitive enteropathy), there are often no associated gastrointestinal complaints [8]. The rash and associated small bowel villous blunting often resolves with the elimination of gluten from the diet.

## VI. DIAGNOSIS OF FOOD ALLERGY

### A. General Approach

In the case of acute reactions, such as acute urticaria or, rarely, flaring of AD, the history may clearly implicate a particular food. In a chronic disorder such as AD, however, it is more difficult to pinpoint causal food(s) from the history. Several factors complicate the diagnosis of food allergy in AD: (1) the immediate response to ingestion of causal foods is downregulated with repetitive ingestion; (2) various environmental factors (other allergens, irritants, infection) may play a role in the waxing and waning course of the rash, obscuring the effect of dietary changes; and (3) patients have a propensity to generate IgE to multiple allergens. A general approach to the diagnosis of food allergy in patients with AD is presented in Figure 1. A thorough history is obtained, and tests for IgE (skin prick tests or RASTs) are performed as indicated. It must be appreciated that most children with AD have positive prick skin tests to several foods, but only about one third of positive skin tests correlate with positive food challenges [5,11]. Another important point to consider is that although virtually any food protein can cause a reaction, only a small number of foods account for over 90% of reactions [4,5,12] (Table 1). In children, the most common foods causing reactions are egg, milk, peanut, soy, wheat, tree nuts, and fish [4,5,12], and in children with AD and food allergy, two thirds are reactive to egg [87]. In adults, peanut, tree nuts, fish, and shellfish are most frequently implicated [88,89]. Although many reports have suggested that children with AD are sensitive to a large number of foods,

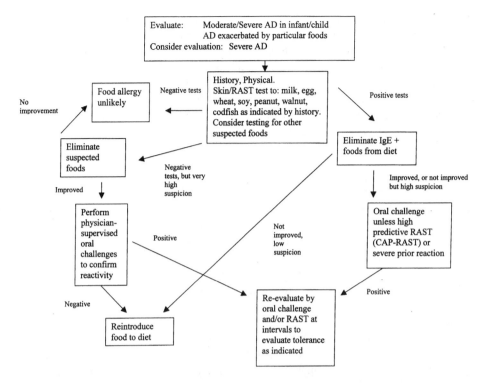

**Figure 1** Scheme for evaluation of food allergy in AD. Double-blind, placebo-controlled food challenges should be used when multiple common foods are implicated; open or single-blind challenges may be used when screening few foods. Oral food challenges should be performed under physician supervision, and foods should be reintroduced under physician supervision if there is any risk for a severe reaction. See text for details. CAP-RAST-Pharmacia CAP System FEIA.®

most patients (80–99%) diagnosed by DBPCFC developed symptoms to only one to three foods [4,11]. A rational approach is to screen children with moderate to severe AD for allergy to egg, milk, peanut, soy, wheat, fish, and a tree nut (walnut, cashew) using prick tests or RAST [4,27], with additional testing for any other suspected foods. When there is a history suggestive of food-related skin disease and tests for IgE antibody to the food

**Table 1** Common Food Allergies

| Infants | Children | Older children/adults |
|---|---|---|
| Cow's milk | Cow's milk | Peanut |
| Egg | Egg | Tree nuts |
| Peanut | Peanut | Fish |
| Soy | Soy | Shellfish |
| | Wheat | |
| | Tree nuts (cashew, walnut, etc.) | |
| | Fish | |
| | Shellfish | |

are positive, the first course of action is to completely eliminate all forms of the suspected food from the diet. Further initial testing is usually not needed in cases of severe, acute reactions or if dramatic improvement occurs. However, if symptoms are chronic as with AD and/or if a large number of foods are implicated, it is generally necessary to perform diagnostic oral food challenges. In addition, certain food additives have been documented to cause the same types of reactions as those caused by IgE-mediated responses (asthma, urticaria, AD, etc.) but with a much lower prevalence [90–92]. Since these reactions are generally not IgE mediated, diagnosis requires trials of dietary elimination and oral challenge testing.

## B. Skin and In Vitro Testing

In the evaluation of AD and acute urticaria, specific tests can help identify, or exclude, suspected foods. One method to determine the presence of specific IgE antibody is prick-puncture skin testing. After the patient has discontinued antihistamines for a sufficient length of time, a device such as a bifurcated needle or lancet is used to puncture the skin through a glycerinated food extract and appropriate positive (histamine) and negative (saline-glycerin) controls. A local wheal and flare response indicates the presence of food-specific IgE antibody. Prick skin tests are most informative when they are negative since the negative predictive value of the tests is very high (over 95%) [10,93]. Unfortunately, the positive predictive value is on the order of under 50% [10,93]. Thus, a positive skin test in isolation cannot be considered proof of clinically relevant food hypersensitivity, while a negative test virtually rules out IgE-mediated food allergy to the food in question. Intradermal allergy skin tests with food extracts give an unacceptably high false-positive rate and a greater risk for adverse reactions to testing and should not be used [93]. The proteins in commercial extracts of some fruits and vegetables are prone to degradation, so fresh extracts of these foods are more reliable [94].

Although slightly less sensitive than prick skin tests, in vitro tests for specific IgE antibodies (RAST) are more practical than prick skin tests in the screening of food allergy in most office settings, can be used while the patient is taking antihistamines, and do not depend on having an area of rash-free skin for testing. Like skin tests, a negative result is very reliable in ruling out an IgE-mediated reaction to a particular food, but a positive result has low specificity. A study by Sampson and colleagues [95] compared the results of DBPCFCs in 196 patients to the levels of food-specific IgE antibody obtained using the Pharmacia CAP System FEIA (reported in kU/liter). As shown in Table 2, levels of food-specific IgE indicating the positive (PPV) and negative (NPV) predictive values for the test were calculated. For egg, milk, peanut, and codfish, levels above which clinical reactivity was highly likely (> 95% PPV) were obtained. Thus, patients with concentrations of food-specific IgE above these values would be likely to react upon ingestion of the food and would not necessarily need further evaluation. An oral challenge would be needed to confirm reactivity for children with levels falling below the 90 or 95% PPV.

While patients frequently have positive skin tests and RASTs to several members of a botanical family or animal species, indicating immunological cross-reactivity, very few patients have symptomatic intrabotanical or intraspecies cross-reactivity. Legume cross-reactivity was evaluated in 69 children with AD utilizing prick skin tests, RASTs, and Western blot analyses [96,97]. Extensive immunological cross-reactivity was demonstrated in many patients. However, only two patients were symptomatic to more than one

**Table 2** Positive Predictive Value (PPV) and Negative Predictive Value (NPV) of Food-Specific IgE Concentrations (kU/liter) for Predicting Reactions Upon Oral Challenge[a]

| Food | >95% PPV | >90% PPV | >95% NPV | >90% NPV |
|------|----------|----------|----------|----------|
| Egg | 6 | 2 | — | 0.6 |
| Milk | 32 | 23 | 0.8 | 1.0 |
| Peanut | 15 | 9 | Best NPV = 85% at <0.35 kU/liter | |
| Fish | 20 | 9.5 | 0.9 | 5 |
| Soy | Best PPV = 50% at 65 kU/liter | 2 | | 5 |
| Wheat | Best PPV = 75% at 100 kU/liter | 5 | | 79 |

[a] No relationship between IgE level and severity.

legume when challenged orally. Both patients had a history of severe allergic reactions to peanut and mild reactions to a soy challenge. In addition, both "outgrew" their reactivity to soy in 1–2 years. Similar studies with cereal grains showed significant IgE antibody cross-reactivity but little (about 20%) clinical cross-reactivity [98]. In our experience, about 50% of egg-allergic children have IgE antibodies to chicken meat but few (about 5%) have clinical reactivity; similarly, about 50% of milk-allergic children have a positive skin prick test or RAST to beef but only about 10% exhibit clinical symptoms. Because of increased severity of reactions and greater possibility of misidentifying similar foods, consideration should be given to eliminating certain "food families" such as shellfish, fish [99,100], and tree nuts [101] once an allergy to one type of these foods is identified. However, the practice of avoiding all foods within a botanical family when one member is suspected of provoking allergic symptoms generally appears to be unwarranted.

As noted above, some workers have documented late-onset eczematous reactions to foods. Studies using both skin prick tests and patch testing with foods have been undertaken by Isolauri and Turjanmaa and have shown value in identifying patients with these late reactions [9], children with immediate reactions generally had positive skin prick tests, while those with late reactions were more likely to have positive patch tests to the relevant foods. Further studies with patch testing are needed to confirm these results prior to making general recommendations. Tests such as measurement of IgG$_4$ antibody, provocation-neutralization, cytotoxicity, and applied kinesiology, among other unproven methods, are not useful [102].

## C. Oral Food Challenges

DBPCFCs are considered the "gold standard" for diagnosing food allergy [10,12,103]. The procedure is labor intensive but can be modified to an office setting [103]. Patients avoid the suspected food(s) for at least 2 weeks, antihistamines are discontinued according to their elimination half-life, and asthma medications are reduced as much as possible. Children with moderate to severe AD usually require several days of in-hospital topical skin care including hydrating baths, moisturizers and topical steroids [104], and, in some cases, antibiotics [105], to establish a clear baseline before challenges. Intravenous access is necessary in some cases prior to challenges. Medical supervision and immediate access to emergency medications, including epinephrine, antihistamines, steroids, inhaled beta-agonists, and equipment for cardiopulmonary resuscitation, are required since reactions can potentially be severe. The authors and colleagues generally perform two challenges each day, one containing the test food antigen and one containing placebo. The taste of the food is camouflaged so the patient is unaware of the contents of the challenge substance. Over a 60- to 90-minute period, up to 10 g of dehydrated powdered food is administered in 100–150 ml of liquid such as juice, blenderized food, or infant formula. The initial challenge dose is generally 100–500 mg and is increased in a stepwise fashion at 10- to 15-minute intervals until the entire 10 g is consumed or a reaction occurs. Each challenge is evaluated and scored using a standardized symptom sheet [26]. Negative challenges are always confirmed with open feedings of larger, meal-sized portions of the food. Patients are also observed for delayed reactions.

If allergy to only a few foods is suspected, single-blind or open challenges may be used to screen for reactivity. These challenges, of course, are subject to observer and patient biases and may overestimate true reactivity. Oral challenges should usually not be performed when there is a clear, recent history of airway reactivity or if there was a history of a severe reaction. The practice of instructing patients to perform "home challenges" should not be undertaken since potentially severe reactions can result [106].

## VII. TREATMENT OF FOOD ALLERGY

In addition to medical management of the manifestations of food allergy (e.g., topical therapy for AD, antihistamines for urticaria), the mainstay of treatment for food allergy is dietary elimination of the offending food. The elimination of food proteins is a difficult task, and incomplete elimination of an incriminated food can lead to confusing results during trials of dietary elimination. In a milk-free diet, for example, patients must be instructed to not only avoid all milk products, but also to read ingredient labels for key words that may indicate the presence of cow's milk protein. Terms such as casein, whey, lactalbumin, caramel color, and nougat may, for example, signify the presence of cow's milk protein. When vague terms such as "high-protein flavor" or "natural flavorings" are used, it may be necessary to contact the manufacturer to determine if a particular protein, such as milk caseinate, is an ingredient. Examples of words used in food labeling are shown in Table 3.

Patients and parents must also be made aware that the food protein, as opposed to sugar or fat, is the ingredient being eliminated. For example, lactose-free milk contains cow's milk protein, and many egg substitutes contain chicken egg proteins. Conversely, peanut oil and soy oil generally do not contain allergenic food protein unless the processing method is one in which the protein is not completely eliminated (as with cold-pressed or "extruded" oil) [107].

Elimination of a particular food can be more difficult than expected. For example, a utensil used to serve cookies both with and without peanut butter can contaminate the peanut-free cookie with enough protein to cause a reaction. Similarly, when a food without cow's milk or peanuts is processed using the same commercial equipment used for making cow's milk–or peanut-containing food, contamination can occur. Hidden ingredients can also cause a problem. For example, egg white may be used to glaze pretzels or peanut butter may be used to seal the ends of egg rolls. The Food Allergy Network (Fairfax, VA;

**Table 3**  Reading Food Labels

1. Milk: artificial butter flavor, butter, butter fat, buttermilk, casein, caseinates (sodium, calcium, etc.), cheese, cream, cottage cheese, curds, custard, Half&Half®, hydrolysates (casein, milk, whey), lactalbumin, lactose, milk (derivatives, protein, solids, malted, condensed, evaporated, dry, whole, low-fat, nonfat, skim), nougat, pudding, rennet casein, sour cream solids, sour milk solids, whey (delactosed, demineralized, protein concentrate), yogurt. MAY contain milk: brown sugar flavoring, natural flavoring, chocolate, carmel flavoring, high protein flour, margarine, Simplesse®.
2. Egg: albumin, egg (white, yolk, dried, powdered, solids), egg substitute, eggnog, gloublin, livetin, lysozyme, mayonnaise, maringue, obalbumin, ovomucin, ovomucoid, Simplesse®.
3. Wheat: bread crumbs, bran, cereal extract, cracker meal, enriched flour, farina, gluten, graham flour, high gluten flour, high protein flour, malt, vital gluten, wheat bran, wheat germ, wheat gluten, wheat starch, whole wheat flour, spelt. MAY contain wheat: gelatinized starch, hydrolyzed vegetable protein, modified food starch, modified starch, natural flavoring, soy sauce, starch, vegetable gum, vegetable starch.
4. Soy: hydrolyzed vegetable protein, miso, shoyu sauce, soy (flour, grits, nuts, milk, sprouts), soybean (granules, curd), soy protein (concentrate, isolate), soy sauce, textured vegetable protein (TVP), tofu. MAY contain soy: hydrolyzed plant protein, hydrolyzed soy protein, hydrolyzed vegetable protein, natural flavoring, vegetable broth, vegetable gum, vegetable starch.
5. Peanut: cold pressed peanut oil, ground nuts, mixed nuts, Nu-Nuts® artificial nuts, peanut, peanut butter, peanut flour. MAY contain peanut: African, Chinese, Thai, and other ethnic dishes, baked goods (pastries, cookies, etc.), candy, chili, chocolate candy, egg rolls, hydrolyzed plant protein, hydrolyzed vegetable protein, marzipan, nougat.

800-929-4040) is a lay organization that provides educational materials to assist families, physicians, and schools in the difficult task of eliminating allergenic foods and in approaching the treatment of accidental ingestions. When multiple foods are eliminated from the diet, it is prudent to enlist the aid of a dietitian in formulating a nutritionally balanced diet.

In addition to elimination of the offending food, an emergency plan must be in place to treat severe reactions (respiratory reactions, anaphylaxis) caused by accidental ingestions. Although anyone may, theoretically, experience a severe allergic reaction, the individuals at higher risk appear to be those with previous severe reactions, underlying asthma [108], and allergy to peanuts, tree nuts, fish, or shellfish [89,101,108–111]. Injectable epinephrine and oral antihistamine should be readily available to treat patients at risk for severe reactions. The prompt administration of epinephrine at the first signs of a severe reaction must be emphasized since delayed administration of epinephrine has been associated with reports of fatal and near-fatal food-allergic reactions [108]. Caregivers must be taught the indications for the use, method of administration of these medications, and the need to seek immediate medical attention in the event of a reaction.

## VIII. NATURAL HISTORY

Most children outgrow their allergies to milk, egg, wheat, and soy [71]. However, patients allergic to peanuts, tree nuts, fish, and shellfish are much less likely to lose their clinical reactivity [88,89,109,112–114], and these sensitivities may persist into adulthood. Approximately one third of children with AD and food allergy "lost" (or "outgrew") their clinical reactivity over 1–3 years with strict adherence to dietary elimination, believed to have aided in a more timely recovery [11]. Elevated concentrations of food-specific IgE may indicate a lower likelihood of developing tolerance in the subsequent few years [115,116]. However, prick skin test results do not correlate with loss of clinical reactivity and remain positive for years after the food had been reintroduced into the diet [11]. Thus, it is recommended that patients be rechallenged intermittently (e.g., egg: every 2–3 years; milk, soy, wheat: every 1–2 years; foods other than peanut, nuts, fish, and shellfish: every 1–2 years) to determine whether their food allergy persists so that restriction diets may be discontinued as soon as possible. The immunological change associated with loss of symptomatic food hypersensitivity is under intensive study. While food allergy and AD may resolve, these infants and children are, unfortunately, likely to develop other allergic sensitivities and atopic diseases. Approximately 90% of children with AD and egg-specific IgE antibody develop asthma and respiratory allergies [117].

## REFERENCES

1. Bruijnzeel-Koomen C, Ortolani C, Aas K, Bindslev-Jensen C, Bjorksten B, Noneret-Vautrin D, Wuthrich B. Adverse reactions to food. Position paper. Allergy 1995; 50:623–635.
2. Hanifin JM. Critical evaluation of food and mite allergy in the management of atopic dermatitis. J Dermatol 1997; 24:495–503.
3. Sicherer SH, Sampson HA. Auriculotemporal syndrome: a masquerader of food allergy. J Allergy Clin Immunol 1996; 97:851–852.
4. Burks AW, James JM, Hiegel A, Wilson G, Wheeler JG, Jones SM, Zuerlein N. Atopic dermatitis and food hypersensitivity reactions. J Pediatr 1998; 132:132–136.
5. Sampson HA, McCaskill CC. Food hypersensitivity and atopic dermatitis: evaluation of 113 patients. J Pediatr 1985; 107:669–675.
6. Geha RS. Regulation of IgE synthesis in humans. J Allergy Clin Immunol 1992; 90:143–150.
7. Mudde G, van Reijsen F, Boland G, de Gast G, Bruijnzeel P, Bruijnzeel-Koomen C. Allergen presentation by epidermal Langerhan's cells from patients with atopic dermatitis is mediated by IgE. Immunology 1990; 69:335–341.
8. Egan CA, O'Loughlin S, Gormally S, Powell FC. Dermatitis herpetiformis: a review of fifty-four patients. Ir J Med Sci 1997; 166:241–244.
9. Isolauri E, Turjanmaa K. Combined skin prick and patch testing enhances identification of food allergy in infants with atopic dermatitis. J Allergy Clin Immunol 1996; 97:9–15.
10. Sampson HA, Albergo R. Comparison of results of skin tests, RAST, and double-blind, placebo-controlled food challenges in children with atopic dermatitis. J Allergy Clin Immunol 1984; 74:26–33.
11. Sampson HA, Scanlon SM. Natural history of food hypersensitivity in children with atopic dermatitis. J Pediatr 1989; 115:23–27.
12. Bock SA, Atkins FM. Patterns of food hypersensitivity during sixteen years of double-blind, placebo-controlled food challenges. J Pediatr 1990; 117:561–567.
13. Hill DJ, Firer MA, Shelton MJ, Hosking CS. Manifestations of milk allergy in infancy: clinical and immunological findings. J Pediatr 1986; 109:270–276.
14. Isolauri E, Virtanen E, Jalonen T, Arvilommi H. Local immune response measured in blood lymphocytes reflects the clinical reactivity of children with cow's milk allergy. Pediatr Res 1990; 28:582–586.
15. Schloss OM. Allergy to common foods. Trans Am Pediatr Soc 1915; 27:62–58.

16. Talbot FB. Eczema in childhood. Med Clin North Am 1918; 1:985–996.
17. Blackfan KD. A consideration of certain aspects of protein hypersensitiveness in children. Am J Med Sci 1920; 160:341–350.
18. Brunner M, Walzer M. Absorption of undigested proteins in human beings: the absorption of unaltered fish protein in adults. Arch Intern Med 1928; 42:173–179.
19. Wilson SJ, Walzer M. Absorption of undigested proteins in human beings. IV. Absorption of unaltered egg protein in infants. Am J Dis Child 1935; 50:49–54.
20. Engman WF, Weiss RS, Engman MF. Eczema and environment. Med Clin North Am 1936; 20:651–663.
21. Hammar H. Provocation with cow's milk and cereals in atopic dermatitis. Acta Dermato Vener (Stockh) 1977; 57:159–163.
22. David TJ, Waddington E, Stanton RHJ. Nutritional hazards of elimination diets in children with atopic dermatitis. Arch Dis Child 1984; 59:323–325.
23. Bock S, Lee W, Remigio L, May C. Studies of hypersensitivity reactions to food in infants and children. J Allergy Clin Immunol 1978; 62:3327–3334.
24. Jones SM, Sampson HA. The role of allergens in atopic dermatitis. In: Leung DYM, ed. Atopic Dermatitis: From Pathogenesis to Treatment. Georgetown, TX: R.G. Landes Company, 1996:41–112.
25. Sampson HA. Atopic dermatitis [review]. Ann Allergy 1992; 69:469–479.
26. Sampson HA. Role of immediate food hypersensitivity in the pathogenesis of atopic dermatitis. J Allergy Clin Immunol 1983; 71:473–480.
27. Eigenmann PA, Sicherer SH, Borkowski TA, Cohen BA, Sampson HA. Prevalence of IgE-mediated food allergy among children with atopic dermatitis. Pediatrics 1998; 101:e8.
28. Hanifin JM, Rajka G. Diagnostic features of atopic dermatitis. Acta Dermatol Venereol 1980; 92(suppl):44–47.
29. Burks AW, Mallory SB, Williams LW, Shirrell MA. Atopic dermatitis: clinical relevance of food hypersensitivity reactions. J Pediatr 1988; 113:447–451.
30. Atherton DJ, Soothill JF, Sewell M, Wells RS, Chilvers CED. A double-blind controlled crossover trial of an antigen-avoidance diet in atopic dermatitis. Lancet 1978; 1:401–403.
31. Neild VS, Marsden RA, Bailes JA, Bland JM. Egg and milk exclusion diets in atopic eczema. Br J Dermatol 1986; 114:117–123.
32. Juto P, Engberg S, Winberg J. Treatment of severe infantile atopic dermatitis with a strict elimination diet. Clin Allergy 1978; 8:493–500.
33. Hill DJ, Lynch BC. Elemental diet in the management of severe eczema in childhood. Clin Allergy 1982; 12:313–315.
34. Lever R, MacDonald C, Waugh P, Aitchison T. Randomised controlled trial of advice on an egg exclusion diet in young children with atopic eczema and sensitivity to eggs. Pediatr Allergy Immunol 1998; 9:13–19.
35. Host A. Cow's milk protein allergy and intolerance in infancy. Some clinical, epidemiological and immunological aspects. Pediatr Allergy Immunol 1994; 5:1–36.
36. Zeiger RS. Development and prevention of allergic disease in childhood. In: Middleton E, Reed C, Ellis E, Adkinson N, Yunginger J, Busse W, eds. Allergy: Principles and Practice. St. Louis: Mosby, 1993:1137–1171.
37. Chandra R, Shakuntla P, Hamed A. Influence of maternal diet during lactation and use of formula feeds on development of atopic eczema in high risk infants. Br Med J 1989; 299: 228–230.
38. Hattevig G, Kjellman B, Bjorksten B, Kjellman N. Effect of maternal avoidance of eggs, cow's milk and fish during lactation upon allergic manifestations in infants. Clin Exp Allergy 1989; 19:27–32.
39. Sigurs N, Hattevig G, Kjellman B. Maternal avoidance of eggs, cow's milk, and fish during lactation: effect on allergic manifestation, skin-prick tests, and specific IgE antibodies in children at age 4 years. Pediatr 1992; 89:735–739.

40. Fergusson DM, Horwood LJ, Shannon FT. Early solid feeding and recurrent eczema: a 10-year longitudinal study. Pediatrics 1990; 86:541–546.

41. Fergusson D, Horwood L, Shannon F. Asthma and infant diet. Arch Dis Child 1983; 58: 48–51.

42. Kajosaari M, Saarinen UM. Prophylaxis of atopic disease by six months; total solid food elimination. Arch Pediatr Scand 1983; 72:411–414.

43. Kajosaari M. Atopy prophylaxis in high-risk infants: prospective 5-year follow-up study of children with six months exclusive breastfeeding and solid food elimination. Adv Exp Med Biol 1991; 310:453–458.

44. Zeiger R. Prevention of food allergy in infancy. Ann Allergy 1990; 65:430–441.

45. Zeiger R, Heller S. The development and prediction of atopy in high-risk children: Follow-up at seven years in a prospective randomized study of combined maternal and infant food allergen avoidance. J Allergy Clin Immunol 1995; 95:1179–1190.

46. Zeiger R, Heller S, Mellon M, Forsythe A, O'Connor R, Hamburger R. Effect of combined maternal and infant food-allergen avoidance on development of atopy in early infancy: a randomized study. J Allergy Clin Immunol 1989; 84:72–89.

47. Zeiger R, Heller S, Mellon M, Halsey J, Hamburger R, Sampson H. Genetic and environmental factors affecting the development of atopy through age 4 in children of atopic parents: a prospective randomized study of food allergen avoidance. Pediatr Allergy Immunol 1992; 3:110–127.

48. Mihm MC, Soter NA, Dvorak HF, Austen KF. The structure of normal skin and the morphology of atopic eczema. J Invest Dermatol 1976; 67:305–312.

49. Solley GO, Gleich GJ, Jordan RE, Schroeter AL. Late phase of the immediate wheal and flare skin reactions: its dependence on IgE antibodies. J Clin Invest 1976; 58:408–420.

50. Lemanske R, Kaliner M. Late-phase allergic reactions. In: Middleton E, Reed C, Ellis E, Adkinson N, Yunginger J, eds. Allergy: Principles and Practice. St. Louis: CV Mosby Company, 1988:12–30.

51. Leiferman K, Ackerman S, Sampson H, Haugen H, Venencie P, Gleich G. Dermal deposition of eosinophil-granule major basic protein in atopic dermatitis. Comparison with onchocerciasis. N Engl J Med 1985; 313:282–285.

52. Hamid Q, Boguniewicz M, Leung DYM. Differential in situ cytokine gene expression in acute versus chronic atopic dermatitis. J Clin Invest 1994; 94:870–876.

53. Hamid Q, Naseer T, Minshall EM, Song YL, Boguniewicz M, Leung DYM. In vivo expression of IL-12 and IL-13 in atopic dermatitis. J Allergy Clin Immunol 1996; 98:225–231.

54. Tsicopoulos A, Hamid Q, Varney V, Ying S, Moqbel R, Durham S, Kay A. Preferential messenger RNA expression of Th-1-type cells [IFN-gamma, IL-2] in classical delayed-type [tuberculin] hypersensitivity reactions in human skin. J Immunol 1992; 148:2058–2061.

55. Bieber T, Kraft S, Jurgens M, Strobel I, Haberstok J, Tomov H, Regele D, de la Salle H, Wollenberg A, Hanau D. New insights in the structure and biology of the high affinity receptor for IgE (Fc epsilon RI) on human epidermal Langerhans cells. J Dermatol Sci 1996; 13: 71–75.

56. Mudde G, Bheekha R, Bruijnzeel-Koomen C. Consequences of IgE/CD23-mediated antigen presentation in allergy. Immunol Today 1995; 16:380–383.

57. Johnson E, Irons J, Patterson R, Roberts M. Serum IgE concentration in atopic dermatitis. J Allergy Clin Immunol 1974; 54:94–99.

58. Sampson HA, Jolie PL. Increased plasma histamine concentrations after food challenges in children with atopic dermatitis. N Engl J Med 1984; 311:372–376.

59. Magnarin M, Knowles A, Ventura A, Vita F, Fanti L, Zabucchi G. A role for eosinophils in the pathogenesis of skin lesions in patients with food-sensitive atopic dermatitis. J Allergy Clin Immunol 1995; 96:200–208.

60. Suomalainen H, Soppi E, Isolauri E. Evidence for eosinophil activation in cow's milk allergy. Pediatr Allergy Immunol 1994; 5:27–31.

61. Abernathy-Carver K, Sampson H, Picker L, Leung D. Milk-induced eczema is associated with the expansion of T cells expressing cutaneous lymphocyte antigen. J Clin Invest 1995; 95:913–918.
62. Van Reijsen FC, Felius A, Wauters AK, Bruijnzeel-Koomen CAFM, Koppelman SJ. T-cell reactivity for a peanut-derived epitope in the skin of a young infant with atopic dermatitis. J Allergy Clin Immunol 1998; 101:207–209.
63. Van Reijsen FC, Bruynzeel-Koomen CA, Kalthoff FS, et al. Skin-derived aeroallergen-specific T-cell clones of the TH2 phenotype in patients with atopic dermatitis. J Allergy Clin Immunol 1992; 90:184–193.
64. Reekers R, Beyer K, Niggemann B, Wahn U, Freihorst J, Kapp A, Werfel T. The role of circulating food antigen-specific lymphocytes in food allergic children with atopic dermatitis. Br J Dermatol 1996; 135:935–941.
65. Werfel T, Ahlers G, Schmidt P, Boeker M, Kapp A. Detection of a Kappa-casein-specific lymphocyte response in milk-responsive atopic dermatitis. Clin Exp Allergy 1996; 26:1380–1386.
66. Kondo N, Fukutomi O, Agata H, Yokoyama Y. Proliferative responses of lymphocytes to food antigens are useful for detection of allergens in nonimmediate types of food allergy. J Invest Allergol Clin Immunol 1997; 7:122–126.
67. Hoffman KM, Ho DG, Sampson HA. Evaluation of the usefulness of lymphocyte proliferation assays in the diagnosis of allergy to cow's milk. J Allergy Clin Immunol 1997; 99:360–366.
68. Sampson HA, Broadbent KR, Bernhisel-Broadbent J. Spontaneous release of histamine from basophils and histamine-releasing factor in patients with atopic dermatitis and food hypersensitivity. N Engl J Med 1989; 321:228–232.
69. Lyczak JB, Zhang K, Saxon A, Morrison SL. Expression of novel secreted isoforms of human immunoglobulin E proteins. J Biol Chem 1996; 271:3428–3436.
70. Guillet G, Guillet MH. Natural history of sensitizations in atopic dermatitis. Arch Dermatol 1992; 128:187–192.
71. Bock SA. The natural history of food sensitivity. J Allergy Clin Immunol 1982; 69:173–177.
72. deMaat-Bleeker F, Bruijnzeel-Koomen C. Food allergy in adults with atopic dermatitis. Monogr Allergy 1996; 32:157–163.
73. Munkvad M, Danielsen L, Hoj L, Povlsen CO, Secher L, Svejgaard E, Bundgaard A, Larsen PO. Antigen-free diet in adult patients with atopic dermatitis. Acta Dermatol Venereol 1984; 64:524–528.
74. Guin JD. The evaluation of patients with urticaria. Dermatol Clin 1985; 3:29–49.
75. Sehgal VN, Rege VL. An interrogitave study of 158 urticaria patients. Ann Allergy 1973; 31:279–283.
76. Nizami RM, Baboo MT. Office management of patients with urticaria: an analysis of 215 patients. Ann Allergy 1974; 33:78–85.
77. Jarmoc LM, Primack WA. Anaphylaxis to cutaneous exposure to milk protein. Clin Pediatr 1987; 26:154–156.
78. Fisher AA. Contact urticaria from handling meats and fowl. Cutis 1982; 30:726–729.
79. Champion R, Roberts S, Carpenter R, Roger J. Urticaria and angioedema: a review of 554 patients. Br J Dermatol 1969; 81:588–597.
80. Champion RH. Urticaria: then and now. Br J Dermatol. 1988; 119:427–436.
81. Volonakis M, Katsarou-Katsari A, Stratigos J. Etiologic factors in childhood chronic urticaria. Ann Allergy 1992; 69:61–65.
82. Freeman S, Rosen RH. Urticarial contact dermattis in food handlers. Med J Aust 1991; 155:91–94.
83. Kanerva L, Estlander T, Jolanki R. Occupational allergic contact dermatitis from spices. Contact Dermatitis 1996; 35:157–162.

84. Maibach H. Immediate hypersensitivity in hand dermatitis. Role of food-contact dermatitis. Arch Dermatol 1976; 112:1289–1291.

85. Fry L, Seah PP. Dermatitis herpetiformis: an evaluation of diagnostic criteria. Br J Dermatol 1974; 90:137–146.

86. Caproni M, Felicani C, Fuligni A, Salvatore E, Atani L, Bianchi B, Mohammad Pour S, Proietto G, Toto P, Coscoine G, Amerio P, Fabbri P. Th2-like cytokine activity in dermatitis herpetiformis. Br J Dermatol 1998; 138:242–247.

87. Sampson HA. Food sensitivity and the pathogenesis of atopic dermatitis. J R Soc Med 1997; 30(suppl):2–8.

88. Bock SA, Atkins FM. The natural history of peanut allergy. J Allergy Clin Immunol 1989; 83:900–904.

89. Yunginger JW, Sweeney KG, Sturner WQ, Giannandra LA, Teigland JD, Bray M, Benson PA, York JA, Biedrzycki L, Squillace DL. Fatal food-induced anaphylaxis. JAMA 1988; 260:1450–1452.

90. Young E, Patel S, Stoneham MD, Rona R, Wilkinson JD. The prevalence of reactions to food additives in a survey population. J R Coll Phys Lond 1987; 21:241–271.

91. Fuglsang G, Madsen C, Halken S, Jorgensen M, Ostergaard PA, Osterballe O. Adverse reactions to food additives in children with atopic symptoms. Allergy 1994; 49:31–37.

92. Schwartz HJ. Asthma and food additives. In: Metcalfe DD, Sampson HA, Simon RA, eds. Food Allergy: Adverse Reactions to Foods and Food Additives. Cambridge: Blackwell Science, 1997:411–418.

93. Bock S, Buckley J, Holst A, May C. Proper use of skin tests with food extracts in diagnosis of food hypersensitivity. Clin Allergy 1978; 8:559–564.

94. Ortolani C, Ispano M, Pastorello EA, Ansaloni R, Magri GC. Comparison of results of skin prick tests (with fresh foods and commercial food extracts) and RAST in 100 patients with oral allergy syndrome. J Allergy Clin Immunol 1989; 83:683–690.

95. Sampson HA, Ho DG. Relationship between food-specific IgE concentrations and the risk of positive food challenges in children and adolescents. J Allergy Clin Immunol 1997; 100:444–451.

96. Bernhisel-Broadbent J, Sampson HA. Cross-allergenicity in the legume botanical family in children with food hypersensitivity. J Allergy Clin Immunol 1989; 83:435–440.

97. Bernhisel-Broadbent J, Taylor S, Sampson HA. Cross-allergenicity in the legume botanical family in children with food hypersensitivity. II. Laboratory correlates. J Allergy Clin Immunol 1989; 84:701–709.

98. Jones SM, Magnolfi CF, Cooke SK, Sampson HA. Immunologic cross-reactivity among cereal grains and grasses in children with food hypersensitivity. J Allergy Clin Immunol 1995; 96:341–351.

99. Bernhisel-Broadbent J, Scanlon SM, Sampson HA. Fish hypersensitivity. I. In vitro and oral challenge results in fish-allergic patients. J Allergy Clin Immunol 1992; 89:730–737.

100. Bernhisel-Broadbent J, Strause D, Sampson HA. Fish hypersensitivity. II: Clinical relevance of altered fish allergenicity caused by various preparation methods. J Allergy Clin Immunol 1992; 90:622–629.

101. Sicherer SH, Burks AW, Sampson HA. Clinical features of acute allergic reactions to peanut and tree nuts in children. Pediatrics 1998; 102:e6.

102. Terr AI, Salvaggio JE. Controversial concepts in allergy and clinical imunology. In: Bierman CW, Pearlman DS, Shapiro GG, Busse WW, eds. Allergy, Asthma, and Immunology from Infancy to Adulthood. Philadelphia: W.B. Saunders, 1996:749–760.

103. Bock SA, Sampson HA, Atkins FM, Zeiger RS, Lehrer S, Sachs M, Bush RK, Metcalfe DD. Double-blind, placebo-controlled food challenge (DBPCFC) as an office procedure: a manual. J Allergy Clin Immunol 1988; 82:986–997.

104. Leung DYM, Hanifin JM, Charlesworth EN. Disease management of atopic dermatitis. Ann Allergy Asthma Immunol 1997; 79:197–211.

105. Leung DY, Harbeck R, Bina P, Reiser RF, Yang E, Norris DA, Hanifin JM, Sampson HA. Presence of IgE antibodies to staphylococcal exotoxins on the skin of patients with atopic dermatitis. Evidence for a new group of allergens. J Clin Invest 1993; 92:1374–1380.

106. David TJ. Hazards of challenge tests in atopic dermatitis. Allergy 1989; 44:101–107.

107. Hourihane JO, Bedwani SJ, Dean TP, Warner JO. Randomised, double blind, crossover challenge study of allergenicity of peanut oils in subjects allergic to peanuts. BMJ 1997; 314: 1084–1088.

108. Sampson HA, Mendelson LM, Rosen JP. Fatal and near-fatal anaphylactic reactions to food in children and adolescents. N Engl J Med 1992; 327:380–384.

109. Kemp SF, Lockey RF, Wolf BL, Lieberman P. Anaphylaxis. A review of 266 cases. Arch Intern Med 1995; 155:1749–1754.

110. Pumphrey RSH, Stanworth SJ. The clinical spectrum of anaphylaxis in north-west England. Clin Exp Allergy 1996; 26:1364–1370.

111. Sampson HA. Peanut anaphylaxis. J Allergy Clin Immunol 1990; 86:1–3.

112. Hourihane JO'B, Dean TP, Warner JO. Peanut allergy in relation to heredity, maternal diet, and other atopic diseases: results of a questionnaire survey, skin prick testing, and food challenges. Br Med J 1996; 313:518–521.

113. Hourihane JO'B, Kilburn SA, Dean P, Warner JO. Clinical characteristics of peanut allergy. Clin Exp Allergy 1997; 27:634–639.

114. Hourihane JO, Roberts SA, Warner JO. Resolution of peanut allergy: case-control study. BMJ 1998; 316:1271–1275.

115. Sicherer SH, Sampson HA. Cow's milk protein-specific IgE concentrations in two age groups of milk-allergic children and in children achieving clinical tolerance. Clin Exp Allergy 1999; 29:507–512.

116. James JM, Sampson HA. Immunologic changes associated with the development of tolerance in children with cow milk allergy. J Pediatr 1992; 121:371–377.

117. Nickel R, Kulig M, Forster G, Bergmann R, Bauer CP, Lau S, Guggenmoos-Holzmann I, Wahn U. Sensitization to hen's egg at the age of twelve months is predictive for allergic sensitization to common indoor and outdoor allergens at the age of three years. J Allergy Clin Immunol 1997; 99:613–617.

# 22

## The Role of Inhalant Allergens in Atopic Dermatitis

**Lisa M. Wheatley and Thomas A. E. Platts-Mills**
*University of Virginia,*
*Charlottesville, Virginia*

## I. INTRODUCTION

The term atopic dermatitis (AD) was introduced not only because of the very strong association between AD and other allergic diseases but also because many investigators at that time were convinced that exposure to common inhalant allergens played an important role in the disease. Patients with AD are more allergic than those with asthma or rhinitis as judged by total IgE, the quantity of IgE to specific allergens, the number of positive skin tests, and peripheral blood eosinophilia. In addition, some patients report seasonal exacerbations or exacerbations on exposure to well-defined sources of allergen, such as a cat. Since adults and older children with AD react to allergens that are ubiquitous in the modern home, allergen avoidance is potentially an important component of disease management. However, the role of allergy in atopic dermatitis remains controversial [1]. It may be helpful to recognize the arguments that are used against a role for allergens in this disease to distinguish those that may be valid from those that have been refuted or at least partially answered (Table 1). For example, the theory that the extremely elevated levels of specific IgE directed against inhalants can be explained by concomitant rhinitis or asthma is unconvincing because the levels are much higher than those seen in allergic respiratory diseases without AD. Additionally, since it is well established that many asthmatics are unaware of their allergy to perennial inhalant antigens, it is not hard to conclude that AD patients may be similarly in the dark. The narrowly focused view that IgE-mediated reactivity in the skin is expressed as urticaria ignores a body of evidence on IgE as a potentiator of T-cell reactivity in delayed hypersensitivity responses. This chapter will present the studies that address the evidence that common inhalant allergens play an important role in causing and exacerbating eczema in atopic individuals. The available data on the response of the skin to experimental exposure and avoidance provide convincing evidence of the importance of aeroallergens in AD. Further, identification of humoral (i.e., IgEab) responses to allergens is a useful approach to identifying those external and modifiable factors that may contribute to disease.

**Table 1**   Arguments Against the Importance of Allergy in Atopic Dermatitis

The elevation of IgE is explained by concomitant respiratory allergy.

''Pure'' AD cases (i.e., AD without other allergic disease) where IgE is often within the normal range suggest that elevated IgE is not essential for expression of disease.

Immediate hypersensitivity in the skin is characterized by an urticarial rather than a eczematous response.

The majority of patients do not complain of worsening of their disease after exposure to house dust.

Allergen avoidance has not been shown to prevent new cases of AD nor fully clear preexisting disease.

Allergen desensitization therapy tends to exacerbate rather than ameliorate disease.

## II. ATOPIC DERMATITIS AND ATOPY

Even before the introduction of the term ''atopy'' by Coca and Cooke in 1923, there had been descriptions of a pruritic skin rash exacerbated by exposure to grass, ragweed, and horse dander [2]. Subsequently in 1933, when Hill and Sulzberger defined the cardinal features of atopic dermatitis, three of the nine criteria were evidences of the allergic nature of the disease (personal or family history of atopy, many immediate positive skin tests, high reaginic [later recognized to be IgE] activity in the serum) [3]. In 1994, the U.K. Working Party defined six minimum criteria to distinguish atopic dermatitis from other inflammatory dermatosis; one of these is a history of atopy in the patient or a first-degree relative [4]. The predictive value of total or specific IgE and eosinophil counts was not evaluated as the report specifically excluded ''invasive'' procedures.

Atopic dermatitis is associated with the other primary atopic disorders of allergic rhinitis and extrinsic asthma in 80% of cases. Atopic dermatitis keeps company with allergic asthma in 35–40% of cases [5,6]. It is generally the first atopic disease to manifest itself in infants, in tandem with the appearance of specific IgE to food antigens. Respiratory allergy generally follows later [7]. This association of allergic respiratory disease with atopic dermatitis is stronger in moderate to severe disease. In addition to the congregation of allergic diseases in individuals, atopic disease, both respiratory and cutaneous, has been rising as a group in several countries [8]. The magnitude of the increase is somewhat harder to judge in AD than it is for allergic respiratory disease. This is because the large epidemiological surveys are questionnaire based and there have been no validated questions that could distinguish AD from other skin disorders, whereas for allergic rhinitis a seasonal history of sneezing and nasal and/or ocular symptoms correlate well with physician evaluation and skin test results. Even physician-based diagnoses of AD are somewhat unreliable in the historical setting as uniform diagnostic criteria did not appear until 1980. However, the data suggest that there has been a substantial rise in the prevalence of atopic dermatitis since World War II.

There is a subset of patients with ''pure'' AD, defined as such because there is no personal or family history of allergic respiratory disease. Even in this subset of patients, the more severe disease was associated with higher levels of serum IgE [9,10]. Only about 10% of people with AD lack evidence of a role for IgE, and as mentioned previously, these patients tend to have milder disease [11]. This suggests that IgE-mediated reactions are required for full expression of the disease. Alternatively, atopic dermatitis may be compared to asthma, where extrinsic (allergic) and intrinsic forms of the disease share many characteristics at the symptomatic, cellular, and molecular level, but the former is IgE initiated and IgE is not obviously involved in the latter. In patients with extrinsic asthma, the association with exposure to perennial indoor allergens is often not obvious to the patient or the physician. This is because exposure is chronic and probably low dose. It is generally easier to recognize a causal association when the response is either immediate, high dose, or episodic, conditions that are common for seasonal allergic rhinitis, occasional in asthma, and rare for AD.

## III.  ATOPIC DERMATITIS AND SERUM IgE

The elevated IgE in atopic dermatitis is polyclonal but not nonspecific. It is directed at a variety of inhalational and food antigens as well as to bacterial and fungal products to which the patient has been exposed. IgE is usually not found to antigens encountered by vaccinations, such as diphtheria toxin, or to allergens to which the patient has not been exposed [12]. (There are exceptions to the latter rule, especially where antigens are cross-reactive or heavily glycosylated. There is extensive cross-reactivity within some food groups and between apparently unrelated pollens and foods.) IgE levels have correlated with disease activity in some studies, but not in others. The level of serum IgE does not vary in concert with disease activity in the short run (i.e., months) for either spontaneous or treatment-induced changes [10,13,14]. For this reason, some have argued that the high levels of IgE are not directly relevant to the pathogenesis of the dermatosis. Of course, it is also true that seasonal exacerbations of hay fever are accompanied by only modest changes in the level of total and specific IgE and that treatment with antihistamines and nasal steroids substantially improve the inflammatory mucosal disease without changing the IgE levels, yet no one seriously doubts the causal role of IgE to pollen in allergic rhinitis. In patients free from dermatitis for prolonged periods (1 or more years) the level of serum IgE can fall by as much as 10-fold [14].

In children less than 5 years of age, AD is usually associated with food sensitization rather than with inhalant allergens. Many of these cases will resolve spontaneously in early childhood, with others having a prolonged remission by 3 years of age [15]. Persistence into adulthood is linked to the severity of disease. Among those cases where infantile eczema required hospitalization, eczema continued to be a problem in adulthood in over 60% of cases; if the disease was moderate, it persisted in 40% [16]. The importance of nonfood allergens increases with age, with most children over the age of 7 years having positive skin tests for inhalant allergens [17]. In addition, approximately 15% of teenage patients with allergic respiratory disease will develop AD [18]. Neither the existence of specific IgE by in vitro testing nor an immediate response to a skin test with an environmental allergen necessarily means that the individual will have disease. Many individuals with strong immediate skin tests live without any allergic manifestations, and equally many patients with allergic disease have specific IgE to antigens that have no clinical relevance. The presence of IgE to any particular antigen does not dictate any specific disease manifestation because a person may be allergic to house dust mites and have rhinitis, asthma, AD, or any combination of the three. It is widely accepted that a positive prick test to food antigens is pertinent to clinical symptoms less than half of the time. The relevance of food is judged by a response to a double-blind, placebo-controlled food challenge.

There are some who argue that the presence of specific IgE to aeroallergens is explained by, and its pathogenic importance limited to, the accompanying atopic respiratory disease. This is a difficult idea to embrace given the allergen specific reactivity of the skin and the presence of cutaneous lymphocyte antigen, the skin homing receptor, on allergen specific T cells [19]. In addition, the levels of total and specific IgE are usually much higher in AD than in rhinitis or asthma. Evidence for the role of inhalant antigens comes from two basic sources: (1) evaluation of exposure and response to challenge or avoidance and (2) the immunological investigations based on the allergen patch test model (APT).

## IV. ATOPIC DERMATITIS AND EXPOSURE TO INHALANT ANTIGENS

Most studies have focused on the house dust mite (HDM) because of the high prevalence of IgE antibodies to allergens derived from this antigen source. Up to 90% of persons with AD have specific IgE to dust mite, with levels over 4000 IU of mite-specific IgE/ml in some cases [12]. In a study of patients with moderate to severe AD at the University of Virginia, 93% of subjects had IgE specific for *Dermatophagoides pteronyssinus*, and it represented a mean of 5% of total IgE and in some cases accounted for over 50% of total IgE. While the overall % is similar in allergic asthmatics, the absolute level of IgE Ab to *D. pteronyssinus* is up 100-fold higher. Additionally, much is known about the component antigens, and exposure to these antigens can be measured with sensitive immunoassays. Dust mites are distributed largely according to environmental characteristics of the home, such as temperature and humidity, and generally without regard to the atopic tendency of the human occupant. AD may be somewhat different from other atopic diseases, as there is speculation that dust mites may actually increase in the homes of patients with scaling skin disease, as epithelial cells are important in the diet of dust mites. Exposure to dust mite in the homes of patients with atopic dermatitis has been measured and compared with those of healthy volunteers and patients with other skin diseases. In one study, there was a higher mite concentration in the homes of patients with AD who were known to be sensitized to mites compared to nonatopic healthy controls, whereas in another, dust mite exposure was somewhat higher but not significantly different for patients with AD, when compared to persons with psoriasis or without skin disease [20,21]. In the second study, many patients in both groups were exposed to levels of HDM antigen higher than 2 µg/g dust, the level often associated with sensitization in predisposed individuals. Interestingly, no difference in exposure to HDM between nonsensitized and sensitized patients with AD was demonstrated. No evaluation of disease severity in reference to exposure was undertaken in the study by Hansen and colleagues [21]. In another study, patients with mild to moderate AD were exposed to more mites than healthy control subjects. When only sensitized AD patients were considered, patients with moderate to severe AD had higher numbers of mites sharing their beds than those with mild disease, although again there was no difference in exposure between sensitized and nonsensitized patients [22].

Several studies have investigated the effect of (often drastic) avoidance of HDM in an uncontrolled way by moving patients to specially built houses, or hospital rooms, or through use of acaricides, etc., and suggested that such measures improved the disease [23–26]. One double-blind, placebo-controlled study using a combination of effective measures in the home (mite-impermeable bed covers, high-filtration vacuums, and aca-

**Table 2** Dust Mite–Avoidance Procedures

| | |
|---|---|
| Priority goals: | Encase matresses and pillows in dust mite–proof coverings (vinyl, plastisized fabric or fabric with pore size of <10 μm). |
| | Wash all bed linens in hot water (≥130°F) weekly. Comforters that cannot be washed should be encased. |
| | Vacuum using a model with "microfiltration" provided either by the bag or extra filtration; damp mop and dust weekly. |
| | Patient should wear a mask while cleaning or avoid the area for 20 minutes. |
| | Reduce clutter in bedroom. |
| | Freeze stuffed animals overnight each week. |
| Intermediate goals: | Maintain relative indoor humidity ≤50% with air-conditioning or dehumidifiers. |
| | Replace draperies with washable fabrics or blinds. |
| Long-term goals: | Replace carpets with smooth flooring (wood, vinyl, ceramic). |
| | Reduce fabric upholstered furniture. |
| | Avoid residences in the basement or built on cement slabs. |

ricides) is in the literature. While both active and control groups decreased Der p 1 concentrations in carpeting, the reduction in the amount of dust was greater on the mattresses in the active group, and the disease improved significantly more in the active treatment group [27]. Another recent study demonstrated that the use of HDM-impermeable mattress covers could reduce the acquisition of sensitization to HDM antigen in infants with AD and food allergy [28]. These studies emphasize the potential efficacy of avoidance measures in the home. We recommend avoidance routinely for HDM-allergic patients (Table 2), concentrating initially on the bedroom but expanding the scope of the avoidance as disease severity and personal finances dictate.

## V. ATOPIC DERMATITIS AND THE ALLERGEN PATCH TEST

Although it is established that patch tests with allergens (APT) can give rise to a patch of eczema, there is enormous variation in the performance and interpretation of these tests. In the APT, allergens are applied to intact or mildly abraded skin and a positive response is read in the same way as standard contact hypersensitivity panels. It might be considered surprising that the APT should be positive at all. AD has long been described as the "itch that rashes," and trauma to the skin is thought to be an integral part of the disease process. Engman et al. published in 1936 a report that preventing scratching could prevent eczema following a food challenge [29]. Nevertheless, positive eczematous responses to patch tests with a purified dust mite antigen were first demonstrated in 1982 [30]. Biopsy of such sites revealed a cellular infiltrate including basophils, eosinophils, and predominantly CD4+ lymphocytes [30–32]. Biopsies of involved skin in AD also show a prominent CD4+ infiltrate but few basophils or eosinophils [33,34]. This difference in the composition of cellular infiltrates is attributed to the stage of the lesions. Eosinophil recruitment into the site of a patch test is evident by 6 hours and wanes after 48–72 hours if a single application is used [35]. When antigen was applied every other day, the eosinophil infiltrate persisted through at least 6 days but was largely absent after 10 days even as antigen application was continued [36]. The finding that eosinophil granule products can be stained in lesional biopsy specimens suggests that eosinophils were present at an earlier time point and presumably degranulated, consistent with the patch test findings [37]. Basophils are involved in only the earliest phases of a traditional delayed-type hypersensitivity (DTH) response to contact sensitizers and are proposed to play a similar role in AD [38].

Since Mitchell et al., there have been numerous studies employing this technique, but with many variations: in the vehicle, the concentration of antigen, the source of antigen, the state of the skin (intact, abraded, or affected), and the duration of the application. Patient selection is another important variable, which is perhaps the hardest to interpret. As might be expected, results have varied considerably. However, a positive patch test rate of between 30 and 45% has been seen consistently in AD. In most studies, APT reactions have correlated well with immediate prick tests or elevated serum IgE antibodies to the same antigen [39]. APT and prick tests have been shown to be concordant for several allergens, including HDM, birch, and cedar [40,41]. In a few studies, APT reactions were unrelated to prick reactions (e.g., approximately 40% reaction rate was reported by Seidenari et al. [42] whether or not there was evidence of immediate hypersensitivity). APT reactions have been found predominantly in AD, although rare positive tests have been recorded in patients with allergic respiratory disease alone, asymptomatic skin test–positive controls, and even in skin test–negative healthy volunteers [43]. The bulk of reports suggest a positive response to APT in a large proportion of AD patients for dust mite–derived proteins, with rare reactivity in persons without this disease. If more antigens were studied, it is possible that an even larger group of AD patients would demonstrate evidence for aeroallergen involvement in their disease. Even when a lack of concordance between prick and patch tests is found, that does not mean that the results of the patch tests are irrelevant. Skin reactivity is depressed in some patients with AD, making a negative prick test less definitive, and a delayed eczematous cutaneous response to HDM or other allergens could be important without an immediate response.

## A.  T Cells and the Immune Response to Allergen Patch Testing

The current thinking on the mechanism of inflammation of the skin involves IgE in the initiation phase. One of the most important findings of the studies using patch tests to induce eczema was the discovery that Langerhans cells carry IgE on their surface [44]. Initially, this was described as the low-affinity IgE receptor (CD23), which showed evidence of upregulation on exposure to cytokines, but later it was recognized that Langerhans cells also express the high-affinity IgE receptor (FcεRI) on their surface [45]. Presentation by Langerhans cells to T cells was then shown in vitro to be dependent on having IgE carried by the FcεRI on their surface [46,47]. This may explain why persons with specific IgE but without AD do not produce an eczematous response to patch testing, because while they have antigen specific T cells, they do not have IgE on the Langerhans cells in their skin. Passive transfer experiments have demonstrated that intradermal injection of specific IgE for Der p 1 followed by patch testing with Der p 1 results in recruitment of eosinophils to the site [36]. Transfer of allergic serum would presumably result in loading of FcεRI on both Langerhans cells and mast cells with specific IgE. Which cell type is responsible for the cellular influx in this situation is unclear. If the host has allergen-specific T cells, Langerhans cells could present antigen and start the cascade to eosinophilic inflammation. Presentation by Langerhans cells is important because they predominantly express B7.2 rather than the B7.1 form of the CD28 ligand on their surface when freshly cultured or in APT sites [48,49]. Signaling through B7.2 (CD86) has been associated with skewing of T-cell responses to a Th2 pattern in mice [50]. Repeated presentation of antigen by Langerhans cells predisposes to a Th2 lymphocyte response characterized by a predominance of IL-4 rather than IFN-$\gamma$ [51]. However, mast cells are known to produce IL-4 and IL-5 after cross-linking of IgE on their surface and may also be able to recruit eosinophils to the site.

Biopsies of patch test sites have also been used as a source of T cells, and this has demonstrated that allergen-specific cells are enriched relative to peripheral blood, although they still only represent a minority of the infiltrating cells as is true in delayed-type hypersensitivity reactions [52]. If the patch test site is biopsied in the first 24 hours, the predominant cytokine by immunohistochemical staining or in situ hybridization is IL-4. After 48 hours, as the number of T cells at the site continue to increase, IL-4 declines and IFN-$\gamma$ becomes the dominant cytokine [35,53,54]. This biphasic pattern in the patch test mimics spontaneous lesions where IL-4 predominates in the acute phase and IFN-$\gamma$ in chronic lichenified skin [55,56].

Atopic dermatitis in early childhood is generally considered to be related to food antigens because of the presence of specific IgE to foods as identified by RAST or skin testing. Generally, there is little evidence of IgE to aeroallergens, but they have been reported in some studies. However, a group in Japan recently investigated responses to house dust mite in infants and children. Instead of standard proliferation assays read as tritiated thymidine incorporation, this group used fluorescence activated cell sorter (FACS) analysis of T cells entering the S phase of the cell cycle after culture in the presence of house dust mite antigen. Even in children less than 1 year of age, the percentage of cells entering the S phase was elevated when compared to either nonatopic infants or the response when *Candida* was used as the stimulant. The stimulation index correlated with severity of disease and with IL-5 in the culture supernatants, as well as with specific IgE after 1 year of age [28].

## B. Route of Exposure

The route by which the environmental allergens generally referred to as inhalants affect AD is still undetermined. Food allergens are presumed to act upon the skin after absorption into the systemic circulation from the gut, so a skin response to antigens that are inhaled is also possible. In 1930, Cohen et al. was able to elicit a Prausnitz-Küstner reaction in the skin 20 minutes after nasal inhalation of ragweed allergen [57]. There are multiple reports of seasonal or, in the case of animals, environmental exposure leading to worsening of disease in correspondingly sensitized individuals [2,40,58]. In 1952, Tuft reported that patients with a positive patch and prick tests to *Alternaria* and ragweed developed eczema after inhalation of relevant antigen but not placebo [59]. The antigens of house dust mite can be inhaled, but given the poor aerodynamic properties of the particles upon which it is carried, it is likely that the majority of contact will be through the skin. Even though the dust mite proteins that induce IgE antibody responses are large (13–29 kDa) compared to contact sensitizers such as nickel or poison ivy (<1 kDa), it has been demonstrated that dust mite antigen will enter the epidermis and dermis through visually uninvolved skin with or without gentle scarification [60,61]. Recently, a double-blind, placebo-controlled challenge on the inhalation of HDM demonstrated both new lesions and exacerbations of existing lesions [62]. In eight of nine cases, the skin reaction was preceded by a bronchial response including dyspnea. This may be interpreted as indicating that inhalation challenge results in eczematous changes predominantly in patients who have bronchial reactivity to dust mite. However, there must be some question of how well blinding could be maintained if patients were having a symptomatic response in the lungs.

Most studies have focused on HDM, but other aeroallergens have been implicated in causing exacerbations. Considerable reservoirs for animal dander, insect debris, pollens, and fungi are found in the home, so that each of these allergens can have contact with the skin as well as the respiratory tract. One interesting observation was a report that patch tests were more commonly positive on areas of the skin that were normally exposed to the air [63]. In addition, allergen-responsive T cells in AD often bear cutaneous lymphocyte antigen (CLA), the skin-homing receptor [19]. These homing receptors are thought to serve to bring T cells back to the site that activated or generated them, suggesting recruitment of T cells from the lymphatic tissue draining cutaneous areas [64]. Finally, the fungus that has most commonly been cited as etiological in AD is not *Alternaria* or *Aspergillus*, fungi strongly associated with allergic asthma, but the skin colonizer *Malassezia furfur* (formerly *Pityrosporum ovale* or *P. orbiculare*). The presence of specific IgE to *Alternaria* and *Aspergillus* is more common in AD than in asthma or nonasthmatic controls, but clinical relevance remains to be proven (64a). The levels of specific IgE to *M. furfur* are not as spectacular as those to *D. pteronyssinus* (Fig. 1), but in our experience as well as reports from others, specific IgE to *M. furfur* is rare outside of AD [65,66]. Positive APT reactions to this yeast have been demonstrated, and T cells specific for *M. furfur* cloned from such patch tests exhibit a Th2-like cytokine profile [67,68]. In addition, some have reported that patients with specific IgE to *M. furfur*, particularly with the head and neck variant of AD, improve substantially when treated with antifungal agents [69].

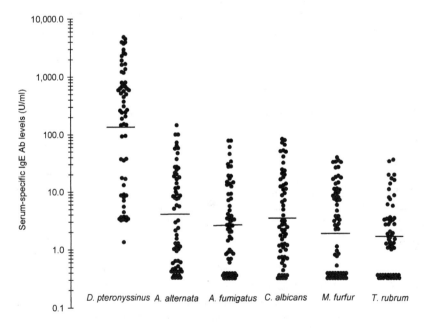

**Figure 1** Specific IgE to house dust mite and fungal antigens in patients with moderate to severe atopic dermatitis. (From Ref. 64a.)

The importance of colonizing fungal organisms may not be limited to *M. furfur* as Kolmer et al. reported improvement in the condition of the skin in atopic dermatitis after treatment for a number of different fungal infections [70].

## VI. CONCLUSION

In conclusion, antigens that are commonly referred to as aeroallergens are implicated in the pathogenesis of atopic dermatitis. The lines of evidence are several:

1. Specific IgE antibodies are often extremely elevated and will decline when the disease is in remission for prolonged periods.
2. Seasonal exacerbation of AD in patients with pollen-specific IgE has been reported.
3. Allergen extracts applied to the skin surface result in an inflammatory response that is similar to involved regions of the skin in AD in terms of cytokine production and cellular infiltrate.
4. Effective avoidance of allergen can improve disease activity.

Whether aeroallergens are important when inhaled or when in contact with the skin remains unresolved. The finding that *M. furfur* is associated with AD predominantly in the same distribution as it colonizes the human body suggests, at least in that case, that the effect is probably directly through the skin. However, it is also clear that antigens that are inhaled or ingested can appear in the skin. This question is important, as specific avoidance requires knowledge about route of exposure so that as little impact on the patient's quality of life and maximum effect on the disease course can be achieved. That atopic dermatitis, particularly the more severe forms, can be affected by many different factors is undeniable. Nonetheless, exposure to inhalant allergens is one exacerbating factor, and exposure can be decreased. The combination of careful skin care, judicious medication usage, and allergen avoidance should be the first line of treatment for moderate to severe atopic dermatitis.

## REFERENCES

1. Halbert AR, Weston WL, Morelli JG. Atopic dermatitis: Is it an allergic disease. J Am Acad Dermatol 1995; 33:1008–1018.
2. Walker IC. Causation of eczema, urticaria and angioneurotic edema by proteins other than those derived from foods. JAMA 1918; 70:897–900.
3. Hill LW, Sulzberger M. Yearbook of dermatology and syphilology. Chicago: Yearbook Medical Publishers, 1933:1–70.
4. Williams HC, Burney PGJ, Hay RJ, et al. The U.K. Working Party's diagnostic criteria for atopic dermatitis. Br J Dermatol 1994; 131:383–396.
5. Leung DYM. Atopic dermatitis: the skin as a window into the pathogenesis of chronic allergic diseases. J Allergy Clin Immunol 1995; 96:302–318.
6. Musgrove K, Morgan JK. Infantile eczema: a long term follow-up study. Br J Dermatol 1976; 95:365–372.
7. Van Asperen PP, Kemp AS. The natural history of IgE sensitization and atopic disease in early childhood. Acta Paediatr Scand 1989; 78:239–245.
8. Schafer T, Ring J. Epidemiology of allergic diseases. Allergy 1997; 52:14–22.

9. Uehara M. Family background of respiratory atopy: a factor of serum IgE elevation in atopic dermatitis. Acta Derm Venereol Suppl (Stockh) 1989; 144:78–82.
10. MacKie RM, Cobb SJ, Cochran REI, Thomson J. Total and specific IgE levels in patients with atopic dermatitis. The correlation between prick testing, clinical history of allergy, and in vitro quantification of IgE during clinical exacerbation and remission. Clin Exp Dermatol 1979; 4:187–195.
11. Johnson E, Irons J, Patterson R, et al. Serum IgE concentration in atopic dermatitis. J Allergy Clin Immunol 1974; 54:94–99.
12. Chapman MD, Rowntree S, Mitchell EB, Di Prisco de Fuenmajor MC, Platts-Mills TAE. Quantitative assessments of IgG and IgE antibodies to inhalant allergens in patients with atopic dermatitis. J Allergy Clin Immunol 1983; 72:27–33.
13. Stone S, Gleich GJ, Muller SA. Atopic dermatitis and IgE. Relationship between changes in IgE levels and severity of disease. Arch Dermatol 1976; 112:1254–1255.
14. Gunnar S, Johansson O, Juhlin L. Immunoglobulin E in ''healed'' atopic dermatitis and after treatment with corticosteroids and azathioprine. Br J Derm 1970; 82:10–13.
15. Queille-Roussel C, Raynaud F, Saurat J-H. A prospective computerized study of 500 cases of atopic eczema in childhood. Acta Derm Venereol Suppl (Stockh) 1985; 114:87–92.
16. Rystedt I. Prognostic factors in atopic eczema. Acta Derm Venereol (Stockh) 1985; 65:206–213.
17. Tuft L. Importance of inhalant allergens in atopic dermatitis. J Invest Dermatol 1949; 12:211–219.
18. Lammintausta K, Kalimo K, Raitala R, Forsten Y. Prognosis of atopic dermatitis. A prospective study in early adulthood. Int. J Dermatol 1991; 30:563–568.
19. Babi LFS, Picker LJ, Solar MTP, et al. Circulating allergen-reactive T cells from patients with atopic dermatitis and allergic contact dermatitis express the skin-selective homing receptor, the cutaneous lymphocyte-associated antigen. J Exp Med 1995; 181:1935–1940.
20. Colloff MJ. Exposure to house dust mites in homes of people with atopic dermatitis. Br J Dermatol 1992; 127:322–327.
21. Hansen SK, Deleuran M, Johnke H, Thestrup-Pedersen K. House dust mite antigen exposure of patients with atopic dermatitis or psoriasis. Acta Derm Venereol (Stockh) 1998; 78:139–141.
22. Beck H-I, Korsgaard J. Atopic dermatitis and house dust mites. Br J Dermatol 1989; 120:245–251.
23. Roberts DLL. House dust mite avoidance and atopic dermatitis. Br J Dermatol 1984; 110:735–736.
24. Sanda T, Yasue T, Oohashi M, Yasue A. Effectiveness of house dust-mite allergen avoidance through clean room therapy in patients with atopic dermatitis. J Allergy Clin Immunol 1991; 89:653–657.
25. Beck H-I, Bjerring P, Harving H. Atopic dermatitis and the indoor climate: the effect from preventive measures. Acta Derm Venereol (Stockh) 1989; 69:162–165.
26. Kort HSM, Koers WJ, van Nes AMT, et al. Clinical improvement after unusual avoidance measures in the home of an atopic dermatitis patient. Allergy 1993; 48:468–471.
27. Tan BB, Weald D, Strickland I, Friedmann PS. Double-blind controlled trial of effect of house-dust-mite allergen avoidance on atopic dermatitis. Lancet 1996; 347:15–18.
28. Kimura M, Tsuruta S, Yoshida T. Correlation of house dust mite-specific lymphocyte proliferation with IL-5 production, eosinophilia, and the severity of symptoms in infants with atopic dermatitis. J Allergy Clin Immunol 1998; 101:84–89.
29. Engman MF, Weiss RS, Engman MEJ. Eczema and the environment. Med Clin North Am 1936; 20:651–663.
30. Mitchell EB, Crow J, Chapman MD, Jouhal S, Pope FM, MIlls TAE. Basophils in allergen-induced patch test sites in atopic dermatitis. Lancet 1982; 1:127–130.
31. Bruijnzeel PLB, Kuijper PHM, Kapp A, Warringa RAJ, Betz S, Bruijnzeel-Koomen CAFM.

The involvement of eosinophils in the patch test reaction to aerollergens in atopic dermatitis: its relevance for the pathogenesis of atopic dermatitis. Clin Exp Allergy 1993; 23:97–109.

32. Reitamo S, Visa K, Kahonen K, Kayhko K, Stubb S, Salo OP. Eczematous reactions in atopic patients caused by epicutaneous testing with inhalant allergens. British Journal of Dermatology 1986; 114:303–309.

33. Braathen L, Forre O, Natvig J, Eeg-Larsen T. Predominance of T-lymphocytes in the dermal infiltrates of atopic dermatitis. Br J Dermatol 1979; 100:511–519.

34. Leung D, Bhan A, Schneeberger EE, Geha RS. Characterization of the mononuclear cell infiltrate in atopic dermatitis using monoclonal antibodies. J Allergy Clin Immunol 1983; 71:47–56.

35. Thepen T, Langeveld-Wildschut EG, Bihari IC, et al. Biphasic response against aeroallergens in atopic dermatitis showing a switch from an initial Th2 response to a Th1 response in situ: an immunocytochemical study. J Allergy Clin Immunol 1996; 97:828–837.

36. Mitchell EB, Crow J, Rowntree S, Webster AD, Platts-Mills TAE. Cutaneous basophil hypersensitivity to inhalant allergens in atopic dermatitis: elicitation of delayed responses containing basophils following local transfer of immune serum but not IgE antibody. J Invest Dermatol 1984; 83:290–295.

37. Leiferman K, Ackerman S, Sampson H, Haugen H, Venencie P, Gleich G. Dermal deposition of eosinophil-granule major basic protein in atopic dermatitis. N Engl J Med 1985; 313:47–56.

38. Dvorak HF, Mihm MC, Dvorak AM. Morphology of delayed-type hypersensitivity reactions in man. J Invest Dermatol 1976; 67:391–401.

39. de Groot AC, Young E. The role of contact allergy to aeroallergens in atopic dermatitis. Contact Dermatitis 1989; 21:209–214.

40. Rasanen L, Reunala T, Lehto M, Virtanen E, Arvilommi H. Immediate and delayed hypersensitivity reactions to birch pollen in patients with atopic dermatitis. Acta Derm Venereol (Stockh) 1992; 72:193–196.

41. Reitamo S, Visa K, Kahonen K, et al. Patch test reactions to inhalant allergens in atopic dermatitis. Act Derm Venereol (Stockh) 1989; 144(suppl):119–121.

42. Seidenari S, Manzini BM, Danese P, Giannetti A. Positive patch tests to whole mite culture and purified mite extracts in patients with atopic dermatitis, asthma, and rhinitis. Ann Allergy 1992; 69:201–206.

43. Manzini BM, Motolese A, Donini M, Seidenari S. Contact allergy to *Dermatophagoides* in atopic dermatitis patients and healthy subjects. Contact Dermatitis 1995; 33:243–246.

44. Bruijnzeel-Koomen C, van Wichen DF, Toonstra J, Berrens L, Bruijnzeel PL. The presence of IgE molecules on epidermal Langerhans cells in patients with atopic dermatitis. Arch Dermatol Res 1986; 278:199–204.

45. Stingl G, Maurer D. IgE-mediated allergen presentation via Fc epsilon RI on antigen-presenting cells. Int Arch Allergy Immunol 1997; 113:24–29.

46. Mudde GC, van Reijsen FC, Boland GJ, De Gast PLB, Bruijnzeel-Koomen C. Allergen presentation by epidermal Langerhans' cells from patients with atopic dermatitis is mediated by IgE. J Immunol 1990; 69:335–341.

47. Maurer D, Ebner C, Reininger B, et al. The high affinity IgE receptor (FcɛR1) mediates IgE-dependent allergen presentation. J Immunol 1995; 154:6285–6290.

48. Rattis FM, Peguet-Navarro J, Staquet MJ, et al. Expression and function of B7-1 (CD80) and B7-2 (CD86) on human epidermal Langerhans cells. Eur J Immunol 1996; 26:449–453.

49. Ohki O, Yokozeki H, Katayama I, et al. Functional CD86 (B7-2/B70) is predominantly expressed on Langerhans cells in atopic dermatitis. Br J Dermatol 1997; 136:838–845.

50. Kuchroo VK, Das MP, Brown JA, et al. B7-1 and B7-2 costimulatory molecules activated differentially the Th1/Th2 developmental pathways: applications to autoimmune disease therapy. Cell 1995; 80:707–718.

51. Hauser C, Snapper CM, Ohara J, Paul WE, Katz SI. T helper cells grown with hapten modified cultured Langerhans cells produce interleukin 4 and stimulate IgE production by B cells. Eur J Immunol 1989; 19:2435–2451.

52. Sager N, Feldmann A, Schilling G, Kreitsch P, Neumann C. House dust mite-specific T cells in the skin of subjects with atopic dermatitis: frequency and lymphokine profile in the allergen patch test. J Allergy Clin Immunol 1992; 89:801–810.

53. Grewe M, Walther S, Gyufko K, Czech W, Schopf E, Krutmann J. Analysis of the cytokine pattern expressed in situ in inhalant allergen patch test reactions of atopic dermatitis patients. J Invest Derm 1995; 105:407–410.

54. Yamada N, Wakugawa M, Kuwata S, Yoshida T, Nakagawa H. Chronologic analysis of in situ cytokine expression in mite allergen-induced dermatitis in atopic subjects. J Allergy Clin Immunol 1995; 96:1069–1075.

55. Hamid Q, Boguniewicz M, Leung D. Differential in situ cytokine gene expression in acute vs. chronic atopic dermatitis. J Clin Invest 1994; 94:870–876.

56. Grewe M, Gyufko K, Schopf E, Krutmann J. Lesional expression of interferon-γ in atopic eczema. Lancet 1995; 343:25–26.

57. Cohen MB, Ecker EE, Breitbart JR, Rudolph JA. The rate of absorption of ragweed pollen material from the nose. J Immunol 1930; 18:419–425.

58. Clark RAF, Adinoff AD. The relationship between positive aeroallergen patch test reactions and aeroallergen exacerbations of atopic dermatitis. Clin Immunol Immunpathol 1989; 53: S132–S140.

59. Tuft L, Heck VM. Studies in atopic dermatitis. IV. Importance of seasonal inhalant allergens, especially ragweed. J Allergy 1952; 23:528–540.

60. Gondo A, Saeki N, Tokuda Y. Challenge reactions in atopic dermatitia after percutaneous entry of mite antigen. Br J Dermatol 1986; 115:485–493.

61. Tanaka Y, Anan S, Yoshida H. Immunohistochemical studies of mite antigen-induced patch-test sites in atopic dermatitis. J Dermatol Sci 1990; 1:361–368.

62. Tupker RA, De Monchy JGR, Coenraads PJ, Homan A, van der Meer JB. Induction of atopic dermatitis by inhalation of house dust mite. J Allergy Clin Immunol 1996; 97:1064–1070.

63. Darsow U, Vieluf D, Ring J. The atopy patch test: an increased rate of reactivity in patients who have an air-exposed pattern of atopic eczema. Br J Dermatol 1996; 135:182–186.

64. Picker LJ, Tree JR, Ferguson-Darnell B, Collins PA, Bergstresser PR, Terstappen LWMM. Control of lymphocyte recirculation in man II. Differential regulation of the cutaneous lympho-cyte-associated antigen, a tissue-selective homing receptor for skin homing T cells. J Immunol 1993; 150:1122–1136.

64a. Scalabrin DMF, Bavbek S, Perzanowski, Wilson BB, Platts-Mills TAE, Wheatley LM. Use of specific IgE in assessing the relevance of fungal and dust mite allergen to atopic dermatitis: a comparison with asthmatic and nonasthmatic control subjects. J Allergy Clin Immunol 1999; in press.

65. Kieffer M, Bergbrandt I-M, Faergemann J, et al. Immune reactions to *Pityrosporum ovale* in adult patients with atopic and seborrheic dermatitis. J Am Acad Dermatol 1990; 22:739–742.

66. Broberg A, Faergemann J, Johansson S, Johansson SGO, Strannegard I-L, Svejgaard E. Pityro-sporum ovale and atopic dermatitis in children and young adults. Acta Derm Venereol (Stockh) 1992; 72:187–192.

67. Rokugo M, Tagami H, Usuba Y, Tomita Y. Contact sensitivity to *Pityrosporum ovale* in pa-tients with atopic dermatitis. Arch Dermatol 1990; 126:627–632.

68. Tengvall Linder M, Johansson C, Bengtsson A, Holm L, Harfast B, Scheynius A. *Pityrosprum orbiculare*-reactive T-cell lines in atopic dermatitis patients and healthy individuals. Scand J Immunol 1998; 47:152–158.

69. Back O, Scheynius A, Johansson SGO. Ketoconazole in atopic dermatitis: therapeutic response is correlated with the decrease in serum IgE. Arch Dermatol Res 1995; 1995:448–451.

70. Kolmer H, Taketomi E, Hazen K, Hughs E, Wilson B, Platts-Mills T. Effect of combined antibacterial and antifungal treatment in severe atopic dermatitis. J Allergy Clin Immunol 1996; 98:702–707.

# 23

## The Atopy Patch Test: Its Role in the Evaluation and Management of Atopic Eczema

**Ulf Darsow and Johannes Ring**
*Technical University Munich, Munich, Germany*

## I. DEFINITION

Atopic eczema (atopic dermatitis) is a chronic inflammatory skin disease characterized by intense pruritus and a typical age-related distribution and skin morphology [1,2]. We have defined atopy as a "familial tendency to develop certain diseases (extrinsic bronchial asthma, allergic rhinoconjunctivitis and/or atopic eczema) on the basis of a hypersensitivity of skin and mucous membranes against environmental substances, associated with increased immunoglobulin E (IgE) production and/or altered nonspecific reactivity" [3,4]. The atopy patch test (APT) is an epicutaneous patch-test with allergens known to elicit IgE-mediated reactions for the evaluation of eczematous skin lesions [5–7].

## II. INTRODUCTION

A frequent finding in patients with atopic eczema is elevated serum IgE (for review, see Ref. 8). Positive correlation between total IgE level and severity of atopic eczema has been described [9,10]. A high proportion of the elevated IgE consists of antibodies against aeroallergens, especially specific IgE to house dust mites, for which a connection of disease severity and specific IgE levels has been described [11]. Patients with atopic eczema and elevated mite-specific IgE show marked improvement of skin lesions in a mite-free room [12,13].

The scientific basis for the concept of aeroallergens as triggers of atopic eczema was sustained by the discovery of IgE and IgE-binding structures on the surface of epidermal Langerhans cells [14–16] together with the major mite allergen Der p I [17]. Allergen-specific T cells have been cloned from atopy patch test biopsies. Depending on the developmental stage of the APT reaction, these T cells showed characteristic Th2 secretion patterns [18,19]. Thus, a role of Langerhans cells in binding and presenting "immediate-type" allergens penetrating the defective epidermal barrier in atopic eczema patients is suggested to explain the development of eczema.

However, there is still marked discrepancy between this theoretical concept and the practical side: the classic skin and in vitro tests of IgE-mediated sensitivity are discussed controversially in their diagnostic value in patients with atopic eczema. A test for the evaluation of the actual clinical relevance of (often multiple) sensitizations is needed to initiate appropriate and economically sensible allergen-avoidance measures.

Following the clinical observation that some patients describe exacerbation of their skin lesions after contact with aeroallergens like animal dander and improve after appropriate avoidance strategies [20], several groups demonstrated that eczematous skin lesions can be induced in some patients with atopic eczema by patch-testing with aeroallergens (mostly house dust mite) [5–7,21–36]. Aeroallergens were included in an early series of patch tests reported by Rostenberg and Sulzberger, in 1937 [37]. "Dermatitis of the Hand Due to Atopic Allergy to Pollen" was published by Rowe in 1946 [38]. In a subgroup of patients with atopic eczema, environmental substances, in most cases aeroallergens, seem to play an important role in exacerbating skin lesions. An epicutaneous patch test with allergens known to elicit IgE-mediated reactions and evaluation of eczematous skin lesions [5–7] seems to be the diagnostic tool in characterizing this subgroup of patients (APT).

Patch tests with aeroallergens in a group of patients with atopic eczema were first published in 1982 by Mitchell et al. [28]. Percentages from 15 to 100% of positive APT results were reported from different groups, obviously due to wide variations in the methodology: skin abrasion [25,28,29], tape stripping [22,36], and sodium lauryl sulfate application [34] were used to enhance allergen penetration. In a preliminary trial, we obtained positive atopy patch test reactions in 30% of tested patients using standard skin prick test solutions without clear-cut correlations to skin prick test or specific IgE measurements [7]. We performed investigations on vehicle, dose-response relationships and clinical covariates of the APT in order to obtain a test for clinical routine with optimal allergen penetration without irritation of the atopic skin.

## III. CLINICAL EXPERIENCE

### A. Materials

APT studies were performed with allergens (lyophilisates) from house dust mite (*Dermatophagoides pteronyssinus*), cat dander, and grass pollen mixture. In a larger multicenter trial, birch and mugwort pollen were also included. Lyophilisates were provided by Allergopharma, Reinbek and different preparations for testing according to our study plans were made by Hermal, Reinbek. Allergen dose varied between 500 and 10,000 protein nitrogen units (PNU) per gram in different trials. Initially, petrolatum and hydrogel (methylcellulose) vehicles were compared.

### B. Methods

All APT studies were performed after discontinuance of antihistamines and systemic and topical (test area) steroids for at least 7 days. Large Finn chambers (12 mm in diameter) were used to apply the test substances on clinically uninvolved, nonabraded and untreated back skin. Grading of positive APT reactions was similar to the criteria used in conventional contact allergy patch testing (ICDRG rules, 39). In control areas, vehicles without allergens were tested; the vehicle additives propylene glycole and isopropyl myristate

(10% each) and a 0.5% solution of sodium lauryl sulfate as irritative model were also included in the test panel. Results were evaluated after 48 and 72 hours and compared with skin prick, total, and specific serum IgE.

Thirty-six patients with atopic eczema, 4 patients with rhinoconjunctivitis only, and 10 healthy controls were included in a methodological trial [6]. APT were performed with 1,000 and 10,000 PNU/g in petrolatum and hydrogel. After 48 hours, the reactions of 17 patients were graded as clear-cut positive (47% ≥ +). An example is given in Figure 1. Allergens in petrolatum elicited twice as many APT reactions as allergens in hydrogel vehicle. This held true for different reaction intensities and allergen concentrations. Thirty-six percent of patients reacted to house dust mite. The reactions to cat dander and grass pollen were seen in 22% and 16% of patients. Control patch test sites with vehicles and additives remained negative in all subjects. Nonatopic controls and patients suffering from allergic rhinoconjunctivitis only presented no positive APT reactions. To evaluate and compare nonspecific irritation, sodium lauryl sulfate was included in the test: 33% of patients and 29% of controls developed a sharp-lined erythema without papules, which was strictly limited to the edges of the Finn chamber containing the irritant. These reactions, clinically distinguishable from aeroallergen test sites, were not correlated with APT reactivity. No influence of a history of allergic rhinoconjunctivitis was seen. In most cases, the peak severity of APT reactions was reached after 48 hours. Thus, the following results describe the APT reactions obtained after this time.

## C. Dose-Response of the APT

In the first study with 36 patients, 72% of clear-cut positive reactions were provoked with 10,000 PNU/g of allergen. In contrast, only 28% were already elicited by 1,000 PNU/g. This difference was independent of the vehicle used, as similar proportions were obtained with hydrogel and petrolatum. The comparison of vehicles and allergen concentrations was performed with regard to the total number of reactions and to the number of patients

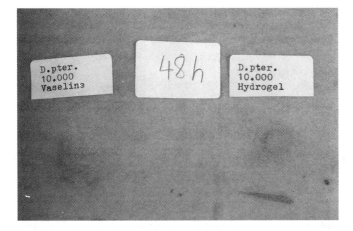

**Figure 1**   Atopy patch test reaction in a patient with atopic eczema after removal of Finn chambers after 48 hours.

showing at least erythematous reactions under certain test conditions. In 15 of 23 patients, a higher rate of reaction was obtained with higher concentrations ($p = 0.0023$, Wilcoxon matched-pairs signed-rank test).

A prospective dose-dependency study with four concentrations of the same three aeroallergens was performed in 57 patients with atopic eczema using the petrolatum vehicle [40]. According to their eczema pattern, patients were divided into two subgroups. Group I ($n = 26$) patients had eczematous skin lesions predominantly on air-exposed areas: hands, lower arms, head and neck area, ankles. In group II, 31 patients were compared as a control group without a conspicious distribution of skin lesions: these patients had lesions exceeding air-exposed areas or only on the trunk. The allergens were used in concentrations of 500, 3,000, 5,000, and 10,000 PNU/g. In 53% of patients, at least one APT reaction was graded as clear-cut positive according to ICDRG guidelines. In this study, control areas with vehicle again remained negative in all subjects. In the same patient the strength of reaction typically increased with the allergen concentration in a dose-dependent manner. The percentage of patients with clear-cut positive reactions was significantly higher in group I patients with eczematous skin lesions predominantly in air-exposed areas (18 of 26 patients = 69%) compared with group II (12 of 31 patients = 39%; $p = 0.02$, Fisher's exact test). A clear dose-response relationship between allergen concentration and number of patients with a positive APT result was obtained in both groups (Fig. 2). However, the mode of this dose-dependent increase in positive results in group I differed from group II ($p = 0.03$, Halton-Freeman test). Both groups were best differentiated with 5,000 PNU/g. In group I, the last concentration step doubling allergen concentration to 10,000 PNU/g increased APT reactivity only in 11%. The effect was independent from reaction intensity or kind of allergen. The results of this study confirmed that aeroallergens are able to elicit eczematous skin lesions in a dose-dependent way in different groups of patients with atopic eczema when applied epicutaneously. A subgroup of patients prone to develop an APT reaction was characterized.

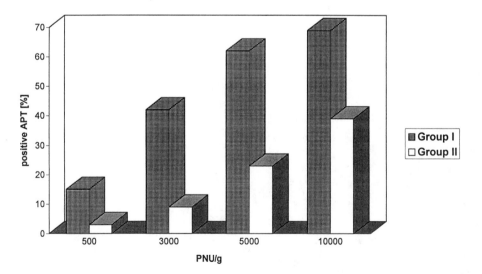

**Figure 2**  Percentage of patients with positive APT reactions and pattern of atopic eczema ($n =$ 57). Group I: Patients with eczematous skin lesions predominantly located in air-exposed areas. Group II: Control patients with atopic eczema.

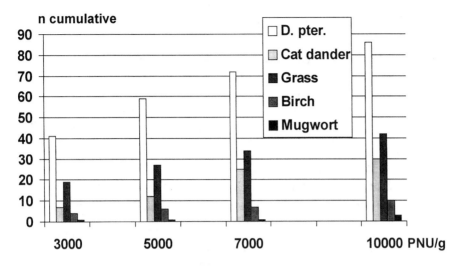

**Figure 3** Dose-response of atopy patch test in 253 patients with atopic eczema (birch and mugwort pollen, $N = 88$).

Generally suitable allergen concentrations for the APT could finally be obtained in a multicenter trial involving 253 adult patients with atopic eczema [41] (Figs. 3 and 4). This time, we focused upon the important allergen concentration range from 5,000 to 10,000 PNU/g. The allergen dose with the most clear-cut results (positive or negative) could be determined for the most frequent aeroallergens by means of a two-step McNemar-statistics. For house dust mite and cat dander, 5,000–7,000 PNU/g gave best results. Grass pollen may be tested with 5,000 PNU/g. We are currently planning a study with biologically standardized allergen preparations with defined major allergen content.

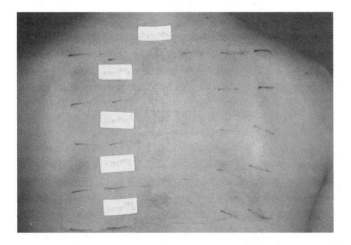

**Figure 4** APT reaction (48 hr) to 3,000–10,000 PNU/g *D. pter.* allergen lyophilisate in petrolatum. Reaction shows dose-dependent increase in intensity.

## D.  Concordance of APT, Skin Prick Test, and Specific IgE

The individual APT allergen pattern of the patients varied with their skin prick and specific IgE results. In the first study, patients with positive APT to D. pter. showed in 62% a corresponding positive skin prick test and in 77% a corresponding elevated specific IgE. This results in allergen-specific concordance of 0.53 (skin prick) and 0.69 (specific IgE). For APT with cat allergen the concordance is 0.5 for skin prick and 0.67 for specific IgE; in grass pollen APT concordances of 0.39 (skin prick) and 0.42 (specific IgE) were observed (the cross-tabulation is shown in Table 1).

These results were corroborated in a large-scale, double-blind multicenter trial [41]. Two hundred and fifty-three adult patients with atopic eczema were tested with 3,000–10,000 PNU/g of house dust mite, cat dander, grass pollen, and (in two study centers, $n = 88$) with birch and mugwort pollen in petrolatum. Forty-eight–and 72-hour readings were done after obtaining skin prick and specific IgE data and a detailed history on aeroallergen-induced eczema flares. Clear-cut positive APT reactions were seen in 34% (44%) with house dust mite, 18% (24%) with grass pollen, 11% (17%) with birch pollen, 12% (15%) with cat dander, and 3% (5%) with mugwort pollen (excluding, respectively, patients with questionable results and 10 dropouts). Positive skin prick and specific IgE results were more frequent (See Table 2). Cross-table analysis and logistic regression revealed significant concordances of APT results with history, skin prick test, and specific corresponding IgE for house dust mite, cat dander, and grass pollen ($p < 0.001$). However,

**Table 1**   Results of Atopy Patch-Test, Skin Prick Test, and Specific IgE in 36 Patients with Atopic Eczema

|  | Number of patients with | | |
|---|---|---|---|
|  | APT+ | APT− | Total |
| *D. pter.* |  |  |  |
| Skin prick+ | 8 | 12 | 20 |
| − | 5 | 11 | 16 |
| Total | 13 | 23 | 36 |
| Spec. IgE+ | 10 | 8 | 18 |
| − | 3 | 15 | 18 |
| Total | 13 | 23 | 36 |
| Cat dander |  |  |  |
| Skin prick+ | 7 | 17 | 24 |
| − | 1 | 11 | 12 |
| Total | 8 | 28 | 36 |
| Spec. IgE+ | 5 | 9 | 14 |
| − | 3 | 19 | 22 |
| Total | 8 | 28 | 36 |
| Grass pollen |  |  |  |
| Skin prick+ | 4 | 20 | 24 |
| − | 2 | 10 | 12 |
| Total | 6 | 30 | 36 |
| Spec. IgE+ | 4 | 19 | 23 |
| − | 2 | 11 | 13 |
| Total | 6 | 30 | 36 |

**Table 2** APT Multicenter Study: Reactivity to Different Allergens in Different Test Systems

| Clear-cut positive results: | | Skin prick (%) | RAST (%) | APT48 (%) |
|---|---|---|---|---|
| *D. pter.* | $n = 253$ | 59 | 56 | 34 |
| Cat dander | $n = 253$ | 54 | 49 | 12 |
| Grass pollen | $n = 253$ | 65 | 75 | 18 |
| Birch pollen | $n = 88$ | 65 | 65 | 11 |
| Mugwort pollen | $n = 88$ | 36 | 53 | 3 |

One allergen 22%; 2 allergens 8%, 3 allergens 5% (APT 48 hr).

the results also showed that high allergen-specific IgE in serum is not mandatory for a positive atopy patch test, and the same holds true for the correlation with skin prick tests. One may conclude that the APT may give further diagnostic information in addition to patient's history and classical tests of IgE-mediated hypersensitivity. On the other hand, a role for IgE in the reaction mechanism of APT is suggested, since in most APT-positive patients elevated specific IgE was found compared to those with negative APT.

## E. Clinical Significance of the APT—Sensitivity and Specificity

In classic contact allergy patch testing with low molecular weight chemicals, the history of allergen-induced eczema exacerbation is used as proof of clinical relevance. With regard to the clinically known phenomenon of "summer eruption of atopic eczema," we tested 79 patients with an APT with 10,000 PNU/g grass pollen allergen mixture in petrolatum and simultaneously with 10 mg dry unprocessed pollen of *Dactylis glomerata* grass [42]. Again, the APT results were compared with history, skin prick tests, specific corresponding IgE, and the eczema pattern. In this study, significantly higher frequencies of positive APT with both methods were seen in patients with corresponding history of exacerbation of their eczema in the summer months of the previous year and/or in direct contact with grass (12 of 79 patients, 75% had positive APT) compared to patients without this history (67 of 79, 16% had positive APT; $p < 0.001$). There was also a significant concordance of standardized and raw grass pollen APT. The standardized allergen mixture also significantly correlated with the other items tested ($p < 0.001$). Controls showed no APT reaction, either to lyophilized grass pollen allergens or to dry unprocessed pollen. The concordances allowed first calculations of precision data of the APT (as described in Table 3). With regard to a predictive history of grass pollen–induced exacerbations of eczema lesions, the APT specificity exceeded the specificity of the classic tests of IgE-mediated

**Table 3** Results of Tests for Grass Pollen Hypersensitivity

| Test | Sensitivity[a] | Specificity[a] |
|---|---|---|
| Skin prick test grass pollen | 1.00 | 0.33 |
| CAP-FEIA grass pollen | 0.92 | 0.33 |
| APT grass pollen allergens petrolatum | 0.75 | 0.84 |
| APT native pollen *D. glomerata* | 0.67 | 0.90 |

[a] Referred to history of exacerbations during grass pollen season.

**Table 4**  APT, Skin Prick Test and Specific IgE in 253
Patients with Atopic Eczema[a]

| Test | Sensitivity (%) | Specificity (%) |
|------|-----------------|-----------------|
| Skin prick | 69–82 | 44–53 |
| Specific IgE | 65–94 | 42–64 |
| APT | 42–56 | 69–92 |

[a] Sensitivity and specificity (allergen-dependent) in a double-blind multicenter trial.

hypersensitivity by far. The calculated positive predictive value (percentage: true positive
compared to all positive) was 0.45 and 0.53 with APT versus 0.21 with skin prick test
and 0.20 with specific IgE (Pharmacia CAP System). The fact that unprocessed pollen
elicited eczematous skin reactions on unpretreated skin of atopic eczema patients (in
healthy and rhinoconjunctivitis controls, no positive reactions were observed) with good
correlation to history suggests that pollen are involved in eczema flares in some patients.

In the blinded multicenter study, 10–52% of patients reported previous eczema flares
after contact with specific allergen. The APT showed a higher specificity (depending on
allergen) with regard to clinical relevance of an allergen as compared to skin prick test
and specific IgE, but also under certain conditions lower sensitivity (Table 4). A predictive
eczema pattern with predominantly face, head, and neck involvement was associated with
a positive 48-hour APT reaction to cat dander ($p = 0.03$).

## IV.  MECHANISMS OF APT REACTIONS

The results of APT studies in several groups of patients with atopic eczema have clearly
given evidence that aeroallergens are able to elicit eczematous skin lesions in at least a
subgroup of these patients through skin contact and without alteration of skin surface
characteristics by using irritants, tape stripping, scratching, or others. The reactions were
allergen-specific and dose-dependent. Regarding the correlation of APT with skin prick
test and specific IgE results, no 100% concordance was observed. This means that with
APT a dimension of atopic skin inflammation is registered that is different from the sensitization demonstrable in the skin prick test or RAST. The allergen-specific nature of atopy
patch test reactions has been shown by several groups. Langeland et al. [27] transferred
APT reactivity to egg performing a Prausnitz-Küstner test. Van Reijsen et al. [18] and
Sager et al. [19] characterized allergen-specific T-cell clones derived from skin specimens
taken from APT sites. Mite allergen has been demonstrated in the epidermis under natural
conditions [17] and in APT sites [25,34] in proximity to Langerhans cells. Langerhans
cells carry all three human IgE-binding structures, namely the high and low-affinity IgE
receptors (FceRI and II) and the epsilon-binding protein [14,15,34]. Thus, they are capable
of binding allergens via specific IgE on their surface. According to their known function
as antigen-presenting cells, they may also internalize, process, and present these allergens
to T cells. We and others described a significant association of positive APT reactions
and specific serum-IgE. This might explain how IgE-associated activation of allergen-
specific T cells can lead to eczematous skin eruptions in the atopy patch test (Fig. 5). One
may speculate that features of the skin barrier contribute to different epicutaneous reaction
patterns in patients with atopic eczema. Recently, increased transepidermal water loss in

# Barrier defect

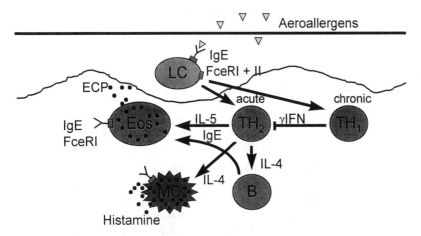

**Figure 5** Mechanism of aeroallergen-triggered atopic eczema. LC, Langerhans cell; FceRI+ II, IgE receptors; Eos, Eosinophil; MC, mast cell; ECP, eosinophil cationic protein; TH1/TH2/B, lymphocyte subsets.

patients with atopic eczema and positive APT reactions was described comparing their APT sites with positive patch test sites after classic contact allergy testing [43].

Within the APT lesions, the inflammatory infiltrate is dominated by T lymphocytes with a T4:T8 ratio of 2–6:1 and, to a lesser degree, of Langerhans and indeterminant T-cells when immunostaining is performed in cryostat sections [44]. A similar situation is found in natural lesions of atopic eczema characterized also by a predominance of CD4-positive T cells [45,46]. Aeroallergen-specific T-cell clones were derived from positive APT reaction sites [19,47]. However, allergen-specific T cells represent always a minority of lesional T cells (2–5%). In a subgroup of our patients of the multicenter trial, specific activation parameters of T cells in peripheral blood were compared with the patients' APT result. Also, specific lymphocyte proliferation was investigated in these patients [48]. APT reactions were significantly more frequent in patients with elevated CD54+ or CD30+ T cells after in vitro stimulation with the corresponding allergen. Positive APT were associated with an allergen-specific lymphocyte proliferation ($p < 0.001$). These data sustain the clinical results on allergen-specificity of APT reactions.

When serial biopsies of APT were performed to analyze the cytokine pattern, marked time-dependent differences were seen: interleukin-4 mRNA as marker of the Th2 response was noted after 24 hours, followed by a switch to a Th1-like cytokine response with increased levels of interferon-gamma mRNA after 48 hours [49]. The increase in interferon-gamma mRNA levels during a late APT reaction confirms earlier findings, in which interferon-gamma, but not interleukin 4 mRNA, is increased in chronic lesions of atopic eczema [50]. Other cell populations may also be involved in the initiation and perpetuation of APT reactions (Fig. 5). Among these are basophils, present in the infiltrate after 48 hours [28], and activated eosinophils [22]. Eosinophil-derived basic proteins (MBP, ECP, EPX) can be detected in atopic eczema lesions by immunohistochemical staining, even with low eosinophil counts in normal HE staining. These eosinophil products may have a role in barrier impairment, thus perpetuating allergen penetration (Fig. 5). The role of mast cells remains to be elucidated. With regard to neutrophil density, marked differences of APT (low) versus experimental late phase reactions (high numbers) were described [51].

## V. POTENTIAL ROLE OF THE APT IN THE MANAGEMENT OF ATOPIC ECZEMA

In patients with an aeroallergen-predictive eczema pattern, positive APT reactions occur with smaller allergen doses compared with other atopic eczema patients. Statistically, there also was a significant correlation with the patient's aeroallergen-specific history. Thus, the APT may provide an important diagnostic tool, especially for these patient subgroups. A preliminary interpretation of the data from larger patient groups (see above for sensitivity and specificity, Table 4) suggests that the APT represents a kind of provocation performed in addition to skin prick test and specific IgE determination. As in bronchial asthma and rhinoconjunctivitis, B. Wüthrich's concept of extrinsic (allergic) versus intrinsic (cryptogenic) atopic eczema seems attractive to explain the heterogenity of disease subgroups. However, open questions remain concerning the clinical relevance of APT results since at the moment no golden standard exists for the provocation of eczematous skin lesions in atopic eczema (in analogy to bronchial or nasal provocation techniques). Controlled studies using specific provocation and elimination procedures in patients with positive and negative APT reactions are desirable to answer these questions. The German multicenter APT study revealed 3–17% (allergen-dependent) APT-positive patients without a corresponding skin prick test and 4–29% positive APT without corresponding elevated specific IgE (CAP class 0 or 1). House dust mite, the allergen where these effects were most frequent, may have additional irritative potential. At the present time, the relevance of these "non-IgE" reactions is unclear. However, the correlation of mite-APT and corresponding specific history was not impaired by this observation.

So far, controlled, double-blind randomized studies examining the impact of preventive measures or active therapeutic interventions based on the results of positive APT reactions on the course of atopic eczema have not been done. Some evidence for the practical relevance of positive APT reactions in the management of the disease can be drawn from Clark and Adinoff's report on 18 patients [23,52], in which a positive APT reaction in combination with the detection of specific IgE antibodies and skin prick tests correlated strongly with aeroallergens identified in the patient's environment, respectively, with their history. Improvement or resolution of skin lesions was documented after avoidance of the identified aeroallergens, followed by an exacerbation after rechallenge [53,54]. Although the final scientific proof for the relevance of aeroallergens identified by positive APT reactions for disease exacerbation or perpetuation still has to be given, the facts described should be considered in clinical management of atopic eczema.

## VI. APT: OUTLOOK

Efforts for standardization of the APT are being coordinated in Europe within the European Task Force on Atopic Dermatitis (ETFAD). This also involves the development of a grading key for APT reactions since these show a somewhat different morphology from classical contact allergy patch test reactions. To date the following key is suggested as a result of two consensus study meetings in Munich on April 11, 1997, and June 30, 1998:

| | |
|---|---|
| − | negative |
| ? | only erythema, questionable |
| + | erythema, infiltration |
| + + | erythema, few papules (up to 3) |
| + + + | erythema, papules from 4 to many |
| + + + + | erythema, many papules or spreading papules |
| + + + + + | erythema, vesicles |

Another goal of future studies is the biological standardization of APT allergen extracts, followed by characterization of the concentration in micrograms of major allergen. More controlled studies are necessary to investigate the diagnostic validity of APT in routine diagnosis of aeroallergen-triggered atopic eczema, but appropriate allergen-specific avoidance strategies are still recommended in patients showing positive APT reactions.

## REFERENCES

1. Hanifin JM, Rajka G. Diagnostic features of atopic dermatitis. Acta Derm Venereol Suppl (Stockh) 1980; 114:146–148.
2. Hanifin JM. Clinical and basic aspects of atopic dermatitis. Semin Dermatol 1983; 2:5.
3. Ring J. Atopy: Condition, disease or syndrome? In: Ruzicka T, Ring J, Przybilla B, eds. Handbook of Atopic Eczema. Berlin: Springer, 1993:3–8.
4. Ring J. Angewandte Allergologie. 2d ed. Munich: MMV Medizin Verlag, 1991.
5. Ring J, Kunz B, Bieber T, Vieluf D, Przybilla B. The "atopy patch test" with aeroallergens in atopic eczema (abstr). J Allergy Clin Immunol 1989; 82:195.
6. Darsow U, Vieluf D, Ring J. Atopy patch test with different vehicles and allergen concentrations—an approach to standardization. J Allergy Clin Immunol 1995; 95:677–684.
7. Vieluf D, Kunz B, Bieber T, Przybilla B, Ring J. "Atopy patch test" with aeroallergens in patients with atopic eczema. Allergo Journal 1993; 2:9–12.
8. Leung DYM, Rhodes AR, Geha RS, Schneider LC, Ring J. Atopic dermatitis (atopic eczema). In: Fitzpatrick TB, Eisen AZ, Wolff K, Freedberg IM, Austen KF, eds. Dermatology in General Medicine. 4th ed. New York: McGraw-Hill, 1993:1543–1563.
9. Jones HE, Inouye JC, McGerity JL, Lewis CW. Atopic disease and serum immunoglobulin-E. Br J Dermatol 1975; 92:17–25.
10. Meneghini CL, Bonifazi E. Correlation between clinical and immunological findings in atopic dermatitis. Acta Derm Venereol (Stockh) 1985; 114:140–142.
11. Barnetson RSC, MacFarlane HAF, Benton EC. House dust mite allergy and atopic eczema: a case report. Br J Dermatol 1987; 116:857–860.
12. Fukuda H, Imayama S, Okada T. Mite-free room for the management of atopic dermatitis. Jpn J Allergol 1991; 40:626–632.
13. Sanda T, Yasue T, Oohashi M, Yasue A. Effectiveness of house-dust mite allergen avoidance through clean room therapy in patients with atopic dermatitis. J Allergy Clin Immunol 1992; 89:653–657.
14. Bieber T, Rieger A, Neuchrist C, Prinz JC, Rieber EP, Boltz-Nitulescu G, Scheiner O, Kraft D, Ring J, Stingl G. Induction of FCeR2/CD23 on human epidermal Langerhans cells by human recombinant IL4 and IFN. J Exp Med 1989; 170:309–314.
15. Bieber T, de la Salle C, Wollenberg A, Hakimi J, Chizzonite R, Ring J, Hanau D, de la Salle C.

Constitutive expression of the high affinity receptor for IgE (FCeR1) on human Langerhans cells. J Exp Med 1992; 175:1285–1290.

16. Bruynzeel-Koomen C, van Wichen DF, Toonstra J, Berrens L, Bruynzeel PLB. The presence of IgE molecules on epidermal Langerhans cells in patients with atopic dermatitis. Arch Dermatol Res 1986; 278:199–205.

17. Maeda K, Yamamoto K, Tanaka Y, Anan S, Yoshida H. House dust mite (HDM) antigen in naturally occurring lesions of atopic dermatitis (AD): the relationship between HDM antigen in the skin and HDM antigen-specific IgE antibody. J Derm Sci 1992; 3:73–77.

18. van Reijsen FC, Bruynzeel-Koomen CAFM, Kalthoff FS, Maggi E, Romagnani S, Westland J, Mudde GC. Skin-derived aeroallergen-specific T-cell clones of Th2 phenotype in patients with atopic dermatitis. J Allergy Clin Immunol 1992; 90:184–192.

19. Sager N, Feldmann A, Schilling G, Kreitsch P, Neumann C. House dust mite-specific T cells in the skin of subjects with atopic dermatitis: frequency and lymphokine profile in the allergen patch test. J Allergy Clin Immunol 1992; 89:801–810.

20. Platts-Mills TAE, Chapman MD, Mitchell B, Heymann PW, Deuell B. Role of inhalant allergens in atopic eczema. In: Ruzicka T, Ring J, Przybilla T, eds. Handbook of Atopic Eczema. Berlin: Springer, 1993:192–203.

21. Adinoff A, Tellez P, Clark R. Atopic dermatitis and aeroallergen contact sensitivity. J Allergy Clin Immunol 1988; 81:736–742.

22. Bruynzeel-Koomen C, van Wichen D, Spry C, Venge P, Bruynzeel P. Active participation of eosinophils in patch test reactions to inhalant allergens in patients with atopic dermatitis. Br J Dermatol 1988; 118:229–238.

23. Clark R, Adinoff A. Aeroallergen contact can exacerbate atopic dermatitis: patch test as a diagnostic tool. J Am Acad Dermatol 1989; 21:863–869.

24. Darsow U, Vieluf D, Ring J. Concordance of atopy patch test, prick test and specific IgE in patients with atopic eczema. J Derm Sci 1993; 6:95.

25. Gondo A, Saeki N, Tokuda Y. Challenge reactions in atopic dermatitis after percutaneous entry of mite antigen. Br J Dermatol 1986; 115:485–493.

26. Imayama S, Hashizume T, Miyahara H, et al. Combination of patch test and IgE for dust mite antigens differentiates 130 patients with atopic dermatitis into four groups. J Am Acad Dermatol 1992; 27:531–538.

27. Langeland T, Braathen L, Borch M. Studies of atopic patch tests. Acta Derm Venereol (Stockh) 1989; Suppl 144:105–109.

28. Mitchell E, Chapman M, Pope F, Crow J, Jouhal S, Platts-Mills T. Basophils in allergen-induced patch test sites in atopic dermatitis. Lancet 1982; 1:127–130.

29. Norris P, Schofield O, Camp R. A study of the role of house dust mite in atopic dermatitis. Br J Dermatol 1988; 118:435–440.

30. Platts-Mills T, Mitchell E, Rowntree S, Chapman M, Wilkins S. The role of dust mite allergens in atopic dermatitis. Clin Exp Dermatol 1983; 8:233–247.

31. Reitamo S, Visa K, Kaehoenen K, et al. Patch test reactions to inhalant allergens in atopic dermatitis. Acta Derm Venereol (Stockh) 1989; Suppl 144:119–121.

32. Seidenari S, Manzini BM, Danese P, Giannetti A. Positive patch tests to whole mite culture and purified mite extracts in patients with atopic dermatitis, asthma and rhinitis. Ann Allergy 1992; 69:201–206.

33. Seifert H, Wollemann G, Seifert B, Borelli S. Neurodermitis: Eine Protein-Kontaktdermatitis? Dtsch Derm 1987; 35:1204–1214.

34. Tanaka Y, Anan S, Yoshida H. Immunohistochemical studies in mite antigen-induced patch test sites in atopic dermatitis. J Derm Sci 1990; 1:361–368.

35. Vocks E, Seifert H, Seifert B, Drosner M. Patch test with immediate type allergens in patients with atopic dermatitis. In: Ring J, Przybilla B, eds. New Trends in Allergy III. Berlin: Springer, 1991:230–233.

36. van Voorst Vader PC, Lier JG, Woest TE, Coenraads PJ, Nater JP. Patch tests with house

dust mite antigens in atopic dermatitis patients: methodological problems. Acta Derm Venereol (Stockh) 1991; 71:301–305.

37. Rostenberg A, Sulzberger MD. Some results of patch tests. Arch Dermatol 1937; 35:433–454.

38. Rowe AH. Dermatitis of the hand due to atopic allergy to pollen. Arch Dermatol Syph 1946; 53:437.

39. Wahlberg JE. Patch testing. In: Rycraft, RJG, Menné T, Frosch PJ, eds. Textbook of Contact Dermatitis. Heidelberg: Springer, 1992:241–367.

40. Darsow U, Vieluf D, Ring J. The atopy patch test: an increased rate of reactivity in patients who have an air exposed pattern of atopic eczema. Br J Dermatol 1996; 135:182–186.

41. Darsow U, Vieluf D, Ring J for the APT study group. Evaluating the relevance of aeroallergen sensitization in atopic eczema with the atopy patch test: a randomized, double-blind multicenter study. J Am Acad Dermatol 1999; 40:187–193.

42. Darsow U, Behrendt H, Ring J. Gramineae pollen as trigger factors of atopic eczema—evaluation of diagnostic measures using the atopy patch test. Br J Dermatol 1997; 137:201–207.

43. Gfesser M, Rakoski J, Ring J. Disturbance of epidermal barrier function in atopy patch test reactions in atopic eczema. Br J Dermatol 1996; 135:560–565.

44. Reitamo S, Visa K, Kähönen K, Stubb S, Salo OP. Eczematous reactions in atopic patients caused by epicutaneous testing with inhalant allergens. Br J Dermatol 1986; 114:303–309.

45. Leung DYM, Bhan AK, Schneeberger EE, Geha RS. Characterization of the mononuclear cell infiltrate in atopic dermatitis using mononuclear antibodies. J Allergy Clin Immunol 1983; 71:47–56.

46. Zachary GB, Allen MH, MacDonald DM. In situ quantification of T-lymphocyte subsets and Langerhans cells in the inflammatory infiltrate of atopic eczema. Br J Dermatol 1985; 112:149–155.

47. Ramb-Lindhauer CH, Feldmann A, Rotte M, Neumann CH. Characterization of grass pollen reactive T-cell lines derived from lesional atopic skin. Arch Dermatol Res 1991; 283:71–76.

48. Wistokat-Wülfing A, Schmidt P, Darsow U, Ring J, Kapp A, Werfel T. Atopy patch test reactions are associated with T-lymphocyte mediated allergen-specific immune responses in atopic dermatitis. Clin Exp Allergy 1999; 29:513–521.

49. Grewe M, Walther S, Gyufko K, Czech W, Schöpf E, Krutmann J. Analysis of the cytokine pattern expressed in situ in inhalant allergen patch test reactions of atopic dermatitis patients. J Invest Dermatol 1995; 105:407–410.

50. Grewe M, Gyufko K, Schöpf E, Krutmann J. Lesional expression of interferon-gamma in atopic eczema. Lancet 1994; 343:25–26.

51. Langeveld-Wildschut EG, Thepen T, Bihari IC, van Reijsen FC, de Vries IJM, Bruijnzeel PLB, Bruijnzeel-Koomen CAFM. Evaluation of the atopy patch test and the cutaneous late-phase reaction as relevant models for the study of allergic inflammation in patients with atopic eczema. J Allergy Clin Immunol 1996; 98:1019–1027.

52. Clark RA, Adinoff AD. The relationship between positive aeroallergen patch test reactions and aeroallergen exacerbations of atopic dermatitis. Clin Immunol Immunpathol 1989; 53:S132–S140.

53. Kubota Y, Imayama S, Hori Y. Reduction of environmental mites improved atopic dermatitis patients with positive mite-patch test. J Dermatol (Tokyo) 1992; 19:177–180.

54. Lau S, Ehnert H, Cremer B, Nasert S, Buettner B, Czarnetzki BM, Wahn U. Häusliche Milben-allergenreduktion bei spezifisch sensibilisierten Patienten mit atopischem Ekzem. Allergo J 1995; 8:432–435.

# 24

## Role of Infection

**Lone Skov and Ole Baadsgaard**
*Gentofte Hospital, University of Copenhagen,
Hellerup, Denmark*

## I. INTRODUCTION

For decades it has been a clinical experience that infection and even colonization of the skin with bacteria and to some extent also with viruses and fungi may lead to the aggravation and even induction of inflammatory skin diseases. Especially in atopic dermatitis, skin colonization with bacteria seems to have a proinflammatory role. However, the role of colonization and the mechanisms for the inflammation induced by infection are not well studied. In this chapter we will focus on the role of colonization and infection in atopic dermatitis.

## II. ATOPIC DERMATITIS

### A. Bacteria

#### 1. Bacterial Skin Flora in Healthy People and Patients with Atopic Dermatitis

Normal skin is colonized by large numbers of bacteria. Those organisms that are found regularly on the skin constitute its normal resident flora. The bacteria live harmlessly in microcolonies on the surface of the stratum corneum and within the outermost layer of the epidermis. The normal flora is part of the defense against potentially pathogenic organisms. The bacteria that belong to the resident human skin flora are Micrococcaceae, including coagulase-negative staphylococci (*Staphylococcus epidermidis*), *Corynebacterium*, *Propionibacterium*, and *Acinetobacter* [1]. The regional variation in the number and type of bacteria is high. On normal skin the number of anaerobic bacteria is higher than the number of aerobic bacteria. In contrast, the skin of patients with atopic dermatitis contains an increased number of aerobic bacteria, especially *S. aureus* and *S. epidermidis* [2–4]. *S. aureus* is not a member of the resident skin flora but is found on the skin in 10% of an unselected population [5]. Several authors have studied the colonization of *S. aureus* on atopic dermatitis skin. In 1974 Leyden et al. [3] found that *S. aureus* could be isolated from 90% of chronic skin lesions in 50 atopic dermatitis patients; the *S. aureus* was isolated at a density of $1 \times 10^6/cm^2$. *S. aureus* was isolated from all patients with exudative lesions at a density of $14 \times 10^6/cm^2$ [3]. Increased numbers of *S. aureus* were also found on clinically normal skin in atopic dermatitis patients [3]. The finding that *S. aureus* is increased in number on atopic skin and that the degree of colonization correlates to the type of skin lesion has been confirmed by several groups [2,4,6,7]. Not only *S. aureus* but also *S. epidermidis* is found in increased number on the skin of patients with atopic dermatitis. It is not known whether *S. epidermidis* has any proinflammatory capacity.

One reason for the increased number of *S. aureus* on atopic skin may be the wet lesions and carry-over due to scratching. Another mechanism may be that *S. aureus* can better adhere to nasal mucosa and corneocytes in patients with atopic dermatitis than in patients with other skin diseases [8–10]. Protein A from *S. aureus* and laminin in the basal membrane may be involved in the adhesion [9,11]. Interestingly, fibronectin, a gluco-protein found in the basal membrane, connective tissue, wounds, and serum, functions as receptor for *S. aureus*, and teichoic acid expressed on *S. aureus* acts as ligand [12–14].

## 2. Staphylococcus aureus *and Atopic Dermatitis*

It is often difficult to determine on clinical grounds whether the skin of patients with atopic dermatitis is colonized with *S. aureus* and, as mentioned above, even skin with a normal appearance may harbor increased numbers of *S. aureus*. Signs of infection are pustules on skin that looks normal, crusting, weeping lesions, increased pruritus, and lymphadenopathy. Usually the patients do not have symptoms of a systemic infection, and the colonization with *S. aureus* does not usually become invasive.

Previously colonization with *S. aureus* was not considered a problem. However, it is now a common clinical experience that infection and even colonization with *S. aureus* may lead to exacerbation of the skin disease. The general opinion has been changed by studies showing that exacerbation was associated with bacterial colonization and that treatment with topical steroid in combination with an antibiotic was more effective than treatment with steroid alone [15].

## 3. *Possible Mechanism for* Staphylococcus aureus–*Induced Aggravation of Atopic Dermatitis*

For years it was believed that the exacerbation following *S. aureus* colonization was due to allergy to the bacteria proteins. Several groups have done skin tests with *S. aureus* antigens, but the results have been inconclusive. The skin test used was primarily a prick test to whole *S. aureus* or to purified *S. aureus* proteins [16,17]. The test methods and the condition of the included patients have not been standardized, and it is therefore impossible to compare the data. In addition, some groups have found strong response to the prick test in normal volunteers [16,17].

*S. aureus* produces enterotoxins including staphylococcal enterotoxins A–E and toxic shock syndrome toxin 1. Ten years ago it was shown that these toxins, like a group of other bacterial and viral proteins, function as a new type of allergens termed superantigens [18]. Superantigens are characterized by their capacity to stimulate a large number of T cells. In contrast to conventional antigens, superantigens bypass intracellular processing and bind directly to the major histocompatibility complex (MHC) class II molecule on the surface of the antigen-presenting cell outside the antigen-binding groove [19–21] (Fig. 1). The superantigen then cross-links the MHC class II molecule on the antigen-presenting cell with T cells according to the composition of the variable region of the T-cell receptor $\beta$ chain (V$\beta$), leading to polyclonal T-cell activation and cytokine release

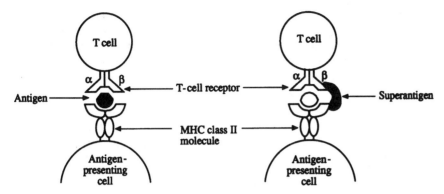

**Figure 1** T-cell activation in the presence of peptide antigens (left) or superantigens (right). The peptide antigen binds in the groove of the major histocompatibility complex (MHC) class II molecule and activates antigen-specific T cells through the T-cell receptor. The superantigen binds to the MHC class II molecule outside the antigen-binding groove and directly cross-links the MHC class II molecule and Vβ chain of the T-cell receptor, leading to polyclonal T-cell activation. (From Ref. 94. Copyright 1995, American Medical Association.)

[22,23]. T cells belonging to both the CD4 and CD8 subtypes are activated. T-cell activation in the presence of superantigens may lead to the activation of several percents of the total T-cell population and thereby activate more than 10–100 times the number of T cells activated in the presence of conventional antigens.

*S. aureus* isolated from the skin of patients with atopic dermatitis releases superantigens [24,25], and it was therefore important to investigate the role of staphylococcal superantigens in atopic dermatitis. We have performed patch tests on the forearm with the superantigen staphylococcal enterotoxin B (SEB) on intact normal and intact atopic skin. In all subjects tested, application of the superantigen induced dermatitis [26]. In addition, three of six subjects suffering from atopic dermatitis experienced a flare of their disease in the elbow flexure ipsilaterally to where the superantigen was applied.

SEB is a relatively large molecule (molecular weight 28 kDa) and may not easily penetrate the skin barrier. The inflammation seen after SEB application was localized to the follicles in many subjects, particularly with the lower doses of SEB. This suggests that SEB may penetrate through sweat gland ducts or hair follicles. Noteworthy, MHC class II molecules are constitutively expressed on the acrosyringial epithelium in the sweat gland ducts [27,28] and have the capacity to bind superantigens. Staphylococcal superantigens probably penetrate the injured skin barrier in patients with atopic skin more easily than they do an intact skin barrier. Keratinocytes, which in healthy epidermis lack MHC class II molecules, are induced to express MHC class II molecules during inflammation [29,30]. Such keratinocytes do not have the capacity to process and present conventional antigens to T cells. In contrast, MHC class II–positive keratinocytes potently activate T cells in the presence of superantigens [31,32]. This may be of special relevance to patients with atopic dermatitis since when keratinocytes that are MHC class II positive present superantigens to T cells, preferentially Th2 type cells are activated [33]. The Th2 cells are thought to be important for the initiation of atopic dermatitis lesions [34,35].

Preliminary data indicate that superantigen-specific T-cell activation is responsible for the dermatitis induced by superantigen application, since biopsies from superantigen-treated skin demonstrated an upregulation of T cells expressing Vβ chains specific for the applied superantigen compared to vehicle-treated skin and peripheral blood mononuclear cells (L. Skov and D. Y. Leung, unpublished). Besides activation of T cells, bacterial superantigens have been shown to induce expression of the skin-homing receptor, the cutaneous lymphocyte-associated antigen (CLA), which may strengthen homing of T cells to the skin [36]. The superantigen-induced expression of CLA may also be responsible for the finding that 14 of 68 patients who survived superantigen-induced toxic shock syndrome subsequently complained of dermatitis [37].

In addition to T-cell activation, superantigens may also directly activate keratinocytes, resulting in the induction of the adhesion molecule ICAM-1 [38] and release of TNF-α [39,40]. After application of SEB on normal human skin, we performed suction blister and found increased release of IL-1β from the blister roofs (L. Skov, unpublished). To summarize, *S. aureus* isolated from atopic skin produces superantigens, superantigens applied on the skin induce dermatitis, superantigens are extremely potent T-cell activators and induce cytokine release from epidermal cells. Superantigens may therefore play an important role in the inflammation seen in patients with atopic dermatitis.

The function of superantigens as allergens has been investigated in one study, in which half of the patients with atopic dermatitis produced IgE directed against staphylococcal superantigens [25]. Basophils from normal subjects and patients with atopic dermatitis who lacked IgE antitoxin failed to release any histamine on exposure to the staphylococcal enterotoxins. In contrast, basophils from patients with atopic dermatitis who produce IgE antitoxin released histamine on exposure to the relevant enterotoxins but not in response to enterotoxins in which there is no IgE response. Not only IgE antibodies directed against staphylococcal enterotoxins but also antibodies to other *S. aureus* antigens have been detected in patients with atopic dermatitis [17,41,42]. The role of IgE antibodies to *S. aureus* may be twofold: (1) IgE specific for *S. aureus* may bind to mast cells or basophils and induce histamine release and thereby induce inflammation and (2) Langerhans cells in atopic skin, compared to normal Langerhans cells, express an increased number of the high-affinity IgE receptor and bind IgE [43–45]. This binding of antigen-specific IgE to the Langerhans cells has been shown to facilitate and amplify the presentation of aeroallergens to the T cells [46,47] and may be involved in the presentation of superantigens as well.

Finally, other staphylococcal toxins may be involved in the exacerbation of atopic dermatitis seen following *S. aureus* colonization. Staphylococcal protein A stimulates release of the proinflammatory cytokine TNF-α from keratinocytes in vitro, and staphylococcal α-toxin, another *S. aureus* toxin, produces profound cytotoxic damage in a keratinocyte cell line [40].

## 4. Treatment

Since it is well documented that the number of *S. aureus* organisms is increased on atopic skin, that the number of bacteria correlates with the intensity of the eczema, and that superantigens from *S. aureus* induce inflammation, it seems rational to reduce the number of *S. aureus* on the skin. Both topical steroids and ultraviolet-B phototherapy have been shown to decrease the density of *S. aureus* on the skin of patients with atopic dermatitis [48–50]. Ultraviolet-B irradiation may have a direct antibacterial effect since, in vitro, the radiation inhibits the growth of *S. aureus* [51,52]. Ultraviolet-B irradiation, like steroids, is known to be effective in the treatment of atopic dermatitis, and this is probably the primary reason for the decreased density of *S. aureus* on the skin. Another way to reduce the number of *S. aureus* is to use disinfectants such as chlorhexidine. The clinical effect of chlorhexidine has not been well studied, but it seems to reduce the number of bacteria on atopic skin [53]. The antibacterial effect is not as strong as with antibiotics, and chlorhexidine can cause irritation. Therefore, many patients are treated with a topical or systemic antibiotic, particularly if the eczema is exudative or extensive.

The beneficial effect of systemic antibiotics in patients with atopic dermatitis has not been investigated in controlled studies. One of the most frequently used antibiotics is erythromycin because it has a lower capacity to sensitized than penicillin. The problem with erythromycin is that an increasing number of *S. aureus* isolated from the skin are resistant to the drug. Since fewer than 5% of *S. aureus* isolates remain sensitive to penicillin, penicillinase-resistant penicillins such as methicillin or cephalosporins are the other drugs of choice if systemic treatment is needed. Methicillin and cephalosporins may lead to sensitization, and the number of methicillin-resistant *S. aureus* is increasing. Alternative drugs are clindamycin, fusidic acid, or the new macrolides. Long-term maintenance therapy should not be used because of the risk of development of resistance.

The efficacy of topical antibiotics seems to be equal to systemic treatment. Leyden et al. compared treatment with topical neomycin and oral erythromycin in patients with atopic dermatitis and found a similar effect on the clinical improvement and decrease in the density of *S. aureus* on the skin following both treatments [3]. In another study gentamycin in combination with steroid was found to be superior to steroid alone [54]. Neomycin and gentamycin are seldom used because of the tendency to induce allergic dermatitis and cross-reactions. Mupirocin, a topical antistaphylococcal agent that is also effective against streptococcus, was found to be effective in atopic dermatitis in a double-blind, placebo-controlled study. Lever et al. found that a combination of topical steroid and mupirocin was more effective than steroid alone judged by both clinical evaluation and the number of *S. aureus* on the skin [15]. Fusidic acid is effective against *S. aureus*, has a low incidence of sensitization, and is often used to treat colonization in atopic dermatitis patients and in impetigo. Treatment with fusidic acid in combination with hydrocortisone acid compared to hydrocortisone acid alone has been investigated in a study including 186 patients with atopic dermatitis [55]. When the authors analyzed only the data from the patients with pathogens on the skin at entry (*S. aureus* and *Streptococcus pyogenes*), they found a significant difference in favor of the combination. In another study the effect of fusidic acid and betamethasone in combination was investigated. Patients with different kinds of eczema including atopic dermatitis were included. The study demonstrated that the combination of fucidic acid and betamethasone was better than betamethasone alone, but the difference was not significant [56]. Problems associated with using topical treatment are sensitization, absorption, and development of resistance.

As noted above, several studies have demostrated that the combination of topical antibiotics and corticosteroids is more effective than corticosteroids alone. These studies strongly corroborate the role of *S. aureus* as an aggravation factor in atopic dermatitis.

## B. Fungi

### 1. Pityrosporum *Yeasts*

In addition to bacteria, the normal human skin is colonized by yeasts. Among the various yeasts, the *Pityrosporum* species seems to be most important. The genus *Pityrosporum* can be divided into several different species, of which the majority are lipophilic. Different names, including *Pityrosporum orbicular*, *Pityrosporum ovale*, and *Malassezia furfur*, have been used for the yeasts cultured from the human skin, but it is not clear whether they are different stages of the same yeast or different species. For practical reasons the term *P. ovale* will be used here.

*P. ovale* is a member of the normal human cutaneous flora and binds to corneocytes [57–59]. The yeast can be cultured from almost all parts of the body, but the highest number is found in the seborrheic areas such as the scalp, face, neck, and upper part of the chest [58]. In most studies *P. ovale* is rarely found before puberty [58,60], but in a study including children under one year, up to 53% of the children were harboring *P. ovale* [61]. The various findings may be due to different culture techniques and culture conditions.

## 2. Pityrosporum *Yeasts and Atopic Dermatitis*

Under special conditions *P. ovale* may become pathogenic. Predisposing factors are increased heat and humidity, occlusive clothing, extensive use of emollients, diabetes, hyperhidrosis, and systemic steroid treatment. *P. ovale* is associated with several skin diseases such as pityriasis versicolor, pityrosporum folliculitis, and seborrheic dermatitis [62,63]. In one study including children and young adults, *P. ovale* could be cultured with the same frequency from patients with atopic dermatitis and healthy age-matched subjects and from involved and uninvolved skin in the patients, indicating that colonization with *P. ovale* is not more frequent on atopic skin [60].

Still, it has been suggested that *P. ovale* plays a role in atopic dermatitis because the findings of positive reactions of prick tests to pityrosporum [64] and a beneficial effect of antifungal treatment [65]. *P. ovale* has especially been associated with a subgroup of atopic patients; patients with itchy, erythematous, dry lesions on the face, scalp, neck, and upper chest termed head-and-neck dermatitis.

## 3. IgE-Mediated Reactions

In a large study of 741 patients prick tested with an aqueous extract of *P. ovale*, 6% of the patients with atopic dermatitis and 28% of the patients with the head-and-neck type of atopic dermatitis had a positive reaction. In contrast, patients with other types of atopic diseases and positive prick tests to aeroallergens had negative prick-test reactions to *P. ovale* extracts. No normal controls were included in the study [64]. These data were confirmed in several other studies including both adults and children [60,66]. The highest percentage of positive prick-test reactions were found by Kieffer et al. in a study including patients with the head-and-neck type atopic dermatitis, other forms of atopic dermatitis, seborrheic dermatitis, and control subjects. They found that 79% of 33 patients with head-and-neck dermatitis and 45% of 22 patients with other types of atopic dermatitis had a positive prick-test reaction to *P. ovale* and only one positive reaction in the two control groups [66].

When ELISA or RAST test was used, patients with atopic dermatitis were found to have specific IgE antibodies against *P. ovale*, and these antibodies were rarely found in patients with atopic conditions in the absence of eczema [67]. A correlation between the presence of atopic dermatitis and specific IgE to *P. ovale* has also been shown in children [60,68].

All together, patients with atopic dermatitis compared with other types of atopic patients and healthy controls have a higher frequency of positive prick test and specific IgE to *P. ovale*. The cause is not known but could be that in patients with atopic dermatitis the cutaneous immune system is skewed towards a Th2-type immune response resulting in IgE production. Furthermore, it has been suggested that the altered skin barrier and scratching in atopic dermatitis patients facilitate the sensitization to *P. ovale* [60].

## 4.  T-Cell–Mediated Reaction

Few groups have made epicutaneous tests with *P. ovale*. Kieffer et al. used a standard patch-test method with an aqueous solution of *P. ovale* and found 12% positive reaction among patients with atopic dermatitis and no positive reaction among healthy subjects and patients with seborrheic dermatitis [66]. Using a chamber scarification test, Rokugo et al. found 64% positive reactions [69]. The relevance of the epicutaneous test is supported by the finding that peripheral blood mononuclear cells and T-cell lines from atopic dermatitis patients demonstrated a significantly higher level of proliferation and Th2 cytokine production, including IL-4 and IL-5, following stimulation with *P. ovale* than healthy controls [70,71].

## 5.  Treatment

If *P. ovale* is involved in atopic dermatitis and especially the head-and-neck form of atopic dermatitis, one would expect that antifungal treatment would be effective. One study has investigated the effect of systemic antifungal treatment using ketoconazole 200 mg/day or placebo for 4 weeks followed by a crossover study after 1 week of washout [65]. Nineteen patients were included all with a positive prick test to *P. ovale* and atopic dermatitis; 14 patients had eczema only in the head-and-neck area. Concomitant topical steroid treatment was allowed. All patients improved, but only following treatment with ketoconazole was the difference significant. When the patients were separated into patients with or without head-and-neck dermatitis, the improvement was seen only in the group with head-and-neck dermatitis.

Recently another double-blind study investigating the effect of topical treatment was published [72]. Sixty patients were included, all with the head-and-neck type of atopic dermatitis, but most also had eczema on other parts of the body; 55% had a positive prick test to *P. ovale*. The patients were separated into two groups: one treated with miconazol-hydrocortisone cream and ketoconazole shampoo and the other treated with hydrocortisone cream and placebo shampoo for 6 weeks. The steroid was included since, in addition to an antifungal effect, ketoconazole has proved to have an antiinflammatory effect. To eliminate the effect of *S. aureus*, all patients were treated with flucloxacillin or erythromycin for the first 2 weeks. After 4 weeks of treatment, all patients improved significantly, but there was no difference between the groups despite the fact that the number of *P. ovale* in the group receiving antifungal treatment was significantly reduced. The improvement in both groups may be due to the treatment with antibiotic. As mentioned, only 55% of the patients in this study were prick-test positive to *P. ovale*, and that may be the reason for the lack of additional improvement in the group treated with antifungal cream and shampoo. However, another explanation is that the beneficial effect seen following systemic ketoconazole treatment may be because ketoconazole has been shown (1) to inhibit several P450-dependent enzymes, (2) to inhibit 5-lipooxygenase activity, and (3) to have some antibacterial effect on gram-positive bacteria such as *S. aureus* [73–75]. The effect of antifungal treatment, especially when given systemically, needs to be further investigated. Whether *P. ovale* is involved in the pathogenesis of atopic dermatitis or whether the positive prick test and elevated specific IgE just reflect the tendency to produce IgE-dominated responses is still not known.

## C.  Viral Infection

### 1.  Herpes Simplex Virus

There is general agreement that patients with atopic dermatitis are more susceptible to severe cutaneous viral infection, in particular herpes simplex infection and formerly vaccinia. Herpes simplex viruses (HSV) belong to the group of double-stranded DNA herpesviruses and are subgrouped into HSV-1 and HSV-2. Characteristic of the herpesviruses is the absence of virus elimination following clinical recovery and thus the risk of recurrent infection.

### 2.  Atopic Dermatitis and Herpes Simplex Virus Infection

In a large retrospective study including 955 patients with past or present atopic dermatitis and 199 healthy controls, the incidence of recurrent cold sore was measured [76]. It was found that the number of cold sores correlated with the severity of the eczema. Patients with severe atopic dermatitis (need of hospitalization) and those with mild atopic dermatitis had a significantly higher incidence of recurrent cold sore ($>5$ episodes/y) than the controls [76]. These data are confirmed by others [77]. In contrast, patients with atopic dermatitis seem not to be more often primarily infected with HSV since serological data from children did not show any difference between atopic dermatitis patients and controls [78].

### 3.  Eczema Herpeticum

Patients with atopic dermatitis, like patients without atopy, may acquire primary herpetic gingivostomatitis followed by the risk of recurrent herpes infection. However, eczema herpeticum, a herpes simplex virus infection with disseminated skin involvement, is usually seen in patients with atopic dermatitis. Formerly eczema herpeticum was primarily described in infants, but newer data indicate that the disease is also common around puberty [79]. Eczema herpeticum is most often associated with the primary HSV infection but may be a dissemination of a recurrent herpes infection. Recurrence of eczema herpeticum is common. Mild cases have been described with localized HSV infection in atopic dermatitis lesions and low-grade fever but no dissemination [80] and may be difficult to recognize. Sudden deterioration of atopic dermatitis and vesicles or failure of infected eczema to respond to antibiotics within 48 hours should lead to suspicion of herpes. Treatment should be initiated immediately with acyclovir or related drugs.

### 4.  Other Types of Virus Infection

It is a clinical experience that molluscum contagiosum, a poxvirus infection, is more widespread in patients with atopic dermatitis, but it has only been described in a few case reports [81,82]. Whether patients with atopic dermatitis are more affected by extracutaneous viral infections is not known. A single study found an increased number of cases with upper airway infection in patients with atopic dermatitis without other types of atopy [76], and atopic patients are said to be more affected by a varicella infection.

### 5.  Possible Mechanism for the Increased Severity of Cutaneous Virus Infection

Overall, patients with atopic dermatitis seem to have a tendency to severe cutaneous virus infection, especially HSV infection. The mechanism for the increased risk of developing eczema herpeticum has often been correlated with the defective skin barrier since eczema herpeticum is also seen in patients with Darier's disease [83], and ichthyosis vulgaris [84].

Other explanations are (1) a reduced number and function of cytotoxic CD8-positive T cells in patients with atopic dermatitis (CD8-positive T cells are involved in virus clearance), (2) atopic dermatitis, at least in the acute phase, is dominated by Th2 cells in the skin. Th2 cells promote an IgE response and via IL-10 inhibit Th1 responses including cell-mediated reactions. Cell-mediated reactions are critically involved in virus clearance and contact allergic reactions, and the Th1/Th2 imbalance in atopic skin may account for the increased susceptibility to cutaneous virus infection as well as the decreased susceptibility to development of contact sensitivity. The potential relevance of the Th1/Th2 imbalance in atopic skin is underscored by the observation that patients with atopic dermatitis experience a temporary remission of their skin disease following measles infection [85]. The clearance of the varicella and measles infection is dependent on Th1-type T cells, which might downregulate the atopic eczema. In support of this hypothesis, conversion from dominance of Th2 to Th1 cells in atopic dermatitis following varicella infection has been described [86]. Finally, a study with children from Guinea-Bissau demonstrated that children who had early measles infection had a lesser degree of atopy than vaccinated children. This suggests that early measles infection and thereby stimulation of Th1 responses may prevent the development of atopy later [87].

## III. CONTACT DERMATITIS

As mentioned in the introduction, the role of infection in contact dermatitis has been investigated in only a few studies. Welbourn et al. found an increased frequency of *S. aureus* on the skin of patients with eczema [88]. In a study including 20 patients with hand eczema, 18 of the patients were colonized with *S. aureus*, but 10 of the patients had atopic dermatitis [89]. Despite the lack of studies, it is a clinical experience that patients with dermatitis, especially hand eczema and nummular eczema, are often superinfected with *S. aureus* and streptococcus. As in the case of atopic dermatitis, superantigens released from the bacteria may lead to aggravation of the eczema because of the potent T-cell activation, cytokine release, and CLA upregulation.

## IV. DERMATOPHYTID

Dermatophytid is a noninfectious eruption seen following a primary dermatophyte infection at a distant site. The diagnosis is based on the following criteria: (1) a proven dermatophyte infection, (2) an eruption at a distant site without dermatophytes, and (3) the eruption subsides after the primary fungus infection has cleared [90]. The dermatophytid reaction usually starts when the patient starts antifungal treatment. Dermatophytid was initially described in combination with kerion but may also be seen following other type of dermatophyte infection, especially tinea pedis. *Trichophyton verrucosum*, *T. mentagophytes*, and *T. rubrum* are frequently mentioned as dermatophytes that may lead to dermatophytid reaction [91]. The typical reaction is an acute vesicular eruption on the hands, distributed symmetrically. Since the eruption usually begins following inflammation of the infection or after the start of treatment, it has been postulated that the reaction is due to release of antigens from the primary infection. In support of this, patients with dermatophyte infection demonstrated an increased number of positive intradermal and patch tests to extracts of dermatophytes and increased stimulation in a lymphocyte transformation test compared to normal controls [90,92,93]. However, whether the dermatophytid is an immunological reaction to the dermatophyte infection is unknown and needs to be further investigated.

## V. CONCLUSION

The skin is colonized by a large number of microorganisms, both as members of the normal flora and as temporary residents. There is strong evidnece that some of these mirroorganisms may lead to aggravation or even induction of inflammatory skin diseases. However, the exact mechanisms of the interactions between such microorganisms and inflammation are not well understood and require further investigation.

## REFERENCES

1. Roth RR, James WD. Microbiology of the skin: resident flora, ecology, infection. J Am Acad Dermatol 1989; 20:367–390.
2. Aly R, Maibach HI, Shinefield HR. Microbial flora of atopic dermatitis. Arch Dermatol 1977; 113:780–782.
3. Leyden JJ, Marples RR, Kligman AM. Staphylococcus aureus in the lesions of atopic dermatitis. Br J Dermatol 1974; 90:525–530.
4. Hauser C, Wuethrich B, Matter L, Wilhelm JA, Sonnabend W, Schopfer K. Staphylococcus aureus skin colonization in atopic dermatitis patients. Dermatologica 1985; 170:35–39.
5. Noble WC, Valkenburg HA, Wolters CH. Carriage of *Staphylococcus aureus* in random samples of a normal population. J Hyg (Lond) 1967; 65:567–573.
6. Hanifin JM, Rogge JL. Staphylococcal infections in patients with atopic dermatitis. Arch Dermatol 1977; 113:1383–1386.
7. Williams RE, Gibson AG, Aitchison TC, Lever R, MacKie RM. Assessment of a contact-plate sampling technique and subsequent quantitative bacterial studies in atopic dermatitis. Br J Dermatol 1990; 123:493–501.
8. Aly R, Shinefield HI, Strauss WG, Maibach HI. Bacterial adherence to nasal mucosal cells. Infect Immun 1977; 17:546–549.
9. Cole GW, Silverberg NL. The adherence of *Staphylococcus aureus* to human corneocytes. Arch Dermatol 1986; 122:166–169.
10. Bibel DJ, Aly R, Shinefield HR, Maibach HI, Strauss WG. Importance of the keratinized epithelial cell in bacterial adherence. J Invest Dermatol 1982; 79:250–253.
11. Lopes JD, dos Reis M, Brentani RR. Presence of laminin receptors in *Staphylococcus aureus*. Science 1985; 229:275–277.
12. Kuusela P. Fibronectin binds to *Staphylococcus aureus*. Nature 1978; 276:718–720.
13. Ryden C, Rubin K, Speziale P, Hook M, Lindberg M, Wadstrom T. Fibronectin receptors from *Staphylococcus aureus*. J Biol Chem 1983; 258:3396–3401.
14. Aly R, Shinefield HR, Litz C, Maibach HI. Role of teichoic acid in the binding of *Staphylococcus aureus* to nasal epithelial cells. J Infect Dis 1980; 141:463–465.
15. Lever R, Hadley K, Downey D, Mackie R. Staphylococcal colonization in atopic dermatitis and the effect of topical mupirocin therapy. Br J Dermatol 1988; 119:189–198.
16. White MI, Noble WC. The cutaneous reaction to staphylococcal protein A in normal subjects and patients with atopic dermatitis or psoriasis. Br J Dermatol 1985; 113:179–183.
17. Hauser C, Wuethrich B, Matter L, Wilhelm JA, Schopfer K. Immune response to *Staphylococcus aureus* in atopic dermatitis. Dermatologica 1985; 170:114–120.

18. Marrack P, Kappler J. The staphylococcal enterotoxins and their relatives. Science 1990; 248: 705–711.

19. Carlsson R, Fischer H, Sjogren HO. Binding of staphylococcal enterotoxin A to accessory cells is a requirement for its ability to activate human T cells. J Immunol 1988; 140:2484–2488.

20. Fleischer B, Schrezenmeier H. T cell stimulation by staphylococcal enterotoxins. Clonally variable response and requirement for major histocompatibility complex class II molecules on accessory or target cells. J Exp Med 1988; 167:1697–1707.

21. Dellabona P, Peccoud J, Kappler J, Marrack P, Benoist C, Mathis D. Superantigens interact with MHC class II molecules outside of the antigen groove. Cell 1990; 62:1115–1121.

22. Kappler J, Kotzin B, Herron L, Gelfand EW, Bigler RD, Boylston A, et al. V beta-specific stimulation of human T cells by staphylococcal toxins. Science 1989; 244:811–813.

23. Choi YW, Kotzin B, Herron L, Callahan J, Marrack P, Kappler J. Interaction of Staphylococcus aureus toxin ''superantigens'' with human T cells. Proc Natl Acad Sci USA 1989; 86: 8941–8945.

24. Mcfadden JP, Noble WC, Camp RDR. Superantigenic exotoxin-secreting potential of staphylococci isolated from atopic eczematous skin. Br J Dermatol 1993; 128:631–632.

25. Leung DY, Harbeck R, Bina P, Reiser RF, Yang E, Norris DA, et al. Presence of IgE antibodies to staphylococcal exotoxins on the skin of patients with atopic dermatitis. Evidence for a new group of allergens. J Clin Invest 1993; 92:1374–1380.

26. Strange P, Skov L, Lisby S, Nielsen PL, Baadsgaard O. Staphylococcal enterotoxin B applied on intact normal and intact atopic skin induces dermatitis. Arch Dermatol 1996; 132:27–33.

27. Murphy GF, Shepard RS, Harrist TJ, Bronstein BR, Bhan AK. Ultrastructural documentation of HLA-DR antigen reactivity in normal human acrosyringial epithelium. J Invest Dermatol 1983; 81:181–183.

28. Carr MM, McVittie E, Guy K, Gawkrodger DJ, Hunter JA. MHC class II antigen expression in normal human epidermis. Immunology 1986; 59:223–227.

29. Volc-Platzer B, Majdic O, Knapp W, Wolff K, Hinterberger W, Lechner K, et al. Evidence of HLA-DR antigen biosynthesis by human keratinocytes in disease. J Exp Med 1984; 159: 1784–1789.

30. Bieber T, Dannenberg B, Ring J, Braun Falco O. Keratinocytes in lesional skin of atopic eczema bear HLA-DR, CD1a and IgE molecules. Clin Exp Dermatol 1989; 14:35–39.

31. Nickoloff BJ, Mitra RS, Green J, Zheng XG, Shimizu Y, Thompson C, et al. Accessory cell function of keratinocytes for superantigens. Dependence on lymphocyte function-associated antigen-1/intercellular adhesion molecule-1 interaction. J Immunol 1993; 150:2148–2159.

32. Strange P, Skov L, Baadsgaard O. Interferon gamma-treated keratinocytes activate T cells in the presence of superantigens: involvement of major histocompatibility complex class II molecules. J Invest Dermatol 1994; 102:150–154.

33. Goodman RE, Nestle F, Naidu YM, Green JM, Thompson CB, Nickoloff BJ, et al. Keratinocyte-derived T cell costimulation induces preferential production of IL-2 and IL-4 but not IFN-gamma. J Immunol 1994; 152:5189–5198.

34. Kay AB, Ying S, Varney V, Gaga M, Durham SR, Moqbel R, et al. Messenger RNA expression of the cytokine gene cluster, interleukin 3 (IL-3), IL-4, IL-5, and granulocyte/macrophage colony-stimulating factor, in allergen-induced late-phase cutaneous reactions in atopic subjects. J Exp Med 1991; 173:775–778.

35. van der Heijden FL, Wierenga EA, Bos JD, Kapsenberg ML. High frequency of IL-4-producing CD4+ allergen specific T lymphocytes in apotic dermatitis lesional skin. J Invest Dermatol 1991; 97:389–394.

36. Leung DY, Gately M, Trumble A, Ferguson Darnell B, Schlievert PM, Picker LJ. Bacterial superantigens induce T cell expression of the skin-selective homing receptor, the cutaneous lymphocyte-associated antigen, via stimulation of interleukin 12 production. J Exp Med 1995; 181:747–753.

37. Michie CA, Davis T. Atopic dermatitis and staphylococcal superantigens. Lancet 1996; 347: 324.

38. Wakita H, Tokura Y, Furukawa F, Takigawa M. Staphylococcal enterotoxin B upregulates expression of ICAM-1 molecules on IFN-gamma-treated keratinocytes and keratinocyte cell line. J Invest Dermatol 1995; 105:536–542.

39. Tokura Y, Yagi J, O'Malley M, Lewis JM, Takigawa M, Edelson RL, et al. Superantigenic staphylococcal exotoxins induce T-cell proliferation in the presence of Langerhans cells or class II-bearing keratinocytes and stimulate keratinocytes to produce T-cell-activating cytokines. J Invest Dermatol 1994; 102:31–38.

40. Ezepchuk YV, Leung DY, Middleton MH, Bina P, Reiser R, Norris DA. Staphylococcal toxins and protein A differentially induce cytotoxicity and release of tumor necrosis factor-alpha from human keratinocytes. J Invest Dermatol 1996; 107:603–609.

41. Abramson JS, Dahl MV, Walsh G, Blumenthal MN, Douglas SD, Quie PG. Antistaphylococcal IgE in patients with atopic dermatitis. J Am Acad Dermatol 1982; 7:105–110.

42. Friedman SJ, Schroeter AL, Homburger HA. IgE antibodies to *Staphylococcus aureus*. Prevalence in patients with atopic dermatitis. Arch Dermatol 1985; 121:869–872.

43. Bruynzeel Koomen C, van Wichen DF, Toonstra J, Berrens L, Bruynzeel PL. The presence of IgE molecules on epidermal Langerhans cells in patients with atopic dermatitis. Arch Dermatol Res 1986; 278:199–205.

44. Bieber T, de la Salle H, Wollenberg A, Hakimi J, Chizzonite R, Ring J, et al. Human epidermal Langerhans cells express the high affinity receptor for immunoglobulin E (Fc epsilon RI). J Exp Med 1992; 175:1285–1290.

45. Wang B, Rieger A, Kilgus O, Ochiai K, Maurer D, Fodinger D, et al. Epidermal Langerhans cells from normal human skin bind monomeric IgE via Fc epsilon RI. J Exp Med 1992; 175: 1353–1365.

46. Maurer D, Ebner C, Reininger B, Fiebiger E, Kraft D, Kinet JP, et al. The high affinity IgE receptor (Fc epsilon RI) mediates IgE-dependent allergen presentation. J Immunol 1995; 154: 6285–6290.

47. Jurgens M, Wollenberg A, Hanau D, de la Salle H, Bieber T. Activation of human epidermal Langerhans cells by engagement of the high affinity receptor for IgE, Fc epsilon RI. J Immunol 1995; 155:5184–5189.

48. Nilsson EJ, Henning CG, Magnusson J. Topical corticosteroids and *Staphylococcus aureus* in atopic dermatitis. J Am Acad Dermatol 1992; 27:29–34.

49. Jekler J, Bergbrant IM, Faergemann J, Larko O. The in vivo effect of UVB radiation on skin bacteria in patients with atopic dermatitis. Acta Derm Venereol 1992; 72:33–36.

50. Stalder JF, Fleury M, Sourisse M, Rostin M, Pheline F, Litoux P. Local steroid therapy and bacterial skin flora in atopic dermatitis. Br J Dermatol 1994; 131:536–540.

51. Faergemann J, Larko O. The effect of UV-light on human skin microorganisms. Acta Derm Venereol 1987; 67:69–72.

52. Yoshimura M, Namura S, Akamatsu H, Horio T. Antimicrobial effects of phototherapy and photochemotherapy in vivo and in vitro. Br J Dermatol 1996; 135:528–532.

53. Stalder JF, Fleury M, Sourisse M, Allavoine T, Chalamet C, Brosset P, et al. Comparative effects of two topical antiseptics (chlorhexidine vs KMn04) on bacterial skin flora in atopic dermatitis. Acta Derm Venereol Suppl 1992; 176:132–134.

54. Wachs GN, Maibach HI. Co-operative double-blind trial of an antibiotic/corticoid combination in impetiginized atopic dermatitis. Br J Dermatol 1976; 95:323–328.

55. Ramsay CA, Savoie JM, Gilbert M, Gidon M, Kidson P. The treatment of atopic dermatitis with topical fusidic acid and hydrocortisone acetate. JEADV 1996; 7(suppl 1):s15–s22.

56. Hjorth N, Schmidt H, Thomsen K. Fusidin acid plus betamethasone in infected or potentially infected eczema. Pharmatherapeutica 1985; 4:126–131.

57. Roberts SO. Pityrosporum orbiculare: incidence and distribution on clinically normal skin. Br J Dermatol 1969; 81:264–269.

58. Faergemann J, Aly R, Maibach HI. Quantitative variations in distribution of *Pityrosporum orbiculare* on clinically normal skin. Acta Derm Venereol 1983; 63:346–348.
59. Faergemann J, Aly R, Maibach HI. Adherence of *Pityrosporum orbiculare* to human stratum corneum cells. Arch Dermatol Res 1983; 275:246–250.
60. Broberg A, Faergemann J, Johansson S, Johansson SG, Strannegard IL, Svejgaard E. *Pityrosporum ovale* and atopic dermatitis in children and young adults. Acta Derm Venereol 1992; 72:187–192.
61. Ruiz-Maldonado R, Lopez-Matinez R, Perez Chavarria EL, Rocio Castanon L, Tamayo L, *Pityrosporum ovale* in infantile seborrheic dermatitis. Pediatr Dermatol 1989; 6:16–20.
62. Faergemann J. Seborrhoeic dermatitis and *Pityrosporum orbiculare*: treatment of seborrhoeic dermatitis of the scalp with miconazole-hydrocortisone (Daktacort), miconazole and hydrocortisone. Br J Dermatol 1986; 114:695–700.
63. Back O, Faergemann J, Hornqvist R. Pityrosporum folliculitis: a common disease of the young and middle-aged. J Am Acad Dermatol 1985; 12:56–61.
64. Waersted A, Hjorth N. *Pityrosporum orbiculare*—a pathogenic factor in atopic dermatitis of the face, scalp and neck? Acta Derm Venereol Suppl 1985; 114:146–148.
65. Clemmensen OJ, Hjorth N. Treatment of dermatitis of the head and neck with ketoconazole in patients with type 1 sensitivity to *Pityrosporon orbiculare*. Semin Dermatol 1983; 2:26–29.
66. Kieffer M, Bergbrant IM, Faergemann J, Jemec GB, Ottevanger V, Stahl Skov P, et al. Immune reactions to *Pityrosporum ovale* in adult patients with atopic and seborrheic dermatitis. J Am Acad Dermatol 1990; 22:739–742.
67. Wessels MW, Doekes G, Van Ieperen-Van Kijk AG, Koers WJ, Young E. IgE antibodies to *Pityrosporum ovale* in atopic dermatitis. Br J Dermatol 1991; 125:227–232.
68. Nordvall SL, Johansson S. IgE antibodies to *Pityrosporum orbiculare* in children with atopic diseases. Acta Paediatr Scand 1990; 79:343–348.
69. Rokugo M, Tagami H, Usuba Y, Tomita Y. Contact sensitivity to *Pityrosporum ovale* in patients with atopic dermatitis. Arch Dermatol 1990; 126:627–632.
70. Tengvall Linder M, Johansson C, Zargari A, Bengtsson A, van der Ploeg I, Jones I, et al. Detection of *Pityrosporum orbiculare* reactive T cells from skin and blood in atopic dermatitis and characterization of their cytokine profiles. Clin Exp Allergy 1996; 26:1286–1297.
71. Tengvall Linder M, Johansson C, Bengtsson A, Holm L, Harfast B, Scheynius A. *Pityrosporum orbiculare*-reactive T-cell lines in atopic dermatitis patients and healthy individuals. Scand J Immunol 1998; 47:152–158.
72. Broberg A, Faergemann J. Topical antimycotic treatment of atopic dermatitis in the head/neck area. A double-blind randomised study. Acta Derm Venereol 1995; 75:46–49.
73. Van Cutsem J, Van Gerven F, Cauwenbergh G, Odds F, Janssen PA. The antiinflammatory effects of ketoconazole. A comparative study with hydrocortisone acetate in a model using living and killed *Staphylococcus aureus* on the skin of guinea-pigs. J Am Acad Dermatol 1991; 25:257–261.
74. Beetens JR, Loots W, Somers Y, Coene MC, De Clerck F. Ketoconazole inhibits the biosynthesis of leukotrienes in vitro and in vivo. Biochem Pharmacol 1986; 35:883–891.
75. Janssen PAJ, Vanden Bossche HFA, Van Wauwe JP, Cauwenbergh GFMJ, Degreef HJ. The role of cytochrome P-450 in dermatology. Int J Dermatol 1989; 28:493–496.
76. Rystedt I, Strannegard IL, Strannegard O. Recurrent viral infections in patients with past or present atopic dermatitis. Br J Dermatol 1986; 114:575–582.
77. David TJ, Longson M. Herpes simplex infections in atopic eczema. Arch Dis Child 1985; 60:338–343.
78. David TJ, Richmond SJ, Bailey AS. Serological evidence of herpes simplex virus infection in atopic eczema. Arch Dis Child 1987; 62:416–417.
79. Bork K, Brauninger W. Increasing incidence of eczema herpeticum: analysis of seventy-five cases. J Am Acad Dermatol 1988; 19:1024–1029.

80. Leyden JJ, Baker DA. Localized herpes simplex infections in atopic dermatitis. Arch Dermatol 1979; 115:311–312.

81. Pauly CR, Artis WM, Jones HE. Atopic dermatitis, impaired cellular immunity, and molluscum contagiosum. Arch Dermatol 1978; 114:391–393.

82. Wolff HH. Eczema herpeticatum, Eczema vaccinatum, Eczema verrucatum, Eczema molluscatum. Der Hautarzt 1977; 28:98–99.

83. Verner E, Shteinfeld M, Zuckerman F. Eczema herpeticum in a patient with Darier's disease during treatment with etretinate [letter]. J Am Acad Dermatol 1985; 13:678–680.

84. Verbov J, Munro DD, Miller A. Recurrent eczema herpeticum associated with ichthyosis vulgaris. Br J Dermatol 1972; 86:638–640.

85. Boner AL, Valletta EA, Bellanti JA. Improvement of atopic dermatitis following natural measles virus infection. Four case reports. Ann Allergy 1985; 55:605–608.

86. Fujimura T, Yamanashi R, Masuzawa M, Fujita Y, Katsuoka K, Nishiyama S, et al. Conversion of the CD4+ T cell profile from T(H2)-dominant type to T(H1)- dominant type after varicella-zoster virus infection in atopic dermatitis. J Allergy Clin Immunol 1997; 100:274–282.

87. Shaheen SO, Aaby P, Hall AJ, Barker DJ, Heyes CB, Shiell AW, et al. Measles and atopy in Guinea-Bissau. Lancet 1996; 347:1792–1796.

88. Welbourn E, Champion RH, Parish WE. Hypersensitivity to bacteria in eczema. I. Bacterial culture, skin tests and immunofluorescent detection of immunoglobulins and bacterial antigens. Br J Dermatol 1976; 94:619–632.

89. Nilsson E, Henning C, Hjörleifsson M. Density of the microflora in hand eczema before and after topical treatment with a potent corticosteroid. J Am Acad Dermatol 1986; 15:192–197.

90. Kaaman T, Torssander J. Dermatophytid––a misdiagnosed entity? Acta Derm Venereol 1983; 63:404–408.

91. Veien NK, Hattel T, Laurberg G. Plantar *Trichophyton rubrum* infections may cause dermatophytids on the hands. Acta Derm Venereol 1994; 74:403–404.

92. Tagami H, Watanabe S, Ofuji S, Minami K. Trichophytin contact sensitivity in patients with dermatophytosis. Arch Dermatol 1977; 113:1409–1414.

93. Stahl D, Svejgaard E. Lymphocyte transformation in vitro in acute dermatophytosis: a follow-up study. Acta Derm Venereol 1982; 62:289–293.

94. Skov L, Baadsgaard O. Superantigens. Do they have a role in skin diseases? Arch Dermatol 1995; 131:829–832.

# 25

## Identifying the Causes of Urticaria

**Richard W. Weber**
*National Jewish Medical and Research Center, and*
*University of Colorado Health Sciences Center,*
*Denver, Colorado*

In defining urticaria, clinicians have traditionally divided presentations into acute and chronic in the belief that there is a greater likelihood of discerning an etiology with an abrupt recent onset. There is also the hope that the urticarial lesions will be self-limited and not require management beyond short-term symptomatic care. Depending on the ease of achieving symptom relief, there may be little impetus to pursuing causal factors, especially in the face of the historically low probability of identifying an etiology. As symptoms persist past 4–6 weeks or require the use of antiinflammatory agents for control, either patient or physician may wish an attempt to delineate causative factors.

## I. HOW USEFUL IS THE TRADITIONAL EVALUATION?

Acute urticaria may be arbitrarily defined as persisting less than 4–8 weeks, and lesions are frequently generalized and explosive in onset. A food or drug may be incriminated, as may a viral syndrome. With IgE-mediated reactions to a food, the term ''recurrent urticaria'' may be more appropriate, since the patient is frequently assured of a reaction if the specific food is again ingested. For some patients, the aggravation of urticaria is worth the enjoyment derived from the ingestion of a favored food.

Although drug reactions are likely to be acute, occasionally onset may be insidious and delayed. Such is the experience with angiotensin-converting enzyme (ACE) inhibitors and angioedema. Several reports document both the magnitude of the association as well as the likelihood of delayed presentation—although symptoms are likely to develop within the first month of therapy, they may be delayed 6 months or more [1–4]. In patients presenting to an emergency department with angioedema, about 40% were found to be due to ACE inhibitors [1,2]. African American males appear to be more affected, with an adjusted relative risk of 4.5 compared to white patients, and the risk could not be attributed to dose, specific ACE inhibitor, or concurrent medications [3].

A more formal definition of ''recurrent urticaria'' has been suggested, episodes of urticaria being shorter than the intervening symptom-free periods [5]. However, the latter classification does not necessarily increase the likelihood of defining an etiology. In one study, the incidence of definable triggers was less in the recurrent group than in either the acute or the chronic group [5].

While Sheldon et al. felt that causes for chronic urticaria could be found in up 50% of cases, more recent papers have estimated the likelihood of identifying the exact cause of urticaria as between 16–25% [6,7,8]. Occasionally, much higher success has been reported. Kauppinen et al. reported in 1984 finding an etiology in 55% of children with acute, chronic, or recurrent urticaria [5]. They attributed their success to being able to hospitalize the children in a specialized unit in order to perform appropriate challenge procedures. Miller et al. in 1968 felt they could explain the etiology of chronic urticaria in almost all of 50 patients evaluated over one year's time [9]. This extraordinary result was due, on the one hand, to persistence in thorough evaluation, but also to attributing a cause to some factors that were accepted on face value. For example, 22% were felt to have urticaria based on inhalant allergy: none of these were challenged. Forty-eight percent had some form of physical urticaria. And while it is common practice in many studies to attribute the description of physical urticaria as an etiology, this is a fallacy, for there may be underlying sensitivities that contribute to such a presentation. Smith and coworkers described a case of dermographism due to penicillin allergy [10]. Similarly, cold urticaria may be secondary to viral infections or a food allergen [11–13]. Therefore, it seems that naming a physical urticaria as such is just classifying an attribute, and not defining a cause. If the physical urticarias are removed from the list of definite etiologies, the success rate in identifying causes of urticaria or angioedema becomes even more dismal. However, the few studies with higher rates of attributing causality suggest that perseverance may occasionally be rewarded.

What then, is worth pursuing? Kaplan, in a recent textbook of allergy and immunology, has suggested that the appropriate initial evaluation of urticaria and angioedema would include the following: history, physical examination, chest x-ray, complete blood count and differential, sedimentation rate, antinuclear antibody (ANA), stool for ova and parasites, and skin biopsy [14]. This may be seen as the traditional approach, but how successful is this? There is no question that a careful history and thorough physical examination may give clues, for example, to triggering factors or the presence of a systemic disease such as lupus erythematosis. Older texts have stressed the importance of infection, often a localized abscess, as a predominant cause of hives. Cooke, in his 1946 text, stated that 35% of urticaria in his practice were due to infection, frequently focal, 10% due to food, another 10% to drugs, and the remaining 45% remained etiologically undiagnosed [15]. He stressed that the infection need not be extensive and cited a case of urticaria caused by a granuloma at the base of a tooth root. The search for the "hidden focus of infection" therefore was a tenet of the textbook approach to the diagnosis of urticaria. While Cooke emphasized the need for a very careful physical examination, more recently this concept has translated into obtaining a series of x-rays and laboratory determinations. But how helpful is the laboratory assessment?

## II. LABORATORY ASSESSMENT

Jacobson et al. reported the lack of value of 11 commonly performed laboratory studies in the work-up of 125 chronic urticaria patients [16]. The tests included and number performed were: urinalysis, 100; urine culture, 56; ANA, 99; eosinophil count, 94; stool for ova and parasites, 120; sedimentation rate, 74; rheumatoid factor, 71; complement C3 and

C4, 70; sinus series, 64; dental series, 44; and cryoglobulins, 33. Twenty-six patients (21%) had reproducible abnormalities. With the exception of 11 abnormal sinus films, the findings were all predictable on the basis of a careful history and physical examination and did not contribute to the management of the patients' urticaria. The authors calculated the cost of the assessments per number of diagnoses achieved and felt that, with the possible exception of sinus series, the routine laboratory evaluation in chronic urticaria was ineffective and expensive. They recommended careful history and physical examination followed by judicious use of laboratory and radiological studies to further evaluate clues from the former assessment. In a follow-up evaluation of the value of routine sinus films, Nelson reported on 128 series obtained in 263 urticaria patients [17]. Only 17 were abnormal, and in only 3 did the urticaria subside coincident with the treatment and clearing of the sinus films. Therefore, it appeared that sinus series were ultimately less helpful than suggested in the first study.

A variety of viral infections have been implicated in urticaria and are significant causes of acute and subacute bouts of urticaria in both children and young adults. Hepatitis A and B viruses have been known to produce urticaria during the prodromal phase, which frequently remits as jaundice ensues. Kanazawa and associates have recently reported on finding evidence for hepatitis C (HCV) in an appreciable percentage of urticaria patients [18]. Anti-HCV antibody was detected in 19 of 79 patients (24%) and HCV RNA in 17 (22%), while being present in only 1.1% of age- and sex-matched controls. Whether such high percentages represent a causative relationship or coincidental infection is uncertain. It does suggest that serology for hepatitis viruses may be a useful procedure.

The association of thyroid autoimmunity and chronic urticaria was first reported by Leznoff and colleagues in 1983 [19]. Seventeen of 140 consecutively seen cases of urticaria (12.1%) demonstrated thyroid autoantibodies, compared to 27 of 477 other patients (5.6%) seen in a family practice setting. In a 1989 follow-up study, Leznoff and Sussman reported that 90 patients from a pool of 624 chronic urticaria and angioedema patients (14.4%) had evidence of thyroid autoimmunity [20]. Turktas and colleagues compared 94 patients with chronic urticaria and angioedema with 80 age- and sex-matched controls [21]. Eleven patients had anti-thyroglobulin antibodies (11.7%), and nine had antithyroid microsomal antibodies (9.6%), with three controls (3.7%) having both antibodies ($p <$ 0.01). Of the 11 patients, 6 had thyroid dysfunction, and 5 were euthyroid, reinforcing that thyroid function tests of themselves are not adequate to rule out thyroid autoimmunity. These positivity rates are strikingly similar, and the latter authors felt the percentages were high enough to warrant checking autoantibodies in all chronic urticaria patients. Patients may have lesions remit with thyroid-suppressive therapy whether or not they are euthyroid [19,22].

## III. SKIN TESTING

As discussed in greater detail elsewhere in this text, intradermal skin testing with autologous serum may give evidence of an autoimmune process involving antibodies to either IgE or the IgE receptor in a significant number of patients with chronic urticaria. However, the usefulness of routine immediate hypersensitivity skin testing in the evaluation of urticaria is in question. Older reports incriminated inhalants in urticaria, but as commented on above, many of these cases were not substantiated. Seasonal urticaria due to inhalants happens but does not appear to be common. In an evaluation of 210 chronic urticaria

**Table 1**  Immediate Skin Testing in Chronic
Urticaria: Results in 210 Patients

| Allergen type | Number positive (%) |
|---|---|
| Food allergens | 33/52 Hx+ (63.5) |
|  | 19/92 Hx− (20.6) |
| Aeroallergens | 54/96 (56) |
| Penicillin battery | 18/95 (18) |
|  | 3/9 PCN Hx+ (33) |
| *Candida albicans* | 11/56 (19.6) |

Hx+ = History positive; Hx− = History negative; PCN = Penicillin.
*Source*: Schkade et al., unpublished.

patients, Schkade et al. (unpublished) found positivity in 54 of 96 patients skin-tested to inhalants, but only 2% of these were felt to be clinically relevant (Table 1). Other ubiquitous allergens may have a role. In 1971, James and Warin suggested the importance of *Candida albicans* in chronic urticaria, finding 26% of 100 patients to be sensitive to the yeast and to respond to anti-*Candida* therapy and a low-yeast diet [23]. Recently, the role of mold spores, either inhaled or ingested, has received little attention. A study of 52 Japanese patients with chronic urticaria revealed skin test positivity to *Dermatophagoides farinae* in 30 (58%), and it was suggested that the dust mite may play an important role [24]. There was no control comparison, and no clinical correlations were made, so it is uncertain whether this observation has clinical relevance.

Skin testing for penicillin sensitivity in the work-up of urticaria is controversial.

**Table 2**  Diet Manipulation in Diagnosis and Management of
Chronic Urticaria

| Diet and Ref. | Number successful (%) |
|---|---|
| Dye and preservative free |  |
|   Gibson and Clancy [49] | 49/65 (75) |
|   Kemp and Schembri [50] | 7/18 (39) |
|   Malanin and Kalimo [52] | 16/18 ST+ (89) |
|  | 17/42 ST− (40) |
|   Schkade et al., unpublished | 3/4 (75) |
| Dairy free |  |
|   Boonk and Van Ketel [25] | 22/42 PCN ST+ (52) |
|  | 2/40 PCN ST− (5) |
|   Schkade et al., unpublished | 5/12 (42) |
| Elemental, lamb/rice, or specific elimination |  |
|   Schkade et al., unpublished | 7/17 (41) |
| Mold free |  |
|   James and Warin [23] | 29/36 ST+ (81) |
|  | 7/18 ST− (39) |
|   Schkade et al., unpublished | 1/2 (50) |

PCN = Penicillin, ST = skin test.

The rationale for its use stems in part from two reports from Europe linking hives and penicillin exposure in dairy products. Boonk and Van Ketel showed positivity to penicillin G and penicilloylpolylysine 24% of 245 patients [25]. Twenty-two of 42 skin-test–positive patients who went on a dairy-free diet remitted, compared to 2 of 40 chronic urticaria patients with negative skin tests to penicillin. Ormerod and coworkers found RAST positivity to penicillin in 30% of 50 recurrent urticaria patients [26]. Thirteen of these were challenged to 0.1 U/cc of penicillin in milk, four had definite reactions, and another three questionable reactions. Those with positive provocations had improvement of their urticaria on dietary avoidance, although the authors raised the possibility that the clearing of the urticaria was coincidental (Table 2).

## IV. SEARCHING FOR INTESTINAL PARASITES

The medical literature has numerous case reports of a large variety of intestinal or invasive parasites causing urticaria or angioedema. A partial list includes *Giardia*, *Ascaris*, *Ancyclostoma*, *Strongyloides*, *Filaria*, *Echinococcus*, *Schistosoma*, *Trichinella*, *Toxocara*, and *Fasciola*. [27–30]. In a number of cases originating in the United States in the absence of foreign travel, a recurring theme is of exposure as a result of camping or hunting [31]. The question is, in the absence of an obvious history, is obtaining stool for ova and parasites helpful? A study by Jacobson and colleagues found no instances of parasitic infestation [16]. A study from New Delhi, India, cast some further light on this question [32]. The authors investigated 78 cases of urticaria and compared these patients with 50 others with nonurticarial dermatoses. Stool specimens were examined for 3 consecutive days; if parasites were found the patients were treated with the appropriate therapeutic agents, followed by 3 more days of specimens. Patients with urticaria were requested to take antihistamines only if necessary; frequency and severity of lesions were compared before and after treatment. Both groups of patients showed similar rates of infestation: 61.5% of the urticaria patients and 72% of the others. Treatment was successful in clearing parasites in 24 of 25 patients who returned for follow-up; of these 12 reported decreased severity of attacks, while 13 reported no change or worsening. In 3 of the successful cases, the urticaria had stopped prior to treatment, and another was found to have food allergy relieved by food elimination. Thus, even in a population where intestinal parasites are pervasive, a link with urticaria could not be convincingly demonstrated. An evaluation of 226 children from Athens, Greece, revealed 1.3% of urticaria due to parasitic infestation [8]. A similar study of 163 children from Helsinki, Finland, found 3% due to parasites [5].

Several recent reports, primarily from Spain, have documented the importance of the nematode fish parasite *Anisakis simplex* in causing acute urticaria or even anaphylaxis [33]. Another report utilized both direct ELISA IgE and inhibitions to document co-sensitization with two nematode larvae, *A. simplex* and *Hysterothylacium aduncum*, as well as varying degrees of cross-reactivity between the two [34]. The authors reported that about 40% of a mackerel sold in the Granada fish market were infested with either *A. simplex* or *H. aduncum* and suggested that other parasites besides *A. simplex* are relevant allergens. Whether this is ultimately a regional phenomenon or is important in other places is uncertain. If urticaria patients have access to fresh fish, this type of fish-ingestion allergic disease needs to be considered.

## V.  FOOD ADDITIVE CHALLENGES AND ADDITIVE-FREE DIETS

In the 1960s a variety of case reports linked food additives to adverse reactions, including asthma and urticaria. An early investigation by Juhlin et al. demonstrated reactivity of aspirin-intolerant patients to *para*-hydroxybenzoic acid (propylparaben) and sodium benzoate [35]. Five of seven urticaria patients responded to *p*-hydroxybenzoic acid. In a further study by the same group, of 52 patients with urticaria or angioedema, they found reactivity to the benzoates in 52% after oral challenge [36]. A number of publications showed reactivity ranging from 17 to 60% [37–39]. Such high prevalence was most likely misleading, in that a number of these studies were single-blinded or did not use appropriate placebos. Many gave placebo on the first day of challenges (when antihistamine effect was still waning) and not again, so as breakthrough urticaria reappeared it was interpreted as positive challenges. More stringently done challenges resulted in lower rates of positivity, such as a study by Ortolani and associates where only 4% of 72 challenged urticaria patients reacted to sodium benzoate [40]. In a challenge battery using more placebo controls, Warin and Smith found 11% of 111 patients reacting to sodium benzoate and 5% to *para*-hydroxybenzoic acid [41].

In a similar vein, tartrazine (FD&C yellow #5) was linked to aspirin sensitivity in asthma and urticaria patients, and many of the studies cited above also evaluated tartrazine and other azo dyes such as sunset yellow (FD&C yellow #6), amaranth (FD&C red #2), or ponceau (FD&C red #4). Similar rates of reactivity were described; as above, the same faults could be entertained [42]. Better designed studies resulted in lower numbers: Ortolani and coworkers found a 7% reactivity to tartrazine and Warin and Smith a 13% rate [40,41].

The synthetic antioxidants butylated hydroxyanisole (BHA) and butylated hydroxytoluene (BHT) came under similar scrutiny. Thune and Granholt found 13–14% reactivity to these antioxidants, and Juhlin found 15% [38,42]. The most thorough documentation of BHA and BHT causing urticaria was reported by Goodman and colleagues [43]. Two patients with chronic urticaria were shown by repeated double-blind testing to respond to these agents, and elimination from the diet resulted in persistent abatement of symptoms. The authors estimated that these two cases compromised less than 1% of 271 chronic urticaria patients evaluated at a tertiary care medical center over a number of years. In the intervening 9 years, the present author has seen two additional patients with positive double-blind challenges to BHT (R. W. Weber, unpublished results).

The controversy, then, is not whether this panoply of food colorants and preservatives can induce urticaria, but how often they do so. Stevenson and colleagues stated in a review of nine urticaria studies that with tartrazine sensitivity ranging from 8 to 100%, false-positive interpretations of reactions constituted a majority of the reported events, and the true prevalence was unknown [44]. A reasonable estimate would be that at most, tartrazine and the benzoates provoke symptoms in 5–10% of chronic urticaria patients. Other azo dyes may be incriminated in lesser percentages, perhaps between 1 and 5% [45,46]. BHA and BHT reactions appear to be uncommon [47].

Even if the prevalence of urticarial responses to food additives is lower than initially estimated, provocative challenges may be worth the effort in protracted cases with poor response to pharmaceutical suppressive therapy. Several issues deserve comment in setting up a challenge protocol. If additives are suspected, a dye- and preservative-free diet should be initiated prior to the onset of challenges. This will accomplish two things: (1) minimize lesional activity, and thereby allow decreasing doses of antihistamines, with a lesser fear of having breakthrough urticaria judged as false positives, and (2) allow recovery from a putative refractory period. It is suspected, although unproven, that reactions to dyes or preservatives may be similar in nature to aspirin and nonsteroidal anti-inflammatory drug reactions, and therefore could likewise induce a refractory period following a reaction. If this is the case, there are implications for the timing of challenges as well. If the patient sustains an obvious flare, 3–5 days should be allowed to pass before proceeding, to decrease the chance of masking other positive reactions.

There is also the question of what constitutes an appropriate challenge dose. A wide range of doses has been utilized, depending on whether the researchers wished to reproduce the amount of the additive found in a single pill or approximate the amount accumulated with a diet rich in processed foods. Based on doses reflecting natural exposure, Bosso and Simon have recommended the following maximum doses for common additive challenges: tartrazine, 50 mg; sulfites, 200 mg; monosodium glutamate, 5 g; aspartame, 150 mg; and parabens and benzoates, 100 mg [45]. Others have recommended higher doses for certain additives, such as 500 mg for sodium benzoate and 200 mg for *para*-hydroxybenzoic acid [41]. The maximum doses given in Table 3 are based on those used in several studies [43,48].

Challenges utilize opaque capsules and may be performed on an outpatient basis after a dye- and preservative-free diet has been instituted. If the patient is not free of urticaria, it is wise to establish baseline activity before starting the challenges. Bosso and Simon have recommended assessing percent body involvement using a "rule of nines" similar to that used in body involvement in burn patients [45]. The lower dose is taken in the morning with breakfast, followed by the larger dose at noon, assuming there has been no obvious exacerbation. If no reactions occur, the challenges can be done on an alternate-day schedule. While some studies have considered positive reactions to occur up to 24 hours, it is difficult to assess causality after that length of time. If a suspected reaction does occur, because of the possibility of a refractory period it may be wise to wait at least 5 days before proceeding further. If challenges are performed under observation in

**Table 3** Food Additive Challenge Protocol: Suggested Agents and Doses[a]

| Agent | Sequential doses |
|---|---|
| Preservatives | |
|   Sodium benzoate | 125 mg, 250 mg |
|   Propylparaben (para-hydroxybenzoic acid) | 125 mg, 250 mg |
| Antioxidants | |
|   Butylated hydroxyanisole (BHA) | 125 mg, 250 mg |
|   Butylated hydroxytoluene (BHT) | 125 mg, 250 mg |
| Azo dyes | |
|   Tartrazine (FD&C yellow #5) | 10 mg, 25 mg |
|   Sunset yellow (FD&C yellow #6) | 10 mg, 25 mg |
|   Amaranth (FD&C red #2) | 10 mg, 25 mg |
| Nonazo dyes | |
|   Erythrosine (FD&C red #3) | 10 mg, 25 mg |
|   Brilliant blue (FD&C blue #1) | 10 mg, 25 mg |

[a] See text for recommended dosing schedule and references.

a clinic setting, it may be possible to truncate the time between capsule doses, but at the risk of having delayed reactions occur during the next capsule cycle. Ideally, challenges should be done in a double-blind fashion, with as many placebo sets as active additive sets, to minimize false positives from random events.

Several authors have commented on the benefit of dye- and preservative-free diets in abating symptoms [49–51]. What is surprising is that a significant number of patients will improve, whether oral challenges have been positive or not (Table 2). Supramaniam and Warner described 43 children who responded to an additive-free diet, but only 24 reacted to a blinded challenge [51]. Kemp and Schembri had 7 of 18 children show marked remission of urticaria within 2 weeks of elimination diet, yet the response rate to tartrazine and sodium benzoate was no different than the 7% reaction to placebo [50]. Similarly, Malanin and Kalimo had 40% of skin test– and challenge-negative patients improve on an additive-free diet [52]. This suggests that cumulative dietary additives may play a potentiating role in urticaria and angioedema, similar to that seen with aspirin and nonsteroidal anti-inflammatory drugs [53].

## VI. EXERCISE CHALLENGES

Several exercise syndromes have been described, the oldest recognized being cholinergic urticaria [54]. Exercise classically causes marked flushing, pruritus, and punctate urticaria; however, systemic symptoms may occur [55]. Cholinergic urticaria with anaphylactic symptoms may be difficult to discern from exercise-induced anaphylaxis [56]. More recently, food-dependent exercise-induced anaphylaxis has been described [55,57]. Exercise challenge, usually a run on a treadmill, is the desired provocation test, but symptoms may be difficult to reproduce, and a negative challenge does not rule out the condition [55]. For those with suspected food triggers, skin testing is appropriate. Conceivably all patients with exercise-induced anaphylaxis deserve immediate hypersensitivity skin testing; the link to a particular food allergen may not be immediately apparent, since the ingestion may precede or follow the exercise.

## VII. SUMMARY: RECOMMENDATIONS FOR EVALUATION

A careful history and physical examination remains the cornerstone for discerning a definitive etiology for urticaria or angioedema. It is possible that with perseverance, more than 15–20% of cases may be clarified and removed from the ''idiopathic'' bin. A larger proportion of cases from the older literature was assigned definite causes, but it is unclear from reading these reports whether they were bona fide determinations or whether a number were relegated to erroneous causes. It is appropriate to discuss with the patient the likelihood of finding a cause, based in part on the longevity of symptoms, and whether it is reasonable to undergo an evaluation of varying intensity or to treat symptomatically. For example, in the face of a defined viral prodrome, it is reasonable to forgo a work-up in the expectation that symptoms will be self-limited in a few weeks or a few months.

Having made the decision to proceed with an evaluation beyond history and physical, the approach should be tiered based on clues, or lack thereof. One such approach is

**Table 4**  Recommended Evaluation of Chronic Urticaria and Angioedema

I. First Tier—Initial Evaluation
  A. Complete history
  B. Careful physical examination
    1. infectious focus
    2. dermatophyte (tinea)
    3. palpable purpura or other evidence for urticarial vasculitis
    4. physical urticaria
  C. Laboratory
    1. complete blood count with differential
    2. sedimentation rate
    3. thyroid function tests, anti-thyroglobulin antibody, anti-thyroid peroxidase (anti-thyroid microsomal) antibody
II. Second Tier—Driven by Positive History or Physical Findings
  A. Skin testing
    1. limited food battery
    2. selected inhalants
  B. Laboratory
    1. ANA, rheumatoid factor, C3, C4, CH50
    2. immune complex assay
    3. skin biopsy
    4. C2, C4, C1 esterase inhibitor functional assay
    5. screening CT of paranasal sinuses
    6. chest x-ray
    7. parasitic serology and/or stool for ova and parasites
  C. Elimination diet—skin test or history directed
III. Third Tier—Driven by Chronicity or Poor Therapeutic Response
  A. Food diary
  B. Dairy-free diet
  C. Skin testing
    1. penicillin battery
    2. selected food battery
    3. *Candida*, yeast, mold spores
  D. Mold-free diet
  E. Dye- and preservative-free diet
  F. dye and preservative blinded challenge

outlined in Table 4. What if the history and physical is unhelpful in pointing toward triggering factors? As discussed above, routine laboratory determinations in the absence of suggestive history or signs are rarely rewarding. What minimum is worthwhile? A complete blood count, with differential, may point to an infectious etiology, or the presence of eosinophilia might suggest a drug reaction. But frequently eosinophilia does not practically help to pin down an etiology. Elevated sedimentation rates are not uncommon and point to an inflammatory perturbation, but unless markedly elevated may not help further. Since 10–14% of chronic urticaria patients may have thyroid autoimmunity, thyroid function tests, antithyroglobulin antibody, and anti-thyroid peroxidase (anti-thyroid microsomal) antibody are worth obtaining routinely. At the present, it is still unclear whether checking for hepatitis B and C viruses, let alone Epstein-Barr virus or *Mycoplasma*, is worthwhile. This may depend on the prevalence of these infections in the community. Routine skin testing, either inhalant or food, is neither cost-effective nor helpful when done as a screening maneuver. Inhalant skin tests may be positive but in the great majority of cases will have no bearing on the skin condition (see Table 1). The role of penicillin skin testing in the absence of a history of adverse reaction to the antibiotic remains at this point uncertain.

The next tier of evaluation is determined by suggestive history or physical findings. Limited inhalant skin testing may be appropriate for histories of seasonal urticaria. Food skin testing may likewise by helpful, followed by elimination of the incriminated items, followed thereafter by challenge with reintroduction. Physical findings suggestive of urticarial vasculitis may be pursued with serology such as ANA and rheumatoid factor, complement C3, C4, and CH50, or assays for immune complexes. A skin biopsy may verify the presence of vasculitis. Angioedema in the absence of urticaria may be due to C1 esterase inhibitor deficiency, either hereditary or acquired, which can be documented by low C2 and C4, and functional C1 esterase inhibitor assay. History of infection should be evaluated and treated as appropriate. Chronic nasal symptoms warrant a screening CT of the paranasal sinuses, but in the absence of such findings is not beneficial. Likewise, chest x-rays are not helpful in the absence of intimations of pulmonary disease. Screening stool for ova and parasites is distinctly unrewarding unless there is a history as discussed above.

The next tier is driven by persistence of symptoms or poor response to medical management. A food diary may give clues to unsuspected food allergens or additives. An empirical dairy-free diet trial may be useful for approximately 2 weeks. A beneficial outcome should be followed by skin testing for milk proteins and penicillin. If *Candida* or yeast skin testing is positive, a trial of an oral antifungal plus a mold avoidance diet historically has been helpful (see Table 2). Since dye- and preservative-free diets are reported to be of frequent benefit (see Table 2), this is a useful maneuver. There is a possibility that symptoms will remit and not return after following the diet for several months [50,51]. Even if symptoms improve on such a diet, provocative challenges for specific additives may not be positive. Blinded capsule challenges may be worthwhile at this level and may identify a factor in about 10% (R. W. Weber, unpublished data) (see Table 3).

If the evaluation at this point remains negative, the management of the patient defaults to symptomatic control with pharmacotherapy. But it is reasonable to periodically assess the work-up that has been performed to date and consider whether something has been missed or if some aspect of the history may shed new light. It is not reasonable, however, to continue to repeat studies that have been unrewarding in the past.

## REFERENCES

1. Agah R, Bandi V, Guntupalli KK. Angioedema: the role of ACE inhibitors and factors associated with poor clinical outcome. Intensive Care Med 1997; 23:793–796.
2. Gabb GM, et al. Epidemiological study of angioedema and ACE inhibitors. Aust NZ J Med 1996; 26:777–782.
3. Brown NJ, Ray WA, Snowden M, Griffin MR. Black Americans have an increased rate of angiotensin converting enzyme inhibitor-associated angioedema. Clin Pharmacol Ther 1996; 60:8–13.
4. Schiller PI, Langauer Messmer S, Haefeli WE, Schlienger RG, Bircher AJ. Angiotensin-converting enzyme inhibitor-induced angioedema: late onset, irregular course, and potential role of triggers. Allergy 1997; 52:432–435.

5. Kauppinen E, Juntunen K, Lanki H. Urticaria in children: retrospective evaluation and follow-up. Allergy 1984; 39:469–472.

6. Sheldon J, Mathews KP, Lovell RG. The vexing urticaria problem: present concepts of etiology and management. J Allergy 1954; 25:525–560.

7. Harris A, Twarog FJ, Geha RS. Chronic urticaria in childhood: Natural course and etiology. Ann Allergy 1983; 51:161–165.

8. Volonakis M, Katsarou-Katsari A, Stratigos J. Etiologic factors in childhood chronic urticaria. Ann Allergy 1992; 69:61–65.

9. Miller DA, Freeman GL, Akers WA. Chronic urticaria: a clinical study of fifty patients. Am J Med 1968; 44:68–86.

10. Smith JA, Mansfield LE, Fokakis A, Nelson HS. Dermographia caused by IgE mediated penicillin allergy. Ann Allergy 1983; 51:30–32.

11. Wu LY, Mesko JW, Petersen BH. Cold urticaria associated with infectious mononucleosis. Ann Allergy 1983; 50:271–274.

12. Doeglas HMG, Rijnten WR, Schröder FP, Schirm J. Cold urticaria and virus infections: a clinical and serological study in 39 patients. Br J Dermatol 1986; 114:311–318.

13. Wanderer AA. Cold urticaria syndromes: historical background, diagnostic classification, clinical and laboratory characteristics, pathogenesis, and management. J Allergy Clin Immunol 1990; 85:965–981.

14. Kaplan AP. Urticaria and angioedema. In: Middleton E Jr, Reed CE, Ellis EF, Adkinson NF Jr, Yunginger JW, Busse WW, eds. Allergy Principles & Practice. 5th ed. St. Louis: Mosby-Yearbook, 1998:1104–1122.

15. Cooke RA. Allergy in Theory and Practice. Philadelphia: WB Saunders, 1946.

16. Jacobson KW, Branch LB, Nelson HS. Laboratory tests in chronic urticaria. JAMA 1980; 243:1644–1646.

17. Nelson HS. Routine sinus roentgenograms and chronic urticaria. JAMA 1984; 251:1680–1681.

18. Kanazawa K, Yaoita H, Tsuda F, Okamoto H. Hepatitis C virus infection in patients with urticaria. J Am Acad Dermatol 1996; 35:195–198.

19. Leznoff A, Josse RG, Denburg J, Dolovich J. Association of chronic urticaria and angioedema with thyroid autoimmunity. Arch Dermatol 1983; 119:636–640.

20. Leznoff A, Sussman GL. Syndrome of idiopathic chronic urticaria and angioedema with thyroid autoimmunity: a study of 90 patients. J Allergy Clin Immunol 1989; 84:66–71.

21. Turktas I, Gokcora N, Demirsoy S, Cakir N, Onal E. The association of chronic urticaria and angioedema with autoimmune thyroiditis. Int J Dermatol 1997; 36:187–190.

22. Rumbyrt JS, Katz JL, Schocket AL. Resolution of chronic urticaria in patients with thyroid autoimmunity. J Allergy Clin Immunol 1995; 96:901–905.

23. James J, Warin RP. An assessment of the role of *Candida albicans* and food yeasts in chronic urticaria. Br J Dermatol 1971; 84:227–237.

24. Numata T, Yamamoto S, Yamura T. The role of mite allergen in chronic urticaria. Ann Allergy 1979; 43:356–358.

25. Boonk WJ, Van Ketel WG. The role of penicillin in the pathogenesis of chronic urticaria. Br J Dermatol 1982; 106:183–190.

26. Ormerod AD, Reid TMS, Main RA. Penicillin in milk—its importance in urticaria. Clin Allergy 1987; 17:229–234.

27. Hamrick HJ, Moore GW. Giardiasis causing urticaria in a child. Am J Dis Child 1983; 137:761–763.

28. Clyne CA, Eliopoulos GM. Fever and urticaria in acute giardiasis. Arch Intern Med 1989; 149:939–940.

29. Leighton PM, MacSween HM. Strongyloides stercoralis: the cause of an urticarial-like eruption of 65 years' duration. Arch Intern Med 1990; 150:1747–1748.

30. Warin RP, Campion RH. Urticaria. London: WB Saunders, 1974.

31. Kramer MH, Eberhard ML, Blankenberg TA. Respiratory symptoms and subcutaneous granu-

loma caused by mesocercariae: a case report. Am J Tropical Med Hygiene 1996; 55:447–448.

32. Pasricha JS, Pasricha A, Prakash OM. Role of gastro-intestinal parasites in urticaria. Ann Allergy 1972; 30:348–351.

33. Del Pozo MD, Audícana M, Diez JM, Muñoz D, Ansotegui IJ, Fernández E, Garcia M, Etxenagusia M, Moneo I, Fernández de Corres L. *Anisakis simplex*, a relevant etiologic factor in acute urticaria. Allergy 1997; 52:576–579.

34. Fernández-Caldas E, Quirce S, Marañón F, Gómez MLD, Botella HG, Román RL. Allergenic cross-reactivity between third stage larvae of *Hysterothylacium aduncum* and *Anisakis simplex*. J Allergy Clin Immunol 1998; 101:554–555.

35. Juhlin L, Michaëlsson G, Zetterström O. Urticaria and asthma induced by food-and-drug additives in patients with aspirin hypersensitivity. J Allergy Clin Immunol 1972; 50:92–98.

36. Michaëlsson G, Juhlin L. Urticaria induced by preservatives or dye additives in food or drugs. Br J Dermatol 1973; 88:525–532.

37. Doeglas HMG. Reactions to aspirin and food additives in patients with chronic urticaria, including the physical urticarias. Br J Dermatol 1975; 93:135–144.

38. Thune P, Granholt A. Provocation tests with antiphlogistic and food additives in recurrent urticaria. Dermatologica 1975; 151:360–367.

39. Ros A-M, Juhlin L, Michaëlsson G. A following study of patients with recurrent urticaria and hypersensitivity to aspirin, benzoates and azo dyes. Br J Dermatol 1976; 95:19–24.

40. Ortolani C, Pastorello E, Fontana A, Gerosa S, Ispano M, Pravettoni V, Rotondo F, Mirone C, Zanussi C. Chemicals and drugs as triggers of food-associated disorder. Ann Allergy 1988; 60:358–366.

41. Warin RP, Smith RJ. Challenge test battery in chronic urticaria. Br J Dermatol 1976; 94:401–406.

42. Juhlin L. Recurrent urticaria: clinical investigation of 330 patients. Br J Dermatol 1981; 104:369–381.

43. Goodman DL, McDonnell JT, Nelson HS, Vaughan TR, Weber RW. Chronic urticaria exacerbated by the antioxidant food preservatives, butylated hydroxyanisole (BHA) and butylated hydroxytoluene (BHT). J Allergy Clin Immunol 1990; 86:570–575.

44. Stevenson DD, Simon RA, Lumry WR, Mathison DA. Adverse reactions to tartrazine. J Allergy Clin Immunol 1988; 78:182–191.

45. Bosso JV, Simon RA. Urticaria, angioedema, and anaphylaxis provoked by food additives. In: Metcalfe DD, Sampson HA, Simon RA, eds. Food Allergy: Adverse Reactions to Foods and Food Additives. 2d ed. Cambridge, MA: Blackwell Science, 1997:397–409.

46. Jacobsen DW. Adverse reactions to benzoates and parabens. In: Metcalfe DD, Sampson HA, Simon RA, eds. Food Allergy: Adverse Reactions to Foods and Food Additives. 2d ed. Cambridge, MA: Blackwell Science, 1997:375–386.

47. Weber RW. Adverse reactions to the antioxidants butylated hydroxyanisole (BHA) and butylated hydroxytoluene (BHT). In: Metcalfe DD, Sampson HA, Simon RA, eds. Food Allergy: Adverse Reactions to Foods and Food Additives. 2d ed. Cambridge, MA: Blackwell Science, 1997:387–395.

48. Weber RW, Hoffman M, Raine DA Jr., Nelson HS. Incidence of bronchoconstriction due to aspirin, azo dyes, non-azo dyes, and preservatives in a population of perennial asthmatics. J Allergy Clin Immunol 1979; 64:32–37.

49. Gibson A, Clancy R. Management of chronic idiopathic urticaria by the identification and exclusion of dietary factors. Clin Allergy 1980; 10:699–704.

50. Kemp AS, Schembri G. An elimination diet for chronic urticaria of childhood. Med J Aust 1985; 143:234–235.

51. Supramaniam G, Warner JO. Artificial food additive intolerance in patients with angio-oedema and urticaria. Lancet 1986; 2:907–909.

52. Malanin G, Kalimo K. The results of skin testing with food additives and the effect of an

elimination diet in chronic and recurrent urticaria and recurrent angioedema. Clin Exp Allergy 1989; 19:539–543.

53. Moore-Robinson M, Warin RP. Effect of salicylates in urticaria. Br Med J 1967; 4:262–264.
54. Duke WW. Urticaria caused specially by the action of physical agents. JAMA 1924; 83:3–8.
55. Casale TB, Sampson HA, Hanifin J, Kaplan AP, Kulcycki A, Lawrence ID, Lemanske RF, Levine MI, Lillie MA. Guide to the physical urticarias. J Allergy Clin Immunol 1988; 82:758–763.
56. Casale TB, Keahey TM, Kaliner M. Exercise-induced anaphylactic syndromes: Insights into diagnostic and pathophysiologic features. JAMA 1986; 255:2049–2053.
57. Dohi M, Suko M, Sugiyama H, Yamashita N, Tadokoro K, Juji F, Okudaira H, Sano Y, Ito K, Miyamoto T. Food-dependent, exercise-induced anaphylaxis: a study on 11 Japanese cases. J Allergy Clin Immunol 1991; 87:34–40.

# 26

## Antihistamines (H₁- and H₂-Receptor Antagonists) in Skin Disease

**F. Estelle R. Simons**

*University of Manitoba, Winnipeg, Manitoba, Canada*

## I. INTRODUCTION

Histamine, an important chemical mediator of itching and of inflammation, is produced and stored in cytoplasmic granules in tissue mast cells and basophils, from which it is released in large quantities by noncytotoxic mechanisms. Acting on $H_1$ receptors in the skin, histamine causes itching via stimulation of thin, nonmyelinated afferent C-fibers, which have low conduction velocity and large ennervation territories (Fig. 1). $H_2$ receptors are not involved in histamine-evoked itching [1–3].

Acting at $H_1$ and $H_2$ receptors in the skin, histamine induces the vascular endothelium to release nitric oxide, which stimulates guanyl cyclase and increases cyclic guanosine monophosphate (cGMP) in the vascular smooth muscle, causing vasodilation and erythema and increased vascular permeability and edema. The vasodilation is enhanced by an axon reflex resulting from the release of substance P by antidromic conduction on afferent C-fibers, and this also augments histamine release. The affinity of histamine for $H_1$ receptors in the vasculature is approximately 10 times its affinity for $H_2$ receptors.

Although $H_3$ receptors, auto-receptors regulating the release and biosynthesis of histamine, are also present in the skin, their role in histamine-mediated itch and inflammation remains to be determined.

The $H_1$ and the $H_2$ receptors have the characteristics of G-protein–coupled receptors, and the genes encoding them have been cloned in human cells. The molecular structure of the $H_3$ receptor has also recently been established.

$H_1$-receptor antagonists are the cornerstone of symptomatic treatment in urticaria and may play some role in relieving histamine-induced pruritus in other skin disorders [1,3]. Old $H_1$ antagonists still used for urticaria treatment include the piperazine hydroxyzine, the piperidines cyproheptadine and ketotifen, the ethanolamine diphenhydramine, and the alkylamine chlorpheniramine. New $H_1$ antagonists recommended include the piperazine cetirizine and the somewhat atypical piperidines azelastine, ebastine, fexofenadine, loratadine, and mizolastine. Astemizole, in use at the time this chapter was written, has recently had regulatory approval withdrawn.

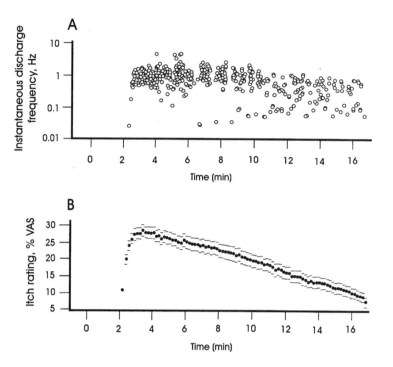

**Figure 1**  Histamine is an important mediator of itching. The cutaneous branch of the peroneal nerve of 21 healthy human volunteers was studied using microneurography. (A) Units were identified with a marking technique as "responsive" or unresponsive" to mechanical stimulation and heat stimulation, then tested for responsiveness to histamine 1 mA, iontophoresed for 20 sec from a 6-mm-diameter probe. (B) Histamine-induced itch sensations lasted several minutes. C-fibers, representing a new class of afferent nerves with extremely thin axons and excessive terminal branching, were found to mediate itch sensations. These fibers were mechanically insensitive and had low conduction velocities. Innervation territories were large (up to 85 mm in diameter) on the lower leg (From Ref. 2.)

## II.  H₁-RECEPTOR ANTAGONISTS: CLINICAL PHARMACOLOGY

The efficacy of $H_1$ antagonists in skin disorders depends primarily on their ability to block the agonist effect of histamine at $H_1$ receptors on afferent C-fibers, resulting in decreased itching, and on histamine blockade at $H_1$ receptors on the smooth muscle of the postcapillary venules, resulting in decreased vascular permeability, exudation, and edema [1,3]. The antiallergic and anti-inflammatory activities of $H_1$ antagonists, which occur independently of $H_1$ blockade, can generally be demonstrated only with high doses and have not yet been convincingly demonstrated to confer additional clinical benefit to that produced by $H_1$ blockade [4] (Table 1).

H₁ antagonists differ considerably in their chemical structures, some of which are shown in Figure 2, and in their pharmacokinetic and pharmacodynamic profiles (Tables 2 and 3). In general, they are well-absorbed after oral administration. They can be divided into two groups: those that are extensively transformed into metabolites in the cytochrome

**Table 1** Antiallergic and Anti-inflammatory Effects[a] of $H_1$-Receptor Antagonists

Decreased release of some chemical mediators of inflammation (e.g., histamine, $PGD_2$, $LTC_4$, kinins, and tryptase) from mast cells and basophils, in vitro and in vivo after immunological stimuli such as specific allergen or anti-IgE; and nonimmunological stimuli such as compound 48/80, substance P, concanavalin A, or calcium ionophore A23187

Decreased migration, accumulation, and activation of eosinophils, neutrophils, basophils, and other inflammatory cells (e.g., decreased chemotaxis of eosinophils stimulated with PAF, fMLP, $LTD_4$, C5a, IL-8, and RANTES)

Decreased pro-inflammatory cell activation and generation of products such as superoxide radicals, $LTB_4$, $LTC_4$, neutrophil elastase, and ECP

Reduced adhesion protein expression (e.g., decreased ICAM-1 expression by epithelial cells)

[a] Antiallergic and anti-inflammatory effects have been best studied for azelastine, cetirizine, ketotifen, and loratadine. Higher doses than used for blockade of histamine at $H_1$ receptors may be required.
*Source*: Adapted from Refs. 1 and 4.

$P_{450}$ system in the liver and gastrointestinal tract (astemizole, azelastine, cyproheptadine, chlorpheniramine, ebastine, hydroxyzine, loratadine, and mizolastine) and those that are eliminated largely unchanged in the urine and/or feces and are not metabolized extensively in the cytochrome $P_{450}$ system (cetirizine and fexofenadine). Terminal elimination half-life values of these $H_1$ antagonists range from 7 to more than 24 hours for the parent compounds and up to 9 days for the metabolites [5–14].

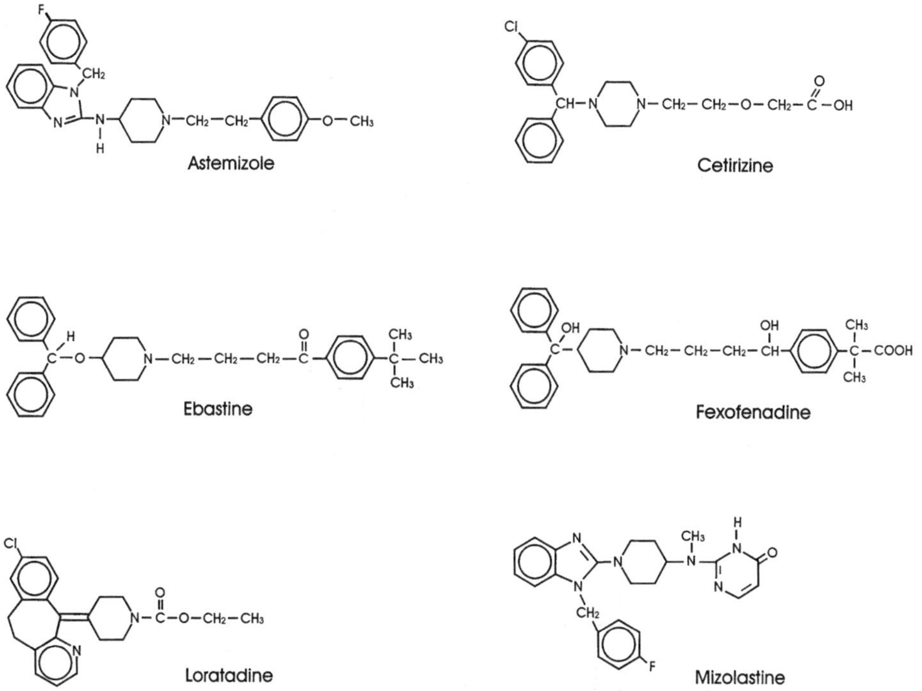

**Figure 2** Chemical structures of selected new $H_1$ antagonists. All the medications shown are piperidines, with the exception of the piperazine cetirizine.

**Table 2** Practical Pharmacokinetics and Pharmacodynamics of Representative Old H₁ Antagonists Used in Urticaria Treatment

| H₁-receptor antagonist (old first-generation H₁ antagonists) | $t_{max}$[a] (hr) after a single dose | Terminal elimination $t_{1/2}$[b] (hr) | % Eliminated unchanged in the urine/feces | Drug interactions | Duration of action (hr) | Population in which dose adjustment is required |
|---|---|---|---|---|---|---|
| Cyproheptadine | 6–9 | 16 | NA | Possible | NA | G |
| Chlorpheniramine | 3 | 21–28 | NA | Possible | 24 | G |
| Diphenhydramine | 2–3 | 9 | NA | Possible | 12 | H, G |
| Doxepin | 2 | 13 | NA | Possible | NA | H |
| Hydroxyzine | 2 | 20 | NA | Possible | 24 | H |
| Ketotifen | 4 | 22 | 1% | Possible | 12 | NA |

Results are expressed as means. Few of the old H₁ antagonists have been optimally studied.
[a] time from oral intake to peak plasma concentration.
[b] terminal elimination half-life.
NA = information not available. bid = twice daily; G = geriatric; R = renal function-impaired; H = hepatic function-impaired.

**Table 3** Practical Pharmacokinetics and Pharmacodynamics of Representative New H₁ Antagonists Used in Urticaria Treatment

| H₁-receptor antagonist (metabolite) | $t_{max}^a$ (hr) after a single dose | Terminal elimination $t_{1/2}^b$ (hr) | % Eliminated unchanged in the urine/feces | Drug interactions | Duration of action (hr) | Once-daily dosing recommended? | Population in which dose adjustment is required |
|---|---|---|---|---|---|---|---|
| Eliminated Largely Unchanged | | | | | | | |
| Cetirizine | 1.0 | 7.4 | 60/0 | Unlikely | 24 | Yes | GRH |
| Fexofenadine | 2.6 | 14.4 | 12/80 | Unlikely | 24 | Yes | none |
| Extensively Metabolized | | | | | | | |
| Astemizole[c] (norastemizole and desmethylastemizole) | 0.5 (0.7) | 1 day (9 days) | NA | Possible | 24 | Yes | H |
| Azelastine[c]; (desmethylazelastine) | 4.5 (3.6) | 25 (54) | NA | Possible | 12 | No (bid) | G |
| Ebastine[c] (carebastine) | | (14) | NA | Possible | 24 | Yes | G |
| Loratadine[d] (descarboethoxyloratadine) | 1.0 (1.5) | 7.8–11.0 (17–24) | Trace | Unlikely[c] | 24 | Yes | RH[c] |
| Mizolastine[e] | 1.9 | 12.9 | Trace | Possible | 24 | Yes | none |

Results are expressed as means.

[a] Time from oral intake to peak plasma concentration.
[b] Terminal elimination half-life.
[c] Not approved in the U.S. at time of publication.
[d] In the presence of CYP3A4 inhibition, loratadine is eliminated via the CYP2D6 metabolic pathway.
[e] No active metabolites identified.
NA = information not available. bid = twice daily; G = geriatric; R = renal function-impaired; H = hepatic function-impaired.

After oral administration in usual doses, $H_1$ antagonists achieve peak concentrations rapidly in the skin [6] (Fig. 3). Suppression of the histamine- or allergen-induced wheal and flare is a useful bioassay for defining dose-response curves and for identifying clinically relevant differences in onset of $H_1$-antagonist activity, maximum activity, and offset of activity. Although the medications in this class are diverse, most produce significant $H_1$-receptor blockade within 1–2 hours and have a duration of action of 24 hours after a single dose [5–14].

During long-term regular administration of an $H_1$ antagonist, there is no decrease in the amount of $H_1$-receptor blockade produced. In studies of 4–12 weeks' duration, subsensitivity or loss of activity of new $H_1$ antagonists such as cetirizine, loratadine, and mizolastine has not been found using objective monitoring of skin wheal and flare suppression, nor has loss of efficacy been found using subjective monitoring of symptom relief in urticaria. The apparent subsensitivity to the antihistaminic effects of the old $H_1$ antagonists reported years ago may have been due to lack of compliance secondary to the relatively poor benefit-to-risk ratio of many of these medications.

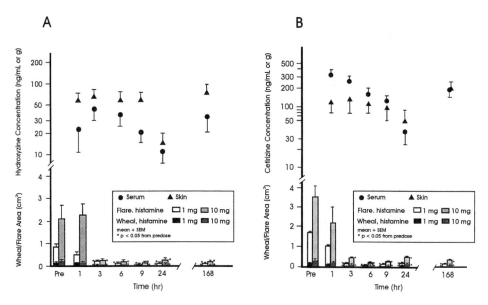

**Figure 3** $H_1$ antagonist concentrations in skin and serum. (A) Skin and serum hydroxyzine concentrations versus time plots and wheal and flare areas after epicutaneous tests with histamine 1 mg/ml and 10 mg/ml. Tests were performed at baseline and 1, 3, 6, 9, and 24 hours after the initial dose of hydroxyzine 50 mg. Subjects then took hydroxyzine 50 mg at 2100 hours for 6 consecutive days, and the tests were repeated at 168 hours (steady-state), exactly 12 hours after the seventh and last dose. (B) Skin and serum cetirizine concentrations versus time plots and wheal and flare areas after epicutaneous tests with histamine 1 mg/ml and 10 mg/ml. Tests were performed at baseline and 1, 3, 6, 9, and 24 hours after the initial dose of cetirizine 10 mg. Subjects then took cetirizine 10 mg at 2100 hours for 6 consecutive days, and the tests were repeated at 168 hours (steady-state), exactly 12 hours after the seventh and last dose. (From Ref. 6.)

## III. H$_1$-RECEPTOR ANTAGONISTS IN CHRONIC URTICARIA

In urticarial lesions, skin tissue fluid histamine concentrations are elevated compared to histamine concentrations in surrounding uninvolved skin [15]. If urticaria is provoked locally by challenge with a relevant stimulus, histamine concentrations in venous blood draining the urticated skin are transiently elevated, peaking at 2–5 minutes after challenge and declining to baseline within 30 minutes. Clinical tolerance to histamine is reduced in patients with chronic urticaria.

The beneficial effects of H$_1$ antagonists in the treatment of urticaria have been well documented, particularly for the symptomatic relief of itching, which is primarily mediated by the action of histamine at H$_1$ receptors, but also for reducing the number, size, and duration of urticarial lesions [16–18] (Figs. 4, 5, and 6). Relief of whealing and flaring (erythema) may be incomplete, as the vascular effects of histamine, increased permeability and vasodilation, are mediated through the action of histamine at H$_2$ receptors as well as at H$_1$ receptors, and also by other vasoactive substances, including proteases, eicosanoids such as prostaglandin E$_1$, and neuropeptides such as substance P [6].

For optimal effectiveness in preventing urticarial lesions from appearing, H$_1$ antagonists should be given on a regular basis, rather than as needed. H$_1$ antagonists have not been optimally studied in patients with chronic urticaria due to cold, delayed pressure, or other physical stimuli. The response to H$_1$-antagonist treatment in urticarial vasculitis is often unsatisfactory.

Old sedating H$_1$ antagonists are still used in urticaria treatment despite their poor benefit-to-risk ratio. Although in time-honored tradition they are often given three or four times daily, this is not necessary as they have long elimination half-life values (Table 2). Combinations of old H$_1$ antagonists (e.g., hydroxyzine plus cyproheptadine) or of old and

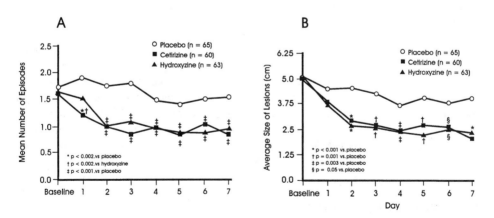

**Figure 4** New and old H$_1$ antagonists have similar efficacy in chronic urticaria. In a 4-week randomized, double-blind, double-dummy, placebo-controlled study, 188 patients with chronic idiopathic urticaria were treated with either cetirizine 10 mg once daily, hydroxyzine 25 mg three times daily, or placebo. Cetirizine and hydroxyzine both significantly improved (A) the number of episodes of urticaria and (B) the size of lesions. The number of lesions and the severity of pruritus were also decreased (not shown). (From Ref. 16.)

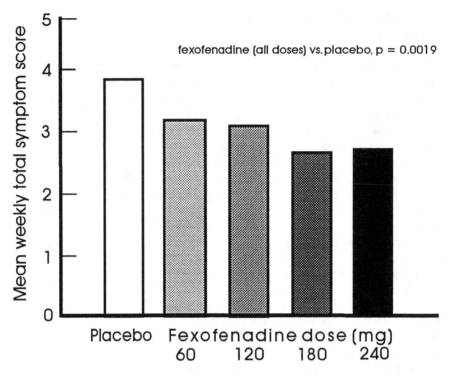

**Figure 5** $H_1$-antagonist dose-response in chronic urticaria. Fexofenadine 60, 120, 180, or 240 mg daily were compared in a double-blind, randomized, placebo-controlled, parallel-group 6-week study in 222 patients with chronic urticaria. In comparison with placebo, all doses decreased itching. Fexofenadine 180 mg ($p = 0.0008$) and 240 mg ($p = 0.0041$) decreased the total symptom score. The recommended dose for urticaria is 180 mg daily. Adverse effects were more common in those receiving placebo than in those receiving fexofenadine. (From Ref. 18.)

new $H_1$ antagonists (cetirizine in the morning and hydroxyzine at night) are recommended on an empirical basis by some highly respected physicians; however, these regimens have not been rigorously tested in randomized, prospective, double-blind, placebo-controlled trials, and they place patients at increased risk for sedation and other adverse effects from the old $H_1$ antagonists administered. In prospective, controlled, double-blind studies, new $H_1$ antagonists have been found to be as effective as the old ones and are significantly less sedating (Fig. 4). Higher doses than those used in allergic rhinitis (Table 4) may be required (Fig. 5).

## IV.  $H_1$-RECEPTOR ANTAGONISTS IN ATOPIC DERMATITIS

The pathogenesis of atopic dermatitis involves antigen-processing Langerhans cells and increased numbers of activated Th2 lymphocytes leading to defective cell-mediated responses, as well as upregulation of B cells, IgE production, and release of histamine and other chemical mediators of inflammation. Histamine is the main pruritogen, and histamine concentrations may be elevated in the skin and plasma in some patients [3].

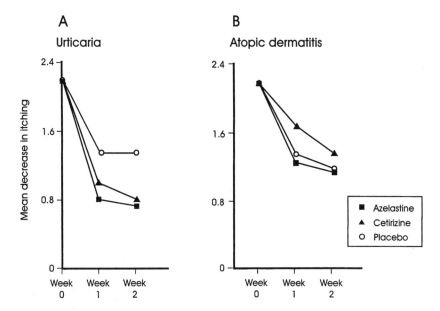

**Figure 6** $H_1$ antagonists are more effective in chronic urticaria than in atopic dermatitis. In a randomized, placebo-controlled, double-blind, parallel-group, 2-week study in 244 subjects with urticaria, atopic dermatitis, and other pruritic dermatoses, azelastine 4 mg was compared with cetirizine 10 mg. Azelastine and cetirizine reduced itching significantly in subjects with urticaria but at these doses had only minor effects on pruritus reduction in patients with atopic dermatitis. (From Ref. 17.)

In atopic dermatitis, relief of itching by $H_1$ antagonists is often incomplete, as the itching produced by proteases and mediators other than histamine is not downregulated. Some physicians consider $H_1$ antagonists to be of little value in atopic dermatitis treatment. Others believe that $H_1$ antagonists relieve itching by central as well as by peripheral $H_1$-blockade mechanisms and that the old sedating $H_1$ antagonists such as hydroxyzine and diphenhydramine are more effective for relief of pruritus in this disorder than the new, nonsedating $H_1$ antagonists. In fact, new medications such as cetirizine, loratadine, and azelastine have been shown to relieve itching in atopic dermatitis; however, high doses are required and efficacy is considerably lower than it is in chronic urticaria [17] (Fig. 6).

Infants with atopic dermatitis and/or elevated serum IgE and a family history of atopy are at increased risk for development of asthma. In placebo-controlled studies of 1–3 years' duration, high-dose cetirizine or ketotifen have been shown to delay the development of asthma in some of these high-risk infants by mechanisms that are not yet completely understood [19].

## V. $H_1$-RECEPTOR ANTAGONISTS IN SKIN DISORDERS OTHER THAN URTICARIA OR ATOPIC DERMATITIS

$H_1$ antagonists relieve histamine-mediated itching, and therefore, not surprisingly, their efficacy has been documented in prospective, randomized, double-blind, placebo-

**Table 4**  Formulations and Dosages of Representative $H_1$-Receptor Antagonists

|  | Formulation | Recommended dose |
|---|---|---|
| Old $H_1$ Antagonists |  |  |
| Chlorpheniramine | Tablets 4 mg, 8 mg,[a] 12 mg[a] | Adult: 8–12 mg bid[a] |
| (Chlortrimeton®) | Syrup 2.5 mg/5 ml | Pediatric[b]: 0.35 mg/kg/24 hr |
|  | Parenteral solution 10 mg/ml |  |
| Cyproheptadine | Tablets 4 mg | 4 mg tid |
|  | Syrup 2 mg/5 ml | 2 mg tid |
| Diphenhydramine | Capsules 25 or 50 mg | Adult: 25–50 mg tid |
| (Benadryl®) | Elixir 12.5 mg/5 ml, Syrup 6.25 mg/5 ml | Pediatric: 5 mg/kg/24 hr |
|  | Parenteral solution 50 mg/ml |  |
| Hydroxyzine (Atarax®) | Capsules 10,25,50 mg | Adult: 25–50 mg qd (hs) or bid |
|  | Syrup 10 mg/5 ml | Pediatric: 2 mg/kg/24 hr |
| Ketotifen (Zaditen®) | Tablets 1 mg; 2 mg[a] | Subjects > 3 yrs: 1 mg bid or 2 mg qd[a] |
|  |  | 4 mg qd[a] is used in urticaria |
| New $H_1$ Antagonists |  |  |
| Astemizole[c] (Hismanal®) | Tablets 10 mg | Adult: 10 mg qd |
|  | Suspension 10 mg/5 ml[c] | Pediatric: 0.2 mg/kg/24 hr |
| Cetirizine (Reactine®, Zyrtec®) | Tablets 10 mg | Adult and pediatric (5–10 yr): 5–10 mg qd |
|  | Syrup 5 mg/5 ml | Pediatric (2–5 yr): 2.5–5 mg |
| Ebastine[c] (Ebastel®) | Tablets 10 mg | Adult: 10 mg qd |
| Fexofenadine (Allegra®) | Tablets 60 mg | Adult: 180 mg qd |
| Loratadine (Claritin®) | Tablets 10 mg | Adult: 10 mg qd |
|  | Syrup 5 mg/5 ml | Pediatric: (2–12 yr): 5 mg/day |
| Mizolastine[c] (Mizollen) | Tablets 10 mg | Adult:10 mg qd |

qd = Once daily; bid = twice daily; tid = three times daily.
[a] Timed-release.
[b] For subjects ≤40 kg (<30 kg or <12 12 yr for loratadine).
[c] Not approved in the United States at time of publication.

controlled trials in mastocytosis and neurofibromatosis, and also for itching caused by insect bites or by medications such as chloroquine [1]. In other skin disorders such as lichen nitidus, evidence for their efficacy consists only of case studies or uncontrolled clinical trials.

Although $H_1$ antagonists are often used to relieve itching in patients with severe hepatic or renal insufficiency, their benefit-to-risk ratio in these disorders is poor. In addition to their inability to relieve itching that is not produced by histamine, their elimination may be significantly decreased, with consequent $H_1$-antagonist accumulation in the central nervous system or in cardiac tissue and a potentially increased risk of adverse effects.

## VI.  $H_1$-RECEPTOR ANTAGONISTS: ADVERSE EFFECTS

Old $H_1$ antagonists potentially cause a wide variety of adverse effects, including anticholinergic effects (dry mouth and mucous membranes, difficulty in micturition, impotence, tachycardia, constipation, and other gastrointestinal symptoms) [1,20]. Cyproheptadine inhibits both histamine and 5-hydroxytryptamine (serotonin) activity and may cause appetite stimulation and inappropriate weight gain. Topical application of diphenhydramine or promethazine to the skin may lead to somnolence and other central nervous system (CNS) effects and may also result in sensitization and contact dermatitis.

Most new $H_1$ antagonists are unlikely to cause dry mouth or other anticholinergic effects, although astemizole and ketotifen may cause inappropriate weight gain. More importantly, many new $H_1$ antagonists are free from both CNS effects and from cardiac toxicity.

## A. Central Nervous System Effects of $H_1$-Receptor Antagonists

In the CNS, histamine is stored in vesicles in histaminergic neurons, from which it is released to play a pivotal role in neurotransmission and maintenance of the waking state [1]. Most old, first-generation $H_1$ antagonists readily penetrate the endothelial lining of the capillaries of the CNS, the so-called blood-brain barrier. In manufacturers' recommended doses, as demonstrated by positron emission tomography, they occupy a major fraction of the $H_1$ receptors in the frontal cortex, temporal cortex, hippocampus, and pons. Their central effects in humans appear to be mediated primarily by a blockade of endogenous histamine, as evidenced by the discovery that the sedative enantiomers (e.g., of chlorpheniramine) are those with the highest $H_1$-receptor affinity.

Use of potentially sedating $H_1$ antagonists is a concern in any patient, but particularly in schoolchildren, employees, the elderly, and those with preexisting CNS disorders [1,20]. The warning contained in the package insert for the old antihistamines—''may cause drowsiness—avoid activities requiring mental alertness''—is increasingly relevant in this high-technology era, in which mental alertness and optimal coordination are needed for most activities and are certainly required for most school- and work-related tasks. Military and commercial pilots are, for obvious reasons, prohibited from using them before or during flights. In other occupations and professions, no rules apply and the old $H_1$ antagonists continue to be implicated as a cause of accidents and injury. The CNS effects produced by the old $H_1$ antagonists are similar to those produced by alcohol or major tranquilizers [21] (Fig. 7). Concomitant ingestion of alcohol or other CNS-active chemicals potentiate the adverse CNS effects of old $H_1$ antagonists. Overdose of an old $H_1$ antagonist can be fatal.

Some physicians recommend giving old $H_1$ antagonists only at bedtime, as somnolence is of no concern during the night and $H_1$ blockade may still be present the next morning [20]. Unfortunately, the day after taking an old $H_1$ antagonist at bedtime, the adverse CNS effects may not have necessarily disappeared and peripheral $H_1$ blockade does not necessarily persist. Other physicians advise regular daytime use, anticipating that tolerance will develop to the adverse CNS effects but not to the peripheral $H_1$ blockade. While anecdotal and subjective reports of tolerance to the CNS effects of old antihistamines are common, tolerance may or may not be evident on objective testing. $H_1$ receptors in the CNS do not differ from $H_1$ receptors in the skin, where tolerance (decreased peripheral $H_1$ blockade over months of treatment) cannot be demonstrated.

The new $H_1$ antagonists do not cross the blood-brain barrier to the same degree that their predecessors did, and they do not interfere with the important neurotransmitter and ''waking'' effects of histamine in the CNS. They differ slightly from each other in their ability to cause adverse CNS effects; however, compared to the old $H_1$ antagonists, they are all relatively free from these effects. Even when administered in high doses, although

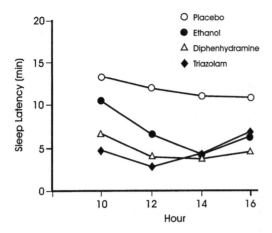

**Figure 7**  Comparative CNS effects of an $H_1$ antagonist, a tranquilizer, and ethanol. Sleep latency was measured 1, 3, 5, and 7 hours after placebo, diphenhydramine 50 mg, triazolam 0.2 mg, or ethanol 0.6 g/kg at 0900 hours, in a double-blind, three-way crossover study in 12 healthy subjects. The sedative effects of diphenhydramine, triazolam, and ethanol were significantly greater than those produced by placebo (diphenhydramine, F = 72.5, $p < 0.0001$; triazolam, F = 40.4, $p < 0.0001$; and ethanol, F = 18.9, $p < 0.001$). Twenty-four–hour clock time is shown on the horizontal axis. (From Ref. 21.)

they may cause some CNS effects, they nevertheless remain relatively nonsedating compared to the old $H_1$ antagonists. Also, in contrast to their predecessors, they do not potentiate the adverse CNS effects produced by alcohol or other CNS-active chemicals.

## B.  Cardiac Toxicity of $H_1$-Receptor Antagonists

The $H_1$ antagonists terfenadine and astemizole have been implicated in prolonging the QTc interval and, rarely, in causing torsade de pointes and other potentially fatal ventricular arrhythmias [22]. Regulatory approval has now been withdrawn for these medications in most countries. The risk of prolonged QTc interval and ventricular arrhythmias from old, sedating $H_1$ antagonists, such as chlorpheniramine, cyproheptadine, diphenhydramine, and hydroxyzine, and from new $H_1$ antagonists, such as azelastiine, cetirizine, fexofenadine, ebastine, loratadine, and mizolastine, is low.

The primary cellular event leading to arrhythmias is the inhibition of repolarization potassium channels, particularly the delayed rectifier potassium current ($I_K$), leading to prolonged duration of the action potential (QT interval) and development of early after-depolarization, which triggers torsade de pointes. Other electrophysiological changes, for example, blockade of the inward rectifier ($I_{k1}$) potassium channel or the transient outward ($I_{TO}$) potassium channel may also lead to prolongation of the action potential. Before new H antagonists enter clinical development, their potential arrhythmogenic effects can be predicted in vitro in human ventricular tissue or in cloned human ion channels. The molecular target in human ventricular for the potassium channel blockade of $H_1$ antagonists may be HERG, the human ether-a-go-go related gene on chromosome 7 that expresses the delayed rectifier $I_{kr}$ channel.

Host variables play an important role in the development of cardiac toxicity from $H_1$ antagonists [1,22]. Factors that increase the risk include a preexisting cardiac disorder including congenital or acquired prolonged QT syndrome or bradycardia, a metabolic problem such as hypokalemia, hypocalcemia, or hypomagnesemia, or concomitant ingestion of another medication which is eliminated in the cytochrome $P_{450}$ system.

## C. Safety of $H_1$-Receptor Antagonists During Pregnancy and Lactation

$H_1$ antagonists cross the placenta. Most are classified as FDA Pregnancy Category C, meaning that there is inadequate information about their use in humans and either no information about their use in animals or documented teratogenicity in animals [23]. These medications should be used during pregnancy only if the expected benefits to the mother exceed the unknown risks to the fetus. Prospective, controlled, observational studies of women taking $H_1$ antagonists during the first trimester of pregnancy are now being performed. Some $H_1$ antagonists, such as cetirizine, chlorpheniramine, diphenhydramine, and loratadine, are classified as lower-risk Pregnancy Category B, meaning that, though adequate studies have not been performed in humans, they are documented to be safe in animals.

In infants whose mothers received large therapeutic doses of old $H_1$ antagonists such as hydroxyzine or diphenhydramine immediately before delivery, withdrawal symptoms, including tremulousness and irritability, may occur. In nursing infants whose mothers have ingested old $H_1$ antagonists, irritability or drowsiness have been reported.

## VII. $H_2$-RECEPTOR ANTAGONISTS: CLINICAL PHARMACOLOGY

$H_2$ antagonists are rapidly absorbed after oral administration, with peak serum concentrations occurring within 1–3 hours [1]. Cimetidine, ranitidine, and famotidine are subject to first-pass hepatic metabolism. Cimetidine and ranitidine, but not famotidine or nizatidine, bind to the heme portion of the hepatic cytochrome $P_{450}$ system and, in a dose-related manner, inhibit hydroxylation, dealkylation, and other mixed-function oxygenase system actions. With cimetidine doses as low as 400–800 mg daily, elimination of many commonly prescribed medications, including many $H_1$ antagonists eliminated in the cytochrome $P_{450}$ system, is reduced by approximately 25%. Ranitidine binds to the cytochrome $P_{450}$ system with 5- to 10-fold less affinity than cimetidine.

In suppression of the histamine-induced cutaneous response, $H_2$ antagonists such as cimetidine and ranitidine administered alone have a variable, weak, dose-related effect. Concomitant oral administration of an $H_2$ antagonist and an $H_1$ antagonist is generally more effective than administration of an $H_2$ antagonist or an $H_1$ antagonist alone; however, the magnitude of the increased suppression is only about 10%, and in some studies it has not been statistically or clinically significant.

The enhanced suppression is due primarily to blockade of histamine action at $H_2$ receptors on the postcapillary venules in the skin and prevention of vasodilation. After cimetidine administration, enhanced suppression may also be due in part to pharmacokinetic inhibition of the hepatic elimination of the co-administered $H_1$ antagonist, resulting in higher $H_1$-antagonist plasma and tissue concentrations, and higher $H_1$-receptor occupancy than when the $H_1$ antagonist is administered alone [24] (Fig. 8).

Doxepin, a tricyclic antidepressant and anxiolytic, has clinically important $H_1$- and $H_2$-antagonist properties. Administered either by mouth or in a topical 5% cream formulation, it is effective in reducing itching and in supressing the histamine-induced wheals and flares in the skin. It is more potent than hydroxyzine or diphenhydramine in blocking $H_1$ receptors and more potent than cimetidine in blocking $H_2$ receptors.

## VIII.  $H_2$-RECEPTOR ANTAGONISTS IN URTICARIA

Although combined $H_1$-/$H_2$-antagonist treatment may enhance relief in some patients with urticaria refractory to treatment with an $H_1$ antagonist alone, this synergistic effect has not been found in all studies [1]. The gain is too small to be worthwhile in many patients and should never be suggested routinely. After a 3- to 4-week trial, if increased efficacy has not been demonstrated, the $H_2$ antagonist should be discontinued. The $H_2$ antagonists generally used are cimetidine 600 mg twice daily or ranitidine 150 mg twice daily. Combinations of $H_1$ and $H_2$ antagonists that have been tested include chlorpheniramine and cimetidine, cyproheptadine and cimetidine, hydroxyzine and cimetidine, and terfenadine and ranitidine. Neither cimetidine nor ranitidine given alone has a significant beneficial effect on itching in chronic urticaria. Combined $H_1$-/$H_2$-antagonist treatment is unlikely to be effective in patients with urticarial vasculitis.

In patients with chronic idiopathic urticaria, doxepin 25 mg three times daily suppresses wheals and pruritus to a significantly greater extent than does placebo, and even a low doxepin dose of 10 mg three times daily is significantly more effective than diphenhydramine. Doxepin, although traditionally given three times daily, has an elimination half-life of 13 hours and is now often administered once daily at bedtime in order to minimize daytime sedation.

## IX.  $H_2$-RECEPTOR ANTAGONISTS IN OTHER SKIN DISORDERS

$H_2$ antagonists have no role in atopic dermatitis treatment. Although topically applied doxepin relieves pruritus in this disorder, the benefit is not worth the risk of local or systemic adverse effects.

Cimetidine and other $H_2$ antagonists have been used for their immunomodulatory effects (not for $H_2$ blockade) in the treatment of recalcitrant warts and other skin disorders; additional randomized, placebo-controlled, double-blind studies are needed in this area [1].

## X.  $H_2$-RECEPTOR ANTAGONISTS: ADVERSE EFFECTS

$H_2$ antagonists have a good safety record and now have nonprescription status in many countries [1]. Doxepin, in addition to being sedating when ingested orally or applied topically, also potentially causes local adverse effects such as burning, sensitization, or contact dermatitis.

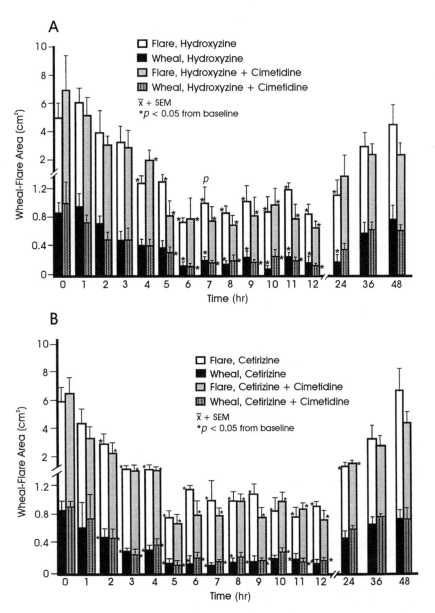

**Figure 8** Coadministration of an $H_1$ antagonist and an $H_2$ antagonist. In a randomized, double-blind, parallel-group study in 16 subjects with chronic urticaria, the suppressive effect of hydroxyzine 25 mg before and after treatment with cimetidine 600 mg q.12.h. for 10 days was examined. (A) When hydroxyzine was given with cimetidine, wheal and flare suppression increased compared with when hydroxyzine was given alone, although the difference was not statistically significant ($p > 0.05$). (B) Coadministration of hydroxyzine with cimetidine resulted in significantly increased plasma hydroxyzine concentrations and a significant increase in the partial hydroxyzine area under the curve from $227 \pm 77$ ng/ml/hr to $303 \pm 92$ ng/ml/hr ($p < 0.05$). This confirms the rationale for a trial of concomitant administration of cimetidine and hydroxyzine in patients with chronic urticaria unresponsive to treatment with an $H_1$ antagonist alone. In the same study, no therapeutic rationale for coadministration of cimetidine with cetirizine was found. (From Ref. 24.)

H$_2$-antagonist ingestion during the first trimester of pregnancy does not represent a major teratogenic risk; however, use of these medications for treatment of urticaria in pregnancy should be restricted to women in whom the modest anticipated benefits outweigh the unknown risks to the fetus. H$_2$ antagonists are excreted in breast milk.

## XI. SUMMARY

H$_1$ antagonists play an important role in the symptomatic treatment of chronic urticaria and a considerably less important role in the treatment of atopic dermatitis and other allergic skin disorders. The potential benefits of each H$_1$ antagonist should be weighed against the potential risks, particularly the common, often subclinical CNS adverse effects produced by the older H$_1$ antagonists.

H$_2$ antagonists play a limited role in the treatment of allergic skin disorders. They may be a useful addition to H$_1$-antagonist treatment in some patients with chronic urticaria.

## REFERENCES

1.  Simons FER. Antihistamines. In: Middleton E Jr, Reed CE, Ellis EF, Adkinson NF Jr, Yunginger JW, Busse WW, eds. Allergy Principles and Practice. St. Louis: Mosby-Year Book, Inc., 1998:612–637.
2.  Schmelz M, Schmidt R, Bickel A, Handwerker HO, Torebjörk HE. Specific C-receptors for itch in human skin. J Neurosci 1997; 17:8003–8008.
3.  Greaves MW, Wall PD. Pathophysiology of itching. Lancet 1996; 348:938–940.
4.  Naclerio RM, Baroody FM. H$_1$-receptor antagonists: antiallergic effects in humans. In: Simons FER, ed. Histamine and H$_1$-Receptor Antagonists in Allergic Disease. New York: Marcel Dekker, Inc., 1996:145–174.
5.  Simons FER, Simons KJ. The pharmacology and use of H$_1$-receptor antagonist drugs. N Engl J Med 1994; 330:1663–1670.
6.  Simons FER, Murray HE, Simons KJ. Quantitation of H$_1$-receptor antagonists in skin and serum. J Allergy Clin Immunol 1995; 95:759–764.
7.  Janssens MM-L. Astemizole. A nonsedating antihistamine with fast and sustained activity. Clin Rev Allergy 1993; 11:35–63.
8.  McTavish D, Sorkin EM. Azelastine: a review of its pharmacodynamic and pharmacokinetic properties, and therapeutic potential. Drugs 1989; 38:778–800.
9.  Spencer CM, Faulds D, Peters DH. Cetirizine. A reappraisal of its pharmacological properties and therapeutic use in selected allergic disorders. Drugs 1993; 46:1055–1080.
10. Wiseman LR, Faulds D. Ebastine. A review of its pharmacological properties and clinical efficacy in the treatment of allergic disorders. Drugs 1996; 51:260–277.
11. Markham A, Wagstaff AJ. Fexofenadine. Drugs 1998; 55:269–274.
12. Haria M, Fitton A, Peters DH. Loratadine. A reappraisal of its pharmacological properties and therapeutic use in allergic disorders. Drugs 1994; 48:617–637.
13. Markham A, Goa KL. Ketotifen. A review of its therapeutic efficacy in dermatological disorders. Clin Immunother 1996; 5:400–411.
14. Simons FER. Mizolastine: antihistaminic activity from preclinical data to clinical evaluation. Clin Exp Allergy 1999; 29(Supplement):3–8.
15. Kaplan AP. Urticaria and angioedema. In: Kaplan AP, ed. Allergy. Philadelphia: W.B. Saunders Company, 1997:573–592.

16. Breneman DL. Cetirizine versus hydroxyzine and placebo in chronic idiopathic urticaria. Ann Pharmacother 1996; 30:1075–1079.
17. Henz BM, Metzenauer P, O'Keefe E, Zuberbier T. Differential effects of new-generation $H_1$-receptor antagonists in pruritic dermatoses. Allergy 1998; 53:180–183.
18. Paul E, Berth-Jones J, Ortonne J-P, Stern M. Fexofenadine hydrochloride in the treatment of chronic idiopathic urticaria: a placebo-controlled, parallel-group, dose-ranging study. J Dermatol Treat 1998; 9:143–149.
19. Wahn U, for the ETAC Study Group. Allergic factors associated with the development of asthma and the influence of cetirizine in a double-blind, randomised, placebo-controlled trial: first results of ETAC. Pediatr Allergy Immunol 1998; 9:116–124.
20. Simons FER. $H_1$-receptor antagonists. Comparative tolerability and safety. Drug Safety 1994; 10:350–380.
21. Roehrs T, Zwyghuizen-Doorenbos A, Roth T. Sedative effects and plasma concentrations following single doses of triazolam, diphenhydramine, ethanol and placebo. Sleep 1993; 16:301–305.
22. Woosley RL. Cardiac actions of antihistamines. Annu Rev Pharmacol Toxicol 1996; 36:233–252.
23. Schatz M, Petitti D. Antihistamines and pregnancy. Ann Allergy Asthma Immunol 1997; 78:157–159.
24. Simons FER, Sussman GL, Simons KJ. Effect of the $H_2$-antagonist cimetidine on the pharmacokinetics and pharmacodynamics of the $H_1$-antagonists hydroxyzine and cetirizine in patients with chronic urticaria. J Allergy Clin Immunol 1995; 95:685–693.

# 27

# Topical Treatment of Allergic Skin Disorders

**John L. Aeling**

*University of Colorado Health Sciences Center, Denver, Colorado*

## I. INTRODUCTION

Dermatitis is a misnomer because the primary pathological process is epidermal inflammation. Even though epidermitis is a more accurate term, it is rarely used. Dermatitis evolves through three stages: acute (epidermal spongiosis with erythema, vesicles, bullae, and weeping), subacute (erythema, scaling, crusts, and excoriations), and chronic (epidermal thickening, scaling, excoriations, lichenification, and prurigo). The differential diagnosis of dermatitis is extensive and includes allergic skin diseases, psoriasiform dermatitis, genodermatosis, neoplastic disease, metabolic diseases, and nonallergic disease (Table 1). A correct diagnosis is imperative for a rational treatment plan.

A skin biopsy is helpful to rule out neoplastic disease, infections, psoriasiform dermatitis, and some drug eruptions. However, a skin biopsy rarely helps to differentiate allergic contact dermatitis, irritant contact dermatitis, or atopic dermatitis.

Dermatitis is a common reason for a patient to see a health care provider. The National Center for Health Care Statistics in 1990 revealed that 1% of all outpatient visits in the United States were for dermatitis and 69% of these patients were seen by nondermatologists [1]. Menne et al. [2] found a history of hand dermatitis in 22% of Danish women in a stratified epidemiological study. It is imperative that all physicians have a basic understanding of dermatitis and are able to diagnose and treat this common skin disease.

## II. IRRITANT CONTACT DERMATITIS

Irritant dermatitis is more common than allergic contact dermatitis. There is a great variability of irritancy threshold from person to person. Atopic patients have a low irritancy threshold, which is the reason wool clothing makes them itch. It has been shown that normal uninvolved skin of patients with atopic dermatitis has several functional abnormalities when compared to normal controls [3]. These patients have decreased epidermal barrier function demonstrated by increased transepidermal water loss in uninvolved skin. Once the skin's barrier function has been breached, repeated exposures to low-grade irritants will prevent healing. This is why recurrence of dermatitis at sites of previous involve-

**Table 1**  Differential Diagnosis of Dermatitis

Allergic skin disease
  Atopic dermatitis
  Allergic contact dermatitis
  Drug eruptions
Nonallergic skin disease
  Irritant dermatitis
  Stasis dermatitis
  Asteototic dermatitis
Metabolic disease
  Phenylketonuria
  Zinc deficiency (acrodermatitis enteropathica)
  Tyrosinemia
  Hartnup disease
  Histidinemia (ahistidasia)
  Pellagra
Psoriasiform dermatitis
  Psoriasis
  Seborrheic dermatitis
  Neurodermatitis
  Psoriasiform drug eruptions
Neoplastic disease
  Cutaneous T-cell lymphoma (mycosis fungoides)
  Langerhans cell histiocytosis
  Glucogonoma syndrome
  Paraneoplastic syndromes
Infectious disease
  Scabies
  Dermatophytosis
  Herpes simplex
  Bacterial infections
Immunodeficiency syndromes
  Agammaglobulinemia
  Wiskott-Aldrich syndrome
  Hyper-IgE syndrome (Job syndrome)
  Ataxia telangiectasia
Ichthyosis
  Ichthyosis vulgaris
  X-linked ichthyosis
  Lamellar ichthyosis
  Netherton's syndrome
  Conradi's disease
  Erythrokeratoderma variabilis
  Miscellaneous ichthyosis syndromes
Exfoliative erythroderma (dermatitis)
  Drug eruptions
  Cutaneous T-cell lymphoma (Sézary syndrome)
  Psoriasis
  Atopic dermatitis
  Seborrheic dermatitis
  Allergic contact dermatitis
  Pityriasis rubra pilaris

ment is common. Chronically inflamed skin has to return to clinical normalcy for at least several weeks or even several months before it will return to its previous irritancy threshold.

Repeated water exposure with resultant wetting and drying damages the barrier function of the skin and makes it more sensitive to irritants. With age the skin becomes drier, irritable, itchy, and even more susceptible to irritants. Dry skin dermatitis (xerosis) is one of the most common forms of irritant dermatitis and is a significant problem in both atopic patients and the elderly. Topical corticosteroid use thins both the epidermis and the dermis, and inappropriate use may prolong a chronic irritant dermatitis. These topical medications, especially the more potent medications, should be used with discretion when treating a patient with chronic dermatitis.

It can be difficult if not impossible to distinguish a low-grade allergic contact dermatitis from a chronic irritant dermatitis on the basis of the clinical presentation. Strong irritants produce immediate stinging and burning, while repeated mild irritant exposures elicit itching and chronic inflammation. It may take days, weeks, or even months for mild irritant exposures to produce a clinical dermatitis. Patch testing for allergic contact dermatitis is indicated in difficult cases. However, positive patch tests may be irrelevant, and both the patient and the treating physician are disappointed when an allergen is identified, the patient is educated regarding allergen avoidance, and the dermatitis persists. This is often seen in atopic patients and in patients with chronic hand and/or foot dermatitis [4].

## A. Irritant and Allergen Avoidance

All patients and parents of children with chronic dermatitis, regardless of the etiology, should be instructed to minimize exposure to irritants and potent contact allergens. The most common low-grade irritants are soaps and detergents. Other commonly encountered irritants include solvents, waxes, cleansers, bubble bath, glues, and many others too numerous to mention. Patients with chronic dermatitis should be instructed to avoid occupations that are typically associated with a high degree of irritant exposure and/or frequent hand washing. It is a common scenario for a patient who had childhood atopic dermatitis to develop a chronic hand or facial dermatitis later in life. This is a common finding in women after the birth of a child and in patients with occupational dermatitis.

Protective gloves and clothing should be recommended when irritant exposure cannot be avoided. Cotton-lined rubber gloves or a dermal cotton glove worn under a commercial rubber glove is mandatory for patients with chronic hand dermatitis who cannot avoid wet work or irritant exposure. A light pair of cotton or leather gloves is recommended for rough outdoor work. Rubber gloves should not be worn for more than 15–20 minutes at a time to minimize perspiration, which increases itching and contributes to the wetting and drying phenomenon. Patients with chronic dermatitis should be encouraged to modify their activities to minimize sweating. The ideal working and home environment has a temperature of 68–72°F and a humidity of 45–50%. Clothing should be loose, open-weaved, and comfortable. Cotton or cotton-blend fabrics are ideal. Fragrance-free washing machine detergents are recommended, and patients should add a second rinse cycle to remove detergent from clothing.

Patients with chronic dermatitis are often frustrated, angry, and desperate. They frequently use many over-the-counter products and medications they see advertised or that are recommended by friends or relatives. The use of some of these products increases the exposure to potential contact antigens. When a patient with a chronic dermatitis devel-

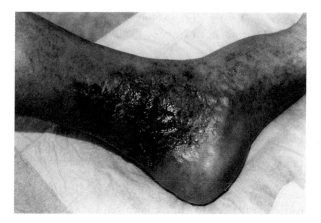

**Figure 1** A patient with chronic stasis dermatitis and secondary allergic contact dermatitis. This patient developed allergic contact dermatitis to both neomycin and Melaleuca (tea tree oil). (Courtesy of John I. Aeling, M.D.)

ops a secondary contact allergy, the problem becomes difficult to evaluate and treat. A typical example is a patient with chronic stasis dermatitis or stasis ulcers who becomes secondarily contact sensitive to a topical antibiotic (Fig. 1). Patients with chronic dermatitis should be instructed to avoid common, potent, over-the-counter contact allergens (Table 2).

## B.  Soaps and Detergents

Patients with chronic dermatitis should be instructed to use nonirritating soaps and dishwashing detergents. Soap should be used sparingly and have minimal defatting activity and a neutral pH. Soap was first discovered by the Phoenicians in 600 B.C. [5]. Today there is a plethora of products available in the marketplace. There are basically two types of skin cleansers: true soaps and synthetic detergents (syndets). True soaps are made by the saponification of animal or vegetable fat, have an alkaline pH, and are either sodium (hard soap) or potassium (soft soap) based. Syndets have a variable pH, and most but not all have a lower irritancy rating. One study rated 18 soaps and syndets for irritancy using Duhring chambers. The study rated erythema, scaling, and fissuring and found Dove to

**Table 2** Common Contact Allergens Found in OTC Products

Neomycin
Fragrance
Caines
Quaternium-15
Vitamin E
Melaleuca (tea tee oil)

**Table 3**  Irritancy Rating for Common Soaps

Mildly irritating: Dove, Aveenobar, Purpose, Dial, Alpha Keri, Fels Naptha
Moderately irritating: Neutrogena, Ivory, Oilatum, Lowila, Jergens, Lubriderm
Most irritating: Cuticura, Basis, Irish Spring, Zest, Camay, Lava

*Source*: Ref. 6

be the mildest [6] (Table 3). A comparison study rating 10 dishwashing liquids for irritancy using a multiple patch-testing technique found Palmolive SS to have the lowest irritancy. The irritancy rating did not correlate with the pH of the product [7].

Most authors think that limited use of a mild skin-cleansing product is permissible for patients with chronic dermatitis. Overuse, even with a mild product, can produce skin irritation.

## III.  HYDRATION AND LUBRICATION

Sixty-two percent of American women use a hand or body lotion on a regular basis, based on a survey of 1500 women screened nationwide across a broad geographic sample [8]. Hydration of the skin should be considered a major part of the treatment plan for any chronic dermatitis. This is especially true when treating atopic, nummular, and irritant dermatitis. This is best accomplished by tub soaks in tepid water for 15–20 minutes. Hot water can exacerbate itching and perpetuate the itch scratch cycle. A skin lubricant must be applied within 3–5 minutes after lightly patting off any excess water. Patients with chronic hand dermatitis should apply a moisturizer after each and every water exposure and hand washing. The recommended lubricant should be available by every sink in the workplace and home to improve compliance. The hydration from bathing also increases the penetration of topical medications, especially topical corticosteroids. Following a tub bath a corticosteroid can be applied to any area of inflammation and a skin lubricant can be applied over the topical steroid and to the uninvolved skin. Bath oils are not recommended because they provide very little occlusion and make the tub slippery.

Dry skin is more than just loss of water from the stratum corneum. Profilaggrin, a high molecular weight phosphorylated protein found in the granular layer of the epidermis, is dephosphorylated to filaggrin, which is further broken down to form a natural moisturizing factor. In ichthyosis vulgaris filaggrin is absent. With aging there is a decrease in all lipid fractions in the stratum corneum. Ceramides that form lipid bilayers are decreased with aging and in both psoriasis and atopic dermatitis [9].

Hundreds of millions of dollars are spent on skin moisturizers each year in the United States. The myriad of products available attest to the fact that no one product meets the needs of all patients and consumers. The ideal moisturizer would be nonirritating, nonsensitizing, easy to apply, cosmetically elegant, and inexpensive. The author tells patients that ''a topical steroid will treat inflammation and lubricating the skin will help to prevent recurrence of the rash. It's like greasing the transmission of your car to prevent a trip to the auto shop.''

Moisturizers include both humectants and occlusives. Humectants bind water in the skin, and occlusives are more effective in preventing evaporation. Table 4 lists common ingredients found in humectants and occlusives. Oil-in-water formulations are the easiest

**Table 4**  Common Occlusives and Humectants

Humectants
   Glycerin
   Propylene glycol
   Pyrrolidone carboxylic acid
   Sodium lactate
   Urea
   Gelatin
   Hyaluronic acid
   Some vitamins
Occlusives
   Petrolatum
   Lanolin
   Jojoba oil
   Cocoa butter
   Paraffin
   Cholesterol
   Olive oil
   Mineral oil

to apply and provide a dose of water to the skin. Patient compliance is usually better with oil-in-water moisturizers than pure occlusives. It is important to recommend an emollient of your choice so the patient thinks it is part of the treatment plan. The science of skin care products has improved greatly in the past 10 years, and there are many excellent products to choose from in the marketplace.

## IV.  ALPHA-HYDROXY ACIDS

Alpha-hydroxy acids are not new. Carl Wilhelm Scheele isolated lactic acid in 1780 [10]. The author first became introduced to lactic acid in a moisturizer while serving as a general medical officer in a military outpatient clinic next door to a Mayo Clinic–trained dermatologist. I was told that this was a favorite moisturizer recommended by the faculty at the Mayo Clinic during his residency in the late 1950s.

    Alpha-hydroxy acids are weak organic acids commonly found in fruits and other natural sources. Of this group, lactic acid found in sour milk and glycolic acid found in sugar cane have been used most frequently in topical preparations. Some other common glycolic acids include malic acid (apples), critic acid (citrus fruits), tartaric acid (grapes), and mandelic acid (bitter almonds). The acidic strength of an acid is expressed as the pKa number. The pKa of the acid represents the proton dissociation and is the negative log of the dissociation constant. The lower the pKa, the stronger the acid. The pKa for glycolic acid is 3.83, for lactic acid 3.86, and for trichloroacetic, a non–alpha-hydroxy acid, 0.52 [11].

    Since the introduction of glycolic acid in a moisturizer by a major cosmetic company in 1992, the public and the cosmetic industry have developed a love affair with these products. As of 1994, 75 manufacturers have marketed more than 100 over-the-counter alpha-hydroxy products [12]. The U.S. Food and Drug Administration continues to monitor these products regarding safety and efficacy. Various over-the-counter products contain 2–10% glycolic acid; unfortunately, most products do not list the concentration of the acid on the product or in the package insert. Alpha-hydroxy acids affect keratinization at the lowest levels of the stratum corneum, at the junction with the stratum corneum. They appear to affect corneocyte cohesion and new stratum corneum formation. In addition they increase dermal mucopolysaccharides and collagen formation [13]. Lavker et al. reported that 12% ammonium lactate mitigates epidermal and dermal atrophy from topically applied potent corticosteroid [14]. There are few studies comparing alpha-hydroxy acids. DiNardo et al. [15] compared 12% ammonium lactate versus 8% glycolic acid in patients with xerosis/ichthyosis of the legs. These patients were graded using the following criteria: skin roughness, skin moisture content, epidermal water binding, transepidermal water loss, stratum corneum thickness, epidermal thickness, dermal glycosaminoglycans, and dermal collagen. Both products improved dry skin and there was no statistical difference between them.

## V. TOPICAL CORTICOSTEROIDS

With the introduction of hydrocortisone as a topical medication in 1952, the first remarkably effective topical drug became available to treat inflammatory skin disease. Since the introduction of hydrocortisone there have been many modifications of this molecule to increase its anti-inflammatory properties. These modifications include halogenation, hydroxylation, modification of side chains, esterification, improvements in the salt molecules, and the development of new bases and formulations. As the potency of this medication has increased, so have the side effects. There are current attempts to engineer products that have the advantage of high potency but are rapidly metabolized to minimize these frustrating side effects. The 1998 PDR lists 80 topical corticosteroid medications. When prescribing one of these medications, consideration should be given to the disease being treated, anatomical site, type of lesion, age of the patient, vehicle, cost, frequency of application, number of refills, side effects, amount of medication, and the specific corticosteroid.

Topical corticosteroids are still the mainstay for the treatment of inflammatory skin disease; however, with a better understanding of the mediators of cutaneous inflammation and the discovery of new anti-inflammatory molecules that modify this response, there are a number of new and exciting therapies on the horizon. Chapter 28 will cover some of these potential new treatments. The anti-inflammatory effects of topical corticosteroids are complex. The steroid molecule can enter a cell nucleus and bind to nuclear DNA, including production of proteins called lipocortins. There is evidence that these proteins inhibit phospholipase $A_2$, an enzyme needed for arachidonic acid production. This inhibition results in the decreased production of prostaglandins, leukotrienes, and platelet-activating factor. The steroid molecule binds to cell membranes and alters cell adherence, phagocytosis, and lysosomal enzyme release. An immediate effect of topical steroids is to induce vasoconstriction, which decreases tissue edema, erythema, and heat. Corticosteroids produce profound effects on inflammatory cells, decreasing their numbers and functions at sites of inflammation. Polymorphonuclear leukocytes, lymphocytes, monocytes, and Langerhans cells all show decreased numbers and function at sites of inflammation when corticosteroid therapy is instituted [16]. The vasoconstrictor assay remains the gold standard for determining the potency of a topical corticosteroid. The assay measures the ability of the steroid to produce blanching when applied to normal human skin under controlled conditions by trained observers. The assay is a reliable, but not infallible, method to measure the clinical efficacy of a topical corticosteroid.

Most authors rank topical corticosteroids into seven groups of potency. The vehicle the product is formulated in can alter the potency of the steroid and move it up or down in this classification. Generic formulations of topical steroids are required to have the same active ingredient and the same concentration as the original product. However, many generics do not have the same formulation of the vehicle and the bioequivalent of the product can vary significantly [17]. In general the same steroid will be most potent in an ointment base, followed by emollients, gels, creams, lotions, and sprays. A simpler way to rank topical steroids is into four classes: superpotent, high-potent, midpotent, and low-potent [18]. Table 5 shows the ranking of some common brand-name corticosteroids.

When possible, the duration of treatment with superpotent topical steroids should not exceed 3 weeks. It is better to start with a high-potency product to gain control of a dermatitis and then downgrade to a lower-potency medication. Low-potency steroids should be recommended for facial, axillary, and groin dermatitis. When writing a prescription for a mid-, high- or superpotent steroid, it is recommended that the prescribing physician add, "Do not apply to face, axilla, or groin" to the prescription instructions. It is common for a patient or family member to use an old prescription for a new skin problem or to forget verbal instructions. Often it is necessary to prescribe more than one topical steroid when a dermatitis is widespread. For example, patients with generalized atopic dermatitis may need a midpotency steroid for the trunk and extremities, a low-potency one for the face, and a solution for the scalp.

The topical steroid vehicle is important when recommending a topical steroid for a patient. Ointments are most effective for chronic, dry, scaly, fissured, and lichenified dermatitis. They also increase skin hydration and steroid penetration. Creams are recommended for acute, subacute, and intertriginous dermatitis. Creams are better tolerated when treating patients in very hot, humid environments. They are more aesthetically acceptable for many patients who do not like the greasy feel of ointments, and patient compliance is usually better. Creams are more drying, contain higher concentrations of propylene glycol, and require preservative systems that may be sensitizing. Some patients with low irritancy thresholds will complain of immediate stinging with cream formulations. Gels, lotions, and sprays are the best vehicles for scalp dermatitis.

Often, the amount of the topical steroid medication is under- or overprescribed. It takes roughly 30 g of medication to treat the entire cutaneous surface. It takes 2 g of medication to treat the hands, face, or groin, 3 g for one arm, and the anterior or posterior trunk, and 4 g to treat one leg. An excellent guideline for dispensing a topical medication is the fingertip unit (FTU) [19]. This is the amount of topical medication that extends from the tip of the index finger to the first joint on the palmar aspect of the index finger. One FTU equals 0.5 g of medication and will treat two palm sizes in the average adult. One palm size is equal to approximately 1% of the skin surface. One FTU will treat the groin or hand, 2 FTUs will treat the face or foot, 3 FTUs will treat the arm, 6 FTUs will treat the leg, and 14 FTUs will treat the trunk.

Topical steroid medications have been used extensively in the United States since the 1950s with remarkably few adverse side effects [20]. However, with the advent of ever-more-potent formulations, the potential for both local and systemic side effects has increased. With a basic understanding of topical therapy and an early recognition of both common and rare adverse effects, many of these problems can be avoided or minimized.

**Table 5**  Ranking of Some Brand-Name Topical Steroids

| |
|---|
| Group I: Superpotent (anti-inflammatory activity > 1500) |
|     Temovate 0.05% |
|     Diprolene 0.05% |
|     Ultravate 0.05% |
|     Psorocon 0.05% |
| Group II: High Potency (anti-inflammatory activity = 100–500) |
|     Lidex 0.05% |
|     Halog 0.05% |
|     Cyclocort 0.05% |
|     Topicort 0.25% |
|     Diprosone 0.05% |
|     Elocon 0.1% |
|     Florone 0.05% |
|     Maxiflor 0.05% |
|     Lotrisone 0.05% |
| Group III: Midpotency (anti-inflammatory activity = 10–100) |
|     Synalar 0.025% |
|     Kenalog 0.1% |
|     Aristocort 0.1% |
|     Cordran 0.05% |
|     Locoid 0.1% |
|     Cutivate 0.05% |
|     Westcort 0.2% |
|     Cloderm 0.1% |
|     Valisone 0.1% |
|     Benisone 0.028% |
| Group IV: Low Potency (anti-inflammatory activity = 1–10) |
|     Hydrocortisone (1% is OTC; >1% is prescription) |
|     Tridesilon 0.05% |
|     DesOwen 0.05% |
|     Aclovate 0.05% |
|     Decadron 0.1% |
|     Medrol 1% |
|     Metiderm 0.5% |

The individual compound can be moved up or down in the potency ranking by changing the base or the concentration of the topical medication.

Superpotent topical steroids are over 1000 times more biologically active than hydrocortisone. These high-potency compounds, when applied topically, can suppress the hypothalamic-pituitary-adrenal (HPA) axis. Infants and children are more at risk for systemic side effects because they have decreased epidermal barrier function, greater surface-to-body ratio than adults, and may not be able to metabolize the steroid molecule efficiently. Systemic side effects include failure to thrive, growth retardation, cataracts, glaucoma, and Cushing's syndrome. Superpotent topical steroids are not recommended for children under the age of 12. Adults can demonstrate HPA suppression, as demonstrated by decreased 8 a.m. cortisol levels, within 3–4 days of using super- and high-potency topical medications. However, it is uncommon for adults to develop clinical Cushing's syndrome.

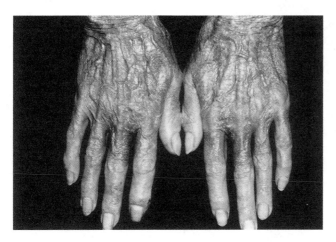

**Figure 2**   A patient with marked epidermal and dermal atrophy of the hands secondary to high-potency topical corticosteroids. (Courtesy of James E. Fitzpatrick, M.D.)

Within 7 days of using a superpotent topical steroid, there is thinning of the epidermis. After 3 weeks of use, all layers of the epidermis are reduced by about one half. Thinning of the epidermis impairs the barrier function of the skin, resulting in increased transepidermal water loss and skin irritancy. Within 2–3 weeks of superpotent topical steroid use, the dermal volume is measurably reduced. This is due to decreased production of dermal ground substance and decreased dermal water content. After many weeks of topical use there is decreased collagen and elastin synthesis resulting in skin fragility, dermal atrophy, striae, telangiectasia, purpura, and poor wound healing (Figs. 2, 3). Other cutaneous side effects include tachyphlaxis, exacerbation of cutaneous infections, acneiform skin lesions, delayed wound healing, hirsutism, topical steroid addiction syndrome, allergic contact dermatitis, and hypopigmentation.

One of the more common side effects is the production or aggravation of acne vulgaris, acne rosacea, and other acneiform eruptions. Perioral dermatitis is frequently associ-

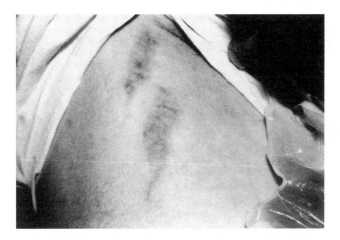

**Figure 3**   A patient with striae of the upper thigh secondary to midpotency topical steroids. (Courtesy of John L. Aeling, M.D.)

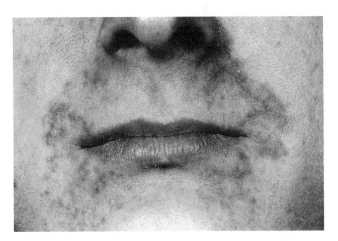

**Figure 4** A woman with perioral dermatitis secondary to inappropriate topical steroid use. (Courtesy of James E. Fitzpatrick, M.D.)

ated with the inappropriate use of topical steroids in adults, and although rare in children it is almost always associated with this complication (Fig. 4). This common skin disease is characterized by erythema, scaling and follicular papules and pustules that occur around the mouth, alar creases, and sometimes on the upper lateral eyelids. It responds well to the discontinuation of the topical steroid and administration of oral tetracycline.

Kligman and Frosch [21] coined the term "topical steroid addiction." This frustrating side effect occurs most commonly on the face of adult women or on the genital skin of adult men when topical steroids are used inappropriately. The patient complains bitterly of burning and irritation of the involved skin, and the clinical findings are subtle and do not explain the symptoms. The patient will often relate a history that the topical medication worked well at first but then stopped working. However, if the patient tries to stop, the symptoms worsen significantly. The treatment is to stop the topical steroid, recommend a bland emollient, and tell the patient that he or she is going to be miserable for several weeks. Many of these patients have low irritancy thresholds, and the topical steroid thins the stratum corneum and epidermis and makes them even more sensitive to low-grade irritants such as soaps, detergents, sunscreens, cosmetics, topical antifungals, etc.

Topical steroids are a remarkably safe and effective therapy for inflammatory skin disease. There are many decisions to be made when prescribing a topical steroid, and there are many opportunities for mistakes (Table 6).

**Table 6** Common Topical Steroid Mistakes

Incorrect diagnosis
Prescribing too much or too little medication
Failure to recognize topical steroid side effects
Recommending a product that is too potent or too weak
Prescribing the steroid in the wrong vehicle
Using the medication for too long or too short a period of time
Skin disease being treated is not topical steroid responsive
Failure to downgrade from a superpotent or high-potency medication
Prolonged air-tight occlusion

Allergic contact dermatitis to a topical steroid is rare and can be due to the vehicle, fragrance, preservative, or the steroid molecule. An allergic contact dermatitis should be suspected when a patient with a steroid-responsive dermatosis worsens or does not respond to appropriate therapy. Cross-reactions can occur within the four major classes of topical corticosteroids.

## VI.   MISCELLANEOUS TOPICAL THERAPY

Tars and tar extracts have been used for many years for their anti-inflammatory effects. Liquor carbonis detergens (LCD), an extract of crude coal tar, can be used in aquaphor or petrolatum at bedtime as adjunctive therapy and is only minimally irritating and cosmetically acceptable to most patients. Many commercial tar preparations are available over the counter, including tar gel preparations (estar gel and psorigel). Tar-based shampoos are helpful for pruritic and scaly scalps. It should be remembered that tars are photosensitizing, produce irritant folliculitis, and can cause contact dermatitis.

Doxepin hydrochloride (Zonalon) is available as a topical antipruritic. The drug has potent H1 and H2 receptor blocking and anticholinergic activity. The topical application can produce drowsiness in some patients, and it is relatively expensive.

Salicylic acid in a concentration of 5% is keratolytic. It is helpful in treating thick, hyperkeratotic, fissured, and lichenified skin lesions. It can be compounded in petrolatum and used at bedtime to treat the hands and/or feet under cotton gloves or stockings.

Acute atopic dermatitis is often excoriated, crusted, weeping, and frequently secondarily infected. Patients with atopic dermatitis are commonly colonized by *Staphylococcus aureus*, and this is the most common etiological agent responsible for secondary infections. When secondary infection is widespread, appropriate systemic antibiotics are indicated. However, mupirocin (Bactroban) can be used for localized cutaneous infections and intranasally to eliminate carrier states [22].

Moist tap water compress therapy is helpful to remove crusts and dry weeping lesions and when used over a topical steroid dramatically increases the percutaneous penetration of the medication. Wet wraps can be used after a tepid bath and the application of a topical steroid. It is not recommended to moist-occlude over superpotent topical medications. For limited areas a wet layer of kerlix gauze covered with two layers of dry kerlix makes an effective dressing. For treating the head and neck area, holes can be cut in the kerlix for the eyes and mouth and the dressing can be held in place with mesh netting. For generalized dermatitis a wet pair of cotton long underwear can be used over wet skin and covered by a dry pair of underwear. The process can be repeated two or three times a day. At night the bed can be covered with plastic and the patient can sleep in the wet wraps. Continual wet wrap therapy should not be continued for more than 3 or 4 days, and the patient should be monitored for chilling. This is very effective treatment for a severe, difficult-to-control dermatitis.

There is a subset of atopic dermatitis patients, usually men, who have had lifelong dermatitis and who develop severe scalp, head, and neck dermatitis later in life and are unresponsive to standard treatment. Some of these patients will respond to systemic antifungal medications such as itraconazole (Sporanox) or ketoconazole (Nizoral). These patients will usually culture a *Candida* species [23]. Maintenance therapy can be provided by topical therapy with topical ketoconazole (Nizoral) shampoo and an appropriate topical antifungal cream.

## VII. CONCLUSION

Slightly over 1% of all outpatient visits in the United States are for dermatitis, and two thirds of these visits are to nondermatologists. All physicians should have a basic understanding of the differential diagnosis and a treatment plan when a patient presents with a chief complaint of dermatitis.

Hydration, lubrication, and irritant avoidance are of utmost importance when treating patients with irritant, atopic, and nummular dermatitis. Detailed written patient instructions are extremely helpful in the management of these patients. Tepid water soaks or tub baths are the most efficient ways to hydrate the skin.

Topical corticosteroids remain the mainstay of treatment for patients with dermatitis. The treating physician should have a thorough understanding of how to use these medications, their cost, and frequently encountered side effects. It is advisable to become familiar with two or three preparations in each group of potency. Hopefully, there will be new, more effective, and exciting topical therapies available in the near future to treat these common and often frustrating skin diseases.

## REFERENCES

1.  Sober AJ, Fitzpatrick TB. Year Book of Dermatology. Philadelphia: Mosby, 1994:35.
2.  Menne T, Borgen O, Green A. Nickle allergy and hand dermatitis in a stratified sample of the Danish female population: an epidemiological study including a statistic appendix. Acta Derm Venereol (Stockh) 1979; 59(suppl 85):47–50.
3.  Seidenari S, Giusti G. Objective assessment of the skin of children affected by atopic dermatitis: a study of pH, capacitance and TEWL in eczematous and clinically uninvolved skin. Acta Derm Venereol 1995; 75:429–433.
4.  Epstein E. Hand dermatitis: practical management and current concepts. J Am Acad Dermatol 1984; 10:395–424.
5.  Conry T. Consumers Guide to Cosmetics. Garden City, NY: Anchor Books, 1980:228–234.
6.  Forsch PJ, Kligman AM. The soap chamber test, a new method for assessing the irritancy of soaps. J Am Acad Dermatol 1979; 1:35–41.
7.  Grammer-West NY, Fitzpatrick JE, Jackson RL, Horton H, Damiano A. Comparison of the irritancy of hand dishwashing liquids with modified patch testing methods. J Am Acad Dermatol 1996; 35:258–260.
8.  Cohen S. Survey indicates consumer perceptions of dry skin and skin care products. Cosmetic Dermatol 1993; April(suppl):4–5.
9.  Rawlings AV. Lipid modulation: promising in combating dry skin. Cosmetic Dermatol 1993; April(suppl):8–10.
10. Hoffer JC. Alpha-keto and alpha-hydroxy branched-chain acid interrelationships in normal humans. J Nutr 1993; 123:1513–1521.
11. Van Scott EJ, Yu RJ. Hyperkeratinization, corneocyte cohesion, and alpha hydroxy acids. J Am Acad Dermatol 1984; 11(5, part I):867–879.
12. Jackson EM. AHA-type products proliferate in 1993. Cosmetic Dermatol 1994; 6(12):29–30.
13. Yu RJ, Van Scott EJ. Alpha-hydroxy acids: Science and therapeutic use. Cosmetic Dermatol 1994; October (suppl):4–11.
14. Lavker RM, Kaidbey K, Leyden JJ. Effects of topical ammonium lactate on cutaneous atrophy from a potent topical corticosteroid. J Am Acad Dermatol 1992; 26:535–544.
15. DiNardo, MS, Grove GL, Moy SM. 12% ammonium lactate versus 8% glycolic acid. J Geriatr Dermatol 1995; 3:144–147.

16. Yohn JJ, Weston WL. Topical glucocorticosteroids. Curr Probl. Dermatol 1990; 2:31–63.
17. Stoughton RB. The vasoconstrictor assay in bioequivalence testing: practical concerns and recent developments. Int J Dermatol 1992; 31:26–28.
18. Aeling JL. Dermatology Secrets. Philadelphia: Hanley & Belfus, Inc./Mosby, 1996:320–326.
19. Finlay AY, Averill RW. The rule of hand: 4 hand areas = 2 FTU = 1 gm. Arch Dermatol 1992; 128:1129–1130.
20. Drake LA, Dinehart S, Farmer ER, Goltz RW, Graham GF, Hordinsky MK, Lewis ICW, Pariser DM, Webster SB, Whitaker DC, Butler B, Lowery BJ. Guidelines of care for the use of topical glucocorticosteroids. J Am Acad Dermatol 1996; 35:615–619.
21. Kligman AM, Frosch PJ. Steroid addiction. Int J Dermatol 1979; 18:23–31.
22. Luber H, Amornsiripanitch S, Lucky AW. Mupirocin and the eradication of *Staphylococcus aureus* in atopic dermatitis. Arch Dermatol 1988; 124:853–854.
23. Kolmer HL, Taketomi EA, Hazen KC. Effect of combined antibacterial and antifungal treatment in severe atopic dermatitis. J Allergy Clin Immunol 1996; 98:702–707.

# 28
## Pharmacotherapy

**Matthew Stiller and David R. Bickers**
*Columbia-Presbyterian Medical Center, New York, New York*

## I. INTRODUCTION

The range of pharmacological agents used to treat allergic skin diseases is extremely broad. Here we provide a sectional overview of such agents. We do not include topical therapy [1–5] and the systemic antihistamines [6–10], which are extensively discussed elsewhere in this text (see Chapters 26 and 27) and in the dermatological and clinical immunological literature. Phototherapy and photochemotherapy [11–14] are modalities employed for allergic skin diseases. Glucocorticosteroids, which have been the centerpiece of therapy for allergic skin diseases for almost a half-century, will be discussed [15–17] as well as the classic cytotoxic immunosuppressive agents azathioprine, cyclophosphamide [18–25], and methotrexate [18,25–28] and the newer immunosuppressive agents cyclosporin [29–36] and tacrolimus (FK506) [1,37]. The antimalarials [19,23,38,39] dapsone [40] and colchicine [41] are also included. The hemorrheologic agent pentoxifylline will be considered because of its use in vasculitis and vasculopathies [19,40–42] and possibly in allergic contact dermatitis [43,44]. Essential fatty acids [1,11] and Chinese herbal therapy [1,11,46] are mentioned briefly because of their currently unsubstantiated role in the management of atopic dermatitis [45]. Thalidomide [47] will be considered because of renewed interest in this controversial drug for use in erythema multiforme and a host of nonallergic dermatoses, most notably erythema nodosum leprosum. Systemic antibiotics and antiviral and antifungal drugs play important roles in the pharmacotherapy of atopic dermatitis because of the superinfection of skin that can occur in severe cases [45,48,49].

The chapter is organized according to categories of therapeutic agents. Atopic dermatitis, allergic contact dermatitis, urticaria, and drug reactions [51] are disorders with an allergic pathogenesis. When considering vasculitis, the distinction is less clear-cut. Urticarial vasculitis, leukocytoclastic vasculitis secondary to drug administration and Henoch-Schoenlein purpura are allergic diseases with skin manifestations. However, classification of leukocytoclastic vasculitis secondary to connective tissue disease [52], polyarteritis nodosa with cutaneous involvement, and Wegener's granulomatosis is murky. Are these allergic skin diseases or immunological skin diseases? In a recent Dohi lecture, Voorhees referred to psoriasis as an ''immunologic disease,'' which, although perhaps true, clearly is beyond the scope of this chapter. No sharp line of demarcation defines allergic and nonallergic immunological skin diseases [53].

## II.  SYSTEMIC CORTICOSTEROIDS

Despite recent advances in pharmacotherapy and in phototherapy, the most widely used class of drugs in dermatology continues to be the corticosteroids. The systemic glucocorticoids were first introduced one-half century ago at the Mayo Clinic by Dr. Miles Hench [54], who subsequently received the Nobel prize. Sulzberger et al. first used systemic cortisone (compound E) in dermatology in the early 1950s [17]. The glucocorticoids are all derivatives of a class of hormones secreted by the zona fasciculata of the adrenal cortex, the basic chemical skeleton of which is the cyclopentanophenanthrene ring. These compounds are important for homeostasis and salt retention. The anti-inflammatory effect of the glucocorticoids can be increased several hundred–fold by modifying the chemical structure, (e.g., adding a fluorine molecule at the 9-α position of cortisol, addition of a 16-α hydroxyl group and a double bond at the 1,2 position, and conversion of the 16- and 17-α hydroxyls into an acetonide moiety) [39].

Systemic glucocorticosteroids exert a wide range of anti-inflammatory and immuno-suppressive effects, including inhibition of release of lysosomal enzymes, reduction in circulating lymphocytes, decreased T-cell responsiveness to selected antigens and mitogens, decreased antibody production by B cells, and decreased response of macrophages to lymphokines and chemotactic factors [1,2,39]. Glucocorticoids modify the distribution of circulating leukocytes, increasing the number of polymorphonuclear leukocytes and concomitantly decreasing the number of lymphocytes, monocytes, and eosinophils. There is a greater reduction of circulating T than of B lymphocytes [38,39].

When used in atopic dermatitis, cutaneous vasculitis, allergic contact dermatitis, and severe urticaria, high doses of prednisone or prednisolone (1 mg/kg) per day should be administered. Initial use of high corticosteroid doses with rapid tapering maximizes the anti-inflammatory/immunosuppressive effects and allows more rapid tapering or conversion to an alternate day regimen when necessary [39,45].

When glucocorticoids are administered to treat acute disease, a single daily dose given in the morning is preferable, as this regimen is thought to minimize hypothalamic-pituitary-adrenal (H-P-A) suppression by mimicking the normal circadian rhythm of adrenal cortisol production. Divided daily dosing of oral corticosteroids increases anti-inflammatory efficacy at the expense of systemic toxicity. When short courses of glucocorticoids are given to treat atopic dermatitis and contact dermatitis, one must be careful not to taper too rapidly so as to minimize the risk of steroid rebound, i.e., post-therapeutic exacerbation of disease to a more severe level, often worse than at the onset of therapy.

The side effects of topical glucocorticoid therapy are well known and include, most prominently, cutaneous atrophy and stria formation, possibly related to the antianabolic properties of glucocorticoids through suppression of proline hydroxylation and cross-linking of collagen [25,39]. Other well-known side effects of topical glucocorticoids include purpura resulting from increased vascular fragility, formation of stellate pseudoscars, steroid acne, rosacea, perioral dermatitis, facial hypertrichosis, and initial masking and then worsening of cutaneous infections including pyodermas, dermatophytoses, viral infections, and scabies [23–25,38,39]. The list of side effects from systemic glucocorticoids is imposing and includes all of the aforementioned adverse events due to topical therapy and multiple more significant sequelae including generalized osteoporosis and aseptic necrosis of the femoral head. There is an increased risk of systemic and cutaneous bacterial, viral, fungal, and parasitic infections. Hypertriglyceridemia, altered lipid metabolism, hyperglycemia, pancreatitis, potassium wasting, myopathy, posterior subcapsular cataracts,

Cushingoid appearance, psychosis, pseudotumor cerebri and growth retardation in children are all possible sequelae of prolonged systemic glucocorticoid administration [23,25,39].

The most useful method of assessing the impact of glucocorticoid therapy on adrenal function is the cosyntropin stimulation test. $\alpha$-1-24-Corticotropin is a synthetic polypeptide identical to the first 24 of the 39 amino acids in naturally occurring corticotropin. In this test of H-P-A axis suppression, 0.25 mg of cosyntropin is parenterally administered. Subsequent determination of plasma cortisol or urinary 17-hydroxycorticosteroids facilitates assessment of adrenal function. Another accurate test of adrenal function is the metapyrone test. Metapyrone, a potent inhibitor of 11-$\beta$-hydroxylation, the terminal step in cortisol synthesis, is administered orally every 4 hours for six doses, each equivalent to 10 mg/kg/day. Subsequent measurement of urinary 17-hydroxycorticosteroids provides an accurate assessment of H-P-A suppression.


## III. CYTOTOXIC/IMMUNOSUPPRESSIVE DRUGS

The plethora of side effects and complications of systemic glucocorticoid use described above have led to a search for less toxic alternatives (steroid-sparing agents). Among these are cytotoxic and immunosuppressive drugs, each with its own distinctive risk/benefit profile. These steroid-sparing agents are frequently useful in the management of chronic cases of vasculitis and atopic dermatitis. They are not helpful in acute allergic contact dermatitis (ACD) and virtually never necessary in urticaria and drug reactions.


### A. Azathioprine

Azathioprine, a purine analog (Fig. 1), is well absorbed after oral intake [23,55]. It is metabolized to 6-mercaptopurine, which is not cytotoxic, and 6-thioinosinic acid and 6-thioguanylic acid, both of which are cytotoxic. After the prodrug azathioprine is metabolized to 6-mercaptopurine, it is activated by the enzyme hypoxanthine-guanine phosphoribosyl transferase. Monophosphate analogs block purine synthesis, and triphosphorylated 6-mercaptopurine is incorporated into DNA causing strand breaks and point mutations [18,56–58]. Conversion to inactive metabolites occurs within approximately 10 hours by erythrocytes and in the liver. Azathioprine is metabolized in part by xanthine oxidase, so simultaneous administration of allopurinol increases xanthine levels [23].

Myelosuppression is the major adverse event caused by azathioprine of concern to clinicians [23,55–58]. Leukocyte counts are primarily decreased, but pancytopenia, thrombocytopenia, and anemia may also occur. Gastrointestinal side effects including nau-

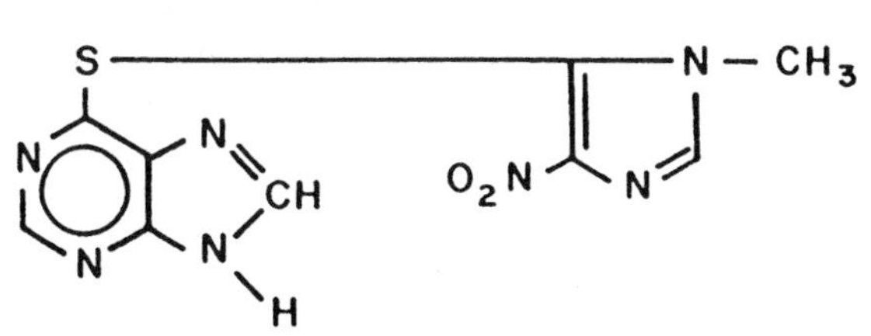

**Figure 1**   Structure of azathioprine.

**Table 1**  Azathioprine Toxicity

Myelosuppression (leukopenia, thrombocytopenia, aplastic anemia, macrocytic anemia)
Predisposition to infection
Predisposition to neoplasia (hematologic malignancy, lymphoma)
Drug fever (headache, chills, malaise, myalgia)
Nausea
Vomiting
Diarrhea (steatorrhea)
Toxic hepatitis
Hepatic veno-occlusive disease
Pancreatitis
Shock
Drug interaction (allopurinol, angiotensin-converting enzyme inhibitors, warfarin,
  cotrimoxazole)
Hypersensitivity pneumonitis
Alopecia

sea, vomiting, diarrhea, and mucosal ulcers may occur (Table 1) [57,58,59]. These can be decreased by administering the drug in two divided doses daily. We favor starting at doses of 1–2 mg/kg/day in patients with recalcitrant atopic dermatitis unresponsive to corticosteroids. The same starting dose can be used in vasculitis. We favor its use in vasculitis only after other drugs such as colchicine, dapsone, indomethacin, antihistamines, antimalarials, and short-course, rapidly tapered prednisone or prednisolone have failed. However, in patients with systemic vasculitis, addition of azathioprine to prednisone can increase therapeutic efficacy and patient survival [60,61]. Azathioprine does not cause gonadal dysfunction, and it is thought to be preferable to other cytotoxic drugs in individuals wishing to conceive after completion of therapy [18]. As previously indicated, azathioprine is a second- or third-line drug in most allergic cutaneous diseases. While its efficacy in allergic contact dermatitis has been demonstrated, this use is still highly experimental. In addition to myelosuppression and gastrointestinal side effects, drug fever, azathioprine-induced shock [59], hepatitis, hepatic veno-occlusive disease, periportal fibrosis, and pancreatitis have been reported [18,56,57]. The hepatitis that occurs in 1% of patients is reversible. The development of cancer is a concern in patients receiving chronic immunosuppressive agents, but in patients with rheumatoid arthritis chronically treated with azathioprine no increase in internal neoplasms has been observed [18,56]. Data indicating an increased risk of skin cancer are controversial [18,56,57]. Clinical data supporting an association is buttressed by laboratory investigations showing an increase in sister chromatid exchange in cells harvested from phytohemagglutinin-stimulated whole blood from azathioprine-treated patients [18]. This effect was augmented when these cells were exposed to ultraviolet radiation over a broad range of wavelengths: visible light, UVC, and UVA (most pronounced effect). Broad-spectrum sunscreens and sunprotective clothing are essential in subjects receiving steroid-sparing cytotoxic agents such as azathioprine [18,57].

## B.  Cyclophosphamide

Cyclophosphamide (Fig. 2) is a highly reactive alkylating agent and a derivative of nitrogen mustard. It is cell cycle nonspecific in its action so that it can act during any stage

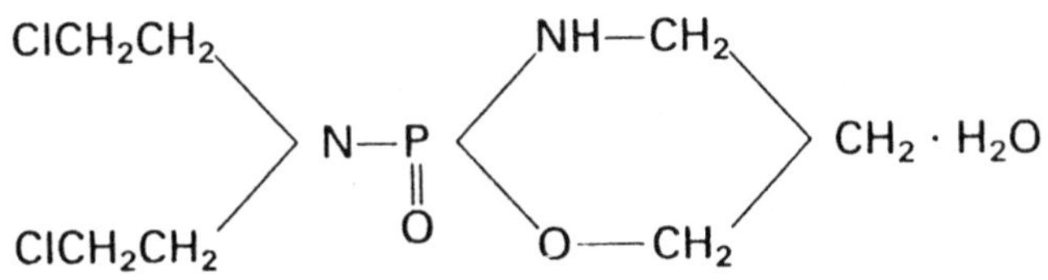

$$ClCH_2CH_2 \diagdown \diagup NH-CH_2 \diagdown$$

CICH₂CH₂     NH—CH₂

N—P     CH₂ · H₂O

CICH₂CH₂     O     O—CH₂

**Figure 2** Structure of cyclophosphamide.

of the cell cycle. The drug binds to DNA covalently as opposed to methotrexate, which is S phase specific. Cyclophosphamide is useful as a steroid-sparing agent and is the drug of choice for Wegener's granulomatosis and lymphomatoid granulomatosis [18]. It can be used in combination with systemic glucocorticoids as a third-line treatment in urticarial vasculitis or Henoch-Schoenlein purpura if antihistamines, indomethacin, colchicine, dapsone, and the antimalarials prove ineffective [19,20]. In contrast to azathioprine, cyclophosphamide has not been used extensively in the management of atopic dermatitis, urticaria, or allergic contact dermatitis.

The side effects of cyclophosphamide are numerous (Table 2) [62–64]. Myelosuppression, chiefly leukopenia and thrombocytopenia, may occur in chronically treated patients. Hematological malignancies have also been reported in chronically treated patients

**Table 2** Cyclophosphamide Toxicity

Urological toxicity
    Hemorrhagic cystitis
    Transitional cell carcinoma of the bladder
    Bladder fibrosis
    Infertility (azospermia, amenorrhea)
Hematologic toxicity
    Leukopenia
    Thrombocytopenia
    Hematological neoplasia (lymphoma)
Dermatologic toxicity
    Alopecia
    Mucocutaneous ulceration
    Skin and nail hyperpigmentation
    Cutaneous squamous cell carcinoma
Cardiac toxicity
    Arrhythmia
    Heart failure
    Cardiomyopathy
    Pericarditis
Gastrointestinal toxicity
    Nausea
    Vomiting
    Abdominal pain
    Anorexia
    Hepatotoxicity
Susceptibility to infection
Pulmonary fibrosis

[64]. Gastrointestinal side effects such as nausea and vomiting are common, as are alopecia and mucocutaneous ulcerations. Hemorrhagic cystitis is a major side effect that occurs in 5–10% of patients, while a similar percentage treated chronically may develop transitional cell carcinoma of the bladder. Bladder carcinoma may occur years after cessation of treatment and appears to be indirectly linked to cystitis [18,63]. The hemorrhagic cystitis may be caused by acrolein, a cyclophosphamide metabolite, and it is minimized by use of the scavenging agent sodium 2-mercaptoethanesulfonate (Mesna) [18]. Severe cardiotoxicity (arrhythmias, cardiomyopathy, pericarditis, acute heart failure) and an increase in skin cancer may also occur.

## C. Methotrexate

Methotrexate (amethopterin) was introduced in 1948 as a cancer chemotherapeutic agent (Fig. 3). It remains one of the most commonly used antimetabolic drugs in cancer therapy and one of the most frequently employed systemic agents in severe, disabling, or recalcitrant psoriasis. Methotrexate is rapidly absorbed from the gastrointestinal tract and also can be administered intravenously or intramuscularly. It is a competitive inhibitor of the enzyme dihydrofolate reductase that catalyzes the formation of tetrahydrofolic acid, which is an essential cofactor in the synthesis of thymidylate and purine nucleotides.

Methotrexate has a decidedly limited role in the management of allergic diseases of the skin. Friedmann et al. [2] list it as a ''second-line treatment'' for atopic dermatitis, although experience with it is limited for this disease. It does have a role in the management of the more severe forms of cutaneous systemic vasculitis, most notably Wegener's granulomatosis [18,26], rheumatoid vasculitis with ulceration and/or systemic involvement [27,28,50], temporal arteritis, and Takayasu's disease.

One approach to reducing the toxicity of methotrexate is to administer the drug either as a single weekly dose or in three divided doses 12 hours apart once weekly. Since the drug is cell cycle–specific and inhibits DNA synthesis in the S phase, the rationale for this strategy relates to timing the cell cycle such that the majority of proliferating epidermal cells are exposed to the drug. The chief side effects of methotrexate are myelosuppression and hepatotoxicity with fibrosis and, less often, cirrhosis (Table 3). Hepatic and hematological functions must be carefully monitored, and periodic percutaneous hepatic needle biopsies are recommended to monitor hepatic status. Weekly doses of 15–35 mg may be required for severe forms of vasculitis. Leucovorin ($N^5$-formyl-tetrahydrofolate) is the antidote for methotrexate toxicity and should be administered parenterally in the event of acute overdosage.

## D. Cyclosporine

Cyclosporine is an 11-amino-acid cyclic peptide with a molecular weight of 1202 daltons [29] (Fig. 4), originally discovered in 1970 at the Sandoz Research laboratories in Basel,

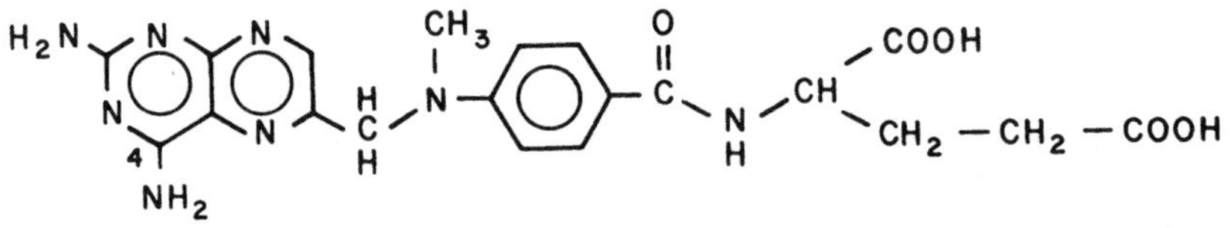

**Figure 3** Structure of methotrexate (amethopterin).

**Table 3** Methotrexate Toxicity

Hepatic
  Transaminemia
  Hepatitis
  Fibrosis
  Cirrhosis
Gastrointestinal
  Nausea
  Vomiting
  Diarrhea
  Stomatitis
  Hemorrhagic enteritis
  Intestinal perforation
Hematopoietic
  Leukopenia
  Anemia
  Thrombocytopenia
  Pancytopenia
Pulmonary
  Hypersensitivity pneumonitis
  Fibrosis
Other systemic effects
  Anaphylaxis
  Opportunistic infections
  Osteoporosis
  Renal tubular necrosis
  Drug interactions (ethanol, probenecid,
      cisplatin, NSAIDs, barbiturates, dilantin)

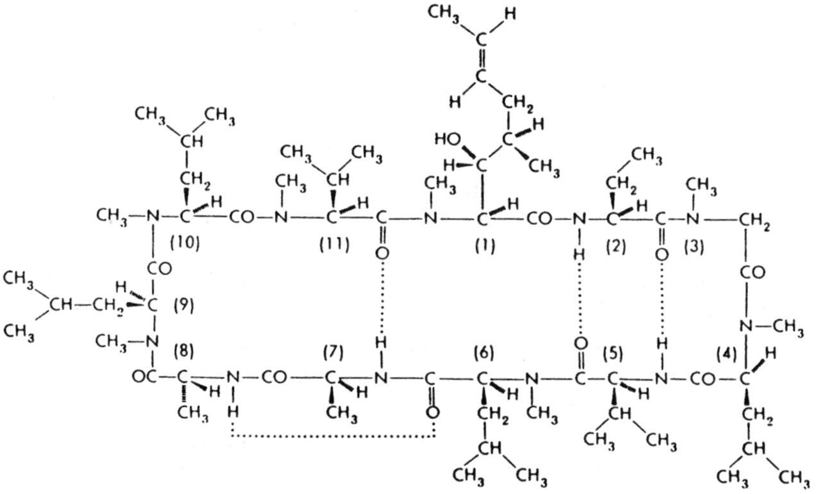

**Figure 4** Structure of cyclosporine.

Switzerland, by scientists searching for novel antifungal agents [65]. The efficacy of this nonmyelosuppressive immunosuppressive agent in the management of severe atopic dermatitis at dosees of 2–6 mg/kg/day was first noted a decade ago [66–68]. Cyclosporine may act by downregulating Th2 cells, which decreases IL-4 and IL-5, thereby lowering peripheral blood eosinophilia.

Eosinophils from patients with atopic dermatitis are thought to be "preactivated" in the circulation as a result of exposure to the T-cell–mediated cytokines IL-3, IL-5, and granulocyte macrophage-colony stimulating factor [1,2,11,67–69]. IL-5 is a particularly potent eosinophil chemotactic factor [1,2,69]. Cutaneous and peripheral blood eosinophilia and the eosinophil cationic protein (ECP) and eosinophil major basic protein (EMB) are increased in atopic skin [7,8]. Shupack et al. demonstrated decreased peripheral blood eosinophil counts in severe psoriatic patients treated with low-dose cyclosprine [69]. Extrapolating this data to atopic patients, one can postulate that cyclosporine may downregulate cytokines responsible for blood and tissue eosinophilia, although this has not been proven.

The usual starting dose of cyclosporine is 2.5–5 mg/kg/day. Such doses can induce remissions in patients with severe recalcitrant atopic dermatitis [11,29,32–34]. Once remission occurs it can be maintained by either decreasing the daily dose of cyclosporine at 2-week intervals or decreasing the number of days per week patients receive cyclosporine to alternate days, biweekly, or even once weekly. Both approaches to dosage reduction frequently can be employed without sacrificing efficacy [11,33].

In some patients gastrointestinal absorption of the drug is unpredictable. This leads to highly variable peak-trough serum levels, which can result in either inadequate therapeutic response or systemic toxicity. Recently a new microemulsion dosage form of cyclosporine known as Neoral® has become available [11,30,31,35,36]. This formulation offers superior bioavailability and reduced variability of absorption and has been tested in patients with severe recalcitrant psoriasis in a double-blind multicenter clinical trial comparing it to the standard formulation of cyclosporine [30,31]. Efficacy and safety of the two are basically similar. In general starting doses of Neoral® should be 20–25% lower than with the standard formulation of cyclosporine. In clinical practice, intra- and interpatient variability in absorption of Neoral® can also be troublesome [30,31]. Rebound flares that occur following abrupt discontinuation of corticosteroids do not occur with cyclosporine. Tachyphylaxis can occur.

While cyclosporine is effective in severe recalcitrant urticaria, it is seldom used for that indication. Cyclosporine does not appear to have a favorable therapeutic index in the management of vasculitis [21]. Topical formulations of the drug are ineffective [23,29].

Cyclosporine is metabolized primarily in the liver via the microsomal cytochrome P450 3A3 and 3A4 isoenzymes [70]. Metabolites of cyclosporine undergo significant enterohepatic circulation and are excreted in the bile. Only 6% of the drug is excreted in the urine. Dosage modification is required for patients with liver disease but not those with renal dysfunction [29,71]. Cyclosporine blood levels may be measured by either whole blood radioimmunoassay or high-performance liquid chromatography [72].

The potential side effects of cyclosporine are substantial. The major limiting side effect is nephrotoxicity. If a patient's glomerular filtration decreases by 25–30%, the drug should be discontinued at least temporarily. Monitoring serum creatinine level seems to be a practical method of evaluating renal function. Creatinine clearance measurements are less desirable due to the inherent difficulty in consistent collection of 24-hour urine specimens. Glomerular filtration rates measured as inulin clearance or radiolabeled diethylene-triamine-penta-acetic acid are time consuming and add only marginally to serum creatinine values. Some believe that peak-trough measurements of cyclosporine should be performed routinely, although they provide limited useful clinical data when Sandimmune® (traditional oral formulation) is prescribed at levels below 5 mg/kg/day or Neoral® below 4 mg/kg/day [73]. While cyclosporine nephrotoxicity is generally reversible if detected early, renal biopsies frequently show changes of interstitial fibrosis and less frequently irreversible glomerulosclerosis [74].

Cardiovascular side effects are of concern in patients receiving cyclosporine for atopic dermatitis. Cyclosporine may worsen hypertension in those with preexisting blood pressure elevation, requiring alterations in antihypertensive regimens. It may also induce hypertension in individuals with no history of the condition. Diet and exercise are often helpful, but antihypertensive drug therapy may be indicated. Angiotensin-converting enzyme inhibitors or calcium-channel blockers are useful [15,29]. Cyclosporine may also cause elevation of serum lipids—triglycerides more so than cholesterol [75]. The potential cardiovascular toxicity of cyclosporine should not be ignored, since some patients have suffered myocardial infarction while ingesting the drug. Table 4 lists adverse effects associated with cyclosporine use. Among the most striking morphologically are hypertrichosis

**Table 4**   Adverse Effects of Cyclosporine

Renal/Electrolyte
   Increase in blood urea nitrogen
   Increase in blood creatinine
   Decrease in glomerular filtration
   Decrease in serum magnesium
Hematological
   Mild normocytic, normochromic anemia
Gastrointestinal
   Nausea
   Vomiting
   Diarrhea
   Bloating
Elevated transaminases
Elevated alkaline phosphatase
Pancreatitis
Cardiovascular
   Hypertension
   Hyperlipidemia
Mucocutaneous
   Hypertrichosis
   Gingival Hyperplasia
Constitutional
   Fatigue
   Weight loss early in therapy
Neurological
   Encephalitis
   Tremor
   Paresthesias

*Source*: Adapted from Ref. 29.

**Table 5**  Drug Interactions with Cyclosporine

Drugs that inhibit cyclosporine metabolism (P-450 3A 3/4 inhibitors)
    Erythromycin
    Ketoconazole
    Itraconazole
    Fluconazole
    Norfloxacin
    Corticosteroids
    Oral contraceptives
    Androgenic steroids
    Calcium-channel blockers
    Cimetidine
    Danazol
Drugs that accelerate cyclosporine metabolism (P-450 3A 3/4 inducers)
    Phenytoin
    Phenobarbital
    Carbamazepine
    Rifampin
    Trimethoprim and sulfadimine
Drugs with which cyclosporine can accelerate nephrotoxicity
    Diuretics
    Nonsteroidal anti-inflammatory drugs, aminoglycosides
    Trimethoprim-sulfamethoxazole
    Amphotericin B
    Melphalan
Miscellaneous drug interactions with cyclosporine
    Lovastatin (rhabdomyolysis)
    Digoxin (digitalis toxicity)

*Source:* Adapted from Ref. 29.

and gingival hyperplasia. Cyclosporine use requires that the clinician be aware of the considerable number of drugs that can interact with it. The group of drugs capable of causing synergistic nephrotoxicity are of particular importance (Table 5).

## E.  Tacrolimus (FK 506)

Similar to cyclosporine, the immunosuppressive macrolide FK 506 is a potent inhibitor of helper T-cell function [11]. The systemic form of the drug is effective in atopic dermatitis [76] but, unlike cyclosporine, does not cause hypertrichosis or gingival hypertrophy [37]. Its oral use is currently limited to immunosuppression in allogeneic transplant recipients. Because it is highly effective topically without known systemic side effects, there is little rationale to use the oral form of the drug for cutaneous disease [37]. Preliminary studies indicate that topical tacrolimus is highly effective in atopic dermatitis.

## Thalidomide

Thalidomide or α-phthalimodoglutarimide, a drug originally produced in West Germany in 1954 for use as an antiemetic, hypnotic, and sedative during the first trimester of pregnancy, has a very restricted niche in the treatment of allergic diseases of the skin. It has been used successfully to treat recurrent erythema multiforme and is the drug of choice in erythema nodosum leprosum [47,77,78]. Thalidomide is notorious for its capacity to produce teratogenic effects (phocomelia), but there has been a resurgence of interest in the drug because of its potential efficacy in AIDS and leprosy. The drug has immunosuppressive properties and prolongs survival of skin homografts in mice. It was also shown to have immunosuppressive properties in primates receiving organ allografts [80]. Barnhill et al. [79] demonstrated inhibition of phagocytosis in cultured polymorphonuclear leukocytes and inhibition of chemotaxis in cultured monocytes [79–81]. In addition to its teratogenicity, thalidomide may produce sensory and motor peripheral neuropathy [47,80,81]. This becomes irreversible if the drug is not discontinued. Thalidomide also produces drowsiness and dizziness in more than one third of patients [47,80]. This is a drug that must be used judiciously. Clear-cut efficacy in allergic diseases currently is limited to erythema multiforme.

## F.  Colchicine

Colchicine is an alkaloid first isolated from a crocus-like plant, *Colchicum autumnale*, in 1820 (Fig. 5). It is a three-ringed compound also known as acetyltermethylcolchicinic acid [39]. Colchicine, which acts on microtubules and arrests mitosis in metaphase, has multiple anti-inflammatory actions, including impairment of polymorphonuclear chemotaxis, blockage of leukocyte adhesiveness, and stabilization of lysosomal membranes. Colchicine also impairs the rolling of leukocytes along the walls of the microvasculature and diminishes the stimulated expression of intercellular adhesion molecule 1 (ICAM-1) on endothelial cells and L-selectin on leukocytes.

Colchicine along with dapsone is thought to be effective in leukocytoclastic vasculitis, although a prospective randomized clinical trial in 41 patients did not confirm this result [41]. The significance of this study is unclear since three patients in the colchicine-treated group relapsed after cessation of therapy. Colchicine can also be combined with other agents in treating vasculitis, including pentoxifylline, dapsone, and indomethacin, increasing the likelihood of therapeutic success.

Even low-dose colchicine inhibits endothelial adhesiveness of neutrophils [79,83,84]. These pharmacological properties support the use of colchicine as an agent directed against leukocytoclastic vasculitis, especially urticarial vasculitis [19,21,82]. Colchicine is usually given at doses of 0.6 mg bid (or tid if tolerated). The limiting factor is usually gastrointestinal irritability including diarrhea, nausea, vomiting, and abdominal

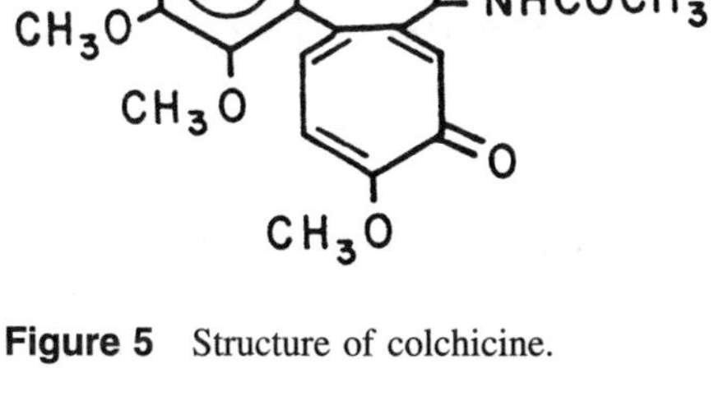

**Figure 5**   Structure of colchicine.

pain. Less common chronic side effects include agranulocytosis, aplastic anemia, myopathy, and alopecia [39,84,85].

## G. Pentoxifylline

Pentoxifylline is a trisubstituted xanthine derivative, a hemorrheologic agent that increases flexibility of erythrocytes and platelets and was originally approved for the treatment of peripheral vascular ischemia. The drug may be useful in urticarial vasculitis [40] and allergic contact dermatitis [43]. The drug is remarkably safe and free of side effects. Nürnberg et al. [40] reported a 40-year-old woman with a 16-year history of urticarial vasculitis unresponsive to $H_1$ and $H_2$ blockers, indomethacin, dapsone, interferon-$\alpha$, and dapsone monotherapy, whereas the combination of dapsone 100 mg/day and pentoxifylline 1200 mg/day was effective.

Immunologically, pentoxifylline decreases transcription of tumor necrosis factor (TNF-$\alpha$) messenger RNA [40]. TNF-$\alpha$ is an important cytokine in the elicitation phase of allergic contact dermatitis. Patch-test reactions in two nickel-sensitive patients were diminished by this drug [86]. Pentoxifylline also downregulates ICAM-1 expression in keratinocytes, providing further support for its potential effectiveness in allergic contact dermatitis and vasculitis [43,87].

## H. Dapsone

Dapsone, the prototypic sulfone, was first synthesized in 1908. Dapsone is diaminodiphenylsulfone (DDS) and has become a first-line drug in the treatment of leukocytoclastic vasculitis [21]. It can be used as monotherapy or in combination with other agents such as pentoxifylline [40], colchicine, or indomethacin. In 1937 this compound was found to be highly effective in treating streptotoccal infections in mice—100 times more effective than sulfanilamide. However, hematopoietic toxicity limited its usefulness. It was subsequently shown to be active against *Mycobacterium leprae*. DDS and the sulfonamide antibiotic sulfapyridine are also remarkably effective in dermatitis herpetiformis and acrodermatitis continua of Hallopeau [21,39]. These indications have created a permanent niche for sulfapyridine and the sulfones in dermatological therapy [39]. Dapsone is particularly useful in leukocytoclastic vasculitis, erythema elevatum diutinum, granuloma faciale, and cutaneous polyarteritis nodosa [21,22].

Both sulfapyridine and dapsone are slowly absorbed following oral administration and acetylated in the liver. With sulfapyridine, patients who are constitutive slow acetylators are at increased risk for adverse events [25,39]. In addition to their antibacterial properties, the sulfones have anti-inflammatory effects [39]. Dapsone is most effective in diseases where polymorphonuclear leukocytes play a pivotal role in pathogenesis, including those cited above. Dapsone inhibits polymorphonuclear leukocyte myeloperoxidase and diminishes generation of toxic oxygen intermediates from $H_2O_2$. Dapsone inhibits the Arthus reaction, adjuvant-induced arthritis, and mitogenic stimulation of lymphocytes [39] and also affects polymorphonuclear leukocyte chemotaxis and stability of lysosomal enzymes. The antibacterial effects of dapsone and sulfapyridine may relate to the competition with para-aminobenzoic acid in folate synthesis.

The most frequent toxic side effects associated with dapsone therapy are hematological, especially hemolysis and methemoglobinemia. Hemolysis is dose-related and much more severe in individuals deficient in glucose-6-phosphate dehydrogenase (G6PD)

[25,38,39]. Rarely leukopenia, hepatic and renal toxicity and, less frequently, agranulocytosis may occur [25,39]. Toxic hepatitis, cholestatic jaundice, renal papillary necrosis, the nephrotic syndrome, and pseudolymphoma have also been reported. Nervous system abnormalities, most notably psychosis and a primarily motor peripheral neuropathy, are serious, if infrequent, occurrences [25,39].

Methemoglobinemia occurs commonly but is seldom a problem, except in individuals with severe preexisting cardiovascular disease. In methemoglobinemia, the iron in hemoglobin is irreversibly oxidized to the ferric state, which ablates its ability to function as an oxygen carrier. In view of the potential toxicity of dapsone, periodic monitoring of laboratory data is essential. This should include blood counts, hepatic and renal function tests, urinalysis, and a baseline G6PD level. Dapsone should not be prescribed in patients with hereditary G6PD deficiency. Laboratory data should be reevaluated every two weeks for one month and every 3 months thereafter. Dapsone is available in 25 and 100 mg tablets. Treatment is initiated with 50–100 mg daily for at least 5 days, increased 50 mg every 5–7 days up to a dose of 300–400 mg daily. Failure to improve with these doses should lead to use of other agents.

## IV. ANTIMALARIALS

The major antimalarials used in dermatology are the two substituted 4-aminoquinolines chloroquine (Fig. 6) and hydroxychloroquine (Fig. 7) and the acridine compound quinacrine. Of these, only chloroquine and hydroxychloroquine are used in leukocytoclastic vasculitis, especially urticarial vasculitis [19,22,88,89,90,91,92].

The antimalarials have multiple pharmacological effects, although their relevance to clinical significance is unclear. The most pharmacologically significant effects relate to accumulation of these drugs in lysosomes, which stabilizes membranes and inhibits chemotaxis and phagocytosis by polymorphonuclear leukocytes. Chloroquine inhibits complement-mediated hemolysis in vitro, which may account in part for its efficacy in rheumatological diseases. It also inhibits eosinophil chemotaxis [39].

The most severe toxicity of the 4-aminoquinoline antimalarials is ocular, so baseline and follow-up ophthalmological examinations with slit lamp every 3–6 months are essential to detect the early, reversible changes of premaculopathy, or preetinopathy. The 4-aminoquinolines can cause visual disturbances due to drug deposition in the basal epithelium of the cornea and ciliary body. True chloroquine (or hydroxychloroquine) retinopathy is extremely uncommon when dermatological doses are prescribed. Chloroquine phosphate is available in 500 mg tablets. The recommended dose is 500–1500 mg daily. Hy-

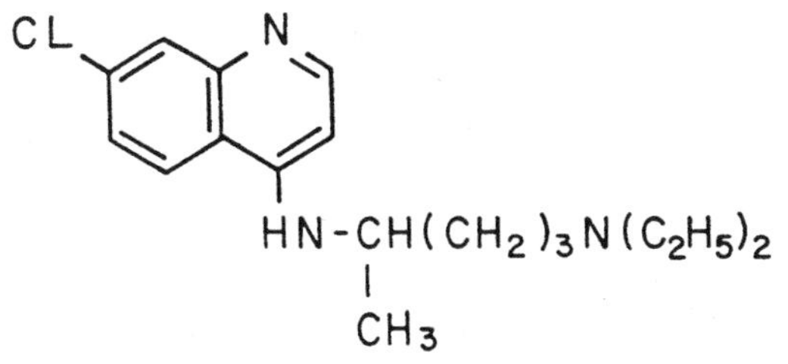

**Figure 6** Structure of chloraquine.

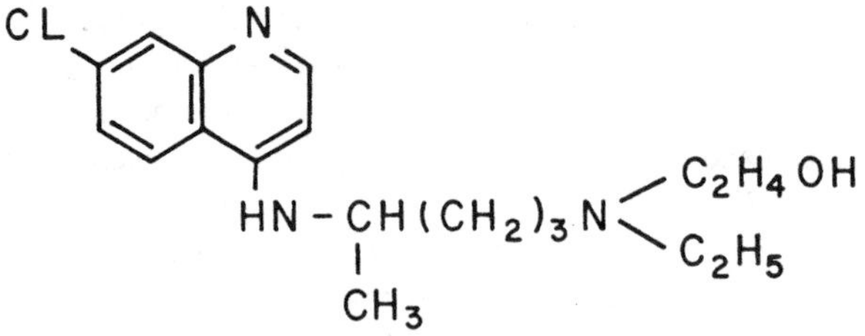

**Figure 7** Structure of hydroxychloroquine.

droxychloroquine sulfate is supplied in 200 mg tablets and the recommended dose is 200–400/day [23,38,39].

In addition to ocular toxicity, the 4-aminoquinolines have other potential side effects. Gastrointestinal toxicity including diarrhea, nausea, and vomiting occur in a small percentage of patients but may be severe enough to necessitate cessation of therapy. Hematological side effects including hemolysis, aplastic anemia, and rarely agranulocytosis can occur [23,39]. Initial and periodic blood counts are advisable, and these drugs should be administered cautiously to patients with glucose-6-phosphate dehydrogenase deficiency [38]. Potential central nervous system toxicity includes psychosis and seizures [23,25]. Antimalarials are traditionally listed among the drugs capable of exacerbating psoriasis, but the risk is probably slight.

## V. MISCELLANEOUS AGENTS

The use of nonsteroidal anti-inflammatory drugs (COX-1 inhibitors), especially indomethacin, has been advocated in the treatment of necrotizing venulitis and urticarial vasculitis [19,22,93,94]. These drugs inhibit the cyclooxygenase or lipoxygenase pathways of arachidonic acid metabolism. The list of potential side effects is lengthy and includes urticaria, anaphylactoid reactions, photosensitivity, purpura, erythema multiforme, and toxic epidermal necrolysis. Hematological adverse events include both blood dyscrasias and episodes of bleeding, usually from gastric irritation/ulceration. Central nervous system side effects include headaches, dizziness, syncope, and seizures. Renal toxicity is an important consideration when these agents are used concomitantly with cyclosporine, a not uncommon phenomenon. Indomethacin is available in 25, 50, and 75 mg capsules. Daily dosage ranges in dermatology vary between 50 and 200 mg. The latter should not be exceeded, as it does not increase drug efficacy [38].

The use of phosphodiesterase inhibitors to treat atopic dermatitis has been advocated for more than 50 years [45,91]. The rationale for their use stems from the finding of decreased cyclic AMP levels in peripheral blood monocytes of patients with atopic dermatitis. Shupack et al. [95] in a double-blind, placebo-controlled clinical trial demonstrated that oral papaverine hydrochloride was ineffective in atopic dermatitis and also potentially hepatotoxic. Short courses of the phosphodiesterase inhibitor theophylline 300 mg bid for 5 days may help selected patients with recalcitrant atopic dermatitis [45].

Essential fatty acid supplementation in the management of atopic dermatitis remains controversial [11,45]. The role of essential fatty acids in the pathogenesis of atopic dermatitis is unclear. Some polyunsaturated fats are precursors of prostaglandins and leukotrienes, which are established pro-inflammatory mediators. Furthermore, increased levels of eicosanoids have been detected in atopic skin [96,97]. However, double-blind, placebo-controlled clinical trials have failed to support the use of inhibitors of prostaglandin and leukotriene synthesis such as evening primrose oil and/or marine fish oil in atopic skin disease [11].

Atopic skin frequently becomes colonized and or infected by bacteria, especially *Staphylococcus aureus* (see Chapter 24). The use of an antibiotic, either a first-generation oral cephalosporin or a penicillinase-resistant agent such as cloxacillin, dicloxacillin, or flucloxacillin, is frequently helpful [3,45]. Atopic skin may be superinfected by dermatophytes and *Pityrosporum ovale* is a proposed triggering agent in flares of atopic skin according to Scandinavian investigators [3–5,48]. Brief courses of oral ketoconazole or fluconazole are sometimes justified in atopic subjects. Atopic skin is also susceptible to viral superinfection. In cases of superinfection with the herpes simplex virus, Kaposi's varicelliform eruption, or eczema herpeticum, a course of therapy with acyclovir, valacyclovir, or famciclovir is mandatory [3–5,48].

## VI. CONCLUSION

Topical and systemic glucocorticoids are the mainstay of pharmacotherapy for allergic skin diseases [1,8,10,15,18]. However, not all patients have significant improvement in skin disease following topical or systemic glucocorticoid therapy. Use of high-potency topical glucocorticoids or systemic glucocorticoids for prolonged periods places these patients at great risk for severe adverse effects. In this chapter, we discussed a number of potent anti-inflammatory/immunosuppressive drugs, which can be steroid sparing or effective in the treatment of allergic skin diseases. In particular, cyclosporine and its more predictably bioavailable newer oral formulation Sandimmun Neoral® are impressive agents for crisis intervention. They also have a niche in the management of severe forms of allergic skin disease [33–36,68]. As with most cytochrome P450–metabolized oral drugs, cyclosporine drug interactions, as well as nephrotoxicity, limit its use [70,71].

The topical application of potent immunosuppressive drugs that do not have significant systemic absorption represents an important approach that has allowed the use of topical steroids in the management of chronic atopic dermatitis and allergic contact dermatitis. In this regard, the recent development of topical tacrolimus (FK506) [98] ointment and SDZ ASM 981 [99] cream appear to be major breakthroughs in the management of chronic eczema. Both drugs are efficacious in the treatment of allergic skin inflammation without significant systemic absorption and do not induce skin atrophy or striae formation. Phototherapy continues to retain an important position in our therapeutic armamemtarium for atopic dermatitis and other allergic skin diseases.

Future developments of safe, effective systemic therapeutic agents will likely need to selectively and effectively intervene in immunologic cascades that lead to allergic skin diseases. Clinical applications in this direction have already been seen with the use of sIL-4 receptor [100] and humanized monoclonal anti-IgE [101] in the treatment of respiratory allergy as well as the use of selective anti-T-cell therapies, such as CTLA4Ig [102] and $DAB_{389}IL$-2 [103], in the treatment of psoriasis. In the new millenium, we face the exciting prospect of using new immunological therapies directed toward correction of the immunological dysfunction observed in allergic skin diseases. This challenge will require physicians caring for patients with allergic skin disease to better understand the immunology of their disease and use new immunological markers for monitoring disease activity.

## REFERENCES

1.   Eckman I, Stiller MJ. Recent developments in the pathogenesis and treatment of atopic dermatitis. Curr Opin Dermatol 1995; 1:3–9.
2.   Friedmann PS, Tan B, Musaba A, Strickland I. Pathogenesis and management of atopic dermatitis. Clin Exp Allergy 1995; 25:799–806.
3.   Leung DYM, Hannifin JM, Charlesworth EN, Li JT, Bernstein IL, Berger WE, Blessing-Moore J, Fineman S, Lee FE, Nicklas RA, Spector SL. Disease management of atopic dermatitis: a practice parameter. Ann Allergy Asthma Immunol 1997; 79:179–211.
4.   Cornell RC, Stoughton RB. Correlation of the vasoconstrictor assay and clinical activity. Arch Dermatol 1985; 121:63–67.
5.   Cornell RC, Stoughton RB. Six-month controlled study of the effect of desoximetasone and betamethasone 17-valerate on the pituitary-adrenal axis. Br J Dermatol 1981; 105:91–95.
6.   Du Buske LM. Clinical comparison of H1-receptor antagonist drugs. J Allergy Clin Immunol 1996; 98:5307–5318.
7.   Simons FER. A new classification of H1-receptor antagonists. Allergy 1995; 50:7–11.
8.   Juhlin L. Nonclassical indications for H1-receptor antagonists in dermatology. Allergy 1995; 50(24 suppl):36–40.
9.   Behrandt H, Ring J. Histamine, antihistamines and atopic eczema. Clin Exp Allergy 1990; 20(suppl 4):25–30.
10.  McHenry PM, Williams HC, Bingham EA. Management of atopic eczema. Br Med J 1995; 310:843–847.
11.  Brehler R, Hildebrand A, Luger T. Recent developments in the treatment of atopic eczema. J Am Acad Dermatol 1997; 36:983–994.
12.  Krutman J, Schöpf E. High-dose UVA 1 phototherapy: a novel and highly effective approach for the treatment of acute exacerbation of atopic dermatitis. Acta Derm Venereal Suppl (Stockh) 1992; 176:120–122.
13.  Falk ES. UV-light therapies in atopic dermatitis. Photodermatology 1985; 2:241–246.
14.  Midelfart K, Stenvold SE, Volden G. Combined UVB and UVA phototherapy of atopic eczema. Dermatology 1985; 171:95–98.
15.  Stiller MJ. The golden age of dermatologic therapy: retrospective and overview (1945–1995). In: Suber AJ, Fitzpatrick TB, eds. Yearbook of Dermatology 1997. St. Louis: Mosby, 1997: 1–7.
16.  Fitzpatrick TB. Dermatology 1945–1995: the golden age of treatment. J Dermatol 1996; 23: 728–734.
17.  Sulzberger MB, Witten VH, Yaffe SN. Cortisone acetate administered orally in dermatologic therapy. Arch Dermatol Syphilol 1951; 64:573–578.
18.  Shupack JL, Kitchin JES, Stiller MJ, Webster GF. Cytotoxic and antimetabolic agents. In: Freedberg IM, et al., eds. Dermatology in General Medicine. 5th ed. New York, McGraw-Hill, Inc.: 1999:2797–2810.
19.  Berg RE, Kantor GR, Bergeld WF. Urticarial vasculitis. Int J Dermatol 1988; 27:468–472.
20.  Gibson LE, Daniel Su Wp. Cutaneous vasculitis. Rheum Dis Clin North Am 1995; 21:1097–1113.
21.  Smith JG. Vasculitis. J Dermatol 1995; 22:822–825.
22.  Kelly RI. Cutaneous vasculitis and cutaneous vasculopathies. Australas J Dermatol 1995; 36:109–119.
23.  Davis IC, Stiller MJ, Shupack JL. Pharmacology of therapeutic agents in photomedicine. In: Lim HW, Soter NA, eds. Clinical Photomedicine. New York: Marcel Dekker: 1993: 59–74.

24. Hannifin JM. Breaking the cycle: how I manage the difficult cases. Fitzpatrick's J Dermatol 1994; 1:13–26.
25. Wolverton SE, Wilkin JK. Systemic Drugs and Skin Disease. Philadelphia: WB Saunders, 1991.
26. Capizzi RL, Berlino JR. Methotrexate treatment of Wegener's granulomatosis. Ann Intern Med 1971; 74:74–78.
27. Upchurch KA, Helkr K, Bress ME. Low-dose methotrexate therapy for cutaneous vasculitis of rheumatoid arthritis. J Am Acad Dermatol 1987; 17:355–359.
28. Exponoza LR, Espinoza CG, Vasey FB, German BF. Oral methotrexate therapy for chronic rheumatoid arthritis ulcerations. J Am Acad Dermatol 1986; 15:508–512.
29. Kauvar AB, Stiller MJ. Cyclosporine in dermatology: pharmacology and clinical use. Int J Dermatol 1994; 33:86–96.
30. Shupack JL. Maintenance therapy with Neoral®. Int J Dermatol 1997; 36(suppl 1):34–36.
31. Lowe NJ. Initiating Neoral® therapy. Int J Dermatol 1997; 36(suppl 1):30–33.
32. Camp RDR, Reitamo S, Friedmann PS, Ho V, Heule F. Cyclosporin A in severe therapy-resistant atopic dermatitis: report of an international workshop. Br J Dermatol 1994; 130: 376–380.
33. Munro CS, Levell NJ, Shuster S, Friedmann PS. Maintenance treatment with cyclosporin in atopic eczema. Br J Dermatol 1994; 130:376–380.
34. Sepp N, Fritsch PO. Can cyclosporin A induce permanent remission of atopic dermatitis? Br J Dermatol 1993; 128:213–216.
35. Freeman D, Grant D, Levy G, Rochon J, Wong PY, Altruif I, Asfar S. Pharmacokinetics of a new oral formulation of cyclosporine in liver transplant recipients. Ther Drug Monit 1995; 17:213–216.
36. Niese D. A double-blind randomized study of Sandimmune Neoral® versus Sandimmune Neoral Study Group. Transplant Proc 1995; 27:1849–1856.
37. Alaiti S, Kang S, Fiedler VC, Ellis CN, Spurlin DV, Fader D, Ulyanov G, Gadgil SD, Tanase A, Lawrence I, Scotellaro P, Raye K, Bekersky I. Tacrolimus (FK 506) ointment for atopic dermatitis: a phase 1 study in adults and children. J Am Acad Dermatol 1998; 38:69–76.
38. Shupack JL, Gold JA, Stiller MJ, Orbuch P. Dermatologic Formulary. Skin and Cancer Unit New York University. New York: McGraw-Hill, 1989.
39. Bickers DR, Hazen PG, Lynch WS. Clinical Pharmacology of Skin Disease. New York: Churchill Livingstone, 1984.
40. Nurnberg W, Gragge J, Czarnetzk BM. Urticarial vasculitis syndrome effectively treated with dapsone and pentoxifylline. Acta Dermatovenereol (Stockh) 1995; 75:54–56.
41. Sais G, Vidaller A, Jucgla A, Gallardo F, Peyri J. Colchicine in the treatment of cutaneous leukocytoclastic vasculitits, results of a prospective randomized controlled trial. Arch Dermatol 1995; 1131:1399–1402.
42. Fleischer AB, Resnick SD. Livedo reticularis. Dermal Clin 1990; 8:347–354.
43. Funk JO, Maibach HI. Horizons in pharmacologic intervention in allergic contact dermatitis. J Am Acad Dermatol 1994; 31:999–1014.
44. Kondo S, Sauder DN. Epidermal cytokines in allergic contact dermatitis. J Am Acad Dermatol 1995; 33:786–800.
45. Hanifin JM. Breaking the cycle. How I manage difficult cases of atopic dermatitis. Fitzpatrick's J Dermatol 1994; 1:13–26.
46. Xu X-J, Banerjee P, Rustin MHA, Poulter LW. Modulation by Chinese herbal therapy of immune mechanisms in the skin of patients with atopic eczema. Br J Dermatol 1997; 136: 54–59.
47. Calderon PA, Anzilotti M, Philps R. Thalidomide in dermatology: new indications for an old drug. Int J Dermatol 1997; 36:881–887.
48. Broberg A, ed. Pityrosporum ovale in healthy children, infantile seborrheic dermatitis and atopic dermatitis. Acta Dermato Venereol (Stockh) 1994; (suppl 191):2–47.

49. Rajka G, ed. Contributions and discussion presented at the 5th International Symposium on Atopic Dermatitis. Acta Dermato Venereol (Stockh) 1994; (suppl 196):3–119.
50. Jorizzo JL. Classification of vasculitis. J Invest Dermatol 1993; 100:1065–1105.
51. Stubb S, Heikkila H, Kauppinen K. Cutaneous reactions to drugs: a series of inpatients during a 5-year period. Acta Dermato Venereol (Stockh) 1994; 74:289–291.
52. Fleischer AB, Resnick SD. Livedo reticularis. Dermatol Clin 1990; 8:347–354.
53. Voorhees J. Psoriasis—an immunologic disease. J Dermatol 1996; 23:854–857.
54. Fitzpatrick TB, unpublished communication.
55. Clements PJ, Davis J. Cytotoxic drugs their clinical application to the rheumatics diseases. Semin Arthrit Rheum 1986; 15:231–254.
56. Singh G, Fried JF, Spitz P, Williams CA. Toxic effects of azathioprine in rheumatoid arthritis. Arthritis Rheum 1989; 32:837–843.
57. Ahmed AR, Moy R. Azathioprine. Int J Dermatol 1981; 20:461–467.
58. Anstey A. Azathioprine in dermatology: a review in the light of understanding methylation pharmacokinetics. JR Soc Med 1995; 88:455–160.
59. Jones JJ, Ashworth J. Azathioprine induced shock. J Am Acad Dermatol 1993; 29:795.
60. Leavitt RY, Fauci AS. Therapeutic approach to vasculitic syndromes. Mt. Sinai J Med 1986; 53:440–448.
61. Leavitt RV, Fauci AS. Pulmonary vasculitis. Am Rev Respir Dis 1986; 134:149–166.
62. Ahmed AR, Hombal S. Use of cyclophosphamide in azathioprine failures in pemphigus. J Am Acad Dermatol 1987; 17:437–442.
63. Stein JP, Skinner EC, Boyd SD, Skinner DG. Squamous cell carcinoma of the bladder associated with cyclophosphamide therapy for Wegener's granulomatosis. J Urol 1993; 149:588–589.
64. Baker GL, Kahl LE, Zee BC, Stolzer BL, Agarwal AK, Medsger TA. Malignancy following treatment of rheumatoid arthritis with cyclophosphamide. Am J Med 1987; 83:1–9.
65. Borel JF, Feurer C, Gubler HV, Stähelin H. Biological effects of cyclosporine A: a new antilymphocytic agent. Agents Action 1976; 6:468–475.
66. Logun RA, Camp RDR. Severe atopic eczema: response to oral cyclosporine A. J R Soc Med 1988; 81:417–418.
67. Motley RJ, Whitaker JA, Holt PJA. Resolution of atopic dermatitis in a patient treated with cyclosporine. Clin Exp Dermatol 1989; 14:243–244.
68. Taylor RS, Cooper KD, Headington JT, Ho VC, Ellis CN, Voorhees JJ. Cyclosporine therapy for severe atopic dermatitis. J Am Acad Dermatol 1989; 21:580–583.
69. Shupack JL, Kenny C, Jondreau L, Eckman I, Gropper C, Stiller MJ. Decreased peripheral blood eosinophil counts in severe patients treated with low-dose cyclosporine A. Dermatology 1992; 185:202–204.
70. Singer MI, Shapiro LE, Shear NH. Cytochrome p. 450 3A: interactions with dermatologic therapies. J Am Acad Dermatol 1997; 37:765–771.
71. Bennett WM. Renal effects of cyclosporine. J Am Acad Dermatol 1990; 23:1302–1311.
72. Mockli G, Kabra PM, Kurtz TW. Laboratory monitory of cyclosporine levels: guidelines for the dermatologist. J Am Acad Dermatol 1990; 23:1275–1279.
73. Furlanit M, Baraldo J, Pea F, Marzocchi V, Croattino L, Galla F. Blood concentrations and clinical effect of cyclosporin in psoriasis. Ther Drug Monit 1996; 18:544–548.
74. Lowe NJ, Wieder JM, Resenbach A, Johnson K, Kunkel R, Bainbridge C, Bourget T, Dimov I, Simpson K, Glass E, Grabie MT. Long-term low-dose cyclosporine therapy for severe psoriasis: effects on renal function and structure. J Am Acad Dermatol 1996; 35:710–719.
75. Stiller MJ, Pak GH, Kenny C, Jondreau L, Davis I, Wachsman S, Shupack JL. Elevation of fasting serum lipids in patients treated with low-dose cyclosporine for severe plaque-type psoriasis: an assessment of clinical significance when viewed as a risk factor for cardiovascular disease. J Am Acad Dermatol 1992; 27:434–438.
76. Tharp M. Unpublished communication.

77. Moisson YF, Janeir M, Civatte J. Thalidomide for recurrent erythema multiforme. Br J Dermatol 1992; 126:92–93.

78. Bahmer FA, Zaun H, Luszpinsi P. Thalidomide treatment of recurrent erythema multiforme. Acta Dermatovener 1982; 62:449–450.

79. Barnhill RL, Doll NJ, Millikan LE, Hastings RC. Studies on the antiinflammatory properties of thalidomide. Arch Dermatol Res 1980; 269:275–280.

80. Tseng S, Pak G, Washenik K, Pomerantz MK, Shupack JL. Rediscovering thalidomide: a review of its mechanism of action, side affects, and potential uses. J Am Acad Dermatol 1996; 35:969–979.

81. Stirling DI. Thalidomide: a pharmaceutical enigma. Pharmaceutical News 1996; 3:17–20.

82. Asako H, Kubes P, Beathage BA, Wolf RE, Granger DN. Colchicine and methotrexate reduce leukocyte emigration and adherence in rat mesenteric venules. Inflammation 1992; 16:45–46.

83. Molad Y, Reibman J, Levin RI, Cronstein BN. A new mode of action of an old drug: colchicine decreases surface expression of adhesion molecules on both neutrophils (PMN) and endothelium (abstr). Arthritis Rheum 1992; 35 (suppl 9):535.

84. Cronstein BN, Weissman G. The adhesion molecules of inflammation. Arthritis Rheum 1993; 36:147–157.

85. Wiles JC, Hansen RC, Lynch PJ. Urticarial vasculitis treated with colchicine. Arch Dermatol 1985; 121:802–805.

86. Schwarz T, Schwarz A, Krone C, Luger TA. Pentoxifylline suppresses allergic patch test responses in humans. Arch Dermatol 1993; 129:513–514.

87. Ely M. Pentoxifylline therapy in dermatology, a review of localized hyperviscosity and its effects on skin. Derm Clinic 1988; 6:585–608.

88. Fromm E, Whittmann J. Derivate des p-nitrophenols. Dtsch Chem Ges 1908; 41:2264–2273.

89. Sulzberger MB. Acrodermatitis continua pustulosa (Hallopeau) treated with sulfapyridine. Arch Dermatol Syph 1939; 40:1019.

90. Callen JP, Kalbleisch S. Urticarial vasculitis: a report of nine cases and review of the literature. Br J Dermatol 1982; 107:87–94.

91. Lopez LR, Davis KC, Kohler PF, Schocket AL. The hypocomplementemic urticarial vasculitis syndrome: therapeutic response to hydroxychloroquine. J Allergy Clin Immunol 1984; 73:600–603.

92. Sanchez NP, Winkelmann RK, Shroeter AL, Dicken CH. The clinical and histopathologic spectrums of urticarial vasculitis: study of 40 cases. J Am Acad Dermatol 1982; 7:599–605.

93. Millns JL, Randle HW, Solley GO, Dicken CH. The therapeutic response of urticarial vasculitis to indomethacin. J Am Acad Dermatol 1980; 3:349–355.

94. Jones RR, Bhogal BO, Dash A, Schifferli J. Urticaria and vasculitis: a continuum of histological and immunopathological changes. Br J Dermatol 1983; 108:695–703.

95. Shupack JL, Stiller MJ, Meola T, Orbuch P. Papaverine hydrochloride the treatment of atopic dermatitis: clinical trial to reassess safety and efficacy. Dermatologica 1991; 183:21–24.

96. Ruzicka T, Simmet T, Peskar BA, Ring J. Skin levels of arachidonic acid-derived inflammatory mediators and histamine in atopic dermatitis and psoriasis. J Invest Dermatol 1986; 86:105–108.

97. Fogh K, Herlin T, Kragballe K. Eicosanoids in skin of patients with atopic dermatitis: prostaglandin E2 and leukotriene B4 are present in biologically active concentrations. J Allergy Clin Immunol 1989; 83:450–455.

98. Boguniewicz M, Fielder VC, Ralmer S, Lawrence ID, Leung DYM, Hanifin JM. A randomized vehicle controlled trial of tacrolimus ointment for treatment of atopic dermatitis in children. J Allergy Clin Immunol 1998; 102(4):637–644.

99. Van Leent EJ, Graber M, Thurston M, Wagenaar A, Spuls PI, Bos JD. Effectiveness of the ascomycin macrolactam SDZ ASM 981 in the topical treatment of atopic dermatitis. Arch Dermatol 1998; 134:805–809.

100. Burchard EG, Silverman EK, et al. Association between a sequence variant in the IL-4 gene promoter and FEV(1) in asthma. Am J Respir Crit Care Med 1999; 160(3):919–922.

101. Corne J, Djukanovic R, Thomas L, Warner J, Botta L, Grandordy B, Gygax D, Heusser C, Patalano F, Richardson W, Kilcherr E, Straehelin T, Davis F, Gordon W, Sun L, Liov R, Wang G, Chang T-W, Holgate S. The effect of intravenous administration of a chimeric anti-IgE antibody on serum IgE levels in atopic subjects: efficacy, safety and pharmacokinetics. J Clin Invest 1997; 99:879–887.

102. Abrams JR, Lebwohl MG, Guzzo CA, Jegasothy BV, Goldfarb MT, Goffe BS, Menter A, Lowe NJ, Krueger JG, Ochs HD, Kelley SL, Kang S. CTLA4Ig-mediated blockade of T-cell costimulation in patients with psoriasis vulgaris. J Clin Invest 1999; 103:1243–1252.

103. Bagel J, Garland WT, Breneman D, Holick M, Littlejohn TW, Crosby D, Faust H, Fivenson D, Nichols J. Administration of $DAB_{389}IL-2$ to patients with recalcitrant psoriasis: a double-blind, phase II multicenter trial. J Am Acad Dermatol 1998; 38:938–944.

# Index